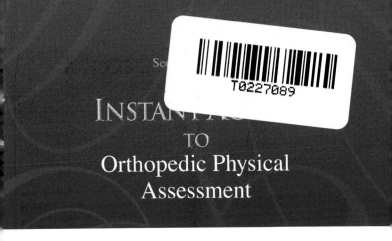

Sec[ond]

INSTANT ACCESS
TO
Orthopedic Physical Assessment

RONALD C. EVANS, D.C., F.A.C.O., F.I.C.C.

Fellow, Academy of Chiropractic Orthopedists
Diplomate, American Board of Chiropractic Orthopedists
Examiner Emeritus, American Board of Chiropractic Orthopedists
Examiner Emeritus, Academy of Chiropractic Orthopedists
Fellow, International College of Chiropractic
Past-Chairman of the Iowa Board of Chiropractic Examiners
    of the Department of Professional Licensure, State of Iowa,
    Des Moines, Iowa (Ret)
Member, Chiropractic Healthcare Benefits Advisory Committee,
    Department of Defense, United States of America
Chief Executive Officer, Iowa Chiropractic Physicians Clinic,
    Des Moines, Iowa
Vice President, Foundation for Chiropractic Education and Research
Chairman, Department of Defense Committee, Foundation for
    Chiropractic Education and Research
Chiropractic Orthopedist, private practice

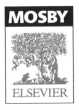

MOSBY

ELSEVIER

MOSBY
ELSEVIER

11830 Westline Industrial Drive
St. Louis, Missouri 63146

INSTANT ACCESS TO ORTHOPEDIC   ISBN: 978-0-323-04533-9
PHYSICAL ASSESSMENT, Second Edition

Notice

ISBN: 978-0-323-04533-9

Vice President and Publisher: Linda Duncan
Senior Acquisitions Editor: Kellie White
Senior Developmental Editor: Jennifer Watrous
Associate Developmental Editor: Kelly Milford
Publishing Services Manager: Julie Eddy
Senior Project Manager: Andrea Campbell
Designers: Renee Duenow, Jessica Williams

Working together to grow
libraries in developing countries

www.elsevier.com | www.bookaid.org | www.sabre.org

ELSEVIER   BOOK AID International   Sabre Foundation

Printed and bound by CPI Group (UK) Ltd, Croydon, CR0 4YY

For Ryan D. and David P.
Men of great integrity, intellect, grace and principle,
who continue to teach me that brevity
is indeed the essence of all important communication...

PREFACE

Instant Access to Orthopedic Physical Assessment, Second Edition, is a companion reference to *Illustrated Orthopedic Physical Assessment, Third Edition*. Much of what makes the Third Edition of *Illustrated Orthopedic Physical Assessment* clinically relevant has been distilled in the *Instant Access* companion reference. *Illustrated Orthopedic Physical Assessment* remains the important desktop and classroom reference useful for both the student and the practicing clinician. *Instant Access to Orthopedic Physical Assessment* is the portable resource. The various lists within *Instant Access* present a range or spectrum of facts or concepts in assessing orthopedic disease. The orthopedic gamuts found in each chapter represent both universal orthopedic precepts and specific regional principles and maxims. The gamuts serve as diagnostic rubric in examining a patient. *Instant Access to Orthopedic Physical Assessment* enhances the use of *Illustrated Orthopedic Physical Assessment*. It is a pocket reference, designed to travel with the clinician for bedside or examination room use.

Each chapter of *Instant Access to Orthopedic Physical Assessment* has a specific format. This format lends to the quick referencing of tests and maneuvers. Each chapter begins with indexing of the tests and procedures found therein. Each chapter also begins with cross-reference tables for the syndromes assessed and by the syndrome suspected. Further, each chapter presents the separate protocols for the regional joint assessment procedures and for assessment of pain in the particular joint or region, presented as testing procedural flow charts. These charts identify the test procedure(s) used to objectify the symptoms of pain, paralysis, weakness, and loss of sensation. The chart provides a plan of examination and selections of tests for the joint.

Each chapter begins with a set of axioms. Axioms are self-evident or universally recognized truths. Axioms are also established rules, principles, or laws. An axiom used in this text is also a principle accepted as true, without proof as the basis for argument.

Each chapter introduction addresses the various unique considerations or pathologies of the focal joint. The introductory section contains the index of the tests presented and illustrated in the chapter.

Gamuts in essential anatomy exist for each region or joint system. The essential anatomy section is not all-encompassing, but rather discusses only the typical tissues that can be examined in orthopedic physical procedures.

Gamuts in essential motion assessment for the joint are included.

Gamuts in essential muscle function for each joint are also included. This section identifies the musculature that is the prime mover of the joint, the innervation, and the action of the muscle, and limited discussion of the muscular anatomy.

Gamuts in essential imaging elements are addressed for the specific region or joint discussed. Not all imaging techniques or modalities are discussed, only those procedures that are germane to the physical orthopedic testing of a patient.

Each test, maneuver, sign, law, or phenomenon is presented separately. The common usage name for the test, as identified in *Stedman's*, *Dorland's*, or *Churchill's* medical dictionaries, is used as the heading for the test. Equally, common synonyms and eponyms follow this name.

Following the name of the test, maneuver, or sign is identification of the specific pathology the test is suited to elicit.

A test is part of the physical examination in which direct contact with the patient is made. It also may be a chemical test, X-ray, or other study. All tests described in this book will relate to the physical examination.

A sign is elucidated by a test or a particular maneuver. A sign can simply be a visual observation (e.g., antalgia) and is an indication of the existence of a problem perceived by the examiner.

A maneuver is a complex motion or series of movements, used either as a test or treatment. A maneuver is also a method or technique.

A phenomenon is any sign or objective symptom, or any observable occurrence or fact.

A law is a description of a phenomenon that is so thoroughly tested and accepted that it is regarded as a principle governing like phenomena.

A bulleted delineation of how to conduct the test or procedure is presented. Each procedure is supported by photo illustrations and legends. When possible, a *"clinical pearl"* identifies the subtle nuances or finesse of the tests that the author has gleaned from empirical practice.

The compiled references for each chapter are listed. The bibliographic listing is new, updated, and extensive. In some instances, the bibliography reflects older volumes or works than is commonly found in scientific literature today. These older references are the original work of the creators of various tests or procedures in this book. Preserving the books in these reference lists is an attempt to preserve a continuum in the development of orthopedic investigation.

Although the various tests and procedures in this book are presented in an anatomical or regional format, the application of the tests are accomplished in a more natural flow of examination procedures. The natural flow of the examination usually moves the patient from the standing position through sitting, supine, and side-lying positions to the prone position.

A listing of tests, alphabetically and anatomically, and a listing of tests according to the position of the patient can be found on the inside front and back covers, respectively. A glossary of abbreviations is also included at the end of the book.

ACKNOWLEDGMENTS

None of this work would exist without the support and encouragement of others. For this revision, Mrs. Linda K. Evans was inexhaustible in her efforts to keep up with the changes in the *Instant Access to Orthopedic Physical Assessment, Second Edition*. Although *Instant Access to Orthopedic Physical Assessment* is a distillation of *Illustrated Orthopedic Physical Assessment*, I am sure she thought the stream of changes would never end. I am grateful for her accuracy and speed at typing and proofreading.

The photographic work of *Illustrated Orthopedic Physical Assessment, Third Edition*, forms the basis of *Instant Access to Orthopedic Physical Assessment, Second Edition*, as pivotal pieces in the depiction of orthopedic physical assessment.

Mr. Jim Visser, primary still photographer, could not have worked harder to achieve any higher degree of excellence with the color photos. He pushed the models to exceed their known abilities, squeezing out every detail of movement or position. His work embodies the constant search for perfection, serving as a guide for me to create prose equal to the illustrations. I look forward to working with him in future endeavors.

In many instances, the clinical photography of Dr. Kim A. Skibsted is unsurpassed in depicting important positions and postures. His clinical photography work is unsurpassed. Dr. Skibsted not only grasped the concept and framing issues of the illustrations, but worked tirelessly to perfect the quality for these books. I am ever indebted.

The primary photographic models include Ms. Kim Alvis, Mr. Sean Brasfield, Ms. Candyse Burns, Mr. Ryan Collart, Mr. Ochuko Ekpere, Ms. Angela Fain, Dr. L.T. Faison, Ms. Sheena Gordon, Mr. John Knott, Mr. Patrick Milford, Ms. Julie Mowczuo, Mr. Gary Taylor, and Ms. Annie Walters. Both Mr. Brasfield and Dr. Faison rose far above the call of duty in providing either specialized and critical equipment for the photos, or in helping recruit suitable models for the shoot. Each of the models demonstrated interminable patience in achieving just the right position or look of a test or procedure. I am grateful for their stamina and physical pliability. It is worthwhile noting that some of these able models subsequently entered successful practice as chiropractic physicians.

Ms. Bailey Schechinger was superb in modeling for the clinical illustrations. She was tireless, well-poised, and eager to learn the meanings and usefulness of the procedures. Because of this, her photographic portrayals are unexcelled.

The Mosby/Elsevier staff for this edition included: Ms. Jennifer Watrous, Senior Developmental Editor, Health Professions I department of Editorial. At the outset, I am pleased that Ms. Watrous elected to engage in the work on my new editions. She worked diligently on the second edition of *Illustrated Orthopedic Physical Assessment*, and it has been exciting to have her working on the third. Her attention to detail perviously made the book into a definitive reference. That same perseverance with editing my writing this time pushed the book yet one notch higher. It is always a pleasure to work with people who truly want to see a project succeed. Ms. Watrous exemplifies this trait. Were it not for Ms. April Falast, Editorial Assistant, Health Professions I department of Editorial, Mosby/Elsevier, we could not have completed the work on time or in an organized fashion. Ms. Falast's creative work in making the photographic masters from the second edition was astounding. The enlarged illustrations were the perfect tool for both the stills and videos. I am sure this was hard work, but the result of the photo catalogs is unsurpassed. I am also grateful for her attention to the needs of the models. Without Ms. Falast's leadership, I am certain the freezing models would simply have left the building, along with Elvis. Ms. Kelly Milford, Associate Developmental Editor, Health Professions I department of Editorial, Mosby/Elsevier, is exceptional in her work. Her attention to detail and dedication to completion of the project kept the manuscripts, models, photographers and the author moving forward. I am ever indebted to her patience in waiting for the several "final" draft(s). Her professionalism is unsurpassed, especially tested in frequent e-mail and teleconference contact from the beginning until the first bound copy. One could not ask for more of an editor. Her activities in compiling the manuscript schedules, arranging the photo shoot, arranging for the models and organizing the video and audio studios, as well as keeping everyone on the same page were invaluable. I could not have done any of the work without her at the "director's table." Ms. Kellie White, Senior Editor, Health Professions I department of Editorial, Mosby/Elsevier, worked with me from the earliest stages of *Illustrated Essentials in Orthopedic Physical Assessment*, through to the *Illustrated Orthopedic Physical Assessment, Second Edition*, and *Instant Access to Orthopedic Physical Assessment*, and now for *Illustrated Orthopedic Physical Assessment, Third Edition*, and

Instant Access to Orthopedic Physical Assessment, Second Edition. Ms. White continues to provide the necessary latitude and unwavering encouragement for the development of both these books to evolve them into nationally recognized definitive works. She embodies the attributes of a senior editor for which every author hopes. She and her excellent staff brought professionalism, interest, and dedication to the project. I have now written two editions under her guidance with great result. The current revisions will surpass both our expectations, which I attribute to her skills at marshaling all the creative elements, models, photographers, and the author, to their best. Doing a book with her and for her is a joy. Elsevier is both astute and fortunate to have Ms. White in its Editorial leadership, and I am fortunate to enjoy her friendship and creative counsel. I will continue to strive to give her the best manuscripts. I look forward to future collaborations. Ms. Andrea Campbell, the project manager, juggled communication with numerous staff constantly. She was the last stop before the "work" becomes a book. She is *the* sous chef for my manuscripts: I gave her the ingredients and she turned them into something everyone will like to look at and want to read. Ms. Campbell sorted out the art problems and kept track of what needed to be redrawn and what needed replacing (according to my seemingly interminable corrections). Quite a task. I am ever grateful for her skills.

INTRODUCTION

For several millennia, physcians have recorded the observations associated with their patients and the diseases they suffered. In the accumulating facts, these same physcians recognized patterns of disordered orthopedic functions and bodily structures. When such constellations of symptoms and signs were recognized, they were termed *disorders* and given specific names.

ORTHOPEDIC GAMUT

Many times during the orthopedic physical assessment of a patient, the physician repeats a pattern of investigation by which is collected and weighed the evidence of disorder or malfunction. This sequence is:
- **Step 1** Acquisition of facts
- **Step 2** Evaluation of facts
- **Step 3** Listing of hypothesis
- **Step 4** Choosing between hypothesis (the differential diagnosis)

In acquisition of the facts, the medical history furnishes the chronology and symptoms of the orthopedic problem. Symptoms are the variations from normal sensations and behavior that enter the patient's activities of daily living. The orthopedic physical assessment discloses the physical signs of the orthopedic disorder or disease.

In evaluation of the facts, the physician repeats procedures and tests for reliability, accuracy, and pertinence to the patient's complaint. The physician must judge if the findings and complaints have been colored by the patient's emotions; whether the patient's motives might lead to distortion; and, from past experience, whether the findings are within normal limits or represent significant abnormalities.

In listing hypotheses, the clinician gathers a list of orthopedic disorders suggested by the clues from the history, physical examination, and supporting tests and imaging. In the four-step sequence of diagnosis, the lists of hypotheses are derived from diseases or disorders called to mind by their key symptoms or signs. Gamuts presented in this text will aid in formulating the differential diagnosis list.

In choosing between the diagnoses (differential diagnosis), each disease in the list of hypotheses is considered in turn and its manifestations are matched with the patient's presentation. Initial comparisons may eliminate some items from the list and retain others. The chronology of events in the patient's orthopedic problem is compared with that of a suspected disorder. Some disorders will be excluded by the duration of symptoms. Sex-linked disorders are promptly excluded from patients of the opposite sex. From the list that survives, the clinician chooses as the diagnosis the orthopedic disorder whose attributes coincide more closely with the patient's presentation. If a good fit does not exist, the clinician must resume the search for more symptoms and signs.

The law of parsimony may prevail in making the differential diagnosis. The law of parsimony is simply the procedure of selecting a single disease to explain all the patient's orthopedic manifestations, rather than explaining them by the coincidence of several diseases. The law of parsimony must be applied *cautiously*. The more experienced clinician realizes that in the process of aging, the patient accumulates more debilitating orthopedic conditions with longer life. Coincidences of orthopedic disease and malfunction often occur.

Solving a patient's health problem can be a demanding exercise of orthopedic medical detection and logical deduction. Each health problem is a new diagnostic jigsaw puzzle for which the pieces must be found and fitted together in a carefully organized manner.

ORTHOPEDIC GAMUT

Success requires an organized thought process in approaching the patient's problem. There must be a clear plan to follow and a particular aim in each stage of the investigation.

- **First**, it must be determined whether a lesion of the musculoskeletal system is present. This determination is accomplished by analysis of the history and physical examination.
- **Second**, the location of the lesion must be determined. Is it possible to locate the lesion at one site, or are multiple sites involved? A system must be developed by the examiner to relate the signs and symptoms to a basic knowledge of musculoskeletal anatomy.
- **Third**, what pathologic conditions are capable of producing the lesions?
- **Fourth**, from careful analysis of the history and examination, and by intelligent use of ancillary tests, which of these suspected conditions is most likely to be present?

Always, the failure to have such an organized plan or approach makes the diagnosis of orthopedic health problems so artificially difficult. Routine steps must be followed, but not blind routine or blunderbuss investigations.

CONTENTS

1   Assessing Musculoskeletal Disorders   1

2   Assessing Cardinal Musculoskeletal
    Symptoms and Signs   37

3   Cervical Spine   63

4   Shoulder   157

5   Elbow   226

6   Forearm, Wrist, and Hand   253

7   Thoracic Spine   302

8   Lumbar Spine   344

9   Pelvis and Sacroiliac Joint   473

10 Hip   516

11 Knee   564

12 Lower Leg, Ankle, and Foot   617

13 Malingering   661

Appendix   763

Glossary of Abbreviations   769

Bibliography   789

Index   877

CHAPTER ONE

ASSESSING MUSCULOSKELETAL DISORDERS

AXIOMS IN ASSESSING MUSCULOSKELETAL DISORDERS

- Eliciting the patient's history is the quintessential skill in orthopedics.
- An examiner needs to learn about the patient's major presenting symptoms, the chronology of the disorder, and its impact on the patient's activities of daily living, as well as ancillary information that includes history and involvement of other systems.
- The orthopedic examination is the focal activity in assessing the patient's musculoskeletal complaint.
- The orthopedic examination process is adapted to the specific needs of the patient's musculoskeletal system, such as inspection, palpation, and observation.

INTRODUCTION

The evaluation for treatment consultation between a physician and a patient is at the center of all orthopedic practice activities.

From the moment of the first encounter with a patient, the physician is simultaneously observing and examining the movements and mannerisms of the patient, as well as listening to what is being said. The physician is trying to piece together the nature of the patient's orthopedic problem.

The purpose of orthopedic evaluation is twofold. First, it allows the patient to present the problem, and second, it enables the physician to triage the nature of the problem and develop a course of action. In this context, the physician must always learn what has brought the patient to the consultation. In some cases a patient visits the orthopedic specialist because of referral by or on the advice of a third party. The diagnostic process is also complex, given that the physician needs to establish the physical issues that are of greatest importance to the patient and that are most disrupting to the activities of daily living, as well as try to differentiate the anatomic and pathologic aspects of any disease that might be present.

The history provides much information about the pathologic process involved and the impact of the condition on the patient, whereas the orthopedic physical examination is essential to define the anatomic structures involved; together these processes allow differentiation of orthopedic disorders into various categories.

ORTHOPEDIC GAMUT 1-1
ORTHOPEDIC EVALUATION PROCESS
The orthopedic *evaluation* process has three phases: 1. History taking 2. Examination 3. Diagnosis

Health care providers assess patients every day in clinical practice. Commonly, clinical practice is impossible without structured assessments and tests. Examination procedures look straightforward; results are either positive or negative. However, all assessment and testing in clinical practice is based on the assumption of uncertainty: Does the patient have a disease? The probability of a particular disease can be established only by performing a test from a chain of tests.

ORTHOPEDIC GAMUT 1-2
CLINICAL ASSESSMENTS
In clinical practice, assessments occur all day every day, including: 1. Elucidating complaints 2. Establishing impact of the complaints 3. Checking the complaint consistency with specific diagnoses 4. Performing a general physical examination 5. Performing special physical examinations 6. Performing laboratory and imaging tests 7. Interpreting test results 8. Formulating a diagnosis 9. Commencing treatment 10. Evaluating treatment efficacy 11. Referring to a specialist, as needed

The accuracy of a test for detecting a disease or a condition is determined by sensitivity and specificity. A high sensitivity (or a high specificity) does not suffice to make a test useful in clinical practice; a test should be as sensitive as possible. The sensitivity and specificity of examination procedures and tests can often be found in the literature. Sensitivity and specificity are important characteristics of evidence-based physical assessment procedures but only in the context of a specific disease or condition.

The probability of a disease or condition after having performed a test (Bayes theorem) is dependent on two factors: (1) the specificity and sensitivity of the procedure (test characteristics) and (2) the probability of the disease or condition before conducting the procedure. Interpretation of Bayes theorem is that the probability of having a disease is not only dependent on the test or examination procedure result and the characteristics of the procedure, but also dependent on how likely the existence of the disease before the procedure is actually conducted. This factor is dependent on the prevalence of the disease.

ORTHOPEDIC GAMUT 1-3

BAYES THEOREM

***Rules of Thumb* Rationale for use in clinical situations:**
1. Highly sensitive and specific tests will not perform well in the clinical context if the *a priori* probability is very low.
2. No single diagnostic test exists that turns an *a priori* risk of disease of less than 10% into a probability that sufficiently convinces a clinician to establish a diagnosis.
3. Testing is most valuable if the *a priori* probability of the disease is somewhere in the range of 40% to 60%.
4. Diagnostic tests can turn such a probability into a sufficiently high posttest probability on which to base further action.

The decision of whether to perform a new test depends on the result of the previous test. Procedures with the lowest burden, risk, and costs for the patient are performed first, and those with the highest burden, risk, or costs are reserved for certain patients in which the prior probability is highest. Examination procedures in the context of a low prior probability of disease are rarely, if ever, informative, with the yield of diagnostic testing that will increase the prior probability approximating 50%. Very experienced clinicians intuitively apply these rules and arrange *their* diagnostic process in such a way that the highest possible yield (a highly probable diagnosis) will be obtained at the lowest possible burden, risk, and cost for the patient. Less-experienced clinicians may learn from experienced colleagues by recalling Bayes theorem and implementing its principles in everyday clinical practice.

Health care providers cannot function adequately without physical examination procedures. In the real world, examiners accomplish clinical practice appropriately *without* a detailed knowledge of the principles of tests. However, the benefits from physical testing can be easily increased by recognizing that these tests do nothing more than increase the probability of a certain condition or diagnosis. Test results are never infallible.

ORTHOPEDIC GAMUT 1-4

PRÉCIS OF PHYSICAL EXAMINATION

- Sensitivity and specificity do not exclusively make a diagnostic test appropriate for clinical use.
- Test results that are considered *normal* or *abnormal* should always be interpreted in the context of the individual patient.
- The probability of having a disease is not totally dependent on the test result and the characteristics of the test.
- The probability of having a disease is also dependent on how prevalent the disease is before the test is actually conducted.
- Testing in the context of a low probability of disease is rarely, if ever, informative.
- Highly sophisticated and costly diagnostic techniques may fail as easily as simple, cheap diagnostic maneuvers.

From the moment of the first encounter with a patient, the examiner is simultaneously observing and examining the movements and mannerisms of the patient, as well as listening to what is being said. The diagnostic process is complex; the examiner needs to establish the physical issues that are of greatest importance to the patient (those most disrupting to the activities of daily living) and try to differentiate the anatomic and pathologic aspects of any disease or injury that might be present.

The **history** provides much information about what difficulties the patient is experiencing and the impact of these on the patient. **Orthopedic examination** is essential to define the structures involved; together, these processes allow differentiation of orthopedic disorders into various **diagnostic categories** (Box 1-1).

BOX 1-1

PRÉCIS IN ORTHOPEDIC DIAGNOSIS

1. History
2. Examination
3. Determination of disability (PILS):
   Preventable causes of disability
   Independent living
   Lifestyle
   Social support

HISTORY

A carefully elicited history is a most crucial element in orthopedic assessment. An experienced examiner can form an idea of the extent and magnitude simply from the patient's history. In the modern era of electronic patient medical record keeping, the examiner has new tools and methods for not only capturing patient information, but also tracking clinically significant changes.

ORTHOPEDIC GAMUT 1-5

ELECTRONIC PATIENT RECORD KEEPING

- An integrated electronic patient record (EPR) is essential for the future of health care services.
- The EPR assists in the sharing of patient information and helps promote efficiency.
- The most important resource for the development of the EPR is the patient.
- Computer systems can take appropriately directed medical histories from patients based on chief complaint.

ORTHOPEDIC GAMUT 1-6

WORKING DIAGNOSIS

Essential steps in formulating a working diagnosis include:

1. History taking
2. Observation
3. Palpation
4. Orthopedic testing
5. Clinical laboratory and imaging procedures

CHIEF COMPLAINT

Patients who have more than one complaint, such as those with pain of spinal origin coupled with other body region symptoms or extremity problems, must be guided in ranking the complaints in priority. Although patients occasionally seek attention for stiffness or some other joint-related complaint, most patients with musculoskeletal conditions do so for reasons related to pain, especially when it compromises the activities of daily living.

OBSERVATION AND INSPECTION

ORTHOPEDIC GAMUT 1-7

OBSERVATION AND INSPECTION

Observation and inspection of the patient occur anytime during the examination or history interview, especially when the patient is not aware of the observation. In this way, the examiner notes:
1. Antalgia or deformities of posture
2. Gait disturbances, especially if the patient needs assistance
3. Spinal symmetry, including prominences or elevations, flattening or depressions, scoliosis, or abnormalities of the anteroposterior curvature
4. Surface scars and wounds

ORTHOPEDIC GAMUT 1-8

PAIN-BASED CLINICAL REASONING

Five main categories of pain-based clinical reasoning are:
- Biomedical (structural-functional source)
- Psychosocial (perception-interpretation of pain)
- Pain mechanisms (underlying pathophysiologic factors)
- Chronicity (temporal aspects of pain)
- Irritability or severity (degree of pain)

A useful approach in clinical examination of the neuromusculoskeletal system is to seek answers to the *Critical 5* questions for an orthopedic specialist. Once all five questions are answered, a differential diagnosis can usually be established (Box 1-2).

BOX 1-2

CRITICAL QUESTIONS IN THE ORTHOPEDIC PHYSICAL EXAMINATION

1. Are any joints abnormal?
2. What is the nature of the abnormality?
3. What is the extent of the involvement?
4. Are other features of diagnostic importance present?
5. Do the answers to questions 1 through 4 provide sufficient data?

ORTHOPEDIC GAMUT 1-9

DETERMINING EXTENT OF INJURY

Other characteristic features of diagnostic importance in determining the extent of the disease or injury include the following questions:
1. Is involvement symmetric or asymmetric?
2. Are large or small joints affected?
3. Is the distribution of the condition peripheral or axial?
4. Does the condition affect upper versus lower limbs, or vice versa?

The physician needs to learn what exacerbates or relieves the symptom pattern. Equally important is how long the complaints have existed (Table 1-1).

PALPATION

Palpation is the process of assessing the physical characteristics of joints and contiguous structures by touching or feeling the patient's body. The purpose of palpation is to locate and substantiate areas of tenderness, swelling, and abnormal muscle tone. Palpation allows the examiner to identify a localized increase or decrease in surface temperature and the presence of induration and mass. Palpation is classically performed with the fingertips, or with the blunt end of a cotton-tip applicator. However, instruments can be used in percussion (gently tapping with a reflex hammer), with vibration (using a C-128 tuning fork), or with the blunt end of a cotton-tip applicator.

TABLE 1-1

JOINT PATTERNS IN ORTHOPEDIC/RHEUMATIC DISORDERS

Diagnosis	Symmetry	Number of Joints Involved*	Large/Small Joints	Peripheral/Central Distribution	Upper/Lower Limb	Predilection
Rheumatoid arthritis	Symmetric	Mono-, oligo-, polyarthritis	Large/small	Peripheral	Upper/lower	MCPs, PIPs, MTPs, DIPs
Ankylosing spondylitis	—	—	—	Central	—	Sacroiliac joints, hip, shoulder
Psoriatic arthritis	Asymmetric	Polyarthritis	Large/small	Peripheral	Upper/lower	DIPs, sacroiliac joints
Reactive arthritis	Asymmetric	Oligo-, polyarthritis	Large	Peripheral	Lower	Sacroiliac joints, DIPs (toes)
Gout	Asymmetric	Mono-, oligoarthritis	Large/small	Peripheral	Lower more often than upper	First MTP, knee, hip

DIPs, Distal interphalangeal joints; *MCPs*, metacarpophalangeal joints; *MTPs*, metarsophalangeal joints; *PIPs*, proximal interphalangeal joints.

*****Monoarthritis** denotes inflammation in a single joint, *oligoarthritis* denotes two to four joints, and *polyarthritis* denotes five or more joints.

ORTHOPEDIC GAMUT 1-10
SPINAL PALPATION

Effective spinal palpation can be accomplished with the patient in the sitting or kneeling variants of Adams position:

- In palpating various structures, the examiner assesses the skin and subcutaneous tissue. Rolling of the skin (Kibler test) can be performed. The examiner observes for surface temperature, hypesthesia, hyperhidrosis, and muscle splinting.
- Tenderness of muscles and tendons and their attachments is assessed in both the anatomic resting position and through various ranges of motion.

NEUROLOGIC EVALUATION

The neurologic evaluation involves locating the lesion; testing deep tendon, superficial, and pathologic reflexes; testing cranial nerve and brainstem function; measuring body parts (mensuration); grading muscular strength; and testing the gross sensory modalities.

ORTHOPEDIC GAMUT 1-11
DEEP-TENDON REFLEXES

1. Scapulohumeral C5–C6
2. Biceps C5–C6
3. Radial C5–C6
4. Triceps C7–C8
5. Wrist C7–C8
6. Ulnar C8–T1
7. Patellar L2–L4
8. Hamstring L4–S1
9. Achilles S1–S2

ORTHOPEDIC GAMUT 1-12
SUPERFICIAL REFLEXES

1. Corneal III, V
2. Upper abdominal T7–T9
3. Lower abdominal T10–T12
4. Cremasteric
5. Gluteal
6. Plantar
7. T12–L2
8. L4–L5
9. S1–S2

ORTHOPEDIC GAMUT 1-13

PATHOLOGIC REFLEXES

1. Hoffmann
2. Babinski
3. Chaddock
4. Oppenheim
5. Bechterew-Mendel
6. Rossolimo
7. Gordon
8. Schaeffer

ORTHOPEDIC GAMUT 1-14

CRANIAL NERVES AND BASIC FUNCTION

I: Smell
II: Vision
III: Light accommodation
III, IV, VI: Eye movement
V: Sensation (wink)
VII: Facial muscle (taste)

VIII: Auditory (balance)
IX: Taste (gag)
X: Voice (swallow)
XI: Shoulder (shrug)
XII: Tongue (motor)

ORTHOPEDIC GAMUT 1-15

COMMONLY ACCEPTED DEEP-TENDON REFLEX GRADING SCHEME

0 = Absent
1 = Diminished or hyporeactive
2 = Average
2+ = Slightly exaggerated (hyperreactive)
3 = Exaggerated (hyperreactive)
4 = Associated with myoclonus

ORTHOPEDIC GAMUT 1-16

COMMON AREAS OF MENSURATION

1. Excursion of the chest during inspiration and expiration
2. Upper-extremity circumference (brachium and antebrachium), measured in the noncontracted and contracted state
3. Lower-extremity circumferences (thigh and calf), measured in the noncontracted and contracted states
4. Leg length (measured standing versus supine or prone); differentiates a functional short leg from an anatomic short leg

ORTHOPEDIC GAMUT 1-17

CERVICAL SPINE EXTRINSIC MUSCULATURE WITH SPECIFIC NERVE ROOTS NOTED

1. Deltoid (C5)
2. Biceps (C6)
3. Wrist extensors (C6)
4. Triceps (C7)
5. Wrist flexors (C7)
6. Finger extensors (C7)
7. Finger flexors (C8)
8. Finger abductors (T1)

ORTHOPEDIC GAMUT 1-18

THORACOLUMBAR EXTRINSIC MUSCULATURE AND SPECIFIC ASSOCIATED NERVE ROOT LEVELS

1. Hip flexors (L2–L3)
2. Knee extensors (L3–L4)
3. Ankle extensors (L4–L5)
4. Hip extensors (L4–L5)
5. Knee flexors (L5–S1)
6. Ankle flexors (S1–S2)

PAIN AND PATTERNS OF PAIN

Pain that arises with activity and decreases with rest is likely to have mechanical causes. The pain may be position dependent; most cases of mechanical spinal pain have both a provocative and a palliative arc of motion.

LOCAL *VERSUS* REFERRED PAIN

Patients with referred pain often point to large generalized areas, whereas patients with localized lesions can be more specific. A patient complaining of unrelenting spinal pain, demonstrating full, pain-free range of motion, presents a problem. The patient likely has either viscerosomatic pain, which mandates further diagnostic testing, or pain resulting from a psychosocial cause. If referred pain from a diseased organ system is mimicking a local orthopedic problem, the examiner should not hesitate to order appropriate tests.

VITAL SIGNS

Vital signs include the brachial blood pressure, peripheral pulse rate, respiration rate, height, weight, and vital capacity. The instrumentation for these measurements includes stethoscopes, spirometers, scales, tape measures, and blood pressure cuffs.

RANGE OF MOTION

Of all the orthopedic tests that an examiner can perform on a patient, none is more crucial than range-of-motion (ROM) testing of the affected articulation. ROM testing often reveals the origin of the patient's discomfort because movement may reproduce the pain. The patient is examined symmetrically for *active* motion of all the joints that may be involved in the dysfunction or injury. The examiner then takes the patient through *passive* ROM, evaluating the *end-feel* (i.e., springiness) of the affected joint.

ORTHOPEDIC GAMUT 1-19

JOINT END-FEEL CATEGORIES

In passive joint motion assessment, the end-feel is important. The accepted end-feel categories are:

- Bone-to-bone: an abrupt halt to movement when two hard surfaces meet
- Capsular end-feel: a *leathery* resistance to movement with a slight amount of give at the very end of the range
- Springy block: a usually pathologic end-feel, generally representing an intraarticular displacement
- Tissue approximation: no further joint movement available
- Empty feel: usually pathologic

STABILITY TESTING

Because clinical examination reveals the degree of ligamentous or joint sprain (Table 1-2), the examiner must be able to test accurately for joint instability. Stability testing moves joint and periarticular structures through their respective arcs and end-range motions. Stability testing involves stressing ligamentous tissues and joint capsules.

MUSCULAR ASSESSMENT

Movement restrictions in a joint's passive ROM are not exclusively articular. Muscular hypertonicity limits passive movement and often occurs in association with articular lesions (joint dysfunction). Chronic joint problems are also commonly associated with myofascitis.

TABLE 1-2
Injured Ligament Residual Function

Extent of Failure	Sprain	Damage*	Joint Motion, Subluxation	Residual Strength	Residual Functional Length	Residual Functional Capacity
Minimal	First degree	Less than one-third of fibers failed; includes most sprains with few to some fibers failed. Microtears also exist.	None	Retained or slightly decreased	Normal	Retained
Partial	Second degree	One-third to two-thirds ligament damage; significant damage, but parts of the ligament are still functional. Microtears may exist.	In general, minimal or no increased motion. Remaining fibers in ligament resist opening.	Marked decrease. At risk for complete failure.	Increased; still within functional range but may later act as a check rein rather than subtle control of joint motions	Marked compromise; requires healing to regain function
Complete	Third degree	More than two-thirds to complete failure; continuity remains in part.	Depends on secondary restraints	Little to none	Lost	Severely compromised or lost
		Continuity lost and gross separation between fibers	Depends on secondary restraints	None	Lost	Lost

*Estimate of damage is often difficult; however, the different types listed can usually be differentiated. Note: Anterior and posterior cruciate tears commonly exist with little to no abnormal laxity. The examination for medial and lateral ligamentous injury is usually more accurate.

From Feagin JA, editor: *The crucial ligaments.* New York, 1988, Churchill Livingstone.

ORTHOPEDIC GAMUT 1-20
RESISTED MUSCLE MOVEMENT

In assessing muscle tissue, resisted movements are the most revealing. Standard interpretations of resisted muscle testing movements include:
- Painful and strong equates with a minor lesion of muscle or tendon.
- Painful and weak equates with a major lesion of the muscle or tendon.
- Painless and weak equates with neurologic injury or complete rupture of the muscular attachment.
- Painless and strong is normal.

CLINICAL LABORATORY

For the examiner concerned with musculoskeletal disorders, differential diagnosis becomes a challenge. Complete blood and urine tests can help determine a diagnosis (Box 1-3). Diseases of the heart, liver, kidney, pancreas, and prostate can mimic back pain of spinal origin.

Most laboratory testing has limited utility for orthopedic diagnosis (Table 1-3). As an example, in **rheumatoid arthritis**, the diagnosis is often established from the history and physical examination; for **systemic lupus erythematosus**, from the laboratory test antinuclear antibody (ANA); for **gout**, from a synovial fluid examination; and for **ankylosing spondylitis**, from a radiograph. In common disorders such as osteoarthritis, fibromyalgia, or muscular strains and sprains, in essence, only a limited diagnostic role exists for laboratory tests, primarily to exclude other diagnostic possibilities.

ORTHOPEDIC GAMUT 1-21
LABORATORY RESULTS INTERPRETATIONS

For laboratory testing in orthopedic evaluations, results interpretation errors usually involve one of four areas:
1. False-positive results
2. False-negative results
3. Measurement error
4. Differences in groups of patients compared with individual patients

TABLE 1-3

LABORATORY STUDIES USEFUL IN DIAGNOSING LOW BACK SYNDROMES

Test	Measurement	Low Back Implication
Complete Blood Count Hematocrit hemoglobin	A measure of volume of circulating red blood cells	May be diminished in systemic diseases (i.e., neoplasm) and in chronic spinal infections.
White blood count and differential	Amount and type of circulating white blood cells	Total white blood cell and shifts in differential may be present in spinal infections or occasionally in spondyloarthropathies.
Sedimentation rate	Nonspecific test of inflammation	Increased in spinal infections; may be increased in neoplasms and spondyloarthropathies.
Chemistry Calcium Phosphorus	A measure of circulating calcium and phosphorus	Calcium is elevated in hyperparathyroidism, may be elevated with primary and secondary osseous tumors, alterations in the distribution of calcium and phosphorus accompany many metabolic disorders but are normal in osteoporosis.
Alkaline phosphatase	Enzyme associated with bone formation; therefore, elevation implies increased bone formation	May be elevated in primary or secondary osseous neoplasms.
Acid phosphatase	An enzyme associated with tumors metastatic to bone	Increased in prostatic tumors.
Serum proteins (albumin globulin protein electrophoresis) protein HLA-B27 antigen	Measurement of amount and type circulating A circulating antigen	Elevations of one fraction of globulin are associated with multiple myeloma. Usually individuals with spondyloarthropathies are HLA-B27 positive. Note 6–8% of men have this antigen and therefore its presence is not confirmatory of a spondyloarthropathy.

HLA, Human leukocyte antigen.
Adapted from Pope ML: *Occupational low back pain, assessment, treatment and prevention,* St Louis, 1991, Mosby.

The simplest orthopedic screen includes rheumatoid factor, ANA, and uric acid, although more elaborate screens are available, which may include erythrocyte sedimentation rate, C-reactive protein (CRP), antistreptolysin O titer, protein electrophoresis, quantitative immunoglobulins, and ANA subsets such as anti-Ro and anti-La, anti-Sm, and anticentromere antibodies.

BOX 1-3

CLINICAL LABORATORY TESTS

Individual Blood and Urine Tests

Acid phosphates
Alkaline phosphatase
Amylase
ANA
Antistreptolysin-O titer
Bence-Jones protein
Bilirubin
Blood urea nitrogen (BUN)
Calcium
Chloride (see Table A-1 in the Appendix)
Cholesterol
Creatinine
Creatinine phosphokinase
Glucose
Heavy metal screens
Hematocrit
Hemoglobin
Human leukocyte antigen (HLA)-B27
Lactic dehydrogenase (LDH) compression test II

Latex agglutination
Leucine aminopeptidase (LAP)
Lipase
Lipids
Lupus erythematosus (LE) cell preparation
Phosphorus
Potassium
Protein-bound iodine
Red blood cell (RBC) counts
Rheumatoid arthritis factor (RA latex) test
Serum glutamate oxaloacetate transaminase (SGOT)
Sodium
Uric acid
Urinalysis
White blood cell (WBC) counts (see Table A-2 in the Appendix)

Blood and Serum Panels Useful in Musculoskeletal Differential Diagnosis

Bone Panel

Alkaline phosphatase
Calcium
Complete blood count (CBC)

BOX 1-3

CLINICAL LABORATORY TESTS—cont'd

Ionized calcium
Serum protein electrophoresis
Total protein

Arthritis Panel
ANA screen
CRP
RA Latex
Uric acid

Liver Function Tests
Alkaline phosphatase
Bilirubin-total and direct
Cholesterol
Gamma-glutamyl transpeptidase (GGT) or peptidase
LDH
Serum glutamate pyruvate transaminase (SGPT)
SGOT
Total protein-albumin and globulin

Parathyroid Function and Calcium Metabolism Tests
Alkaline phosphatase
Serum calcium
Serum phosphorus
Total protein
Urine calcium

Pancreas Function Tests
Amylase
CBC
Glucose tolerance
Lipase

Joint Pain or Swelling Tests (see Table A-3 in the Appendix)
ANA screen
CBC
Heavy metal screen
RA latex
Sedimentation rate
Synovial fluid analysis, including culture
Uric acid

Continued

BOX 1-3

CLINICAL LABORATORY TESTS—cont'd

Thyroid Profile
Free thyroxine index (FTI)
Thyroid-stimulating hormone (TSH) (see Table A-4 in the Appendix)
Thyroxine (T4) (see Table A-5 in the Appendix)
Triiodothyronine (T3) (see Table A-6 in the Appendix)

Prostate Profile
Prostate-specific antigen
Prostatic acid phosphatase

Hypertension (Coronary Risk Profile)
Cholesterol
Coronary risk indicator
High-density lipoprotein (HDL) cholesterol
Low-density lipoprotein (LDL) cholesterol
Triglycerides

Health Screen
Albumin
Albumin-globulin (A/G) ratio
Alkaline phosphatase
Anion gap
Bilirubin-total
BUN
BUN-creatinine ratio
Calcium
Calculated LDL
CBC
Chloride
Cholesterol
Cholesterol-HDL ratio
Creatinine
GGT
Globulin
Glucose
HDL
Ionized calcium
LDH
Phosphorus

BOX 1-3

CLINICAL LABORATORY TESTS—cont'd

Potassium
SGOT
SGPT
Sodium
T4 radioimmunoassay (RIA)
Total carbon dioxide
Total protein
Triglycerides
Uric acid

Synovial Fluid Testing

Normal synovial fluid is a hypocellular, avascular connective tissue. In disease, the synovial fluid increases in volume and can be aspirated. Synovial fluid is a transudate of plasma supplemented with high–molecular-weight, saccharide-rich molecules. The most notable of these is hyaluronan, which is produced by fibroblast-derived type B synoviocyte (Box 1-4). Variation in the volume and composition of synovial fluid reflects pathologic processes within the joint.

BOX 1-4

NORMAL SYNOVIAL FLUID

Osmolarity	296 mOsm/L
pH	7.44
Carbon dioxide pressure	6.0 kPa (range 4.7–7.3)
Oxygen pressure	<4.0 kPa
Potassium	4.0 mmol/L
Sodium	136 mmol/L
Calcium	1.8 mmol/L
Urea	2.5 mmol/L
Uric acid	0.23 mmol/L
Glucose	100 mmol/L
Chondroitin sulfate	40 mg/L
Hyaluronate	2.14 g/L
Cholesterol	Small amounts
Total protein	~25 g/L
Albumin	~8 g/L

Continued

BOX 1-4

NORMAL SYNOVIAL FLUID—cont'd

α_1-antitrypsin	0.78 mcg/L
Ceruloplasmin	~43 mg/L
Haptoglobin	~90 mg/L
α_2-macroglobin	0.31 g/L
Lactoferrin	0.44 mg/L
IgG	2.62 g/L
IgA	0.85 g/L
IgM	0.14 g/L
IL-1β	20 pg/mL
IL-2	15.1 U/mL
TNF-α	1.38 hg/mL
INF-α	350 U/mL
INF-δ	13.7 U/mL

IgA, Immunoglobulin A; *IgG,* immunoglobulin G; *IgM,* immunoglobulin M; *IL,* interleukin; *INF,* interferon; TNF, tumor-necrosis factor.
Adapted from Klippel JH, Dieppe PA: *Rheumatology, vol 1-2,* ed 2, London, 1998, Mosby.

ORTHOPEDIC GAMUT 1-22

SYNOVIAL FLUID

For three significant aspects, analysis of synovial fluid differs from other body fluids:
1. Neoplastic processes rarely affect synovial joints.
2. Recognition of noncellular particulate material, such as microorganisms and crystals and cartilage fragments, is essential for defining the disease process affecting the joint.
3. Diagnostic information comes not only from recognition of cell types, but also from their quantification.

ORTHOPEDIC TESTS

In the orthopedic physical examination, a test is positive or a sign is present when the procedure duplicates the patient's complaint or symptom. Tests are based on joint, muscle, or nerve function. If testing causes different pain or symptoms, it may indeed be significant, but the result is not positive for the findings that the test was designed to elicit.

DIAGNOSTIC IMAGING MODALITIES IN ORTHOPEDICS

Imaging procedures are important to the diagnosis and management of an orthopedic condition. The decision to use any diagnostic imaging procedure, especially ionizing imaging procedures, should be based on a demonstrated need and should be used only after an adequate medical history is obtained and a physical examination is conducted. The decision to use any imaging procedure must also be based on the assumption that the results of the examination, even if negative, will significantly affect the treatment of the patient. The value of the information gained from the imaging examination must be worth the possible detrimental effects of the procedure. In imaging modalities that use ionizing radiation (plain-film radiography, fluoroscopy, and computed tomography [CT]), the possible effect of radiation on the patient or future offspring must be considered.

Plain-Film Radiography (Conventional Radiography)

Plain-film radiography, or conventional radiography, provides a wide and diverse array of diagnostic data about musculoskeletal problems, such as soft-tissue injury, bony malalignment, loss of integrity of the osseous structures, and joint space abnormality.

Plain-film X-ray examination is an efficient way to discover dislocations, fractures, the static component of anatomic subluxations, certain types of stress injuries, metastatic disease, some types of primary tumors, metabolic disease, degenerative arthropathic diseases (Table 1-4), and abnormalities in the growth plate.

A radiologic evaluation of the traumatized sites should include films of the adjacent joints. If a need rises for special projections, other radiologic investigation may be necessary (Table 1-5).

TABLE 1-4

PLAIN-FILM EVALUATION IN DEGENERATIVE ARTHROPATHIC DISORDERS

Diagnosis	Site of Plain-Film Findings
Psoriatic arthritis	Hand, sacroiliac joints (common); pubis symphysis, hip, knee (less common)
Rheumatoid arthritis	Wrist and hand, shoulder, knee, cervical spine, hip
Spondyloarthropathy	Sacroiliac joints, thoracolumbar spine
Osteoarthritis	Lumbosacral spine, hip, knee, foot and ankle, hand

TABLE 1-5

PREFERRED RADIOGRAPHIC VIEWS IN SKELETAL TRAUMA

Area	Specific Views
Skull	Posteroanterior or anteroposterior Caldwell Townes
	Lateral (one lateral should be upright)
Facial bones	Waters
	Modified Waters
	Caldwell
	Lateral
Cervical spine	Anteroposterior
	Coned odontoid or orthopantogram
	Odontoid
	Lateral (cross-table or upright)
	Swimmer lateral (cross-table)
	Both obliques, when possible
Thoracic spine	Anteroposterior
	Lateral (cross-table or routine)
	Swimmer (coned to upper thoracic spine)
Lumbar spine	Anteroposterior
	Lateral (cross-table or upright)
	Lateral (coned to L5–S1)
Sacrum	Anteroposterior (tube-angled cephalad)
	Lateral
Chest	Posteroanterior or anteroposterior
	Left lateral (may not be possible in trauma)
	Lateral decubitus (pneumothorax, pleural fluid)
Ribs	Anteroposterior or posteroanterior
	Oblique
Shoulder	Anteroposterior (internal rotation)
	Anteroposterior (neutral)
	Transscapular lateral (Neer)
	Axillary
Humerus	Anteroposterior (to include elbow and shoulder)
	Lateral (to include both joints)
Clavicle	Anteroposterior or posteroanterior (to include both joints with and without weight bearing)
Sternum, sternoclavicular joints	Posteroanterior
	Right and left anterior obliques with cephalad angle of tube
	Lateral
Radioulnar joints (forearm)	Anteroposterior or posteroanterior
	Lateral

TABLE 1-5

PREFERRED RADIOGRAPHIC VIEWS IN SKELETAL
TRAUMA—cont'd

Area	Specific Views
Wrist and hand	Posteroanterior
	Oblique internal, external, or both
	Lateral
	Navicular views, if needed
Pelvis, acetabulum	Anteroposterior
	Obliques (Judet)
Hip, proximal part of femur	Anteroposterior pelvis
	Frog-leg or cross-table lateral
	Obliques
Femur	Anteroposterior (to include hip and knee)
	Lateral (to include hip and knee)
Distal part of femur and knee	Anteroposterior
	Lateral
	Tunnel
	Internal oblique
Tibia, fibula	Anteroposterior (to include ankle and knee)
	Lateral (to include both joints)
Ankle	Anteroposterior
	Oblique (mortise)
	Lateral
Calcaneus	Tangential
	Lateral
Foot	Lateral
	Anteroposterior
	Oblique
	Lateral

From Gustilo RB, Kyle RF, Templeman DC: *Fractures and dislocations, vol 1*, St Louis, 1993, Mosby.

Care must be taken to investigate the possibility of associated injuries in trauma victims (Table 1-6). Patients may not realize that such injuries have occurred.

TABLE 1-6

Injuries Associated with Skeletal Trauma

Fracture	Associated Injury
Bone and Bone	
Spine	Remote additional spinal fracture
Chest wall	Scapula fracture
Anterior pelvic arch	Sacrum fracture or dislocated sacroiliac joint
Femoral shaft	Fracture or fracture-dislocation of hip
Tibia (severe)	Dislocated hip
Calcaneus	Fractured thoracolumbar spine
Bone and Viscera	
Chance fracture of spine	Ruptured mesentery or small bowel
Lower ribs	Laceration of liver, spleen, kidney, or diaphragm
Pelvis	Ruptured bladder or urethra
Pelvis	Ruptured diaphragm
Bone and Vascular	
Ribs 1, 2, or 3	Ruptured aorta
Sternum	Myocardial contusion
Pelvis	Laceration of pelvic arterial tree
Distal third femur	Laceration of femoral artery
Knee dislocation	Popliteal artery laceration

Adapted from Rogers LF, Hendrix RW: Evaluating the multiple injured patient radiographically, *Orthop Clin North Am* 21(3):444, 1990.

ORTHOPEDIC GAMUT 1-23

ARTHRITIDES: DIAGNOSIS AND CLINICAL PROGRESSION ASSESSMENT STEPS IN RHEUMATOID ARTHRITIS, PSORIATIC ARTHRITIS, ANKYLOSIS SPONDYLITIS, AND OSTEOARTHRITIS

Rheumatoid arthritis
- Serial radiographs (posteroanterior [PA] view) of hands, wrists, and feet at baseline and at 6-month intervals for a minimum of 2 years after onset
- Monitoring frequency decreased after 2 years in patients without erosions at 2 years

ORTHOPEDIC GAMUT 1-23

ARTHRITIDES: DIAGNOSIS AND CLINICAL PROGRESSION ASSESSMENT STEPS IN RHEUMATOID ARTHRITIS, PSORIATIC ARTHRITIS, ANKYLOSIS SPONDYLITIS, AND OSTEOARTHRITIS—cont'd

- Distinguishing radiographic features: bilateral symmetrical involvement of the small joints (hands, wrists, and feet), juxtaarticular osteopenia, lack of proliferative bone response, marginal erosions, joint space narrowing

Psoriatic arthritis
- Serial radiographs (PA view) of hands, wrists, and feet (and spine and other joints if symptoms are present) at baseline and at 6-month intervals for a minimum of 2 years after onset
- Distinguishing radiographic features: asymmetric and possibly oligoarticular joint involvement, initially marginal erosions that become irregular and ill defined, distal interphalangeal joint involvement, abnormalities in phalangeal tufts and at sites of attachments of tendons and ligaments to the bone, possible spondylitis, paramarginal syndesmophytes in nonconsecutive vertebrae, *sausage digits,* proliferative bone changes, and ankylosis

Ankylosing spondylitis
- Serial radiographs (anteroposterior [AP] view) of pelvis, sacroiliac joints, and axial spine
- If early ankylosing spondylitis is suspected, repeat pelvic radiographs 6 months from baseline; otherwise, serial radiographs of pelvis, sacroiliac joints, and axial spine annually or every other year
- Serial radiographs (lateral and AP views) of cervical, thoracic, and lumbar spine annually or every other year
- Radiographs (PA view) of hands and feet at baseline; follow-up radiographs based on clinical features
- Distinguishing radiographic features: cervical lesions not typically associated with instability and subluxations of the lower five vertebrae, as in rheumatoid arthritis, less-severe hip lesions than in rheumatoid arthritis without protrusions, osteophytes along the margin of articular cartilage of the femoral head, marginal syndesmophytes in consecutive vertebrae, sacroiliitis,

Continued

ORTHOPEDIC GAMUT 1-23

ARTHRITIDES: DIAGNOSIS AND CLINICAL PROGRESSION ASSESSMENT STEPS IN RHEUMATOID ARTHRITIS, PSORIATIC ARTHRITIS, ANKYLOSIS SPONDYLITIS, AND OSTEOARTHRITIS—cont'd

bamboo spine, smaller and more localized erosions and less-frequent joint space narrowing, and osteopenia compared with rheumatoid arthritis

Osteoarthritis

- Radiographs (PA view) of the hands and feet annually
- Radiographs of the hips (AP pelvic in supine position) and knees (standing, weight-bearing AP with full knee extension) annually
- Distinguishing radiographic features of osteoarthritis: osteophytes, subchondral sclerosis
- Distinguishing radiographic features of erosive osteoarthritis: distribution in distal joints of fingers similar to that of psoriatic arthritis, centrally located erosions, erosions typically absent in metacarpophalangeal joints

Adapted from Ory PA: Radiography in the assessment of musculoskeletal conditions, *Best Pract Res Clin Rheumatol* 17(3):495-512, 2003.

ORTHOPEDIC GAMUT 1-24

ASSESSMENT ABILITIES AND LIMITATIONS OF PLAIN-FILM RADIOGRAPHY

1. Plain-film radiography is the least expensive and most widely available imaging technique.
2. Radiography offers higher spatial resolution than any other modality, providing extremely high contrast for cortical and trabecular bone.
3. Radiography affords only a projectional viewing perspective.
4. Projection of three-dimensional anatomy onto a two-dimensional film results in morphologic distortion and superimposition of overlapping structures.
5. The sensitivity for trabecular bone loss is relatively poor.

ORTHOPEDIC GAMUT 1-24

1

ASSESSMENT ABILITIES AND LIMITATIONS OF PLAIN-FILM RADIOGRAPHY—cont'd

6. As much as 30% to 50% of trabecular bone must be lost before the change becomes perceptible on conventional radiographs.
7. The contrast for soft tissues that are not calcified or fatty is relatively poor.
8. Radiography cannot directly visualize the articular cartilage, inflamed synovial tissue, joint effusion, bone marrow edema, or intraarticular fat pads.

Tomography

Conventional tomography is also known as *thin-section radiography, planigraphy,* and *linear tomography.* Conventional tomography is largely replaced by CT. However, some circumstances, such as evaluating subtle alterations of bone density and ruling out fracture, necessitate conventional tomography. CT scans are used for more detailed appreciation of skeletal pathologic processes, which can help evaluate suspected intervertebral disc protrusions or herniations, facet disease, or central canal and lateral recess stenosis. If spinal disease is suspected and is not well identified on plain films and the patient is not responding to care, a CT scan is indicated. A CT scan is especially useful for the appreciation of bone and calcifications and surpasses magnetic resonance imaging (MRI) in this regard.

ORTHOPEDIC GAMUT 1-25

ASSESSMENT ABILITIES AND LIMITATIONS OF COMPUTED TOMOGRAPHY

1. The greatest advantage of CT over conventional radiography is its tomographic nature.
2. CT provides high contrast between bone and adjacent tissues and is excellent for evaluating osseous structures.
3. CT offers slightly greater soft-tissue contrast than radiography.

ORTHOPEDIC GAMUT 1-25

ASSESSMENT ABILITIES AND LIMITATIONS OF COMPUTED TOMOGRAPHY—cont'd

4. Image contrast is insufficient to visualize the articular cartilage or synovial tissue or to discriminate between tendonitis and tendon rupture.
5. CT reveals only the surfaces of these structures; it does not disclose intra substance changes that may precede gross morphologic disruption.

Discography

Although effective, discography has been a controversial imaging modality for spinal disc disease. Clinicians use discography for specific cases of spinal pain that are recalcitrant to conventional therapy.

ORTHOPEDIC GAMUT 1-26

USES OF DISCOGRAPHY

- To rule out disc involvement, especially as a cause of post-operative pain
- To determine the appropriate level for spinal fusion
- To test the potential effectiveness of chemonucleolysis
- To visualize internal disc anatomy

Magnetic Resonance Imaging

MRI is a computerized, thin-section imaging procedure that uses a magnetic field and radio-frequency waves rather than ionizing radiation. MRI can produce thin-section images in the sagittal, coronal, or axial planes, as well as any other oblique plane desired. The MRI can image neurologic structures and other soft tissues and can reveal disc degeneration before any other imaging method. Indications for MRI are similar to those for CT. MRI is superior to CT for evaluating possible spinal cord tumors or damage, intracranial disease, and various types of central nervous system disease (e.g., multiple sclerosis). MRI is especially useful in identifying small differences among similar soft tissues and surpasses CT in this regard.

For patients who have sustained head trauma with skull fractures, MRI is an efficient way to identify the early signs of cerebral edema. The test procedure of choice for diagnosing metastatic disease is an MRI scan (Table 1-7).

TABLE 1-7

MAGNETIC RESONANCE IMAGING VERSUS COMPUTED TOMOGRAPHY

Anatomic Area	Indications	Recommended Procedure
Brain (including brainstem)	Initial evaluation (e.g., demyelination disease seizures)	MRI
		MRI
	Previous normal CT	CT or MRI*
	Previous abnormal CT	MRI
	Unchanged abnormal CT with increase in symptoms	MRI
	Contrast allergy	CT
	Acute trauma	MRI
	Pituitary tumors	
Ear, nose, throat, and eye	Neurosensory hearing loss (e.g., to rule out acoustic neuroma)	CT
		CT
	Conductive hearing loss	CT or MRI*
	Cancer staging (including laryngeal cancer)	CT
		CT
	Cholesteatoma of temporal bone	MRI
	Fractures of facial bones	CT or MRI*
	Thyroid or parathyroid dysfunction (after US)	MRI or CT*
	Sinus conditions	MRI
	Orbital disease	MRI
	Disease of optic tracts and chiasm	
	Internal derangement of temporomandibular joint	
Musculoskeletal spine	Lower back or radicular pain in younger person	MRI
		MRI or CT*
	Lower back or radicular pain in older person	MRI
		MRI
	Cervical disk disease	CT or MRI*
	Spinal stenosis	MRI
	Cervical	MRI
	Lumbar	
	Tumors	
	Metastatic disease	
Hips	Early detection of aseptic necrosis	MRI
	Congenital hip dislocation or reduction	US
Extremities	Tumors, disease, or injury to muscle, ligaments, or cartilage	MRI
		CT
	Confirmation of calcification or fracture	

TABLE 1-7

MAGNETIC RESONANCE IMAGING VERSUS COMPUTED
TOMOGRAPHY—cont'd

Anatomic Area	Indications	Recommended Procedure
Chest	Diseases of the hila	MRI
	Diseases of the mediastinum	MRI or CT*
	Lung disease	CT
Abdomen and pelvis	General survey (e.g., to rule out tumor)	CT
		CT or MRI*
	Liver disease	MRI
	Renal cell cancer staging	MRI, CT, or US
	Prostate disease	MRI or CT
	Bladder disease	MRI*
	Abdominal aortic aneurysm	
	Other	

CT, Computed tomography; *MRI,* magnetic resonance imaging; *US,* ultrasonography.
*Consult radiologist for imaging options.
From Brier SR: *Primary care orthopedics,* St Louis, 1999, Mosby; originally courtesy
of Robert Goodman, MD, South Suffolk MRI, PC, Bayshore, New York.

ORTHOPEDIC GAMUT 1-27

FOR CERTAIN PATHOLOGIC CONDITIONS, MAGNETIC RESONANCE IMAGING IS THE DIAGNOSTIC PROCEDURE OF CHOICE

1. Spinal disc disease
2. Medullary tumor
3. Multiple sclerosis
4. Cerebral edema
5. Spinal stenosis
6. Metastatic disease
7. Herniated disc
8. Discitis (or infection)
9. Meniscal tear (fibrocartilage abnormalities)
10. Central nervous system tumor
11. Soft-tissue tumor

| ORTHOPEDIC GAMUT 1-28 | 1 |

ASSESSMENT ABILITIES AND LIMITATIONS OF MAGNETIC RESONANCE IMAGING

1. Diarthrodial joints are particularly suitable for MRI.
2. MRI is unparalleled in its ability to depict soft-tissue detail.
3. MRI is the only modality that can examine all components of the joint simultaneously.

Contrast Arthrography

The conventional use of arthrography in musculoskeletal disease involves the use of air to distend a synovial joint and a radiopaque contrast agent to outline anatomic structures. The injection of contrast material into the joint space results in a radiographic outline of the cartilage, menisci, ligaments, or synovium. Conventional arthrography is used in diagnosis of the scope and magnitude of orthopedic trauma to the shoulder, wrist, knee, and ankle (Table 1-8).

TABLE 1-8

JOINTS TYPICALLY STUDIED WITH COMPUTED TOMOGRAPHIC ARTHROGRAPHY AFTER TRAUMA

Joint	To Observe
Knee	Meniscus, cruciate and collateral ligaments, hyaline cartilage tears, osteochondral defects
Shoulder	Rotator cuff, glenoid labrum disruption
Hip	Hyaline cartilage integrity and tears, prosthetic joint loosening
Wrist	Triangular fibrocartilage, intercarpal ligament integrity
Elbow	Hyaline cartilage integrity, osteochondral defects
Ankle	Ligamentous tears, osteochondral defects
Temporomandibular	Disc and condylar integrity

Adapted from Gustilo RB, Kyle RF, Templeman DC: *Fractures and dislocations, vol 1,* St Louis, 1993, Mosby.

Radionuclide Scanning

Examinations conducted with the use of nuclear medicine techniques, including bone scans, positron emission tomography (PET) scans, and single-photon emission computed tomography (SPECT) scans, are valuable in diagnostic imaging because of their highly sensitive and noninvasive nature. Whole-body scanning for metastatic and infectious diseases, as well as inflammatory and ischemic processes, is possible with scintigraphy.

ORTHOPEDIC GAMUT 1-29

ASSESSMENT ABILITIES AND LIMITATIONS OF RADIONUCLIDE SCANNING

1. The principal advantage of scintigraphy over other imaging modalities is its ability to help in identifying tissues or organs with abnormal physiologic or biochemical properties.
2. Increased skeletal uptake is observable at sites of elevated blood flow or increased bone metabolism.
3. Scintigraphy is a convenient way of surveying the entire skeleton for multifocal processes.

Video Fluoroscopy

Video fluoroscopy is used when a function study of the joint is warranted. Video fluoroscopy should be used when a biomechanical abnormality is present but is not adequately demonstrated by plain film stress surveys or other examination methods.

Diagnostic Ultrasound

Diagnostic ultrasound, a sound wave echo study, is particularly useful for evaluating soft tissues. The diagnostic ultrasound does not provide the same quality of image as CT or MRI.

ORTHOPEDIC GAMUT 1-30

ASSESSMENT ABILITIES AND LIMITATIONS OF ULTRASONOGRAPHY

1. Ultrasonography offers direct multiplanar tomography without any need for image reformatting.
2. Ultrasonography can also provide images in real time, without any exposure to ionizing radiation.

ORTHOPEDIC GAMUT 1-30

ASSESSMENT ABILITIES AND LIMITATIONS OF ULTRASONOGRAPHY—cont'd

3. The modality is inexpensive and widely available.
4. Ultrasonography offers relatively good soft-tissue contrast and is particularly effective at helping to identify fluid collections such as bursitis and abscesses.
5. Ultrasound waves cannot penetrate bone.

Myelography

Traditional myelographic techniques involve the introduction of small amounts of water-soluble contrast medium into the subarachnoid space, either through a lumbar approach below the level of the conus medullaris or at the level of C1–C2 through a posterolateral approach. Standard films of the spinal canal are made to determine the presence or absence of a filling defect. In cases of acute spinal trauma, myelography may be used in conjunction with CT. Myelography remains valuable in evaluating intrinsic spinal cord lesions, nerve root lesions, and dural tears associated with severe trauma (Box 1-5).

BOX 1-5

STRENGTHS AND LIMITATIONS OF MYELOGRAPHIC STUDIES

Strengths

Studies of the subarachnoid space are possible.
Intraarachnoid lesions are shown.
Demarcation of multi-disc levels is shown.
Information on surgical scars is provided.
Assessment of flexion and extension dynamic are possible.

Limitations

Lesions removed from outside of the thecal sac can be missed.
Study variations are problematic.
Detail shown in the dorsal spine is poor.
Postoperative studies are impossible to read with accuracy.
Testing procedure is invasive.

From Brier SR: *Primary care orthopedics,* St Louis, 1999, Mosby.

Thermography

Using temperature differentials of the body, thermography illustrates neurovascular changes in injury or disease. Thermograms do not provide specific information regarding the cause of nerve fiber irritation (e.g., herniated disc, scar tissue, myospasm).

ORTHOPEDIC GAMUT 1-31

ASSESSMENT ABILITIES AND LIMITATIONS OF THERMOGRAPHY

1. The thermographic examination is performed with the use of contact liquid crystal detectors or electronic infrared sensors.
2. Thermography is extremely sensitive to microvascular changes in the skin.
3. Thermography is excellent for differentiating between a neurologic and vascular abnormality.
4. Thermography has a greater degree of sensitivity in documenting neurovascular abnormality than any other imaging system.
5. Thermography has a greater degree of specificity of image than radionuclide bone scan.
6. Thermography has a lesser degree of specificity of image resolution than CT or MRI.

Electrodiagnostic Testing

Although electrodiagnostic testing provides valuable information, it does not stand alone as a diagnostic entity (Table 1-9). The data obtained must be correlated with the physical examination findings and case history.

TABLE 1-9

STRENGTHS AND LIMITATIONS OF ELECTRODIAGNOSTIC TESTING

Testing Modality	Strengths	Limitations
Nerve conduction velocity	Helpful in ruling out peripheral entrapment neuropathic conditions (e.g., prolonged latencies exhibited in carpal tunnel syndrome, tarsal tunnel syndrome) and ulnar neuropathic variations	Provides imperfect sensitivity; limited localization and determination of injury severity; timing of study an important factor

TABLE 1-9

STRENGTHS AND LIMITATIONS OF ELECTRODIAGNOSTIC
TESTING—cont'd

Testing Modality	Strengths	Limitations
F waves	Provides screening for late motor response with distal sweeps starting at the foot	Evaluates motor reflex only; possibly evaluates abnormal findings only in the presence of multiple-level injury
H reflex	Equivalent of ankle joint reflex; evaluates monosynaptic reflex with sensory and motor S1 function	Provides assessment of S1 nerve root only
SSEPs	Helpful in documenting sensory pathway disturbances in proximal neural injury and central conduction delays, as in myopathies and multiple sclerosis	Offers imperfect localization; findings are rarely abnormal if results of other electrodiagnostic tests are within normal limits
Needle EMG	Useful in assessing conductivity of neural tissues; helpful in determining site and severity of lesion; may be helpful in early assessment of recovery, screening for fibrillation potentials, and signs of denervation from nerve root compression disorders	Unable to detect denervation potentials for 14 to 28 days after injury; provides imperfect sensitivity; study timing an important factor; proximal lesions sometimes inaccessible anatomically; effectiveness reduced after surgery

EMG, Electromyography; *SSEPs,* somatosensory-evoked potentials.
Adapted from Brier SR: *Primary care orthopedics,* St Louis, 1999, Mosby.

ORTHOPEDIC GAMUT 1-32

ASSESSMENT ABILITIES AND LIMITATIONS OF NERVE CONDUCTION VELOCITY TESTING

1. Studies of nerve conduction velocity (NCV) can rule out peripheral neuropathic conditions.
2. Routine NCV tests are not specific for conditions such as radiculopathy, but they may be helpful in cases of chronic pain that have a questionable spinal origin.

ORTHOPEDIC GAMUT 1-33

ASSESSMENT ABILITIES AND LIMITATIONS OF ELECTROMYOGRAPHY

1. Electromyography (EMG) shows fibrillation potentials and possible motor unit changes in denervated muscles.
2. Denervation of paraspinal muscle, indicates that the patient has a lesion at the nerve root level.
3. The usual finding of needle EMG in a patient who has dorsal root disease is normal.
4. EMG does not provide any information with respect to the locus of injury (e.g., root, nerve, muscle) and, in fact, often reflects associated tissue injury rather than neurovascular dysfunction.

Doppler Ultrasonic Vascular Testing

Doppler vascular testing allows the assessment of pulses in noisy environments or when pulses are weak. This test is efficient when palpation of a pulse is questionable or not possible. The Doppler instrument aids in the assessment of circulation distal to fracture sites, burns, and other injuries that potentially compromise vascular tissue, quickly determining the extent of injury.

CHAPTER TWO

ASSESSING CARDINAL MUSCULOSKELETAL SYMPTOMS AND SIGNS

AXIOMS IN ASSESSING CARDINAL MUSCULOSKELETAL SYMPTOMS AND SIGNS

- The important symptoms in neuromusculoskeletal disease or injury include pain, stiffness, locking, swelling, weakness or difficulty moving, and fatigue.
- *Pain* is the most common presenting symptom.

INTRODUCTION

The actual technique of examination varies according to individual preference. Nevertheless, developing and adhering to a particular routine can be useful. Familiarity with such a routine ensures that an examiner does not overlook any step in the examination.

The part or region under evaluation must be adequately exposed and in good lighting. Many mistakes are made simply because the examiner does not insist on removing enough of the patient's clothing to allow proper evaluation and inspection (Fig. 2-1). When examining the involved extremity, the uninvolved extremity is always used for comparison.

ORTHOPEDIC GAMUT 2-1

VISUAL INSPECTION

Systematically, visual inspection focuses on four areas:
1. Bones: Observe the general alignment and position of the parts to detect any deformity, shortening, and unusual posture.
2. Soft tissues: Observe the soft-tissue contours, comparing bilaterally and noting any visible evidence of general or local swelling and muscle wasting.

Continued

ORTHOPEDIC GAMUT 2-1

VISUAL INSPECTION—cont'd

3. Color and texture of the skin: Look for rubor, cyanosis, pigmentation, shininess, loss of hair, and other changes.
4. Scars or tissue sinuses: If a scar is present, determine from its appearance whether it was caused by operation (linear scar with suture marks), injury (irregular scar), or suppuration (broad, adherent, puckered scar).

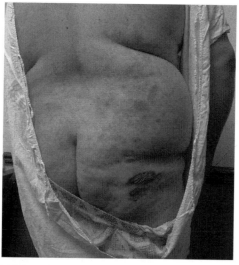

FIG. 2-1 Male patient with chronic piriformis syndrome and sciatica. Examination revealed healed third-degree burns and scarring over the right lower lumbar spine and the right gluteal region secondary to splash injury with molten brass in a foundry. Customary hyperalgesia associated with burn recovery complicated the examination.

ORTHOPEDIC GAMUT 2-2

PALPATION

Four elements are the focus of palpation:

1. Skin temperature: By careful bilateral comparison, determine whether an area of increased warmth or unusual coolness is present. An increase in local temperature denotes increased blood flow; the usual cause is an inflammatory reaction. A rapidly growing tumor also may cause marked local hyperemia.
2. Bones: Investigate the general shape and outline of the bone. Palpate in particular for thickening, abnormal prominence, and disturbed relationship of the normal landmarks. Spinal palpation accuracy is clinically acceptable for noninvasive therapeutic intervention because any given vertebra obviously articulates with vertebra above and below.
3. Soft tissue: Direct attention is given to the muscle (spasm, atrophy), joint tissue (synovial membrane, joint distension), and the detection of any local and general swelling of the part.
4. Local tenderness: The exact borders of any local tenderness should be delineated. An attempt is made to relate this tenderness to a particular structure.

ORTHOPEDIC GAMUT 2-3

PRESENTING MUSCULOSKELETAL SYMPTOMS AND SIGNS

Symptoms and signs will differentiate musculoskeletal complaints into five main types:

1. Inflammatory disease
2. Mechanical articular or periarticular disorder
3. Systemic disease characterized by musculoskeletal symptoms or signs
4. Idiopathic disorder
5. Functional disorder

CARDINAL SYMPTOMS

Pain and Sensibility

Among presenting symptoms, pain is usually most important for the patient. Among presenting signs, swelling of a joint or periarticular tissue is important. With regard to pain, the examiner must be certain of the site of origin and distribution. The patient's verbal description may be misleading. The patient should be able to point to or define the site of maximal intensity and map out the area over which pain is experienced.

Factors that exacerbate or ameliorate the pain are important. Pain during an activity suggests a mechanical problem, particularly if it worsens during use and quickly improves when resting. Pain while at rest, and pain that is worse at the beginning rather than at the end of use, implies a marked inflammatory component. Night pain is a distressing symptom that reflects intraosseous hypertension and accompanies serious problems, such as avascular necrosis, bone neoplastic activity, or bone collapse adjacent to a severely arthritic joint. Persistent bony pain is characteristic of neoplastic invasion. The activities that create a mechanical pain may provide clues as to the appropriate diagnosis. Periarticular problems are often induced by a specific type of activity but are also divided by region (Table 2-1).

TABLE 2-1

REGIONAL PERIARTICULAR SYNDROMES

Region	Periarticular Syndrome
Jaw	Temporomandibular joint dysfunction (myofascial pain syndrome)
Shoulder	Subacromial bursitis
	Long-head bicipital tendinitis
	Rotator cuff tear
Elbow	Olecranon bursitis
	Epicondylitis
Wrist	Extensor tendinitis (including de Quervain tenosynovitis)
	Gonococcal tenosynovitis
Hand	Palmar fasciitis (Dupuytren contracture)
	Ligamentous or capsular injury
Hip	Greater trochanteric bursitis
	Adductor syndrome
	Ischial bursitis
	Fascia lata syndrome
Knee	Anserine bursitis
	Prepatellar bursitis
	Meniscal injury
	Ligamentous tear-laxity
	Baker cyst

TABLE 2-1

REGIONAL PERIARTICULAR SYNDROMES—cont'd

Region	Periarticular Syndrome
Ankle	Peroneal tendinitis
	Achilles tendinitis
	Retrocalcaneal bursitis
	Calcaneal fasciitis
	Sprain
	Erythema nodosum
Foot	Plantar fasciitis
	Pes planus *(fallen arches)*

Adapted from Kelley WN, et al: *Textbook of rheumatology*, ed 5, Philadelphia, 1997, WB Saunders.

Peripheral Nociceptors

The skin, joint structures, arterial walls, and periosteum are richly supplied with nociceptors that are activated by a variety of mechanical (stretching), thermal (heat and cold), and chemical stimuli. The main neurotransmitters involved in pain inhibitory pathways are serotonin, norepinephrine, and the endogenous opioids.

Weakness

Weakness of limbs or of the whole body can be an important clue. The pattern of asymmetric or symmetric muscle weakness and its central or peripheral distribution may give vital clues to the diagnosis. *Weakness* may describe the difficulty that the patient has with movement because of joint disease or the feeling of insecurity that is associated with a loss of proprioception that accompanies many forms of joint disease. Patients may also use the term *weakness* to describe general fatigue rather than loss of muscle power. True generalized muscular weakness often affects gait and stance. Ankle, knee, and hip movements and strength need to be assessed.

Stiffness

Stiffness is a subjective sensation of resistance to movement that probably reflects fluid distension of the limiting boundary of the inflamed tissue. Stiffness resulting from this phenomenon is most noticeable when arising from bed and after inactivity or rest. As normal use resumes, fluid clears from the inflamed structures, and stiffness wears off. The duration and severity of early-morning stiffness (or stiffness after sleep) and inactivity stiffness reflect the degree of local inflammation.

BOX 2-1

ABILITY DEPRECIATION ASSESSMENT

Question the patient's...
Ability to perform key task
Loss of work capacity
Adequacy for job
Adequacy for occupation
Maximal dependable ability

Compared with...
Preinjury ability
Normal values
Specific job demands
General occupational demands
General employment standards

Adapted from Demeter SL: *Disability evaluation*, St Louis, 1996, Mosby.

Disability and Handicap

Disability is present when a tissue, organ, or system cannot function adequately. A handicap exists when disability interferes with a patient's daily activities or social or occupational performance. A marked disability does not necessarily cause a handicap. Conversely, minor disability may produce a major handicap. Both states of disability and handicap require separate assessment, with the evaluation of disability being a purely medical activity, whereas handicap assessment is often a medicolegal function. Patients' perceptions of their problems is a product of their adaptation to the depreciated tissue, as well as aspirations for recovery (Box 2-1).

ORTHOPEDIC GAMUT 2-4

ASSESSING DISABILITY

An aid in assessing the more important aspects of disability is the PILS mnemonic, which considers four issues:
1. **P**reventable causes of disability (e.g., falls, direct trauma)
2. **I**ndependence (e.g., self-care)
3. **L**ifestyle (roles, goals)
4. **S**ocial factors (e.g., family, friends, shelter)

ORTHOPEDIC GAMUT 2-5

SPECIFIC ELEMENTS TO CONSIDER IN ACTIVITIES OF DAILY LIVING ASSESSMENT

Feeding
- Utensil, cup, and plate management and napkin use
- Tidiness and organization
- Awareness of problems in swallowing, chewing, and pocketing
- Ability to handle different food consistencies (e.g., finger foods versus soups)
- Mouth care after eating

Bathing
- Assembling of items and appropriate equipment
- Management of caps, lids, sprays, etc.
- Facial cleansers and cosmetic applications
- Shaving foam or soap application versus electric razor
- Shaving face, underarms, or legs
- Hair care
- Deodorant application
- Tooth or denture care
- Nail care
- Replacement of care items
- Location of bath facilities in hospital or home
- Transfer ability to bathtub or shower

Dressing
- Selection of clothing
- Assembling of clothing
- Application of underwear
- Management of fasteners
- Application of trousers or slacks and belts or suspenders
- Management of pullover tops
- Application of shirt, jacket, dress (front opening), or tie
- Management of buttons
- Application of socks or stockings
- Application of shoes or tying laces
- Location of dressing activities: while in bed, sitting, or standing
- Ability to care for and wear eyeglasses, contact lenses, or hearing aid

Continued

ORTHOPEDIC GAMUT 2-5

SPECIFIC ELEMENTS TO CONSIDER IN ACTIVITIES OF DAILY LIVING ASSESSMENT—cont'd

Toileting and Elimination Management
- Transfer ability
- Clothing management
- Cognitive function
- Bowel and bladder control
- External devices; assembly, application, removal, and care of equipment
- Suppository insertion (include preparation of suppository and cleaning of insertion device, if used)
- Hygiene after toileting
- Timing of bowel program (morning or evening)
- Employment, school, home, or environment considerations
- Colostomy or ileal conduit care
- Performance of bladder management programs
- Accident management

Sleep
- Lying still
- Turning over at night in bed
- Getting up and walking in the morning

Movement and Transfer
- Standing upright
- Sitting
- Walking on a flat surface
- Walking on uneven ground
- Ascending stairs
- Descending stairs

Grasp and Lifting
- Performing overhead work
- Scratching own back
- Lifting light objects
- Carrying out chores at home or at work
- Lifting heavy objects
- Throwing objects

Miscellaneous
- Having sexual intercourse
- Participating in athletics

ORTHOPEDIC GAMUT 2-6

FUNCTIONAL ASSESSMENT

A complete functional assessment includes evaluation of the following:
1. Self-care: ability to wash, bathe, attend to toilet needs, dress, cook, and feed oneself
2. Mobility: ability to stand, transfer, walk, negotiate stairs, drive, and use public transportation
3. Lifestyle: nature of occupation, work capacity, and Social Security benefits

---

SYSTEMIC ILLNESS

Inflammatory musculoskeletal disease may trigger a marked acute-phase response and cause nonspecific symptoms of systemic upset. Symptoms may include fever, reduced appetite, weight loss, fatigue, lethargy,and irritability. The patient might not volunteer specific complaints but might report feeling ill. Florid, acute inflammation may cause confusion, especially in older adults.

Sleep Disturbance

Several factors may interfere with normal sleep patterns and cause anxiety and depression. These factors include chronic pain, triggering of the acute-phase response, unreasonable anxiety concerning deformity and morbidity, central nervous system (CNS) side effects from pain-relieving drugs, and severe arthropathy. Features of masked or overt depression should be sought, particularly in patients with severe musculoskeletal disease. A poor sleep pattern is also a feature of fibromyalgia.

Fatigue

Fatigue is sometimes functional or the result of overexertion. It can be prominent in noninflammatory conditions such as fibromyalgia. Fatigue can be a good indicator of the systemic activity of the disease. In fibromyalgia, most patients report profound fatigue. Seemingly, minor activities aggravate the pain and fatigue, although prolonged inactivity also heightens fibromyalgic symptoms.

Emotional Lability

Patients with emotional lability are usually anxious to the extent that they may have some severe disease or injury that will cause permanent disfigurement or disability. Pain is a potent cause of anxiety. Much of the important information regarding the patient's perception of pain and accommodation is gleaned during the clinical evaluation from the history, either during the examination or from a health assessment questionnaire.

Referred Symptoms

When the source of the symptom is still in doubt after thorough examination of the part, attention must be directed to possible extrinsic disorders. Determination of extrinsic disorders requires examination of other regions of the body that might be responsible. For instance, in a case of pain in the shoulder, examining the neck might be necessary for evidence of a lesion interfering with the brachial plexus. For pain in the thigh, the examination often includes a study of the spine, abdomen, pelvis, and genitourinary system, as well as the local examination of the hip and thigh.

The afferent pain fibers originating from the same area demonstrate extensive convergence onto the dorsal horn relay cells. In certain cases, the convergence may take place by fibers from different areas, causing relay cell activation by pain originating in different body parts. This mechanism underlies the phenomenon of referred pain (e.g., pain originating in the heart is often felt at the inner aspects of the left arm). Referred pain is either caused by convergence of pain fibers from both zones onto the same spinal relay cell or caused by facilitation of somatic signals during excessive pain traffic from a visceral source. Classic examples of this phenomenon include the referral of neck or shoulder pain to the upper arm (Table 2-2).

TABLE 2-2

CERVICAL SPINE SYNDROMES REFERRING PAIN TO THE UPPER EXTREMITY

Lesions Producing Neck and Shoulder Pain	Lesions Producing Predominantly Shoulder Pain
Postural disorders	Rotator cuff tears and tendinitis
Rheumatoid arthritis	Calcareous tendinitis
Fibrositis syndromes	Subacromial bursitis
Musculoligamentous injuries to neck and shoulder	Bicipital tendonitis
	Adhesive capsulitis
Osteoarthritis (apophyseal and Luschka)	Reflex sympathetic dystrophy
	Frozen shoulder syndromes
Cervical spondylosis	Acromioclavicular secondary osteoarthritis
Intervertebral osteoarthritis	

TABLE 2-2		
CERVICAL SPINE SYNDROMES REFERRING PAIN TO THE UPPER EXTREMITY—cont'd		2
Lesions Producing Neck and Shoulder Pain	**Lesions Producing Predominantly Shoulder Pain**	
Thoracic outlet syndrome	Glenohumeral arthritis	
Nerve injuries (serratus anterior, C3–C4 nerve root, long thoracic nerve)	Septic arthritis Tumors of the shoulder	

Modified from Kelley WN, et al: *Textbook of rheumatology*, ed 5, Philadelphia, 1997, WB Saunders.

CARDINAL SIGNS

Posture

The way the patient positions an affected region or joint is important. A joint with synovitis has **intraarticular hypertension** and is most comfortable in the position that minimizes any pressure increases. Usually, the part is adducted and held in internal rotation or flexion. The opposite movements—abduction and external rotation or extension— are the earliest movements affected and the most uncomfortable because they maximize intraarticular hypertension. The attitude of the body part and pattern of restricted movement may suggest the underlying problem.

Changes in Dimension of the Part

Measurement of the circumference of an extremity provides an index of muscle atrophy, soft-tissue swelling, or bony thickening. Signs of active current inflammation and abnormal tissue responses are crucial in distinguishing arthritides from arthralgia of noninflammatory origin (e.g., mechanical defects, hypermobility).

Decreased Circulation

Symptoms in a region or joint may be associated with impairment of the arterial circulation. Time should be spent in assessing the state of the circulation by examining the color, temperature, and texture of the skin and the nails and in measuring the arterial pulses. This examination is particularly important in the extremities and extremely important in the lower extremities. An important point to remember is that position, exertion, and endogenous blood pressures all play a role in tissue health.

TABLE 2-3	
JOINT AND SOFT-TISSUE EDEMA	
Tissue	**Indicative of**
Joint synovium/effusion	Inflammatory joint diseases
Subcutaneous tissue	Inflammatory joint disease
Bursa/tendon sheath	Inflammation of structure
Articular ends of bone	Osteoarthritis

Diffuse Joint Swelling

Soft-tissue swelling is pathognomonic of inflammation (Table 2-3). Joint, bursal, or tenosynovial inflammation is almost invariably accompanied by the presence of an inflammatory exudate. An important step in confirming inflammation is the detection of effusion. In small joints, cross-fluctuation is applied with the examiner's index finger pressing dorsally while the joint is gently squeezed from the sides between the examiner's index finger and thumb.

ORTHOPEDIC GAMUT 2-7
DIFFUSE JOINT SWELLING
Diffuse swelling of a joint as a whole can have only three causes: 1. Thickening of the bone end 2. Fluid within the joint 3. Thickening of the synovial membrane

Skin Changes

Overlying scars or skin disease may be important clues to causation of deeper rheumatic symptoms. Erythema, commonly followed by desquamation, is an important sign reflecting periarticular inflammation. Although erythema may occur in several conditions, a red joint or bursa should always raise suspicion of sepsis or crystal deposition disorders.

2

ORTHOPEDIC GAMUT 2-8

CAUSES OF ERYTHEMA OVERLYING A JOINT

- Sepsis
- Crystals (gout, pseudogout, calcific periarthritis)
- Rheumatoid arthritis
- Acute Reiter or reactive arthropathy
- Early Heberden or Bouchard nodes
- Inflammatory (erosive) osteoarthritis of the hands
- Rheumatic fever

Erythema

Redness is uncommon but is encountered in gout, especially around the big toe, and sepsis in any joint. The primary lesion of erythema migrans, which is nearly pathognomonic of acute Lyme disease, is usually found at the site of the tick bite.

Discoid lupus has a virtually diagnostic appearance and distribution (Table 2-4) but may require histopathologic and immunofluorescence studies. Misdiagnosis of acute lupus can occur in patients expressing other photosensitive eruptions and in patients with conditions that produce vascular dilation (Table 2-5). A clinical history and examination are usually sufficient to discriminate acute lupus from other photosensitive eruptions.

Features of dermatomyositis rash allow discrimination from lupus. These features include occasional nasolabial fold involvement, prominent heliotrope and extrafacial involvement, erythema following the course of extensor tendons, and scaling and fissuring of lateral aspects of the fingers (mechanic's hands). A heliotrope rash and Gottron papules are characteristic and possibly pathognomonic cutaneous features

---

TABLE 2-4

FACIAL DISEASES CONFUSED WITH LUPUS

Polymorphous light eruption (occasional)
Benign lymphocytic infiltration of Jessner (rare)
Seborrheic dermatitis (common)
Acne rosacea (common)
Tinea faciei (occasional)
Lupus vulgaris tuberculous (rare)
Lupus pernio sarcoid (rare)

TABLE 2-5

Revised Criteria for the Classification of Systemic Lupus Erythematosus (1982)

Criterion	Definition
1. Malar rash	Fixed erythema, flat or raised, over the eminences, tending to spare the nasolabial folds
2. Discoid rash	Erythematous raised patches with adherent keratotic scaling and follicular plugging; atrophic scarring may occur in older lesions
3. Photosensitivity	Skin rash as a result of unusual reaction to sunlight, revealed by patient history or physician observation
4. Oral ulcers	Oral or nasopharyngeal ulceration, usually painless, observed by a physician
5. Arthritis	Nonerosive arthritis involving two or more peripheral joints, characterized by tenderness, swelling, or effusion
6. Serositis	a. Pleuritis—convincing history of pleuritic pain or rub heard by a physician or evidence of pleural effusion or b. Pericarditis—documented by ECG or rub or evidence of pericardial effusion
7. Renal disorder	a. Persistent proteinuria greater than 0.5 g/day or greater than 3+ if quantification not performed or b. Cellular casts—may be red cell, hemoglobin, granular, tubular, or mixed
8. Neurologic disorder	a. Seizures: in the absence of offending drugs or known metabolic derangements (e.g., uremia, ketoacidosis, electrolyte imbalance) or b. Psychosis—in the absence of offending drugs or known metabolic derangements (e.g., uremia, ketoacidosis, electrolyte imbalance)
9. Hematologic disorders	a. Hemolytic anemia—with reticulocytosis or b. Leukopenia—less than 4000/mm³ total on two or more occasions or c. Lymphopenia—less than 1500/mm³ on two or more occasions or d. Thrombocytopenia—less than 100,000/mm³ in the absence of offending drugs
10. Immunologic disorder	a. Positive LE cell preparation or b. Anti-DNA; antibody to native DNA in abnormal titer or c. Anti-Sm: presence of antibody to Sm nuclear antigen or d. False-positive serologic test for syphilis known to be positive for at least 6 months and confirmed by Treponema pallidum immobilization or fluorescent treponemal antibody absorption test

TABLE 2-5

Revised Criteria for the Classification of Systemic Lupus Erythematosus (1982)—cont'd

Criterion	Definition
11. Antinuclear antibody	An abnormal titer of antinuclear antibody by immunofluorescence or an equivalent assay at any point in time and in the absence of drugs known to be associated with drug-induced lupus syndrome

ECG, Electrocardiogram; *LE*, lupus erythematosus.
From Tan EM, et al: The 1982 revised criteria for the classification of SLE, *Arthritis Rheum* 25:1271, 1982.

of dermatomyositis. The heliotrope rash consists of a violaceous to dusky erythematous rash, with or without edema, in a symmetrical distribution involving periorbital skin.

Tenderness

Precise localization of tenderness is the most useful sign in determining the cause of the problem. Joint line or capsular tenderness signifies arthropathy or capsular disease around the whole margin. Localized joint line tenderness suggests intracapsular pathologic processes. Periarticular point tenderness, away from the joint line, usually signifies bursitis or enthesopathy.

The only reliable finding on examination in fibromyalgia is the presence of multiple tender points. The diagnostic utility of a tender point evaluation has been objectively documented with the use of a dolorimeter or algometer, pressure-loaded gauges that accurately measure force per area, and with manual palpation. The criteria of at least 11 of 18 tender points are recommended for classification purposes but should not be considered essential in individual patient diagnoses. Patients with fewer than 11 tender points can be diagnosed with fibromyalgia, provided other symptoms and signs are present. An investigation must be made to determine whether the fibromyalgia is primary or secondary. The Leeds Assessment of Neuropathic Symptoms and Signs helps differentiate neuropathic pain and fibromyalgic pain (Box 2-2).

Warmth

Warmth is one of the cardinal signs of inflammation. The back of the examiner's hand is a sensitive area for comparing skin temperature above, over, and below an inflamed structure.

BOX 2-2

LEEDS ASSESSMENT OF NEUROPATHIC SYMPTOMS AND SIGNS
(THE LANSS PAIN SCALE)

A. Pain questionnaire
- Think about how your pain has felt over the last week.
- Please say whether any of the descriptions match your pain precisely.

1. Does your pain feel like strange, unpleasant sensations in your skin? Words such as *pricking, tingling,* and *pins and needles* might describe these sensations.
   - a. NO ☐ (0)
   - b. YES ☐ (5)

2. Does your pain make the skin in the painful areas look different from normal? Words such as *mottled* or *looking more red or pink* might describe the appearance.
   - a. NO ☐ (0)
   - b. YES ☐ (5)

3. Does your pain make the affected skin abnormally sensitive to touch? Getting unpleasant sensations when lightly stroking the skin or getting pain when wearing tight clothes might describe the abnormal sensitivity.
   - a. NO ☐ (0)
   - b. YES ☐ (5)

4. Does your pain come on suddenly and in bursts for no apparent reason when you are still? Words such as *electric shocks, jumping,* and *bursting* describe these sensations.
   - a. NO ☐ (0)
   - b. YES ☐ (5)

5. Does your pain feel as if the skin temperature in the painful area has changed abnormally? Words such as *hot* and *burning* describe these sensations.
   - a. NO ☐ (0)
   - b. YES ☐ (5)

B. Sensory testing
   Skin sensitivity can be examined by comparing the painful area with a contralateral or adjacent nonpainful area for the presence of allodynia and an altered pinprick threshold (PPT).

BOX 2-2

LEEDS ASSESSMENT OF NEUROPATHIC SYMPTOMS AND SIGNS (THE LANSS PAIN SCALE)—cont'd

1. Allodynia
   Examine the response to lightly stroking cotton wool across the nonpainful area and then the painful area. If normal sensations are experienced in the painful site, but pain or unpleasant sensations (tingling, nausea) are experienced in the painful area when stroking, then allodynia is present.
   a. NO, normal sensation in both areas ☐ (0)
   b. YES, allodynia in painful areas only ☐ (5)
2. Altered pin-prick threshold
   If a sharp pin-prick is felt in the nonpainful area, but a different sensation is experienced in the painful area, for example, none or blunt only (raised PPT) or a very painful sensation (lowered PPT), altered PPT is present.
   a. NO, equal sensation in both areas ☐ (0)
   b. YES, altered PPT in painful area ☐ (5)

Scoring:
Add values in parentheses for sensory description and examination findings to obtain overall score.
Total score (maximum 20) _____
Score <12: Neuropathic mechanisms are *unlikely* to be contributing to the patient's pain.
Score ≥12: Neuropathic mechanisms are *likely* to be contributing to the patient's pain.

This pain scale can help determine whether the nerves that are carrying the patient's pain signals are working normally. The examiner should know this information in case different treatments are needed to control the patient's pain.
Adapted from Kaki AM, El-Yaski AZ, Youseif E: Identifying neuropathic pain among patients with chronic low-back pain: use of the Leeds Assessment of Neuropathic Symptoms and Signs Pain Scale, *Reg Anesth Pain Med* 30(5):422.e1-422.e9, 2005.

Painful Arc of Movement

Ligament injuries are detected by eliciting tenderness over the damaged portion of the affected tendon. Injuries are also detected in attempting to distract the bony structures held together by the ligament of interest.

When the tendon is subjected to disease or excessive load, it may rupture. In tendon disease or injury less than rupture, tendon inflammation usually results. Tendinopathy is detected by eliciting a *painful*

TABLE 2-6

DIAGNOSTICALLY USEFUL CLINICAL FEATURES IN THE INITIAL EVALUATION OF THE PATIENT WITH ACUTE MUSCULOSKELETAL SYMPTOMS

	Tendinopathy/ Bursitis	Noninflammatory Joint Problems*	Systemic Rheumatic Disease
Symptoms			
Morning stiffness	Focal, brief	Focal, brief	Significant, prolonged
Constitutional symptoms	Absent	Absent	Present
Peak period of discomfort	With use	After prolonged use	After prolonged inactivity
Locking or instability	Unusual, except rotator cuff tear, trigger finger	Implies loose body, internal derangement, or weakness	Uncommon
Symmetry	Uncommon	Occasional	Common
Signs			
Tenderness	Focal, periarticular, or tender points (fibromyalgia)	Unusual	Over entire exposed joint spaces
Inflammation (fluid, pain, warmth, erythema)	Over tendon or bursa	Unusual	Common
Instability	Uncommon	Occasional	Uncommon
Multisystem disease	No	No	Often

From Kelley WN, et al: *Textbook of rheumatology*, ed 5, Philadelphia, 1997, WB Saunders.
*For example, osteoarthritis or internal derangement.

arc of active movement in the plane of action of the affected tendon. Passive movement in the same plane is almost pain free (Table 2-6).

Fixed Deformity

Although articular deformity may be observed at rest, most become more apparent when the limb is bearing weight or being used. The examiner

2

ORTHOPEDIC GAMUT 2-9

COMMON TERMS TO DESCRIBE PERIPHERAL JOINT DEFORMITIES

1. Dislocation: Articulating surfaces are displaced to the degree that they are no longer in contact with each other.
2. Fixed flexion: Joint extension is lost, resulting in permanent flexion.
3. Valgus: The distal part of the joint is directed laterally from the midline.
4. Varus: The distal part of the joint is directed medially toward the midline.

---

should determine whether the deformity is correctable or noncorrectable. Many conditions are associated with characteristic deformities, but no deformity is pathognomonic of any single disease (Table 2-7). Shorthand terms are used for combined deformities, such as *swan-neck finger deformity* for hyperextension at the proximal and fixed flexion at the distal interphalangeal joints.

TABLE 2-7

SPECIFIC MUSCULOSKELETAL DEFORMITIES

Lower Limb	Upper Limb
Hallux abductovalgus	Fixed flexion of DIPs, PIPs, MCPs
Genu varum	*(prayer sign)*
Genu valgum	Ulnar deviation
Dislocation of the patella	Swan neck deformity of finger
Valgus deformity of the heel	Boutonnière deformity
Coxa vara	Z-shaped thumb
Pes planovalgus	Volar subluxation of wrist
Fixed flexion of the knee	Dorsal subluxation of inferior
Fixed flexion of the hip	radioulnar joint
	Fixed flexion of elbow
	Cubitus valgus
	Upward subluxation of shoulder
	Anterior dislocation of shoulder
	Posterior dislocation of shoulder

DIPs, Distal interphalangeal joints; *MCPs*, metacarpophalangeal joints; *PIP*, proximal interphalangeal joints.

TABLE 2-8		
Joint Plane Motion Characteristics		
Type	**Planes**	**Joints**
Hinge	One	Elbow, knee, ankle, MCP, PIP, DIP, MTP
Two-way hinge	Two (circumduction)	Wrist, trapeziometacarpal
Ball and socket	All planes	Shoulder, hip

DIP, Distal interphalangeal; *MCP*, metacarpophalangeal; *MTP*, metatarsophalangeal; *PIP*, proximal interphalangeal.

Movement

Every joint has a normal range of motion. The range of motion for any joint varies with age, gender, and ethnic origin. A range of movement that is beyond the upper limit represents hypermobility. Ranges below the lower limit represent hypomobility. The normal joint range of motion is diminished by joint inflammation or by irreversible damage to the joint structures. In trauma or disease, movement is first lost from the extreme end ranges. Increasing joint damage results in more profound loss of range of motion. The complete loss of movement of a joint is known as *fixation ankylosis* or *joint ankylosis*, depending on soft-tissue versus bony involvement, respectively. Fixation or joint ankylosis is further complicated by the involvement or loss of multiple planes of motion (Table 2-8).

ORTHOPEDIC GAMUT 2-10

RANGE OF MOTION

Range of motion is assessed as follows:
1. Range of active movement
2. Passive versus active movement
3. Pain during movement
4. Movement crepitation

Hypermobility is recognized by a series of passive maneuvers collectively known as the **9-point scale of Beighton** (Box 2-3). The Beighton modification of the Carter and Wilkinson scoring system has been used for many years as an indicator of widespread hypermobility. A high Beighton score by itself does not mean that an individual has HMS. It simply means that the individual has widespread hypermobility. Diagnosis of Hypermobility Syndrome or HMS should be made using the ***Brighton Criteria***. The Beighton score is an easy to administer 9-point scale where points are given for the performance of five maneuvers. It is generally considered that hypermobility is present if 4 out of 9 points are scored. The scale was not designed for clinical use and has been criticized because it only samples a few joints and gives no indication of the degree of hypermobility.

ORTHOPEDIC GAMUT 2-11

BRIGHTON CRITERIA (DIAGNOSTIC CRITERIA FOR HYPERMOBILITY SYNDROME)

Major criteria
1. A Beighton score of 4/9 or greater (either currently or historically)
2. Arthralgias for longer than 3 months in four or more joints.

Minor criteria
1. A Beighton score of 1,2, or 3/9 (0,1,2,or 3 if aged 50+).
2. Arthralgias (for 3 months or longer) in one to three joints or back pain for (for 3 months or longer), spondylosis, spondylolysis/spondylolisthesis.
3. Dislocation/subluxation in more than one joint, or in one joint on more than one occasion.
4. Soft tissue rheumatism: three or more lesions (e.g., epicondylitis, tenosynovitis, bursitis).
5. Marfanoid habitus (tall, slim, span/height ration >1.03 upper: lower segment ration <0.89, arachnodactyly (positive Steinberg/wrist signs).
6. Abnormal skin striae, hyperextensibility, thin skin, papyraceous scarring.
7. Eye signs: drooping eyelids or myopia or antimongoloid slant.
8. Varicose veins or hernia or uterine/rectal prolapse.

BJHS is diagnosed in the presence of **two major criteria** or **one major** and **two minor criteria**, or **four minor criteria**. Two minor criteria will suffice where there is an unequivocally affected first-degree relative. BJHS is excluded by the presence of Marfan or Ehlers-Danlos syndromes other than the EDS hypermobility type (formerly EDS III). Criteria Major 1 and Minor 1 are mutually exclusive, as are Major 2 and Minor 2.

From R. Grahame, Pain distress and joint hyperlaxity, *Joint Bone Spine* **67** (2000), pp. 157–163

BOX 2-3

MODIFIED BEIGHTON MOBILITY INDEX

1. Hyperextension of the elbows
2. Hyperextension of the knees
3. Apposition of the thumb to the flexor aspect of the forearm
4. Passive dorsiflexion of the metacarpophalangeal joints to 90 degrees
5. Passive dorsiflexion of the ankle past 90 degrees
6. Dorsolumbar flexion, placing hands flat on floor with knees fully extended

1 point is awarded for each side of the body for each extremity clinically involved.
1 point is awarded for dorsolumbar flexion hypermobility.
Total points available for indexing is 11.

Stability

The stability of a joint depends partly on the integrity of its articulating surfaces and partly on its intact ligaments. When a joint is unstable, mobility is abnormal. When testing for abnormal mobility, the examiner must ensure that the muscles controlling the joint are relaxed. A muscle in strong contraction can often conceal ligamentous instability (Table 2-9).

Crepitation

Crepitation is a palpable crunching sensation present throughout the movement of the involved joint or enthesis structure. Fine crepitation

---

TABLE 2-9

JOINT INSTABILITY FINDINGS

Passive side-to-side movement of the tibia on the femur (collateral knee ligaments)
Passive anteroposterior movement of the tibia on the femur (cruciate ligaments)
Gross genu recurvatum
Positive Trendelenburg sign
Arthritis mutilans—flail interphalangeal joints
Spontaneous dislocation of the shoulder or patella
Pes planus (collapse of the longitudinal arch)

TABLE 2-10

CREPITATION GRADING SCALE

	None	Mild	Moderate	Severe
Palpable	Smooth, silky motion	Fine-grade sandpaper	Medium-grade sandpaper	Bone-on-bone grinding
Audible	Quiet	Barely audible	Consistent squeak	Popping-cracking-crunching

Adapted from Lancaster AR, Nyland J, Roberts CS: The validity of the motion palpation test for determining patellofemoral joint articular cartilage damage, *Phys Ther Sport* 8(2):59-65, 2007.

may be audible only by stethoscope and is not transmitted through the adjacent bone. Fine crepitation may accompany inflammation of the tendon sheath, bursa, or synovium. Coarse crepitation may be audible at a distance and is palpable through the bone. Coarse crepitation usually reflects cartilage or bone damage (Table 2-10).

ORTHOPEDIC GAMUT 2-12

CREPITUS NOISES (OTHER THAN FINE OR COARSE)

1. Ligamentous snaps—usually single, loud, and painless—that are common around the upper femur as a clicking hip
2. Cracking by joint distraction, which is common at the finger joints and is caused by production of an intraarticular gas bubble (e.g., cracking cannot be repeated until the bubble has reformed)
3. Reproducible clunking noises that occur at irregular surfaces, such as when the scapula moves on the ribs

---

Muscular Atrophy

Muscle atrophy is a common sign but can be difficult to detect, particularly in older adults. Synovitis quickly produces local spinal reflex inhibition of muscles acting across the joint. Atrophy can be rapid (within several days) in septic arthritis. Severe arthropathy produces widespread periarticular wasting. Localized atrophy is more characteristic of a mechanical tendon or muscle problem or nerve entrapment. Disuse atrophy is complex and highly regulated biochemical process (Table 2-11).

TABLE 2-11

SIGNALS INVOLVED IN DISUSE-INDUCED MUSCLE ATROPHY

Signals	Finding	Function
PI3K, Akt	Decreased	Promotes protein degradation Inhibits protein synthesis
FOXO1, FOXO3	Increased	Promotes protein degradation Downregulates type I fiber genes?
mTOR, p70S6K, eIF4B	Decreased	Inhibits protein synthesis
PHAS-I	Increased	Inhibits protein synthesis
p50, c-Rel, Bcl-3	Increased	Promotes protein degradation
Myostatin, ActIIB	Increased	Inhibits protein synthesis?
p38	Increased	Promotes protein degradation
Erk	Increased	Promotes glucose uptake?
JNK	Increased	Increases insulin resistance
Calcineurin	Increased	Compensatory mechanism?
ROS	Increased	Promotes protein degradation
MAFbx, MuRF1	Increased	Promotes protein degradation

Signal abbreviations: *ACTIIB*, Myostatin receptor; *Akt*, serine/threonine kinase; *Bcl-3*, transcriptional coactivtor; *Calcineurin*, serine/threonine phosphatase; *c-REL*, NF-kB family transcription factor; *E1F4B*, eukaryotic translation initiation factor 4B (homo sapiens); *ERK*, extracellular signal-regulated kinase; *FOXO*, Forkhead family of transcription factor; *JNK*, c-JUN N-terminal kinase; *MAFbx*, muscle atrophy f-box ubiquitin ligase; *mTOR*, mammalian target of rapamycin; *MuRF1*, muscle ring finger 1 ubiquitin ligase; *Myostatin*, inhibitor of skeletal muscle mass; *p38*, p38 isoform mitogen activated protein; *p50*, NF-kB family transcription factor; *p70S6K*, 70-kDa ribosomal protein s6 kinase; *PHAS-I*, eukaryotic initiation factor 4E-binding protein; *PI3K*, phosphatidylinositol 3-OH kinase; *ROS*, reactive oxygen species. Adapted from Zhang P, Chen X, Fan M: Signaling mechanisms involved in disuse muscle atrophy, *Med Hypoth* 70(2):314–316, 2008.

Fasciculations

Fasciculations are visible, spontaneous contractions of muscle fibers supplied by a single motor nerve filament. Visible dimpling or twitching may occur. Fasciculations occurring during muscular contraction (twitching) are associated with conditions of irritability, resulting in poorly coordinated contraction of small and large motor units (spasmophilia). Benign fasciculation occurs in normal individuals and in muscle of normal strength and size. Fascicular twitches noted during rest, with exaggerated muscular weakness and atrophy, are characteristic of peripheral motor neuron disorders. Acute denervation of skeletal muscles results in spontaneous contractions of muscle fibers.

TABLE 2-12

TREMOR CLASSIFICATION

Cause	Type and Rate of Movement	Description
Anxiety	Fine, rapid, 10 to 12/sec	Irregular, variable Increased by attempts to move part; decreased by relaxation of part
Parkinsonism	Fine, regular, or coarse, 2 to 5/sec	Occurs at rest May be inhibited by movement Involves flexion of finger and thumb *pill rolling* Accompanied by rigidity, *cogwheel* phenomena, bradykinesia
Cerebellar tremor	Variable rate	Evident only on movement (most prominent on finger-to-nose test) Dysmetria (seen when patient is asked to pat rapidly; pats are of unequal force and do not all arrive at same point)
Essential or senile	Coarse, 3 to 7/sec	Involves the jaw, sometimes the tongue, and sometimes the entire head Disappears on complete relaxation or in response to alcohol
Metabolic		Variable Patient is obviously ill; if illness is a result of hepatic failure, patient will have other signs, such as palpable liver, spider nevi

From Barkauskas VH et al: *Health & physical assessment*, ed 2, St Louis, 1998, Mosby.

Cramps and Spasm

Muscular spasm, or tremor (Table 2-12), may occur at rest or with movement. Spasms and tremors occur in the normal individual with metabolic and electrolyte alterations. Cramping is a common complaint after excessive sweating and subsequent *hyponatremia, hypocalcemia, hypomagnesemia*, or *hyperuricemia* (electrolyte imbalance).

Tetany

Hypocalcemia and hypomagnesemia often cause the involuntary spasms of skeletal muscle, which resemble cramping. Tetanic cramps can be elicited by repeatedly percussing the motor nerve that leads to a muscle group contraction-cramp-spasm at frequencies of 15 to 20 per second. Chvostek sign is the spasm of facial muscles produced by tapping over the facial nerve near its foraminal exit. Chvostek sign may also occur with normocalcemia, as well as with hypocalcemia.

Impairment of Gait

Finding a spinal or lower extremity orthopedic or neurologic disorder that does not produce abnormalities of gait at some time during its course can be difficult.

ORTHOPEDIC GAMUT 2-13

GAIT

Gait impairments of predominantly neurologic origin include the following (in descending order of frequency):
1. Disorders of the corticospinal pathways (spasticity)
2. Basal ganglia (parkinsonism)
3. Cerebellum and connections (ataxia)
4. Cerebral cortex (gait apraxia)
5. Neuromuscular system (weakness)
6. Sensation (ataxia)

Bladder Control

Incontinence and other disturbances of urinary bladder function are occasionally the first manifestation of disease of the spinal cord, as well as the rest of the nervous system. The physiologic mechanism of micturition is complex. The terms *atonic bladder* and *spastic bladder* are no longer useful in describing different levels of neurologic involvement because they are related mainly to local factors in the bladder wall.

ORTHOPEDIC GAMUT 2-14

IMPAIRED MICTURITION

Localization of impaired micturition depends on the following:
1. Loss of bladder sensation
2. Perineal sensory loss
3. Patulous anal sphincter
4. Absence of the bulbocavernous and anocutaneous reflexes
5. Sensory, motor, and reflex changes in the lower extremities

---

CHAPTER THREE

CERVICAL SPINE

AXIOMS IN ASSESSING THE CERVICAL SPINE

- Cervical spine syndromes are extremely common and are probably the fourth most common cause of musculoskeletal pain.
- At any given time, 9% of men and 12% of women have neck pain with or without arm and hand pain, and 35% of the population can remember having had neck pain at some time.
- The cervical spine is the origin of a large proportion of shoulder, elbow, hand, and wrist disorders.
- Most people who develop pain in the neck do not seek medical attention because they regard such pain as a part of life, and they simply wait for it to disappear.

INTRODUCTION

Neck discomfort commonly appears after sudden and unusual motion of the neck because the cervical spine is the most mobile segment of the spine. Many delicate and vital structures pass through the cervical spinal column, including the carotid and vertebral arteries, the spinal cord, and the spinal nerves, all of which require great protection.

Normal function of the cervical spine requires that all movements be accomplished without injury to the spinal cord and the millions of nerve fibers that pass through it. The spinal cord has the capacity to adapt itself to marked alteration in the length of the cervical spinal canal. Flexion of the neck lengthens the spinal canal, and extension shortens it. The thickness of the cervical spinal cord and the diameter of the spinal canal vary considerably from person to person.

The nerve roots in the neck are particularly vulnerable to injury because of their relatively horizontal position in comparison with those of the lumbar spine. Stretching of the spinal cord itself is greatest at the cervical spine, which also predisposes the cord and nerve roots to trauma (Tables 3-1 and 3-2).

Many provocative tests can be used for the cervical spine. The anatomic structures commonly tested are dural tension, foraminal and

---

ORTHOPEDIC GAMUT 3-1

CERVICAL SPINE PAIN

Differential diagnostic possibilities of cervical spine pain include:

- Cardiovascular disease
- Myocardial infarction
- Aortic dissection
- Meningitis
- Cervical osteoarthritis
- Hypertension
- Temporal arteritis
- Polymyalgia rheumatica
- A spectrum of neurologic diseases and syndromes
- Various metabolic bone diseases
- Primary and metastatic cancer
- Infection
- Lymphoma
- Myeloma

---

vertebral canal patency, and muscle, tendon, or ligamentous injuries (Table 3-3). During investigation of the upper extremity, the examiner must differentiate between canal or nerve root lesions by physical examination and, if necessary, electrodiagnostic studies. Cervical spine canal stenosis, whether of bony or soft-tissue origins, can cause lower-extremity signs and symptoms. Most notable is long tract pain, or rhizalgia, appearing in an ipsilateral leg with a cervical nerve root lesion (Table 3-4).

TABLE 3-1
CERVICAL SPINE CROSS-REFERENCE TABLE BY SYNDROME OR TISSUE

Cervical Spine	Disease Assessed												
Test/Sign	Arthritis	Subluxation	Myospasm	Facet	Sprain	Dural Irritation	Fracture	Tumor	IVD Syndrome	Meningitis	Brachial Plexus	VBA Syndrome	Nerve Root
Bakody sign													●
Barré-Liéou sign												●	
Bikele sign										●	●		
Brachial plexus tension test							●	●	●		●		●
Dejerine sign													●
DeKleyn test												●	
Distraction test			●	●									●
Foraminal compression test													●
Hallpike maneuver												●	

Continued

3

TABLE 3-1

CERVICAL SPINE CROSS-REFERENCE TABLE BY SYNDROME OR TISSUE—cont'd

Test																
Hautant test								•								
Jackson compression test	•	•								•	•					
Lhermitte sign			•			•										
Maximum cervical compression test			•	•					•							
Naffziger test	•	•		•						•						
O'Donoghue maneuver			•	•	•											
Rust sign	•			•	•		•	•								
Shoulder depression test	•															
Soto-Hall sign	•	•	•		•			•		•	•					
Spinal percussion test			•					•			•					
Spurling test	•															
Swallowing test										•	•					
Underburg test													•			
Valsalva maneuver	•									•	•					
Vertebrobasilar artery functional maneuver																•

IVD, Intervertebral disc; VBA, vertebrobasilar artery.

TABLE 3-2

CERVICAL SPINE CROSS-REFERENCE TABLE BY SYNDROME OR TISSUE

Arthritis	Jackson cervical compression test
	Rust sign
	Soto-Hall sign
	Swallowing test
Brachial plexus	Bikele sign
	Brachial plexus tension test
Dural irritation	Lhermitte sign
	Shoulder depression test
Facet	Distraction test
	Jackson cervical compression test
	Maximum cervical compression test
	Shoulder depression test
Fracture	Brachial plexus tension test
	Rust sign
	Soto-Hall sign
	Spinal percussion test
Intervertebral disc syndrome	Brachial plexus tension test
	Jackson cervical compression test
	Naffziger test
	Soto-Hall sign
	Spinal percussion test
	Swallowing test
	Valsalva maneuver
Meningitis	Brachial plexus tension test
	Soto-Hall sign
Myospasm	Distraction test
	Maximum cervical compression test
	Naffziger test
	O'Donoghue maneuver
	Soto-Hall sign
	Spinal percussion test
Nerve root	Bakody sign
	Brachial plexus tension test
	Dejerine sign
	Distraction test
	Maximum cervical compression test
	Naffziger test
	Shoulder depression test
	Spurling test
Sprain	Naffziger test
	O'Donoghue maneuver
	Rust sign
	Soto-Hall sign

Continued

TABLE 3-2

CERVICAL SPINE CROSS-REFERENCE TABLE BY
SYNDROME OR TISSUE—cont'd

Subluxation	Jackson cervical compression test
	Rust sign
	Soto-Hall sign
Tumor	Brachial plexus tension test
	Jackson cervical compression test
	Swallowing test
	Valsalva maneuver
Vertebrobasilar artery syndrome	Barré-Liéou sign
	DeKleyn test
	Hallpike maneuver
	Hautant test
	Underburg test
	Vertebrobasilar artery functional maneuver

ORTHOPEDIC GAMUT 3-2

ORTHOPEDIC EXAMINATION

An orthopedic examination of the cervical spine includes the following:
1. History
2. Vital signs
3. Inspection
4. Palpation of superficial and deep tissues and joint play
5. Percussion
6. Instrumentation (other physical measurement)
7. Range-of-motion evaluation
8. Orthopedic maneuvers
9. Neurologic examination
10. Imaging
11. Laboratory evaluation

TABLE 3-3
COMMON PROVOCATIVE TESTS TO EVALUATE THE SPINE

Provocative Test	Anatomic Structures Being Tested	Positive Finding(s)
Cervical Spine		
Jackson compression test	Dural sheath, nerve root, spinal nerve	Radicular pain
Spurling compression test	Dural sheath, nerve root, spinal nerve	Radicular pain
Maximal foraminal compression test	Dural sheath, nerve root, spinal nerve	Radicular pain
Distraction test	Dural sheath, nerve root, spinal nerve	Relief of radicular pain
Shoulder depression test	Dural sheath, nerve root, spinal nerve, brachial plexus	Radicular pain to one or more dermatomes
E.A.S.T. test	Subclavian artery	Vascular compromise
Eden test	Scalene musculature	Radiculopathy to multiple dermatomes or vascular compromise
Thoracic Spine		
Wright hyperabduction test	Pectoralis minor	Vascular compromise, subclavian artery, TOS
Tests for anterior thoracic wall	Peripheral nerve, muscles	Radicular pain, dull ache
Lumbar Spine		
Straight leg raise	Dural sheath, nerve root, spinal nerve	Radiculopathy to one dermatome usually
Braggard test	Dural sheath, nerve root, spinal nerve	Radiculopathy to one dermatome usually
Bekhterev (Bechterew) test	Dural sheath, nerve root, spinal nerve	Radiculopathy to one dermatome usually
Neri bow string test	Dural sheath, nerve root, spinal nerve	Radiculopathy to one dermatome usually

E.A.S.T., Elevated arm stress test; *TOS,* thoracic outlet syndrome.

From Greenstein GM: *Clinical assessment of neuromusculoskeletal disorders,* St Louis, 1997, Mosby.

TABLE 3-4	
CLASSIFICATION OF POST–SPINAL CORD INJURY PAIN STATES	
Acute Phase Pains	**Chronic Phase Pains**
Acute nociceptive (spinal injury site)	Nociceptive (musculoskeletal, spasm)
Early neurogenic	Neurogenic
Early burning	Peripheral
Transitional zone pain	Transitional zone pain
	Double lesion syndrome pain
	Visceral pain (?)
	Central
	Central dysesthesia syndrome pain
	Syringomyelia pain
	Visceral pain (?)
	Psychogenic

Adapted from Beric A: Post-Spinal Cord Injury Pain States, *Anesthesiol Clin North Am* 15(2):445-463, 1997.

ESSENTIAL CLINICAL ANATOMY

ORTHOPEDIC GAMUT 3-3

CATEGORIES OF INTRACTABLE SPINAL CORD INJURY PAIN

1. **Above-level pain,**
   a. At dermatomes rostral to the injury site in areas where normal sensation persists after injury
2. **At-level pain,**
   a. In dermatomes near the spinal injury, develops shortly after spinal cord injury, and is often characterized as either stabbing pain or a stimulus-independent type that is accompanied by allodynia (nonnoxious stimuli become noxious)
3. **Below-level pain,**
   a. Localized to dermatomes distal to the injury site, develops more gradually than does at-level pain, and is often classified as a stimulus-independent continuous, burning pain

---

ORTHOPEDIC GAMUT 3-4

NEURAL RESPONSES

Pathologic neural responses to cervical injury can be grouped into four categories:

1. Transient neurologic deficit (lasting less than 8 weeks) involving the nerve roots, trunk or the brachial plexus, or motor unit
2. Longstanding, consistent neurologic deficit (lasting more than 8 weeks)
3. Cervical myelopathy (clonus, lower or upper limb findings)
4. Gross spinal cord impairment (quadriplegia)

The atlas consists of a pair of strong lateral masses that are linked by the anterior arch and the posterior arch. The posterior arch of the atlas is attached to the posterior rim of the foramen magnum by the atlantooccipital membrane.

Children often have lax ligaments, which increases spinal motion. This characteristic most commonly occurs in the cervical region. Increased motion seen during physical or X-ray examination should be differentiated from pathologic subluxation. On imaging of the cervical spine, the predental space should not exceed 3 mm. A predental space greater than 3 mm has been found in 20% of normal patients younger than 8 years and can be tracked on patients into early adulthood.

Pathologic subluxation of the atlas on the axis that compromises the spinal cord (compressive myelopathy) is associated with rheumatoid arthritis and ankylosing spondylitis. The common characteristic of these disorders is the destructive weakening of the atlantooccipital ligament system, with resultant translation of the structures.

The costal element in C7 is one of the most common from which accessory ribs may form (e.g., a *cervical rib*). Abnormal positioning of a cervical rib heightens the risk of compression of the nerves and vessels.

The articulations of the vertebral column are of great importance. The vertebral column supports much weight; serves as an axis for movement of the limbs, trunk, head, and neck; and protects the spinal cord from trauma.

The intervertebral discs are fibrocartilaginous flattened structures interposed between adjacent vertebral bodies. Each disc consists of a gelatinous inner region (i.e., the nucleus pulposus), surrounded by a solid ring of stiffer material (i.e., the annulus fibrosus).

The vertebral artery is closely related to the cervical spine and is the first branch of the subclavian artery. It enters the foramen of the transverse process of C6 and ascends through the remaining foramina of the tops of the cervical vertebrae. The vertebral artery passes beneath the posterior atlantooccipital membrane. The union of the two vertebral arteries forms the basilar artery.

ESSENTIAL MOTION ASSESSMENT

ORTHOPEDIC GAMUT 3-5

VERTEBRAL MUSCLES

The vertebral muscles are divided into two large groups:
1. Extrinsic muscles, which are important in the attachment of limbs and limb girdles to the vertebrae and contribute to motions of the trunk
2. Intrinsic muscles, which stabilize and carry out motions of the vertebral column itself

---

During a cervical spine range-of-motion assessment, the examiner should examine active then passive movements. For flexion, the patient brings the chin onto the chest; for extension, the patient bends the head backward as far as possible. For lateral flexion, the patient brings an ear toward the shoulder, first on one side and then on the other. For rotation, the patient looks over one shoulder and then the other. Repeating the movements while applying gentle pressure over the vertex of the skull may trigger pain or paresthesia in the arm if a critical degree of narrowing exists at an intervertebral foramen. In evaluating cervical spine range of motion, the examiner observes not only the total range of movement, but also the smoothness and comfort with which the patient accomplishes the motions (Figs. 3-1 to 3-8).

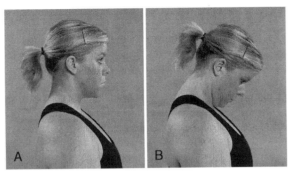

FIG. 3-1 Flexion. **A,** To assess cervical range of motion, the examiner has the patient sit with the head upright. **B,** The examiner then instructs the patient to tuck the chin in toward the chest. The expected range of motion is 80 to 90 degrees. Excessive range is when the chin can reach the chest while the patient's mouth is closed. Two finger widths' distance between the chin and the chest can be considered normal. Forty degrees or less of retained cervical flexion is an impairment of neck function in the activities of daily living.

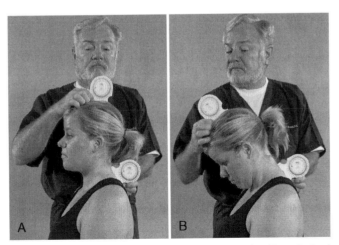

FIG. 3-2 Flexion assessed with an inclinometer. The patient flexes the head and neck forward. The examiner records both angles. The T1 inclination is subtracted from the cranial inclination to determine the cervical flexion angle. The expected range of motion is 60 degrees or greater from the neutral position.

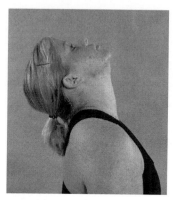

FIG. 3-3 Extension. Extension range of motion is 70 degrees. In extension, the plane of the nose and forehead should be nearly horizontal. Fifty degrees or less of retained cervical extension is an impairment of neck function in the activities of daily living.

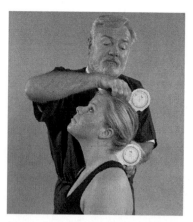

FIG. 3-4 Extension assessed with an inclinometer. The T1 inclination is subtracted from the occipital inclination to determine the cervical extension angle. The expected range of motion is 75 degrees or greater from the neutral position.

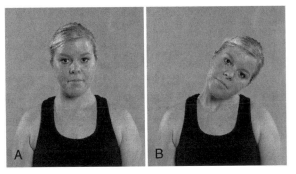

FIG. 3-5 Lateral flexion. Lateral flexion of the cervical spine is normally approximately 20 to 45 degrees to the right and left. Most lateral flexion occurs between the occiput and C1 and between C1 and C2.

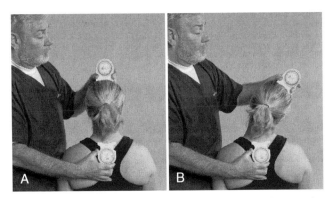

FIG. 3-6 Lateral flexion assessed with an inclinometer. **A,** With the patient seated and the cervical spine in a neutral position, the examiner places one inclinometer on the T1 spinous process in the coronal plane. The examiner places the second inclinometer at the superior aspect of the occiput, or on top of the head, also in the coronal plane. Both instruments are then zeroed. **B,** The patient laterally flexes the head and neck to one side. The examiner records the angles of both instruments. The T1 inclination is subtracted from the occipital inclination to determine the cervical lateral flexion angle.

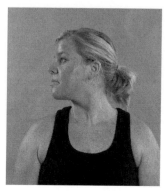

FIG. 3-7 Rotation. Normal rotation of the cervical spine is 70 to 90 degrees. The patient's chin does not often reach the plane of the shoulder.

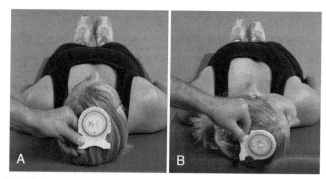

FIG. 3-8 Rotation assessed with an inclinometer. **A,** With the patient in a supine position, the examiner places the inclinometer at the crown of the head in the coronal plane. The instrument is zeroed. **B,** The patient rotates the head to one side, and the examiner records the angle indicated on the instrument.

ESSENTIAL MUSCLE FUNCTION ASSESSMENT

The muscles of the vertebral column are often in an increased state of contraction, which stiffens the vertebral column to serve as a platform for movement of the head or limbs.

ORTHOPEDIC GAMUT 3-6

CERVICAL SPINE MUSCLE STRENGTH

To evaluate cervical spine muscle strength, the patient takes the following actions:
1. Pushes a cheek against the examiner's hand (This maneuver also tests the motor function of cranial nerve XI [sternocleido-mastoid muscle].) (Fig. 3-9)
2. Pushes the back of the head against the examiner's hand
3. Pushes the forehead against the examiner's hand (Figs. 3-10 to 3-12)

3

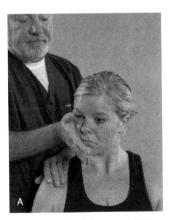

FIG. 3-9 Examining the strength of the sternocleidomastoid and trapezius muscles. **A,** Rotation against resistance.

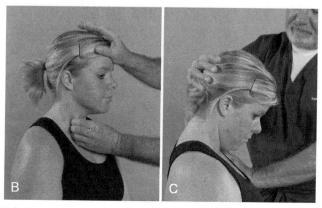

FIG. 3-9, cont'd **B,** Flexion with palpation of the sternocleidomastoid muscle. **C,** Extension against resistance.

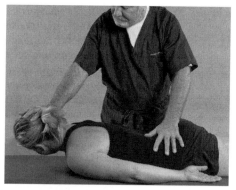

FIG. 3-10 Posterolateral head and neck extensors. The patient tries a posterolateral extension with the face turned toward the side tested. The examiner applies pressure in an anterior direction against the posterolateral aspect of the head.

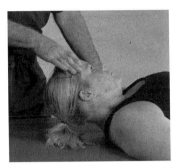

FIG. 3-11 Anterolateral head and neck flexors. The patient attempts anterolateral neck flexion. The examiner applies pressure to the temporal region of the head in an obliquely posterior direction.

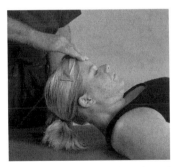

FIG. 3-12 Anterior head and neck flexors. The patient tries to flex the cervical spine by lifting the head from the table toward the sternum while keeping the mouth closed and the chin depressed. The examiner applies pressure to the forehead in a posterior direction.

The intrinsic longitudinal vertebral muscles, placed more superficially, are collectively called the *erector spinae*. The cervical region contains elongated muscles originating from the spinous process (the splenius muscles) and others from the transverse processes (the semispinalis muscles). The suboccipital muscles are a special group of muscles linking the atlas, the axis, and the base of the skull.

ESSENTIAL IMAGING

Plain-Film Imaging

The minimal set of films for the cervical spine includes the anteroposterior (AP), lateral, open-mouth, and odontoid views. The vertebra C7 must be visualized on the lateral projection when the cervical spine is being examined because many fracture-dislocations occur in the lower cervical spine or at the cervicothoracic junction.

ORTHOPEDIC GAMUT 3-7

CERVICAL SPINE INSTABILITY

Plain-film, lateral, flexion, or extension views reveal evidence of cervical spine instability, which includes the following:

1. Anterolisthesis (sagittal displacement of vertebral body more than 3.5 mm)
2. Increased spinous spacing
3. Subluxation of facet joints
4. Acute angular deformity at level of injury (11-degree angulation of adjacent vertebral bodies)
5. Sagittal diameter of spinal canal less than 13 mm
6. Fracture or dislocation
7. Atlantodental interval greater than 3 mm in adults and 4 mm in children

---

ORTHOPEDIC GAMUT 3-8

CERVICAL SPINE PLAIN FILM SERIES

The typical cervical spine plain-film series consists of the following:

1. AP open-mouth (APOM) view
2. AP lower cervical (APLC) view
3. Lateral cervical view
4. Oblique views

3

   Specific views are used to evaluate complex regions of anatomy or spinal placement at extremes of motion (Box 3-1).

BOX 3-1

ACCEPTED ADDITIONAL CERVICAL SPINE PLAIN-FILM IMAGING

- Anteroposterior lower cervical view (APLC)
- Anteroposterior open-mouth view (APOM)
- Lateral view
- Anterior oblique views (right and left)
- Additional views:
  - Flexion and extension lateral view
  - Fuch view
  - Pillar or Boyleston view

Data from Greenstein GM: *Clinical assessment of neuromusculoskeletal disorders,* St Louis, 1997, Mosby.

   In assessing the sagittal diameter of the spinal canal, on a lateral view, the shortest distance from the posterior aspect of the vertebral body to the spinolaminar line is measured. The distance between the posterior aspect of the dens and the posterior cervical line is measured at C1. The ranges for diameter by level are listed in Table 3-5.

TABLE 3-5

ACCEPTED SAGITTAL CANAL DIAMETER OF THE CERVICAL SPINE

Level	Diameter (mm) Minimum	Maximum
C1	16	31
C2	14	27
C3	13	23
C4 to C7	12	22

Adapted from Greenstein GM: *Clinical assessment of neuromusculoskeletal disorders*, St Louis, 1997, Mosby.

BAKODY SIGN

SHOULDER ABDUCTION RELIEF SIGN/TEST— CERVICAL FORAMINAL COMPRESSION TEST

Assessment for Cervical Nerve Root Compression

3

Comment

Cervical radiculopathy is more common than cervical myelopathy. Cervical radiculopathy consists of pain and neurologic dysfunction produced by irritation or injury to a spinal nerve. The injury may be caused by a herniated cervical disc, cervical foraminal stenosis, tumors, fractures, or dislocations. The pathognomic characteristic of cervical radiculopathy is pain in the distribution of nerve (Table 3-6).

ORTHOPEDIC GAMUT 3-9

CERVICAL NERVE ROOT COMPRESSION SYMPTOMS

- Proximal (root) pain and neck pain
- Distal paresthesia in dermatome patterns
- Muscle weakness in one or several muscles supplied by a single root
- Loss of deep-tendon reflexes
- Muscle fasciculation
- Radiating pains that are further aggravated by movements of the neck

---

TABLE 3-6

Clinical Findings Associated with the Cervical Nerve Roots

Root	Disc	Muscle	Reflex	Sensation	Myelogram/CT/MR Deficit
C5	C4–C5	Deltoid biceps	Biceps	Lateral arm Deltoid area Axillary nerve	C4–C5
C6	C5–C6	Biceps Wrist extensors	Brachioradialis	Thumb, index, ring fingers Lateral forearm Musculocutaneous nerve	C5–C6
C7	C6–C7	Triceps Wrist flexors Finger extensors	Triceps	Middle finger, ring finger, or both	C6–C7
C8	C7–T1	Hand intrinsics Finger flexors		Ring and fifth fingers Medial forearm Medial anterior brachial cutaneous nerve	C7–T1
T1	T1–T2	Hand intrinsics		Medial arm Medial brachial cutaneous nerve	

CT, Computed tomography; *MR,* magnetic resonance.
Adapted from Watkins RG: *The spine in sports,* St Louis, 1996, Mosby.

PROCEDURE

- While in the seated position, the patient actively places the palm of the affected extremity on top of the head, raising the elbow to a height approximately level with the head.
- By elevating the suprascapular nerve, traction of the lower trunk of the brachial plexus is relieved (Fig. 3-13).
- Overall, this maneuver decreases stretching of the compressed nerve root.
- The sign is present when the radiating pain is lessened or disappears with this maneuver.
- The test is as reliable as Spurling test and is less painful for the patient to endure.
- Cervical nerve root compression is indicated by a positive Bakody sign.

3

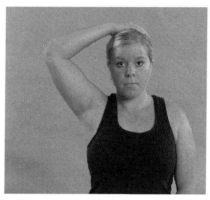

FIG. 3-13 The hand is placed on top of the head. If this position relieves radicular pain, it suggests a nerve root syndrome.

CLINICAL PEARL

Patients with moderate to severe radicular symptoms usually do not have to be directed into the Bakody sign position because it also is an antalgic pain–relieving posture. The more difficult the task is for the patient to lower the arm, the more difficult the condition will be to treat conservatively. If the patient cannot lower the arm without severe exacerbation of pain, surgery is probably indicated. Patients with moderate to severe cervical nerve root compression find the most comfortable sleeping positions to be those that involve abduction and elevation of the arm. Again, this position relieves the traction of the neural elements and is an antalgic position for someone experiencing cervical nerve root compression. A patient often voluntarily assumes the Bakody sign position while in the examination room.

BARRÉ-LIÉOU SIGN

Assessment for Vertebral Artery Syndrome

ORTHOPEDIC GAMUT 3-10

VERTEBRAL ARTERY COMPRESSION

Three mechanisms of vertebral artery compression are:
1. Osteophytes from the lateral disc margin
2. Anteriorly extending osteophytes from the facet joint
3. Compression from the inferior facet as a result of posterior subluxation and a scissoring effect by the adjacent superior facet

3

ORTHOPEDIC GAMUT 3-11

TRAUMA TO THE VERTEBRAL ARTERY

Three areas in which the vertebral artery is most susceptible to trauma:
1. The posterior atlantooccipital membrane, which is dense and inelastic and may become calcified (firmly attached to the artery)
2. The space between the occiput and posterior arch of the atlas, especially during extension
3. Between the lateral mass of the atlas and the transverse process of the axis, especially during extension and rotation

ORTHOPEDIC GAMUT 3-12

CLASSIFICATION OF LOCKED-IN SYNDROME

Locked-in syndrome is subdivided based on the extent of motor impairment:

A. Classical locked-in syndrome (LIS) is characterized by total immobility except for vertical eye movements or blinking.
B. Incomplete LIS permits remnants of voluntary motion.
C. Total LIS consists of complete immobility including all eye movements combined with preserved consciousness.

ORTHOEPDIC GAMUT 3-13

THE AMERICAN CONGRESS OF REHABILITATION MEDICINE (1995) DEFINITION OF LOCKED-IN SYNDROME

1. The presence of sustained eye opening (Bilateral ptosis should be ruled out as a complicating factor.)
2. Preserved basic cognitive abilities
3. Aphonia or severe hypophonia
4. Quadriplegia or quadriparesis
5. A primary mode of communication that uses vertical or lateral eye movement or blinking of the upper eyelid

ORTHOPEDIC GAMUT 3-14

LOCKED-IN SYNDROME

Locked-in syndrome characteristics include:

1. Retained consciousness
2. No volitional movement of the body
3. Nuclei of cranial nerves V to XII destroyed, resulting in their paralysis
4. Loss of sensations carried in the medial lemniscus
5. Normal hearing
6. Sparing of cranial nerve IV nucleus and the superior colliculus of the quadrigeminal plate

PROCEDURE

- The examiner instructs the patient to rotate the head slowly from side to side while in a seated position (Fig. 3-14).
- Rotating the head causes compression of the vertebral arteries.
- Vertigo, dizziness, visual disturbances, nausea, syncope, and nystagmus are signs of a positive test.
- A positive finding strongly indicates a buckling of the ipsilateral vertebral artery and indicates vertebrobasilar insufficiency.

3

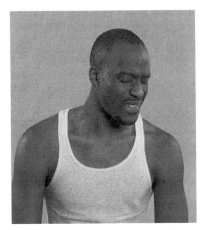

FIG. 3-14 A VA syndrome is suggested by vertigo, blurred vision, nausea, syncope, or nystagmus. These symptoms may occur singly or in combination.

CLINICAL PEARL

The patient with a positive Barré-Liéou sign is a poor risk for aggressive cervical spine manipulation. Such manipulation should not be undertaken until all vascular causes have been investigated. Aggravation of the *sympathetic ganglia* of the cervical spine can produce many, if not all, of these symptoms (vertigo, dizziness, visual disturbances, nausea, syncope, and nystagmus), in which case cervical spinal manipulation is not contraindicated. The examiner absolutely must distinguish between vascular and neural origins before manipulation is performed.

In 1926, Barré studied and established a syndrome that was further described in 1928 by his student Liéou. So diverse and widespread is the combination of symptoms and signs that some people no longer regard the syndrome as a disorder associated with the cervical spine; rather, they view the syndrome as one caused by vertebral artery insufficiency and its multivariate characteristics. The symptoms of this syndrome include pain in the head, neck, eyes, ears, face, sinuses, and throat; sensory disturbances in the pharynx and larynx; paroxysmal hoarseness and aphonia; tinnitus that is synchronous with the pulse; various auditory hallucinations, such as whistling and humming; deafness; visual disturbances, such as blurring, scintillating scotomata, photophobia, blepharospasm, squinting sensations, and a peculiar pulling at the back of the eyes; flushing; sweating; salivation; lacrimation; nausea; vomiting; and rhinorrhea.

BIKELE SIGN

Assessment for Brachial Plexus Neuritis and Meningitis

PROCEDURE

- With the arm held upward and backward and the elbow fully flexed, the patient extends the elbow.
- If this movement meets with resistance and increases radicular pain from the cervicodorsal region, the test is positive (Fig. 3-15).
- This finding indicates brachial plexus neuritis or meningitis because this maneuver stretches the brachial plexus nerve roots or their coverings.

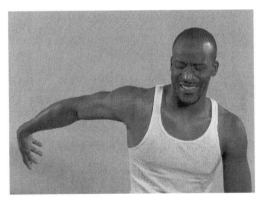

FIG. 3-15 The arm is fully extended at the elbow, and the patient attempts to reach behind. In the presence of radiculopathy or plexopathy, this maneuver produces the radicular pain.

CLINICAL PEARL

Injury to the C8 and T1 roots, the lower trunk, or the medial cord of the brachial plexus may be caused by tumors, disease of the pulmonary apex, or a fractured clavicle or cervical rib. Aneurysm of the arch of the aorta, fracture or dislocation of the humeral head, or unusually abrupt and severe upward traction of the arm may also injure the nerves.

Although Bikele sign does not usually produce a profound finding in minor cervical nerve root compression syndromes, the maneuver often produces startling results in lower brachial plexopathy in the thoracic outlet. Reflex sympathetic changes may be present with the plexopathy and should be correlated with other physiologic findings.

BRACHIAL PLEXUS TENSION TEST

Assessment for Cervical Nerve Root Syndrome or Compression (C5)

ORTHOPEDIC GAMUT 3-15

SLEEP PALSY OF THE BRACHIAL PLEXUS FINDINGS

- Positive neurologic examination
  - Winging of the scapula is usually caused by weakness of either serratus anterior (long thoracic nerve; C5–7) or rhomboids (dorsal scapular nerve; C4–5)
- Positive MRI
  - Increased T2 signal on the MRI in supraspinatus, infraspinatus (suprascapular nerve; C5–C6), and teres minor (axillary nerve; C5–C6)
- Positive nerve-conduction study or electromyographic findings
  - More severe in the upper trunk as exhibited by prominent proximal arm weakness and electromyographic evidence of denervation in the shoulder muscles

---

PROCEDURE

- The examiner passively elevates the patient's shoulders through abduction.
- The elbows are extended to a point just short of the onset of pain and are maintained in this position.
- The shoulders are externally rotated to the point just short of the onset of pain and maintained.
- The examiner supports the shoulders and forearms in this position as the patient flexes the elbows (Fig. 3-16).
- Reproduction of symptoms suggests cervical spine disorders, most likely the C5 nerve root.
- In addition, from this challenge position, symptoms increase when the cervical spine is flexed.

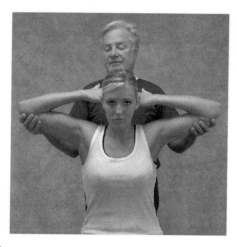

FIG. 3-16

CLINICAL PEARL

Although the brachial plexus tension test involves shoulder joint movement, it also provides maximal stretch on the brachial plexus, which affects the lower branches of the cervical spine (C5) the most. If this test is positive, the early stages of a C5 nerve root disorder may be present along with the subtle signs of a positive *doorbell sign* (pain that occurs at the superior scapulovertebral border and radiates with deep palpation to the C5 segment) and pain in the deltoid area. The deltoid pain is often misconstrued as an articular problem of the shoulder.

DEJERINE SIGN

DEJERINE TRIAD
TRIAD OF DEJERINE

Assessment for Herniated or Protruding Intervertebral Disc and Spinal Cord Tumor or Spinal Compression Fracture

3

PROCEDURE

- Coughing, sneezing, and straining during defecation may aggravate radiculitis symptoms (Fig. 3-17).
- This aggravation results from the mechanical obstruction of spinal fluid flow.
- Dejerine sign is present when one of the following exists: herniated or protruding intervertebral disc, spinal cord tumor, or spinal compression fracture.
- The course of the radiculitis helps identify the location of the lesion.

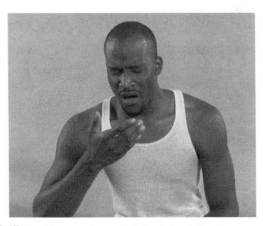

FIG. 3-17 Coughing, sneezing, or straining during defecation causes a reproduction of radicular symptoms, which suggests a space-occupying mass that is creating neurologic compression.

CLINICAL PEARL

Patients with radicular symptoms and pronounced Dejerine sign, especially if it is in the lumbar spine, should be told to bend the knees and lean into a wall during a cough or sneeze. This maneuver reduces intradiscal pressure and minimizes the effect of the cough or sneeze on the nerve root. A more worrisome situation is the sudden, unexpected absence of Dejerine sign when all other clinical findings indicate an active nerve root compression. The loss of the sign indicates fragmentation of the disc with momentary decompression of the nerve.

DEKLEYN TEST

Assessment for Vertebral Artery Syndrome

ORTHOPEDIC GAMUT 3-16

VERTEBRAL ARTERY PATENCY TESTS

Several variations of the vertebral artery patency tests include:
1. Houle test
2. DeKleyn test
3. Smith and Estridge maneuver
4. Modified Adson maneuver
5. Extension rotation test
6. Maigne test
7. Wallenberg test
8. Reclination test

ORTHOPEDIC GAMUT 3-17

POTENTIAL SITES OF COMPRESSION OR INJURY DURING SPINAL MOVEMENT

At least eight potential sites have been identified in the cervical spine at which arterial structures can be compressed or injured by spinal movement:
1. Between C1–C2 transverse processes (Rotation tends to produce stretching of the vertebral artery at this site.)
2. At the level C2–C3 as a result of compression of the vertebral artery by the superior articular facet of C3 on the ipsilateral side to head rotation
3. By the C1 transverse process compressing the internal carotid artery
4. At the C4–C5 or C5–C6 levels as a result of osteoarthrosis of the uncovertebral joints, which can displace the vertebral artery anteriorly and laterally (Compression of the artery is ipsilateral to the side of head rotation.)

ORTHOPEDIC GAMUT 3-17

POTENTIAL SITES OF COMPRESSION OR INJURY DURING SPINAL MOVEMENT—cont'd

5. As a result of compression before entering the C6 transverse process, by traction over a prominent longus colli muscle, or by tissue communicating between the longus colli and scalenus anticus muscles

6. By constriction of the vertebral artery by the ventral ramus of the second cervical nerve during head rotation

7. At the atlantooccipital aperture, on extension:
   - By compression between the posterior arch of atlas and the foramen magnum
   - By folding of the atlantooccipital joint capsule anteriorly and the atlantooccipital membrane posteriorly

8. By compression by the oblique capitis inferior muscle or intertransversarii muscle between the transverse foramina of C1 and C2

Note 1: Maigne and Smith and Estridge Maneuvers

The patient's head is maintained for several seconds in a position of rotation and extension. The patient is asked to comment on the development of any symptoms of vertebrobasilar insufficiency, and the examiner observes for nystagmus. If vertebrobasilar insufficiency signs or symptoms occur, the head is immediately returned to a neutral position.

Note 2: Reclination Test (Sitting)

With the patient sitting, the examiner moves the patient's head into extreme positions of extension and rotation. If threatening signs or symptoms occur, the head is returned to the neutral position.

PROCEDURE

- Coughing, sneezing, and straining during defecation may aggravate radiculitis symptoms (Fig. 3-18).
- This aggravation results from the mechanical obstruction of spinal fluid flow.
- Dejerine sign is present when one of the following exists: herniated or protruding intervertebral disc, spinal cord tumor, or spinal compression fracture.
- The course of the radiculitis helps identify the location of the lesion.

3

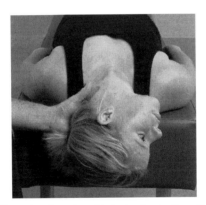

FIG. 3-18 The patient is supine with the head extending off the end of the examination table. The patient rotates and hyperextends the neck to one side and holds this position for 15 to 45 seconds. The examiner may provide minimal support for the weight of the skull. The maneuver is repeated for the opposite side. The production of vertigo, visual disturbance, nausea, syncope, or nystagmus indicates vertebrobasilar circulation compromise.

DISTRACTION TEST

Assessment for Cervical Nerve Root Compression, Intervertebral Foraminal Encroachment, and Facet Capsulitis

---

ORTHOPEDIC GAMUT 3-18

ZYGAPOPHYSEAL JOINT MENISCI

Four distinct types of cervical zygapophyseal joint (Z-joint) menisci exist:

Type I: Menisci are thin and protrude far into the Z-joints, covering approximately 50% of the joint surface (found only in children).

Type II: Menisci are relatively large wedges that protrude a significant distance into the joint space (found almost exclusively at the lateral C1–C2 Z-joints).

Type III: Folds are rather small nubs (found throughout the C2–C3 to C6–C7 cervical Z-joints of most healthy adults).

Type IV: Menisci are quite large and thick (found in degenerative Z-joints).

Pain and stiffness may result from weather changes or unexplained causes. Radiculopathy is not always present. Hyporeflexia, motor weakness, and sensory disturbance (especially paresthesia) are common (Table 3-7).

TABLE 3-7

COMMON CLINICAL FEATURES OF CERVICAL DISC SYNDROMES

Disc	Pain	Sensory Change	Motor Weakness, Atrophy	Reflex Change
C4–C5 (C5 root)	Base of neck, shoulder, anterolateral aspect of arm	Numbness in deltoid region	Deltoid, biceps	Biceps
C5–C6 (C6 root)	Neck, shoulder, medial border of scapula, lateral aspect of arm, dorsum of forearm	Dorsolateral aspect of thumb and index finger	Biceps, extensor pollicus longus	Biceps, brachioradialis
C6–C7 (C7 root)	Neck, shoulder, medial border of scapula, lateral aspect of arm, dorsum of forearm	Index and middle fingers, dorsum of hand	Triceps	Triceps

Adapted from Mercier LR: *Practical orthopedics*, ed 4, St Louis, 1995, Mosby.

TABLE 3-8

CLINICAL PRESENTATIONS IN CERVICAL RADICULOPATHIES

	C5	C6	C7	C8
Pain	To parascapular area, shoulder, and upper arm	To shoulder, arm, forearm, and thumb or index finger	To posterior arm, forearm, and index and middle fingers	To medial arm, forearm, and little and ring fingers
Sensory	Upper arm	Lateral arm, forearm, and thumb and index fingers	Index and mçiddle fingers	Medial arm, forearm, and little finger

Continued

TABLE 3-8

CLINICAL PRESENTATIONS IN CERVICAL
RADICULOPATHIES—cont'd

	C5	C6	C7	C8
Motor	Scapular fixators, shoulder abduction, and elbow flexion	Shoulder abduction, elbow flexion, and forearm pronation	Elbow extension, wrist and fingers extension	Hand intrinsics, long flexors and extensors of fingers
Hyporeflexia/ areflexia	Biceps or brachioradialis reflexes or both	Biceps or brachioradialis reflexes or both	Triceps reflex	None

Adapted from Katirji B: *Electromyography in clinical practice: a case study approach,*
St Louis, 1998, Mosby.

ORTHOPEDIC GAMUT 3-19

**INDIRECT SIGNS OF CERVICAL
TRAUMA OR INJURY**

Abnormal Soft Tissue

Hemorrhage caused by injury of the paracervical soft tissues
displaces certain physiologic spaces that are appreciated radiographically, representing a space-occupying lesion:

- Widened retropharyngeal space (in excess of 7 mm)
- Widened retrotracheal space (in excess of 21 mm)
- Displacement of the prevertebral fat stripe
- Tracheal deviation and laryngeal dislocation

Abnormal Vertebral Alignment

Injury of soft tissue (a strain or sprain of muscle, tendon, ligament,
and capsule) produces spasm, identified by the following:

- Loss of lordosis
- Acute kyphotic hyperangulation
- Torticollis
- Widened interspinous space
- Rotation of vertebral bodies (one spinous process significantly
  rotated, suggesting unilateral facet dislocation)
- Widened middle atlantoaxial joint (the atlantodental interspace)
  (in excess of 2 mm in adults or 5 mm in children)
- Abnormal intervertebral disc
- Widening of apophyseal joints

PROCEDURE

- With the patient seated, the examiner exerts upward pressure on the patient's head.
- This removes the weight of the patient's head from the neck.
- Generalized, increased pain indicates muscle spasm.
- Relief of pain indicates intervertebral foraminal encroachment or facet capsulitis.
- The examiner continues the distraction for up to 30 to 60 seconds to completely relax the involved tissues (Fig. 3-19).
- This test provides some prediction of the effect of cervical spine traction in relieving pain or paresthesia.
- Nerve root compression may be relieved, with disappearance of the symptoms and signs, if the intervertebral foramina are opened or the disc spaces extended.
- Pressure on the joint capsules of the apophyseal joints is also decreased by distraction.

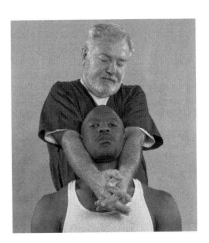

FIG. 3-19

CLINICAL PEARL

The distraction test not only indicates the nature of the patient's complaint but also identifies the merit of cervical traction in the treatment regimen. Notably, the higher the poundage of *static* cervical traction required for relief is, the more unstable the nerve compression syndrome will be. Indeed, the higher poundage requirement is often an indicator of the need for surgical resolution.

FORAMINAL COMPRESSION TEST

Assessment for Cervical Nerve Root Encroachment

3

ORTHOPEDIC GAMUT 3-20

INTERVERTEBRAL FORAMEN

An intervertebral foramen may enlarge as a result of various pathologic conditions:

- Neurofibroma (most common)
- Meningioma
- Fibroma
- Lipoma
- Herniated meningocele
- Tortuous vertebral artery
- Congenital absence of the pedicle with malformation of the transverse process
- Chordoma

PROCEDURE

- With the patient in the seated position, the examiner rotates the patient's neck while exerting strong downward pressure on the head (Fig. 3-20).
- The test is then repeated bilaterally with the head in a neutral position.
- When the neck is rotated and downward pressure is applied, closure of the intervertebral foramen occurs.
- Localized pain indicates foraminal encroachment.
- Radicular pain indicates pressure on the nerve root.
- If nerve root involvement is suspected, the neurologic level must be evaluated.

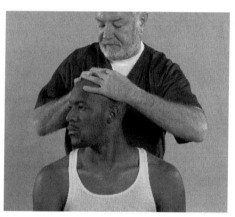

FIG. 3-20

CLINICAL PEARL

This test, as well as other compression maneuvers, often produces a *cervical collapse sign* in addition to radicular complaints. In the presence of capsular sprain with radicular components, compression overcomes the modicum of muscular strength that remains in the neck and is required for postural control. This condition means that the neck will collapse or buckle during the test. This collapse is found in grade II or greater sprain syndromes.

HALLPIKE MANEUVER

Assessment for Vertebrobasilar Artery Insufficiency

ORTHOPEDIC GAMUT 3-21

COMMON VERTEBROBASILAR ARTERIAL ISCHEMIC SYMPTOMS

Ischemic attacks that involve the section of the brain that is supplied by the vertebral and basilar arteries have an extremely wide range of symptoms:

- Vertigo
  - Dizziness is the most common complaint with transient ischemic attacks that are caused by vertebrobasilar insufficiency. However, dizziness is commonly associated with other physiologic disturbances and is rarely the only symptom of brainstem ischemia.
- Tinnitus
  - Tinnitus, hearing loss, and ataxia may be present.
- Diplopia
- Dysarthria
- Dysphagia
- Dysphonia
- Patients may complain of unilateral or bilateral face, arm, and leg weakness and unilateral or bilateral sensations of numbness and tingling in the face, arms, or legs.
- In addition, patients with brainstem ischemia experience drop attacks in which they suddenly lose postural tone and fall to the ground without losing consciousness; they then immediately regain postural control and rise quickly.

3

PROCEDURE

- The Hallpike maneuver is an enhanced DeKleyn test and must be performed with extreme caution.
- The patient lies in the supine position, with the head extending off the end of the examination table.
- The examiner provides support for the weight of the skull.
- The examiner brings the patient's head into positions of reclination (extension), rotation, and lateral flexion.
- The patient's eyes are open so that the examiner may look for nystagmus and other neurovascular signs.
- The test is repeated for the opposite side.
- These positions are held for 15 to 45 seconds.
- In a final maneuver the patient's head is allowed to hang freely in extreme extension (hyperextension) off the end of the examination table (Fig. 3-21).
- Vertigo, blurred vision, nausea, syncope, and nystagmus are signs of a positive test.

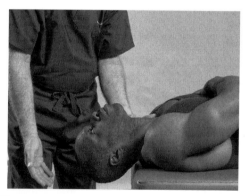

FIG. 3-21

CLINICAL PEARL

Cervical spine manipulation and adjunctive therapeutic techniques are safe to use. Nevertheless, the patient's welfare is always of prime concern, and screening tests will help identify patients who may be predisposed to cerebrovascular problems. During these procedures, symptoms of vertigo, nystagmus, dizziness, fainting, nausea, vomiting, visual blurring, headache (onset), or other sensory disturbances may identify a possible vertebrobasilar insufficiency. Problems in the cervical spine apart from the vertebral arteries may cause the same signs and symptoms. In suspected vertebral artery constriction, resisted neck extension may be painful, and prolonged cervical extension may produce a feeling of faintness. The transverse processes of the atlas are often tender on the side of involvement. These symptoms may improve significantly by using manipulative procedures. Therefore manipulation should not necessarily be abandoned; rather, the manipulative technique should be modified so that simultaneous extension and rotation are not used.

3

HAUTANT TEST

Assessment for Vertebral Artery Syndrome

ORTHOPEDIC GAMUT 3-22

WALLENBERG SYNDROME

Wallenberg syndrome characteristics:

1. Dysphagia, ipsilateral palatal weakness, and vocal cord paralysis (involvement of the nucleus ambiguous of the vagus)
2. Impairment of sensation to pain and temperature on the same side of the face (involvement of the descending root and nucleus of the fifth cranial nerve)
3. Horner syndrome in the homolateral eye (involvement of the descending sympathetic fibers)
4. Nystagmus (involvement of the vestibular nuclei)
5. Cerebellar dysfunction in the ipsilateral arm and leg (interference of the function of the midbrain and cerebellum)
6. Impairment of sensation to pain and temperature on the side of the body opposite (involvement of the spinothalamic tract)

PROCEDURE

- While seated, the patient extends the arms out in front with the palms up.
- With eyes closed, the patient extends and rotates the head to one side (Fig. 3-22).
- The patient repeats this maneuver with the head extended and rotated to the opposite side.
- Drifting of the arms, vertigo, blurred vision, nausea, syncope, and nystagmus are signs of a positive test.
- The test indicates vertebral, basilar, or carotid artery stenosis or compression.

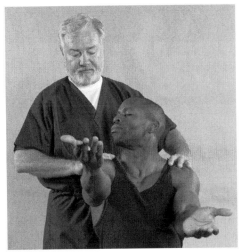

FIG. 3-22

JACKSON COMPRESSION TEST

Assessment for Cervical Nerve Root Compression Resulting from a Space-Occupying Lesion, Subluxation, Inflammatory Edema, Exostosis of Degenerative Joint Disease, Tumor, or Intervertebral Disc Herniation

---

ORTHOPEDIC GAMUT 3-23

CERVICAL NERVE ROOT COMPRESSION SYNDROME

Clinical axioms regarding cervical nerve root compression syndrome:

1. When sensory manifestations occur in C7 radiculopathy, the index or middle finger always is involved.
2. When sensory manifestations occur in C8 radiculopathy, the little or ring finger always is involved.
3. The thumb is never involved exclusively in C7 radiculopathy.
4. Significant triceps weakness is seen only in C7 radiculopathy.
5. Significant supraspinatus and infraspinatus weakness is seen only in C5 radiculopathy.
6. Significant interossei and hand intrinsic weakness is seen only in C8 radiculopathy.

TABLE 3-9

MODIFIED QUEBEC TASK FORCE CLASSIFICATION SYSTEM FOR ACUTE WHIPLASH ASSOCIATED DISORDERS (WAD)

Proposed Grade	Classification	Physical and Psychological Impairments Present
WAD 0		No complaint about neck pain No physical signs
WAD 1		Neck complaint of pain, stiffness or tenderness only No physical signs

TABLE 3-9

MODIFIED QUEBEC TASK FORCE CLASSIFICATION SYSTEM FOR
ACUTE WHIPLASH ASSOCIATED DISORDERS (WAD)—cont'd

Proposed Grade	Classification	Physical and Psychological Impairments Present
WAD II A		Neck pain
		Motor Impairment
		Decreased ROM
		Altered muscle recruitment patterns (CCFT)
		Sensory Impairment
		Local cervical mechanical hyperalgesia
WAD II B		Neck pain
		Motor Impairment
		Decreased ROM
		Altered muscle recruitment patterns (CCFT)
		Sensory Impairment
		Local cervical mechanical hyperalgesia
		Psychological Impairment
		Elevated Psychological distress (GHQ-28, TAMPA)
WAD II C		Neck pain
		Motor Impairment
		Decreased ROM
		Altered muscle recruitment patterns (CCFT)
		Increased JPE
		Sensory Impairment
		Local cervical mechanical hyperalgesia
		Generalised sensory hypersensitivity (mechanical, thermal, BPPT)
		Some may show SNS disturbances
		Psychological Impairment
		Psychological distress (GHQ-28, TAMPA)
		Elevated levels of acute posttraumatic stress (IES)
WAD III		Neck pain
		Motor Impairment
		Decreased ROM
		Altered muscle recruitment patterns (CCFT)
		Increased JPE
		Sensory Impairment
		Local cervical mechanical hyperalgesia
		Generalised sensory hypersensitivity (mechanical, thermal, BPPT)
		Some may show SNS disturbances

Continued

TABLE 3-9

MODIFIED QUEBEC TASK FORCE CLASSIFICATION SYSTEM FOR
ACUTE WHIPLASH ASSOCIATED DISORDERS (WAD)—cont'd

Proposed Grade	Classification	Physical and Psychological Impairments Present
		Psychological Impairment
		Psychological distress (GHQ-28, TAMPA)
		Elevated levels of acute posttraumatic stress (IES)
		Neurological signs of conduction loss including:
		Decreased or absent deep tendon reflexes
		Muscle weakness
		Sensory deficits
WAD IV		Fracture or dislocation

BPPT, Brachial plexus provocation test; *CCFT,* cranio-cervical flexion test; *GHQ,*
general health questionnaire; *IES,* impact of events scale; *JPE,* joint positioning error;
TAMPA, Tampa scale of kinesophobia.
Adapted from Sterling M. A proposed new classification system for whiplash associated
disorders—implications for assessment and management, *Man Ther* 9(2):60-70, 2004.

Comment

Despite the variability in sensory and motor presentations of cervical
radiculopathies, certain classic symptoms and signs exist and are
extremely helpful in localizing the compressed root (Table 3-9).

PROCEDURE

- Cervical compression is commonly performed by having the
  patient sit up and bend the head obliquely backward while the
  examiner applies downward pressure on the vertex.
- However, with the Jackson cervical compression test, the head is
  only slightly rotated to the involved side (Fig. 3-23).
- In either case, the sign is positive if localized pain radiates down
  the arm.
- A positive sign indicates nerve involvement from a space-occupying
  lesion, subluxation, inflammatory swelling, exostosis of degenerative
  joint disease, tumor, or disc herniation.

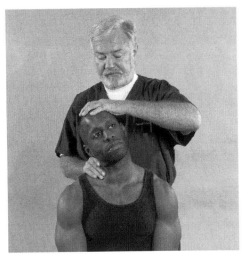

FIG. 3-23

CLINICAL PEARL

Closure of the intervertebral foramina occurs on the side of flexion in this maneuver. This test should be performed without excessive discomfort. The *cervical collapse sign* may be present.

LHERMITTE SIGN

Assessment for Myelopathy of the Cervical Spine

Comment

Peripheral neuropathy is a disorder that affects the peripheral motor, sensory, or autonomic nerves to a variable degree. If only one nerve is affected, mononeuropathy is indicated. If several nerves are involved in a distal symmetric or asymmetric fashion, polyneuropathy is indicated. A patter with multiple, single-peripheral nerves or their branches are involved is considered mononeuritis multiplex (Table 3-10).

ORTHOPEDIC GAMUT 3-24

CAUSES OF PROGRESSIVE DEGENERATIVE NARROWING OF THE CERVICAL SPINAL CANAL

- Osteophytic growth from the edge of the end plates of the vertebral bodies
- Disc herniation

ORTHOPEDIC GAMUT 3-25

OTHER COMMON CAUSES OF CERVICAL MYELOPATHY

- A focus of multiple sclerosis
- Intra- and extraaxial tumor
- Huge cervical disc herniation
- Hydrosyringomyelia

TABLE 3-10

CLINICAL SIGNS OF CERVICAL RADICULOPATHY AND MYELOPATHY*

	Cervical Radiculopathy	Myelopathy
Muscle wasting	Path, unilateral	Path, bilateral
Sensory deficit radicular	Path	Norm
Vibratory sense diminished	Norm	Path, lower extremities
Muscle stretch reflexes	Path (weak)	Path (hyper)
Abdominal reflexes	Norm	Path (absent)
Spurling	Path	Norm
Babinski sign	Norm	Path
Hypertonicity	Norm	Path
Gait	Norm	Path

*Classic findings include limitations in cervical range of motion, spasticity (with increased muscle tendon reflexes below the level of canal compromise), a positive Babinski sign, absent abdominal reflexes, decreased joint position and vibratory sensation, and an abnormal gait.

Norm, Normal; *Path*, pathologic.

Adapted from Salvi FJ, Jones JC, Weigert BJ: The assessment of cervical myelopathy, *Spine J* 6(6, suppl 1):S182-S189, 2006.

ORTHOPEDIC GAMUT 3-26

NEUROPATHY

Neuropathy evolving over many weeks or months suggests several possibilities:
1. Exposure to toxic agents or drugs
2. Nutritional deficiencies
3. Chronically abnormal metabolic state
4. Remote effect of a malignant disease
5. Genetic polyneuropathy, which may have an insidious onset at any age

PROCEDURE

- The patient is seated on the examining table.
- The patient's head is passively flexed.
- A sharp pain radiating down the spine and into the upper or lower limbs is a positive finding (Fig. 3-24).
- Dural irritation in the spine is indicated.
- The test is similar to a combination of other meningeal irritation challenges.

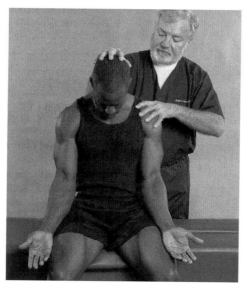

FIG. 3-24

CLINICAL PEARL

Although Lhermitte sign is often construed as a pathognomonic test for multiple sclerosis, it is not. However, Lhermitte sign *does reveal or suggest* myelopathy resulting from multiple sclerosis, stenosis, tumor, or disc herniation.

MAXIMUM CERVICAL COMPRESSION TEST

ASSESSMENT FOR CERVICAL NERVE ROOT SYNDROME OR FACET SYNDROME (CONCAVE TESTING) AND CERVICAL MUSCULAR STRAIN (CONVEX TESTING)

3

Comment

The vulnerability to injury of the cervical region is so great that even low- to moderate-intensity trauma can compromise a multitude of systems. As a result, a variety of signs and symptoms may develop. As is known, the secondary effects of whiplash are sometimes as disabling, if not more so, than the soreness and muscular stiffness of the initial symptoms (Table 3-11).

ORTHOPEDIC GAMUT 3-27

MYOFASCIAL INVOLVEMENT

Two common areas of myofascial involvement of the cervical spine are:
1. Levator scapulae
2. Scalenes

TABLE 3-11

SYMPTOMS EXPERIENCED WITH CERVICAL ACCELERATION-DECELERATION SYNDROMES

Symptom	Lesion Site
Headache	Suboccipital muscles, greater occipital nerve, myofascial trigger points, facet point irritation
Disorientation, irritability	Brain
Visual disturbances	Vertebrobasilar artery network, brainstem, cervical spinal cord
Memory and concentration disturbances	Brain

Continued

TABLE 3-11

SYMPTOMS EXPERIENCED WITH CERVICAL ACCELERATION-DECELERATION SYNDROMES—cont'd

Symptom	Lesion Site
Vertigo	Cervical sympathetic nerves, vertebral artery, inner ear
Arm and hand numbness	Brachial plexus, scalenes
Thumb, index finger, middle finger numbness; weakness; temperature changes	Median nerve, carpal tunnel
Difficulty swallowing	Pharynx
Ringing in ears	Temporomandibular joint, vertebral and basilar arteries, cervical sympathetic chain, inner ear
Dizziness, light-headedness	Cervical sympathetic nerves, brain, inner ear
Neck and shoulder pain	Paravertebral muscles, apophyseal joints, cervical nerve roots, cervical disc
Poor balance, proprioception, and posture	Inner ear

Adapted from Brier SR: *Primary care orthopedics*, St Louis, 1999, Mosby.

ORTHOPEDIC GAMUT 3-28

TESTS OF DIFFERENTIATION

Three tests help in differentiating other thoracic outlet syndrome causes from the scalene trigger point hyperirritability:

1. The cramp test: The patient fully rotates the head to the affected side and drops the chin to the clavicle. The test is positive if a firm contraction or cramp of the scalene muscles occurs.
2. The finger-flexion test: A positive finding is present when all of the medial fingertips cannot press tightly against the metacarpophalangeal joints when the proximal phalanges are extended.
3. The scalene relief test: Elevation of the arm and clavicle lifts the clavicle from the underlying scalenes. To accomplish this task, the patient places the forearm of the involved side across the forehead (similar to reverse Bakody sign); this action produces pain relief within minutes.

PROCEDURE

- While in the seated position, the patient is instructed to approximate the chin to the shoulder and extend the neck (Fig. 3-25).
- The test is performed bilaterally.
- Pain on the concave side indicates nerve root or facet involvement.
- Pain on the convex side indicates muscular strain.

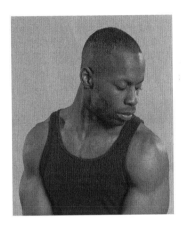

FIG. 3-25

CLINICAL PEARL

The patient with lower cervical nerve root compression syndrome has already discovered that looking up or down with the head rotated is uncomfortable and produces neck and arm pain. If these positions are already producing pain, then attempts to use manipulative procedures incorporating these positions will be difficult for the patient to tolerate.

NAFFZIGER TEST

Assessment for Space-Occupying Mass in the Cervical Spine or Canal

PROCEDURE

- Naffziger compression test is performed by having the patient sit erect while the examiner holds digital pressure over the jugular veins for 30 to 40 seconds.
- The patient is then instructed to cough deeply.
- Pain along the distribution of a nerve may indicate nerve root compression (Fig. 3-26).
- Although this test is more commonly used for lower back involvement, cervical or thoracic root compression may also be aggravated.
- Local pain in the spine does not positively indicate nerve compression but may indicate the site of a strain or sprain injury or other lesion.
- The sign is always positive in the presence of cord tumors, particularly spinal meningiomas.
- The resulting increased spinal fluid pressure above the tumor causes the growth to compress or pull on certain sensory nerve structures, which produces radicular pain.
- The test is contraindicated for a geriatric patient, and extreme care should be taken when performing this test on anyone suspected of having atherosclerosis.
- In all cases, the patient should be alerted that jugular pressure may result in light-headedness or dizziness.

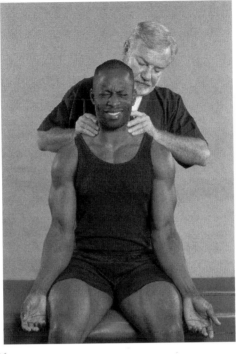

FIG. 3-26

CLINICAL PEARL

This test is *not* a good one for a geriatric or atheromatous patient to endure. The resulting increase in cerebrospinal fluid pressure is uncomfortable, and the momentary circulatory obstruction may result in significant syncope.

O'DONOGHUE MANEUVER

Assessment for Cervical Muscular Strain (Isometric) and Cervical Ligamentous Sprain (Passive Range of Motion)

Comment

Most patients with cervical strain complain of paraspinal muscular aches and stiffness that may extend as far cephalad as the suboccipital region (Table 3-12). Chronic muscular strain of the cervical spine can affect distant organ systems. Pain may be referred to the head, orbits, or scapula.

TABLE 3-12	
CERVICAL STRAIN ASSESSMENT	
Physical examination findings	Paravertebral muscle tenderness
	Intermittent stiffness
	Loss of cervical mobility
	Headaches and alterations of postural reflexes in chronic sufferers
	Normal neurologic signs
	No instability; screening for postural distortion
	Intersegmental posterior joint dysfunction
X-ray findings	Findings generally normal
	Possible decrease in cervical lordosis

Adapted from Brier SR: *Primary care orthopedics*, St Louis, 1999, Mosby.

ORTHOPEDIC GAMUT 3-29

CERVICAL SPINE MUSCULAR INJURY

The mechanism of cervical spine muscular injury is usually one of the following:
1. Athletic participation, which is by far the most frequent means of sustaining a strain injury
2. Overuse
3. Overstretching
4. Contraction of the muscle against resistance
5. Direct blow

ORTHOPEDIC GAMUT 3-30

STRAINS

Strains are divided into three categories according to the degree of muscle tissue damage:
1. A mild strain is a low-grade inflammatory reaction accompanied by no appreciable hemorrhage, minimal amounts of swelling and edema, and some disruption of adjacent fibers.
2. A moderate strain involves laceration of fibers and appreciable hemorrhaging into the surrounding tissue (hematoma), followed by an inflammatory reaction with swelling and edema.
3. A severe strain is the consequence of a single, violent incident that results in complete disruption of the muscle unit. These strains occur when a tendon is torn from the bone or pulled apart, when the musculotendinous junction ruptures, or when the muscle ruptures through its belly.

ORTHOPEDIC GAMUT 3-31

SPRAINS

Sprains are divided into four categories according to the severity of the ligamentous injury:

1. A mild sprain describes an injury in which only a few of the ligamentous fibers are severed.
2. A moderate sprain is a more severe tearing but less than a complete separation of the ligament.
3. A severe sprain is a complete tearing of a ligament from its attachments or a complete separation within its substance.
4. A sprain-fracture has occurred when the ligamentous attachment pulls loose with a fragment of bone (avulsion).

ORTHOPEDIC GAMUT 3-32

CERVICAL ACCELERATION-DECELERATION INJURY

Five types of cervical acceleration-deceleration injury:

Type I: Patients can have severe injuries as a result of seemingly small degrees of acceleration trauma. The symptoms include mild discomfort and stiffness of the cervical spine and loss of small increments in range of motion.

Type II: Injury with palpable muscle splinting, restriction of motion, and mild to moderate spasm. No neurologic deficits or evidence of radiculopathy is observed.

Type III: Injury symptoms include moderate ligamentous sprain, advanced musclea swelling, and muscle spasm. Loss of range of motion in all planes is observed.

Type IV: Injury produces radicular symptoms that may be bilateral or unilateral. Motor and reflex changes are common.

Type V: Injury usually produces signs of neurologic instability. Cervical fracture or facet dislocation are common. Myelopathy and frank disc herniation commonly occur. Swelling and disc fragmentation are possible at the level of the spinal canal.

Separating various grades of cervical whiplash injury is possible according to the degree of external trauma, orthopedic, and neurologic findings, as well as patient disability (Table 3-13).

TABLE 3-13

CERVICAL ACCELERATION-DECELERATION INJURY TYPES

	Type I	Type II	Type III	Type IV	Type V
Physical examination findings	Cervical stiffness or discomfort No motor or sensory deficits No nerve root traction signs No instability Intersegmental fixation, spinal subluxation Results of compression tests normal	Palpable tenderness and muscle guarding No motor or sensory deficits Sympathetic nerve irritation (mild) consisting of headache, dizziness, or light-headedness intermittent for the first week Mild instability Mild to moderate muscle spasm	Swelling and spasm Loss of range of motion in all planes Sympathetic nerve injury with deficit for 7-10 days Moderate signs of instability Possible radiculopathy without motor or reflex loss Results of orthopedic testing abnormal Evaluation for cervical disc lesion and craniomandibular injury	Pain, spasm, and disability Severe restriction of motion in all planes Sympathetic nerve injury involving head, face, and eye disturbances Moderate to severe instability Concomitant disk and articular and soft-tissue injury Severe generalized pain and spasm produced by orthopedic testing; abnormal nerve root traction signs Unilateral or bilateral radicular symptoms	Severe spinal trauma, frank disc herniation with fragmentation common Loss of motor function common Myelopathy and spinal cord compromise Multiple injury sites, often with deformity

Continued

3

TABLE 3-13

CERVICAL ACCELERATION-DECELERATION INJURY TYPES—cont'd

	Type I	Type II	Type III	Type IV	Type V
X-ray findings	Normal	Unremarkable, except for hypolordosis	Soft-tissue swelling and loss of lordotic curve No osseous abnormality	Secondary soft-tissue swelling Loss of lordotic curve Need to rule out ligamentous disruption, fracture, and anatomic subluxation (anterior vertebral translation)	Ligamentous instability usually seen on lateral projection Need to rule out fracture or facet dislocation Immediate follow-up with CT scan to evaluate for occult fractures, disc injury, and spinal cord compromise

Adapted from Brier SR: *Primary care orthopedics*, St Louis, 1999, Mosby.

PROCEDURE

- While the patient is sitting, the cervical spine is actively moved through resisted range of motion and then through passive range of motion.
- Pain during resisted range of motion, or isometric contraction, signifies muscle strain (Fig. 3-27).
- Pain during passive range of motion signifies ligamentous sprain (Fig. 3-28).

3

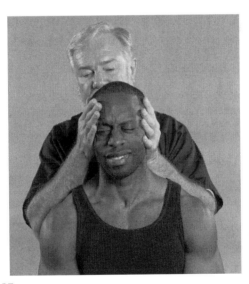

FIG. 3-27

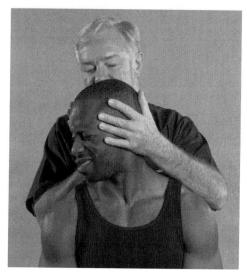

FIG. 3-28 If isometric testing is negative, the examiner passively rotates the patient's head and neck to one side to the limit of joint play. Pain produced in this maneuver suggests ligamentous injury. The maneuver is performed bilaterally.

CLINICAL PEARL

This maneuver can be applied to any joint or series of joints to determine ligamentous or muscular movement. By remembering that resisted range of motion stresses mainly muscles and passive range of motion stresses mainly ligaments, the examiner should be able to differentiate between strain and sprain and should be able to determine whether a combination of both is present.

RUST SIGN

Assessment for Severe Cervical Spine Sprain, Upper Cervical Rheumatoid Arthritis, Upper Cervical Spine Fracture, and Severe Upper Cervical Spine Subluxation

3

ORTHOPEDIC GAMUT 3-33

ODONTOID PROCESS FRACTURES

The Anderson/D'Alonzo classification of odontoid process fractures:

Type I: Fractures of the odontoid are thought to represent an avulsion injury of the tip of the dens by the alar ligament. This injury is very rare, and because it is located above the transverse ligament, no associated atlantoaxial instability occurs.

Type II: Fractures through the body or base of the odontoid have a reported prevalence of nonunion of up to 64%.

Type III: Fractures that extend into the cancellous bone of the axis have an excellent prognosis with adequate reduction and external immobilization.

Comment

Atlantoaxial subluxation is the most common and significant manifestation of rheumatoid involvement of the cervical spine. Long duration of disease, advanced patient age, and peripheral joint erosive instability are associated with more common and severe C1–C2 instabilities, affecting the activities of daily living (Tables 3-14 and 3-15).

TABLE 3-14

NURICK CLASSIFICATION GRADES OF MYELOPATHIC DISABILITY*

Grade	Root Involvement	Cord Involvement	Ambulatory Status	Employable
Grade 0	Present	Absent	Normal	Yes
Grade I	Present	Present	Normal	Yes
Grade II	Present	Present	Mildly abnormal	Yes
Grade III	Present	Present	Severely abnormal	No
Grade IV	Present	Present	Assist dependent	No
Grade V	Present	Present	Nonambulatory	No

*Based on the patient's ability to ambulate and perform daily activities.
Adapted from Gurley JP, Bell GR: The surgical management of patients with rheumatoid cervical spine disease, *Rheum Dis Clin North Am* 23(2):317-332, 1997.

TABLE 3-15

ZEIDMAN AND DUCKER MODIFICATION OF NURICK CLASSIFICATION

Grade	Root Involvement	Cord Involvement	Ambulatory Status	Hand Function
Grade 0	Present	Absent	Normal	Normal
Grade I	Present	Present	Normal	Slightly abnormal
Grade II	Present	Present	Mildly abnormal	Abnormal, functional
Grade III	Present	Present	Severely abnormal	Unable to button
Grade IV	Present	Present	Assist dependent	Severe dysfunction
Grade V	Present	Present	Nonambulatory	Useless

Adapted from Gurley JP, Bell GR: The surgical management of patients with rheumatoid cervical spine disease, *Rheum Dis Clin North Am* 23(2):317-332, 1997.

ORTHOPEDIC GAMUT 3-34

ATLANTOAXIAL INSTABILITY

Atlantoaxial instability caused by rheumatoid arthritis results from a combination of the following:
1. Local arthritic and mechanical instability and pain
2. Neurologic dysfunction of brainstem, cord, and peripheral nerve (root)
3. Vertebral artery insufficiency

PROCEDURE

If the patient spontaneously grasps the head with both hands when lying down or when arising from a recumbent position, this action is a positive sign that indicates severe sprain, rheumatoid arthritis, fracture, or severe cervical subluxation (Figs. 3-29 and 3-30).

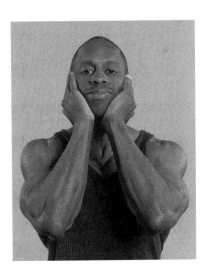

FIG. 3-29

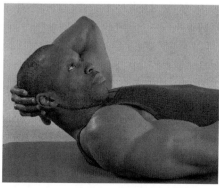

FIG. 3-30 No less significant is the patient who cannot rise from the supine position without lifting the head manually, suggesting gross upper cervical spine instability as a result of fracture or severe sprain.

CLINICAL PEARL

No other physical finding is as important or as revealing as Rust sign. The presence of this sign mandates that (1) no further passive or active testing be undertaken, (2) imaging be performed immediately, and (3) the neck be adequately supported by using a cervical collar. Rust sign has never been observed in conditions of minor consequence.

SHOULDER DEPRESSION TEST

Assessment for Cervical Dural Sleeve Adhesion (Nerve Root) and Shoulder Adhesive Capsulitis

---

ORTHOPEDIC GAMUT 3-35

ADHESION DEGREES BETWEEN DURA MATER AND FIBROUS TISSUE

- Grade 0: when the dura mater is free of the fibrous tissue
- Grade 1: when only thin fibrous band or bands between dura mater and fibrous tissue is observed
- Grade 2: when continuous adherence is observed but less than two thirds of the laminectomy defect
- Grade 3: when fibrous tissue adherence is large, more than two thirds of the laminectomy defect, or extends to the nerve roots

ORTHOPEDIC GAMUT 3-36

MATERIALS USED FOR PREVENTION OF EPIDURAL FIBROSIS

- Fat grafts
- Steroid application and injection
- Silastic membrane and polytetrafluoroethylene barrier
- Polyvinyl alcohol hydrogen membrane
- Polylactic acid membrane
- Vicryl mesh
- Sodium hyaluronate
- Methyl metacrilate
- Gel recombinant tissue plasminogen activator
- Gelatin
- Aprotinine
- Dextran 70
- Gore-Tex®
- Urocynase
- Gel foam and microfibrillar collagen
- Dexametasone
- Fibrin glue
- CO_2 laser
- Mitomycin-C

PROCEDURE

- With the patient seated, the examiner depresses the patient's shoulder on the affected side and laterally flexes the cervical spine away from that shoulder (Fig. 3-31).
- The sign is positive if radicular pain is produced or aggravated.
- A positive sign indicates adhesions of the dural sleeves, spinal nerve roots, or adjacent structures of the joint capsule of the shoulder.

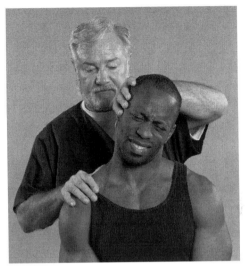

FIG. 3-31

CLINICAL PEARL

As with cervical distraction testing, this maneuver helps predict the viability of cervical traction in therapy. A sharply positive finding usually means that the patient will not tolerate cervical traction. The traction may aggravate the dural sleeve adhesion instead of relieving it.

SOTO-HALL SIGN

Assessment for Cervical Spine Subluxation, Exostoses, Intervertebral Disc Lesion, Muscular Strain, Ligamentous Sprain, Vertebral Fracture, or Meningeal Irritation (Febrile)

ORTHOPEDIC GAMUT 3-37

RISK FACTORS FOR NOSOCOMIAL MENINGITIS

1. History of neurosurgery
2. CSF leakage or recent head trauma
3. Distant focus of infection
4. An immunocompromised state

ORTHOPEDIC GAMUT 3-38

GLASGOW OUTCOME SCALE

1: death
2: vegetative state
3: severe disability
4: moderate disability
5: mild or no disability

PROCEDURE

- The patient is placed supine.
- The examiner places one hand on the sternum of the patient and exerts slight pressure so that no flexion can take place at either the lumbar or thoracic regions of the spine.
- The examiner places the other hand under the patient's occiput and flexes the head toward the chest.
- The test is primarily used when fracture of a vertebra is suspected.
- The flexion of the head and neck on the sternum progressively produces a pull on the posterior spinous ligaments.
- When the spinous process of the injured vertebra is reached, the patient experiences a noticeable local pain.
- A positive result indicates subluxation, exostoses, disc lesion, sprain or strain, vertebral fracture, or meningeal irritation (an elevated temperature must be present for corroboration) (Fig. 3-32).

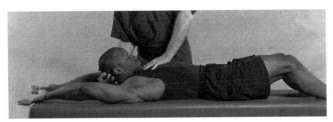

FIG. 3-32

CLINICAL PEARL

Soto-Hall sign is often misapplied in the assessment of fractures and sprains for the entire spine. The sign is a nonspecific test with limited capacity to localize conditions of the cervical and upper thoracic spine. The use of this sign to draw conclusions below T8 is largely guesswork.

With the Kernig or Brudzinski phenomena in this test, the patient's temperature must be assessed. A febrile patient with Kernig or Brudzinski sign—a variation of Soto-Hall sign—is a high-risk candidate for meningitis.

SPINAL PERCUSSION TEST

Assessment for Osseous or Soft-Tissue Injury

ORTHOPEDIC GAMUT 3-39

ATLANTOAXIAL INJURIES

The radiographic signs of atlantoaxial injuries are often subtle:
1. The prevertebral soft-tissue shadow on the lateral radiograph should be less than 5 mm wide at C2 and 5 to 10 mm wide in front of the ring of the atlas.
2. The lateral C-spine view will reveal fractures of the posterior ring of the atlas.
3. The open-mouth odontoid view helps in detecting subtle displacement of the lateral masses in relation to the facets of the axis.

ORTHOPEDIC GAMUT 3-40

CERVICAL SPINE FLEXION-EXTENSION RADIOGRAPHS

The following are prerequisites for cervical spine flexion-extension radiographs:
1. A neurologically intact patient
2. Performance of all movements actively by the patient
3. No altered state of consciousness (including intoxication)
4. Direct physician supervision of the radiographic study

Comment

Pain or discomfort that is nonarticular may be myofascial in origin. The patient with myofascial pain typically has multiple sites of trigger points that refer pain to a distant site (Table 3-16).

TABLE 3-16

REFERRAL ZONES ASSOCIATED WITH TRIGGER POINTS IN MYOFASCIAL PAIN SYNDROME

Localized Trigger Points	Referral Zone
Suboccipital muscles	Temporal region
	Vertex of head
	Temporalis muscle via greater occipital nerve
Levator scapula	Inferior or superior scapula border, occiput
Greater or lesser rhomboid muscles	Cervical spine, shoulder, or scapula region
Infraspinous or teres minor muscles	Arm, shoulder, hand
Sternocleidomastoid muscles	Supraorbital region
	Temporal region
	Forehead, ear
Scalene muscles	Shoulder, arm or hand, chest, scapula
Masseter muscle	Ear, suboccipital region, temporal region
Trapezius muscle	Suboccipital region, shoulder, orbit or temporal area

From Brier SR: *Primary care orthopedics*, St Louis, 1999, Mosby.

PROCEDURE

- With the patient seated and the head slightly flexed, the examiner percusses the spinous processes and associated musculature of each of the cervical vertebra with a neurologic reflex hammer (Fig. 3-33).
- Evidence of localized pain indicates a possible fractured vertebra.
- Evidence of radicular pain indicates a possible disc lesion.
- Because of the nonspecific nature of this test, other conditions will also elicit a positive pain response.
- A ligamentous sprain will cause pain when the spinous processes are percussed.
- Percussing the paraspinal musculature will elicit a positive sign for muscular strain (Fig. 3-34).

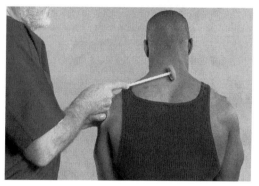

FIG. 3-33

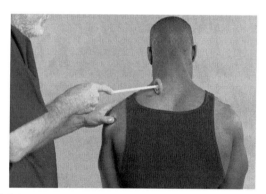

FIG. 3-34

CLINICAL PEARL

When soft-tissue percussion reproduces the pain, the examiner may expect the same phenomenon from applications of ultrasound to the tissue. This pain represents spasmophilia, and the uses of such therapies may need to be delayed until the soft tissue is no longer reactive to percussion.

SPURLING TEST

Assessment for Cervical Nerve Root Compression Syndrome

Comment

All patients who sustain sufficient injury to the cervical spine to make the examiner suspect cervical disc compromise should have a standard three-view, plain-film X-ray film series (Table 3-17).

3

TABLE 3-17

CERVICAL DISC SYNDROMES

Type	Acute Herniated Cervical Disc	Chronic Degenerative Disc Disease
Physical examination findings	Paravertebral myospasm Limited range of motion with signs of instability Radicular signs with possible arm, hand, or scapula referral Often motor, sensory, or reflex changes Nerve root traction signs Abnormal results on compression tests	Chronic cervical stiffness, hypertonicity Upper-extremity referral Possible bilateral or unilateral intermittent radiculopathy, progressive motor changes or atrophy, prolonged cervical instability Possible nerve root traction signs Abnormal results on compression tests
X-ray findings	Standard three-view series (i.e., anteroposterior, open-mouth, lateral), if antecedent trauma Decreased intervertebral disc spacing or spondylosis possible Altered cervical lordosis	Same as for acute conditions, plus oblique films, if neuroforaminal pathologic abnormality or fracture suspected Decreased intervertebral disc space, osteophytes, possible anterior subluxation secondary to anterior longitudinal ligament buckling Hypolordosis

Continued

TABLE 3-17		
CERVICAL DISC SYNDROMES—cont'd		
Type	**Acute Herniated Cervical Disc**	**Chronic Degenerative Disc Disease**
Secondary diagnoses	Cervical radiculopathy, radiculitis; cervical myelopathy; cervical spinal stenosis; acute cervical myospasm	Cervical radiculopathy, radiculitis; cervical myelopathy; cervical spinal stenosis; acute cervical myospasm

Adapted from Brier SR: *Primary care orthopedics*, St Louis, 1999, Mosby.

ORTHOPEDIC GAMUT 3-41

MAGNETIC RESONANCE IMAGING SCANS

Follow-up with an MRI scan of the cervical spine is appropriate for the following patients:
1. Patients who do not respond to conservative measures of care within 2 to 4 weeks and have abnormal neurologic findings
2. Patients who have persistent radiculopathy and loss of motion in multiple planes
3. Patients who exhibit signs of myelopathy and stenosis
4. Patients who have progressive symptoms with motor or sensory deficits
5. Patients who have a cervical spinal canal of questionable patency
6. Patients who have equivocal findings on routine radiography

PROCEDURE

- The test is performed with the patient seated.
- The examiner places one hand on top of the patient's head and gradually increases downward pressure.
- The patient notes any pain or paresthesia and the distribution thereof.
- Pressure may also be applied while the head is laterally flexed to either side and extended (Fig. 3-35).
- Pressure should be maintained.
- This maneuver closes the intervertebral foramina on the side of the flexion and reproduces the familiar pain or paresthesia
- A vertical blow is delivered to the uppermost portion of the cranium. The test will stimulate any nerve root irritation or other pain-sensitive structures related to disc disease and cervical spondylosis. Use of this modification should not be a surprise to the patient (Fig. 3-36).

3

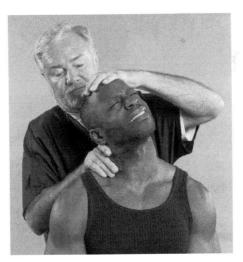

FIG. 3-35

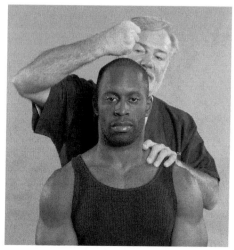

FIG. 3-36

CLINICAL PEARL

Spurling test is an aggressive cervical compression test, and the patient should be informed of each step as it is introduced. However, the examiner should not cue the patient for pain responses. Spurling test elicits *cervical collapse sign* quite easily.

SWALLOWING TEST

Assessment for Space-Occupying Mass, Ligamentous Sprain, Muscular Strain, Fracture, Cervical Intervertebral Disc Lesion, Tumor, or Osteophyte at the Anterior Portion of the Cervical Spine

PROCEDURE

- While seated, the patient is instructed to swallow (Fig. 3-37).
- Presence of pain or difficulty swallowing indicates a space-occupying lesion, ligamentous sprain, muscular strain, or fracture, such as disc protrusion, tumor, or osteophyte at the anterior portion of the cervical spine.

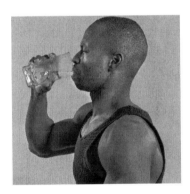

FIG. 3-37

CLINICAL PEARL

Dysphagia is often observed after hyperextension trauma of the cervical spine. Coupled with other sympathetic nervous system phenomena, the patient attributes the sore throat or hoarseness to a cold. The dysphagia is fleeting but serves as a more conclusive sign as to the extent of soft-tissue involvement in the injury.

UNDERBURG TEST

Assessment for Vertebrobasilar Artery Syndrome

ORTHOPEDIC GAMUT 3-42

BRAINSTEM ISCHEMIA

In vertebrobasilar artery insufficiency, brainstem ischemia is the result of:
1. Trauma to the arterial wall producing damage to the arterial wall
2. Trauma to the arterial wall producing vasospasm

ORTHOPEDIC GAMUT 3-43

ARTERIAL WALL (INTIMAL) DAMAGE

In vertebrobasilar syndrome, damage to the artery wall is the result of:
1. Compression or stretching (or both) of the vertebral artery wall that applies enough force to disrupt the vasovasorum, resulting in subintimal hematoma. Vertebral artery blood flow is decreased by occlusion of the lumen.
2. The intima is the most likely tissue to tear when the vessel is stretched, compressed, or both. Exposure of the subendothelial tissue leads to the cascade mechanism, resulting in clot formation (thrombosis). The clot remains adherent to the tear and may lead to vessel occlusion.
3. The propagating clot extends into the lumen. The blood flow may *break off* part of the clot and form an embolus. The embolus causes arterial occlusion distally, leading to infarction.
4. When blood dissects the intima and the internal elastica, a dissecting aneurysm is formed.

ORTHOPEDIC GAMUT 3-44

VASOSPASM

Arterial wall intimal trauma producing vasospasm follows Virchow triad:

1. Change in vessel wall: Within the vertebrobasilar artery (VBA) system neck rotation causes the artery to be momentarily compressed or stretched, which may result in spasm, without vertebral artery damage.
2. Change in blood flow: Within the VBA system, even after the removal of the arterial compression, the spasm may persist, which reduces the blood supply to tissue. Blood flow may stagnate within the involved vessel.
3. Change in blood constituents: Within the VBA system the vertebral arteries can be sufficiently compromised (stasis) to initiate a propagating thrombus and subsequent embolism.

PROCEDURE

- The patient is standing and is instructed to outstretch the arms, supinate the hands, and close the eyes.
- The patient marches in place and extends and rotates the head while continuing to march (Fig. 3-38).
- The test is repeated with the head rotated and extended to the opposite side.
- The examiner watches for a loss of balance, dropping of the arms, and pronation of the hands.
- If any of these actions occurs, the examiner should suspect vertebral, basilar, or carotid artery stenosis or compression.

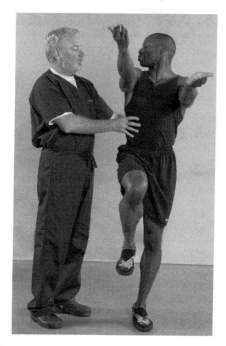

FIG. 3-38

CLINICAL PEARL

If the patient loses equilibrium at any time while the eyes are closed, cerebellar circulation must be evaluated. In this procedure, the patient may lose equilibrium as soon as the head is rotated to one side. The examiner must be prepared to prevent the patient from falling.

VALSALVA MANEUVER—NEURO-ORTHOPEDIC APPLICATION

Assessment for Space-Occupying Lesion, Tumor, Intervertebral Disc Herniation, or Osteophytes

ORTHOPEDIC GAMUT 3-45

CERVICAL SPINE SPONDYLOSIS

Assessment of cervical spine spondylosis includes the following:
1. Plain-film roentgenograms are usually performed first, within the first few weeks of onset of symptoms. AP and lateral views are sufficient.
2. Myelography, sometimes followed by CT, will demonstrate loss of the normal root *sleeve*, and indentation of the dural sac is often seen.
3. MRI is performed.
4. Electromyography and discography are performed. However, the diagnosis can usually be well established based on the history, physical examination, and myelogram alone.

ORTHOPEDIC GAMUT 3-46

NERVE ROOT INVOLVEMENT

Guidelines for quick localization of nerve root involvement:
1. If the deltoid muscle is spared, the lesion is likely to be at C4–C5.
2. If the biceps are spared, the lesion is likely to be at C5–C6.
3. If the triceps are spared, the lesion is likely to be at C6–C7.
4. If the hands are spared, the level is likely to be C7–T1 or below.

PROCEDURE

- The patient takes a deep breath and holds it while bearing down abdominally (Fig. 3-39).
- A positive test is indicated by increased pain caused by increased intrathecal pressure.
- Increased intrathecal pressure is usually caused by a space-occupying lesion (herniated disc, tumor, osteophytes).
- The test should be performed with care and caution because the patient may become dizzy and pass out while or shortly after performing this test because the procedure can block the blood supply to the brain.

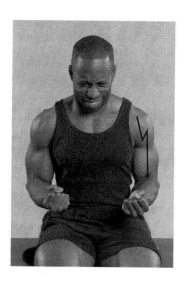

FIG. 3-39

VERTEBROBASILAR ARTERY FUNCTIONAL MANEUVER

Assessment for Vertebral, Basilar, or Carotid Artery Stenosis or Compression

---

ORTHOPEDIC GAMUT 3-47

VERTEBROBASILAR INSUFFICIENCY

The major signs and symptoms of vertebrobasilar insufficiency are as follows:

1. Dizziness, vertigo, giddiness, light-headedness
2. Drop attacks, loss of consciousness
3. Diplopia (or other visual problems, amaurosis fugax)
4. Dysarthria (speech difficulties)
5. Dysphagia
6. Ataxia of gait (walking difficulties, incoordination of the extremities, ataxia, falling to one side)
7. Nausea (with possible vomiting)
8. Numbness on one side of the face or body or both
9. Nystagmus

ORTHOPEDIC GAMUT 3-48

DIFFERENTIAL DIAGNOSES OF FACIAL PURPURA

Bilateral (usual)
- Traumatic origin
- Viral infection
- Scurvy

Unilateral
- Sneddon syndrome, characterized by the association of livedo racemosa and ischemic neurologic events (requires neurologic deficit and abnormal brain CT)
- Harlequin syndrome (autonomic dysfunction affecting sweating and flushing of the face and less commonly the upper limb and upper chest)

ORTHOPEDIC GAMUT 3-49

VERTEBROBASILAR ISCHEMIA

Three types of vertebrobasilar ischemia are:

1. Transient ischemic attacks (TIAs) are brief episodes of neurologic dysfunction most commonly caused by embolic showers from an atheromatous carotid artery to the ipsilateral cerebral hemisphere. Patients experience paresthesia or anesthesia in an arm or leg. When a motor abnormality is prominent, weakness, paralysis, or incoordination on the involved side of the body is present. Brief aphasic or dysphasic symptoms occur with involvement of the dominant hemisphere. Attacks are brief, lasting for a few seconds to minutes. Rarely do the attacks extend beyond 3 hours. TIAs occur on the side opposite the involved area of the brain and carotid artery.

2. Reversible ischemia neurologic deficits (RINDs) persist for longer than 24 hours and disappear completely. When the symptoms of RINDs occur and are identical to those of TIA, the patient may have sustained a small area of cerebral infarction. Neurologic symptoms that persist for long periods are diagnosed as a completed stroke.

3. *Stroke in evolution* and crescendo TIAs may occur. A patient with a stroke in evolution experiences acute neurologic deficit, which progresses over hours or days and ultimately results in a fixed deficit caused by cerebral infarction. Crescendo carotid TIAs is a syndrome of multiple TIAs occurring within a short time. Each attack is followed by complete recovery. These syndromes indicate high-grade carotid artery stenosis with embolization and are an urgent indication for further evaluation.

ORTHOPEDIC GAMUT 3-50

RESIDUAL EFFECT OF CAROTID OCCLUSION

When serious residual effects of carotid occlusion occur, the symptoms will conform to one of the following syndromes:
1. Wallenberg (occlusion of the posterior inferior cerebral artery)
2. Locked-in (occlusion of the basilar artery)
3. Other brainstem syndromes
4. Occipital lobe injury
5. Cerebellar injury
6. Thalamus injury

PROCEDURE

- With the patient in a seated position, the examiner palpates the carotid and subclavian arteries and auscultates for pulsations and bruits (Fig. 3-40).
- If neither of these situations exists, the patient is instructed to rotate and hyperextend the head to one side and then the other (Fig. 3-41).
- This second maneuver should be performed only if initial palpation and auscultation did not reveal bruits or pulsations.
- The test is considered positive if either maneuver reveals pulsations or bruits.
- The rotation and hyperextension portion of this test places motion-induced compression on the vertebral arteries.
- Vertigo, dizziness, visual blurring, nausea, faintness, and nystagmus are all signs of a positive test, which indicates vertebral, basilar, or carotid artery stenosis or compression.

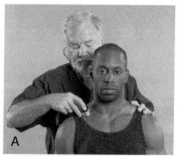

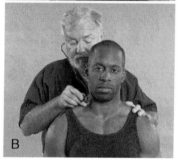

FIG. 3-40

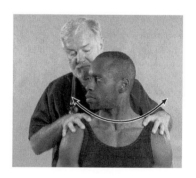

FIG. 3-41

CHAPTER FOUR

SHOULDER

AXIOMS IN ASSESSING THE SHOULDER

- Shoulder motion involves four primary articulations: the gleno-humeral, acromioclavicular, sternoclavicular, and scapulo-thoracic.
- Common shoulder disorders include rotator cuff tendonopathy, rotator cuff tears, capsulitis (frozen shoulder), glenohumeral arthritis, and acromioclavicular syndromes.
- In early capsulitis and glenohumeral arthritis, all active and passive motions are painful, resisted motion produces no pain, and passive motion is decreased.

INTRODUCTION

The shoulder is a system of joints, and many movements of this system involve the neck. Completely independent action of the shoulder is possible, but independent, simultaneous action of the shoulder and neck is not.

The glenohumeral joint may be affected as part of widespread joint disease (i.e., a polyarthropathy such as rheumatoid arthritis, crystal deposition disease arthropathy, other inflammatory arthropathies, or generalized osteoarthritis). Periarticular conditions can be grouped into categories with and without capsulitis. In the absence of capsular involvement, passive joint motion is largely unaffected, whereas active movement may be limited by pain or weakness or both. In the presence of capsulitis, multidirectional restriction of passive motion is seen. Clinical and radiologic studies differentiate these conditions from articular conditions.

Referred pain to the shoulder can occur with cervical disorders, Pancoast tumor of the lung, a subphrenic pathologic condition, entrapment neuropathies, myofascial pain syndromes, and brachial neuritis (Table 4-3).

Identification of the primary cause of shoulder pain is not always easy. Referred pain to the shoulder girdle region occurs from multiple sources other than the neck. With diaphragmatic irritation, pain is

TABLE 4-1

SHOULDER JOINT CROSS-REFERENCE TABLE BY ASSESSMENT PROCEDURE

Shoulder

Disease Assessed

Test/Sign	Abbott-Saunders test	Adson test	Allen maneuver	Apley test	Apprehension test	Bryant sign	Calloway test	Codman sign
Transverse Humeral Ligament								
Adhesive Capsulitis								
Subclavian Arterial Stenosis								
Subacromial Bursa								
Supraspinatus Tendon								●
Posterior Dislocation					●	●	●	
Anterior Dislocation					●	●	●	
Rotator Cuff				●				●
Thoracic Outlet Syndrome		●	●					
Scalenus Anticus Syndrome		●						
Biceps Tendon	●							

Test	1	2	3	4	5	6	7	8	9	10	11
Costoclavicular maneuver									•		
Dawbarn sign				•							
Dugas test						•	•				
George screening procedure			•								
Halstead maneuver						•	•		•		
Hamilton test					•						
Impingement sign											•
Ludington test											•
Mazion shoulder maneuver		•				•	•	•			
Reverse Bakody maneuver									•	•	
Roos test									•		
Shoulder compression test			•						•		
Speed test											•
Subacromial push-button sign					•			•			
Supraspinatus press test					•						
Transverse humeral ligament test	•										•
Wright test											•
Yergason test	•										•

4

TABLE 4-2

SHOULDER JOINT CROSS-REFERENCE TABLE BY SYNDROME OR TISSUE

Adhesive capsulitis	Mazion shoulder maneuver	Scalenus anticus syndrome	Adson test Reverse Bakody maneuver
Anterior dislocation	Apprehension test Bryant sign Calloway test Dugas test Hamilton test Mazion shoulder maneuver	Subcromial bursa	Dawbarn sign
Biceps tendon	Abbott-Saunders test Impingement sign Ludington test Speed test Transverse humeral ligament test Yergason test	Subclavian arterial stenosis	George screening procedure Shoulder compression test
Posterior dislocation	Apprehension test Bryant sign Calloway test Dugas test Hamilton test Mazion shoulder maneuver	Supraspinatus tendon	Codman sign Impingement sign Subacromial push-button sign Supraspinatus press test
Rotator cuff	Apley test Codman sign Mazion shoulder maneuver Subacromial push-button sign	Thoracic outlet syndrome	Adson test Allen maneuver Costoclavicular maneuver Halstead maneuver Reverse Bakody maneuver Roos test Shoulder compression test Wright test
		Transverse humeral ligament	Transverse humeral ligament test Yergason test

TABLE 4-3

COMMON CAUSES OF SHOULDER PAIN

Periarticular Disorders	Regional Disorders	Glenohumeral Disorders
Rotator cuff tendinitis/ impingement syndrome	Cervical radiculopathy	Inflammatory arthritis
Calcific tendinitis	Brachial neuritis	Osteoarthritis
Rotator cuff tear	Nerve entrapment syndromes	Osteonecrosis
Bicipital tendinitis	Sternoclavicular arthritis	Cuff arthropathy
Acromioclavicular arthritis	Reflex sympathetic dystrophy	Septic arthritis
	Fibrositis	Glenoid labrum tears
	Neoplasms	Adhesive capsulitis
	Miscellaneous:	Glenohumeral instability
	Gallbladder disease	
	Splenic trauma	
	Subphrenic abscess	
	Myocardial infarction	
	Thyroid disease	
	Diabetes mellitus	
	Renal osteodystrophy	

From Kelley WN, et al: *Textbook of rheumatology*, ed 5, Philadelphia, 1997, WB Saunders.

referred along the phrenic nerve to the supraclavicular region, the trapezius, and the superomedial angle of the scapula. Gastric and pancreatic diseases may refer pain to the interscapular region. The rare superior sulcus lung tumor, or Pancoast tumor, occasionally coincident with Horner syndrome, may have shoulder pain as its initial symptom.

The arm as a lever is useless unless it has a fixed base. The fixed base comes largely from the layers of flat muscles piled one on top of another and attached to all surfaces of the scapula.

Paralytic disorders implicating these muscles come into clinical focus when weakness in the fixation mechanism is demonstrated. The serratus anterior, when paralyzed, allows the scapula to swing backward and loosen its attachment to the chest. The trapezius allows the scapula to spin like a pinwheel, which contributes to the loss of fixation.

The mobility of this part of the body results from the configuration of the bony parts and the mechanically advantageous attachment of the multiple muscles. The shallow socket and ball head favor frictionless spinning, and the main joint has four accessory articulating zones that complement and enhance the action of the shoulder.

Everyday activities are made up of acts such as lifting, holding, pushing, turning, and shoving. Through such common and accepted motions, clinical disorders are manifested. These activities are combined pattern motions with contributions from many parts of the shoulder complex. Individual joint and muscle contribution may be analyzed in these acts to aid localization and understanding of injury and disease. Consideration must also be given to the part that the elbow and hand play in shoulder function. Shoulders are used unconsciously during actions of the hand, wrist, and elbow. Injury or disease may hamper normal action of any of these areas; therefore, increased replacement effort is sought from the shoulder. For example, loss of rotatory range, as in arthrodesis of the wrist or elbow, unconsciously results in increased rotation at the shoulder. Weakness or disorder of one muscle group evokes replacement effort in another group. For example, the hunching motion by the trapezius that follows attempted abduction is a replacement effort associated with paralysis of the deltoid. Scrutiny of these purposeful patterns is of great help in understanding disability in this region.

Chronic overuse syndromes with repetitive stretching, as in rowing, swimming, or throwing, are injuries of repetitive microtrauma. Atraumatic disorders generally result from ligamentous laxity or congenital hypoplasia of the glenoid. Impact injuries may be divided into direct and indirect trauma. For direct trauma, the injury force is in direct contact with the shoulder complex. Indirect forces injuring the shoulder usually pass up through the hand, wrist, or elbow and result in a rotational or longitudinal force directed along the humerus.

ORTHOPEDIC GAMUT 4-1

DIRECT SHOULDER TRAUMA

Direct trauma to the shoulder consists of:
1. Posterior dislocations of the sternoclavicular joint
2. Acromioclavicular subluxations or dislocations after a fall on the posterior superior shoulder
3. Direct blows to the supraclavicular brachial plexus at the base of the neck or axillary nerve as it courses under the deltoid
4. Clavicular fractures
5. Muscle contusions

ORTHOPEDIC GAMUT 4-2

MECHANISMS OF AXILLARY ARTERY INJURY CAUSED BY BLUNT TRAUMA

- Compression with contusion
- Forceful repeated stress
- Direct trauma by a sharp bony fragment
- Avulsion
- Traction

4

ESSENTIAL ANATOMY

The shoulder joint is a ball-and-socket joint that is the articulation of the humerus and the glenoid fossa of the scapula. To describe the anatomy of the shoulder joint, the term *shoulder joint complex* may be more accurate. The shoulder joint complex really consists of four joints: the glenohumeral, the acromioclavicular, the sternoclavicular, and the scapulothoracic articulation. The acromioclavicular joint is formed by the lateral end of the clavicle and acromion. The acromioclavicular joint is reinforced by the surrounding capsule and ligaments, containing an anterior, posterior, superior, and inferior component, in addition to the coracoclavicular ligaments, which are made up of two individual ligaments: the coracoid and trapezoid ligaments. The short head of the biceps arises with the coracobrachialis from the scapular coracoid process and runs down the medial side of the long head of the biceps. The two bellies join as a common distal tendon just above the elbow joint as a flattened tendon, only to separate into two distal insertions.

ESSENTIAL MOTION ASSESSMENT

Shoulder motion is interpreted through excursion of the arm from the body and is recorded according to the anatomic planes (Fig. 4-1).

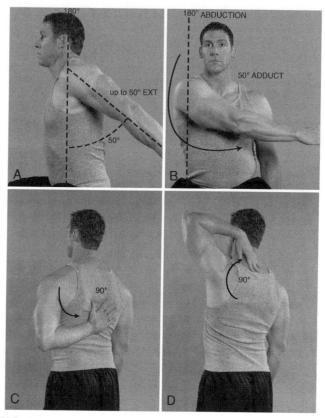

FIG. 4-1 Range of motion of the shoulder. **A**, Forward flexion and extension.
B, Abduction and adduction. **C**, Internal rotation. **D**, External rotation.

ORTHOPEDIC GAMUT 4-3

SHOULDER MOVEMENTS

Primary shoulder movements are:
1. Elevation in the coronal (frontal) plane (abduction and adduction)
2. Flexion and extension in the sagittal plane (Figs. 4-2 and 4-3)
3. Horizontal adduction and abduction in the transverse (horizontal) plane (Figs. 4-4 and 4-5)
4. Internal and external rotation (torque around the humerus) (Figs. 4-6 and 4-7)

4

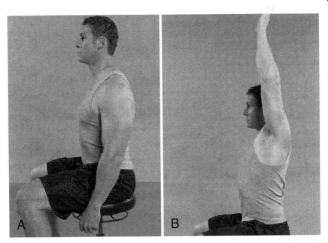

FIG. 4-2 Flexion is accomplished by the anterior deltoid, pectoralis major, coracobrachialis, and biceps. A retained flexion range of motion that is 160 degrees or less is an impairment of the shoulder in the activities of daily living.

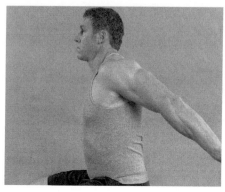

FIG. 4-3 Forty degrees or less of retained extension range of motion is an impairment of the shoulder in the activities of daily living.

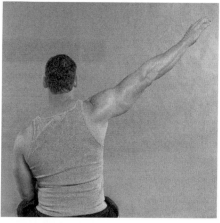

FIG. 4-4 Less than 160 degrees of retained abduction range of motion is an impairment of the shoulder in the activities of daily living.

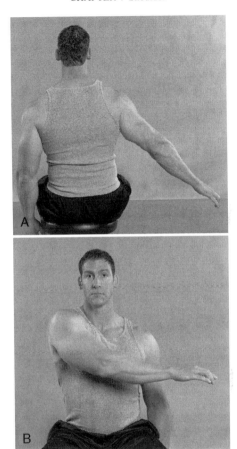

4

FIG. 4-5 A retained adduction range of motion of 30 degrees or less is an impairment of the shoulder in the activities of daily living.

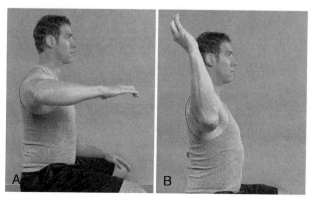

FIG. 4-6 External rotation is the most important action; and when this rotation is lost, shoulder action is seriously compromised. Sixty degrees or less of retained external rotation is an impairment of the shoulder in the activities of daily living.

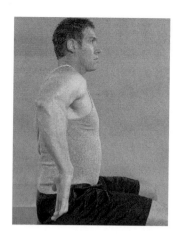

FIG. 4-7

ESSENTIAL MUSCLE FUNCTION ASSESSMENT

The muscles surrounding the shoulder joint complex provide the ability to generate motion while simultaneously providing dynamic stability to the glenohumeral joint.

The teres major muscle arises from the lower third of the lateral border of the scapula and travels around the anterior aspect of the humerus and in front of the long head of the triceps to insert onto the crest of the lesser tubercle. The teres minor and deltoid receive their innervation by the axillary nerve, whereas the teres major is supplied by the lower subscapular nerve (Figs. 4-8 to 4-13).

4

ORTHOPEDIC GAMUT 4-4

MUSCLES OF THE SHOULDER JOINT COMPLEX

Muscles of the shoulder joint complex fall into three categories:
1. Those attaching to the scapula with their origin from the axial skeleton
2. Those that have their origin from the scapula and insert onto the humerus
3. Those that have their origin from the axial skeleton and insert onto the humerus

---

ORTHOPEDIC GAMUT 4-5

MUSCLE ATTACHMENTS

The scapula to spine muscle attachments are as follows:
1. Trapezius
2. Levator scapula
3. Rhomboid major
4. Rhomboid minor
5. Serratus anterior

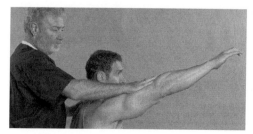

FIG. 4-8 The examiner achieves immobilization by grasping and holding the lower border with one hand. The patient flexes the arm anteriorly to 90 degrees while the forearm is pronated and the elbow slightly flexed.

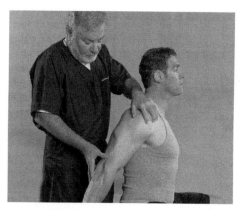

FIG. 4-9 Extension of the shoulder is tested with the patient's elbow straightened and the forearm fully pronated (palm posterior) to prevent lateral rotation and adduction. The examiner fixes the scapula as described for testing flexion, and the patient extends the arm posteriorly through the range of motion.

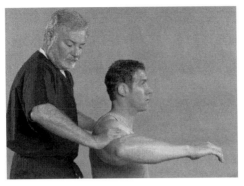

FIG. 4-10 The patient abducts the arm to 90 degrees. This abduction occurs against graded resistance applied by the examiner's other hand, which is placed proximal to the patient's elbow.

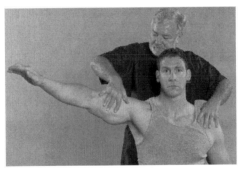

FIG. 4-11 The patient adducts the arm anteriorly through the horizontal plane of motion and against graded resistance. This resistance is applied by the examiner's other hand, which is placed over the front of the arm and proximal to the patient's elbow.

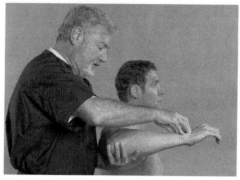

FIG. 4-12 The external rotation of the shoulder is assessed with the patient's arm abducted to 90 degrees (or at the patient's side if abduction is not possible), with the elbow flexed to 90 degrees, and with the hand and fingers pointing forward.

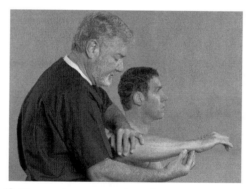

FIG. 4-13 The examiner supports the patient's elbow with one hand, as described previously, while the patient rotates the arm downward (or inward if the shoulder abduction is not possible) against graded resistance that is applied by the examiner's other hand, which is placed on the patient's forearm proximal to the wrist.

ESSENTIAL IMAGING

The shoulder girdle consists of the two bones that attach the upper limb to the thoracic wall: the scapula and the clavicle. The glenoid fossa of the scapula forms the articulation of the shoulder girdle with the head of the humerus.

The most important films to obtain are the true anteroposterior (AP) and the modified West Point views. Both of these projections provide an excellent view of a glenohumeral joint. The examiner is able to appreciate the characteristic posterior glenoid wear. The acromioclavicular joint can be radiographically evaluated and correlated with the physical examination. The AP view should include the proximal two thirds of the humeral shaft so that the physician can safely estimate the appropriate humeral component diameter. When clinically indicated, the radiographic examination of the shoulder must include a cervical spine series.

ABBOTT-SAUNDERS TEST

Assessment for Biceps Tendinitis

ORTHOPEDIC GAMUT 4-6

BICEPS TENDON

The biceps tendon may luxate medially out of the groove and over the lesser medial tuberosity in one of two patterns:

1. Rupture of the transverse ligament and subluxation of the biceps tendon out of the groove, with the tendon lying anterior to the subscapularis muscle

2. Tendon subluxation beneath the subscapularis muscle belly

PROCEDURE

- With the patient in the seated position, the examiner fully abducts and externally rotates the patient's arm.
- The examiner then lowers the arm to the patient's side (Fig. 4-14).
- A palpable or audible click indicates a subluxation or dislocation of the biceps tendon.
- While the examiner's finger or fingers palpate for the point of maximal tenderness within the bicipital groove, the shoulder is alternately rotated.
- A positive test occurs in biceps tendinitis when the patient feels pain as the tendon glides beneath the examiner's finger.

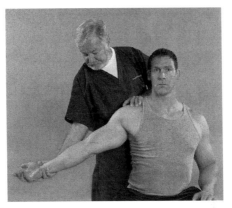

FIG. 4-14

4

CLINICAL PEARL

The biceps tendon will not rupture or dislocate under ordinary stresses unless it is already weak. The predisposing factor to rupture or dislocation is age degeneration, which is probably accelerated by often-repeated friction and angulation at the point where the tendon enters the bicipital groove of the humerus.

ADSON TEST
(ALSO KNOWN AS SCALENE MANEUVER AND SCALENUS ANTICUS TEST)

Assessment for Neurovascular Compression of the Subclavian Artery and Brachial Plexus Caused By Scalenus Anticus or Cervical Rib Thoracic Outlet Syndromes

---

ORTHOPEDIC GAMUT 4-7

THORACIC OUTLET SYNDROME

Even though the first thoracic rib forms the floor of the thoracic compression compartment, trapping or scissoring the brachial plexus and subclavian vessels between the first ribs, other local structures contribute to the problem:

- The clavicle
- A cervical rib
- A anomalous cervical band from an elongated C7 transverse process
- The subclavius muscle
- Bony callous or exostosis

PROCEDURE

- The examiner locates the radial pulse of the involved extremity.
- The patient's head is rotated to the involved extremity.
- The patient extends the neck as the examiner externally rotates and extends the shoulder.
- The patient takes a deep breath and holds it (Fig. 4-15).
- Loss of the pulse is a positive test.
- If the test is negative, it is repeated by having the patient rotate the head to the uninvolved extremity.

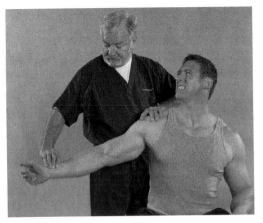

FIG. 4-15

4

CLINICAL PEARL

Radiographic demonstration of a cervical rib does not prove that it is the cause of the symptoms. The condition has to be distinguished (1) from other causes of pain and paresthesia in the forearm and hand, (2) from other causes of muscle atrophy in the hand, and (3) from other causes of peripheral vascular changes in the upper extremity.

ALLEN MANEUVER

Assessment for Thoracic Outlet Syndrome

ORTHOPEDIC GAMUT 4-8

THORACIC OUTLET SYNDROME CLASSIFICATIONS

Thoracic outlet syndrome (TOS) is categorized in three types:

- Vascular (vTOS). Unilateral arm swelling without thrombosis, when not caused by lymphatic obstruction, may be caused by subclavian vein compression at the costoclavicular ligament because of compression by either that ligament or the subclavius tendon most often because of congenital close proximity of the vein to the ligament. Patients with compression of the subclavian artery and vein are classified into two other groups as vascular TOS: arterial TOS or venous TOS.
- Neurogenic (nTOS) compromises the majority of these symptomatic individuals with brachial plexus and T1 nerve palsy. Neck trauma is also the most common cause of nTOS in patients with abnormal ribs. Involvement of the brachial plexus causes the nTOS that comprises two groups: one corresponding to patients harboring the true or classic signs and symptoms and electromyographic (EMG) findings (nTOS) and the other corresponding to patients with nonspecific clinical and EMG findings (nonspecific nTOS).
- Disputed neurogenic TOS (dnTOS). Upper extremity arterial compromise caused by this compacted thoracic outlet may also occur with a resulting limb ischemia. Patients often complain of a painful upper extremity after exercise albeit limb claudication symptoms. Discolored, pale, underperfused arms with absent or decreased arterial pulse is a common finding in these individuals with an arterial form of TOS. This group includes patients with signs and symptoms of posttraumatic neurovascular compression (Paget-Schroetter syndrome).

PROCEDURE

- The patient's elbow is flexed to 90 degrees.
- The shoulder is abducted and externally rotated.
- As the examiner palpates the radial pulse, the patient rotates the head away from the involved extremity (Fig. 4-16).
- If the pulse disappears when the head is rotated, the test is positive for thoracic outlet syndrome.

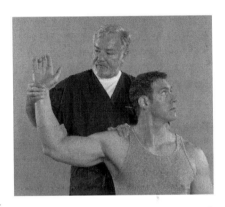

FIG. 4-16

4

CLINICAL PEARL

Altered relative position of the shoulder girdle to the neurovascular bundle, or vice versa, is a common element of thoracic outlet syndrome. However, a group of symptoms may be separated in which a static or gradual process may be underway that appears as a more general development without specific, separate, irritating incidents. Such a condition is labeled *postural* because of the alteration of the normal girdle relationship to the rest of the body.

APLEY TEST
(ALSO KNOWN AS APLEY SCRATCH TEST)

Assessment for Degenerative Tendinitis of One of the Tendons of the Rotator Cuff, Usually the Supraspinatus Tendon

PROCEDURE

- The patient is seated and is instructed to place the affected hand behind the head and touch the opposite superior angle of the scapula (Fig. 4-17).
- The patient is then instructed to place the hand behind the back and attempt to touch the opposite inferior angle of the scapula (Fig. 4-18).
- Exacerbation of the patient's pain indicates degenerative tendinitis of one of the tendons of the rotator cuff, usually the supraspinatus tendon.

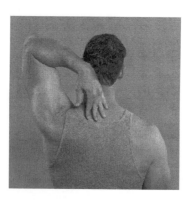

FIG. 4-17

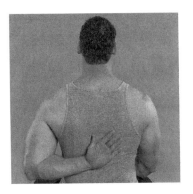

FIG. 4-18

CLINICAL PEARL

Apley inferior is a useful test of internal rotation and extension. With severe restriction, the patient will not be able to get the hand behind the back at all. This movement is commonly affected in adhesive capsulitis.

APPREHENSION TEST

Assessment for Anterior Shoulder Dislocation Trauma and Posterior Dislocation of the Humerus

PROCEDURE

- The patient's shoulder is abducted and externally rotated.
- If the patient shows apprehension or alarm and resists further motion, the test is positive (Fig. 4-19).
- This test may elicit a feeling that resembles the pain felt when the shoulder was previously dislocated.
- This test is performed slowly and cautiously; if the action is performed too quickly, the humerus may dislocate.
- Anterior shoulder dislocation trauma is suggested by a positive test.
- To evaluate posterior shoulder dislocation, the shoulder is flexed and internally rotated (Fig. 4-20).
- A posterior force is applied on the patient's elbow.
- If the patient exhibits apprehension and resists further motion, the test is positive.
- A posterior dislocation of the humerus is suggested by a positive test.

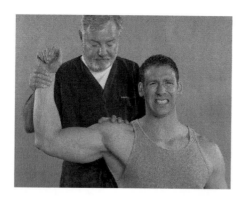

FIG. 4-19

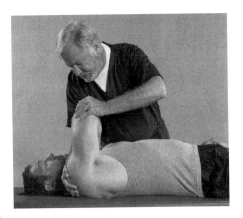

FIG. 4-20

4

CLINICAL PEARL

These maneuvers are also known as the *drawer tests of Gerber and Ganz.* Any movements, clicks, or patient apprehension support the diagnosis of recurrent shoulder dislocation. Axial diagnostic images are made to confirm the diagnosis.

BRYANT SIGN

Assessment for Dislocation of the Glenohumeral Articulation

ORTHOPEDIC GAMUT 4-9

SHOULDER DISLOCATIONS

Shoulder dislocation classification relative to:
1. The degree of instability (dislocation or subluxation)
2. The cause of the instability (traumatic or atraumatic)
3. The direction of the instability (anterior, posterior, or multi-directional)

ORTHOPEDIC GAMUT 4-10

AXILLARY PSEUDOANEURYSM

Accurate detection and diagnosis of axillary pseudoaneurysm after anterior glenohumeral joint dislocation presents difficulties:
- Limited abduction of the arm, as a result of pain and muscle spasm, prevents appropriate and full clinical examination of the axillary region.
- The gradual onset of clinical changes and the delayed radiologic evidence of a pseudoaneurysm may prevent attribution of clinical findings being associated with traumatic glenohumeral joint dislocation.
- An axillary hematoma may be concealed by bone and muscle tissue or bruising mistakenly attributed to the dislocation itself.
- Pulsation of the pseudoaneurysm may be obscured by overlying tissues.
- The motor and sensory disturbances related to ischemia may be mistakenly attributed to brachial plexus damage, which is a more common complication of glenohumeral joint dislocation.
- The robust collateral circulation may maintain the radial pulse, allowing ischemia to go undetected.
- Where recurrent dislocation is experienced, limited hemorrhage may result caused by scar tissue from previous dislocation.

PROCEDURE

The examiner views the characteristic lowering of the axillary fold (anterior and posterior pillars of the armpit) that is seen after trauma when dislocation of the glenohumeral articulation ensues (Fig. 4-21).

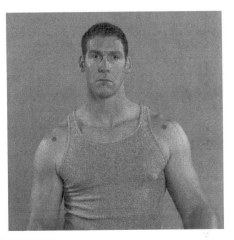

FIG. 4-21

CLINICAL PEARL

With dislocations of the shoulder, the axillary nerve may be injured. The patient is unable to contract the deltoid muscle, and a small patch of anesthesia over the muscle may be noted. This anesthesia is usually a neurapraxia, which recovers spontaneously after a few weeks or months. The posterior cord of the brachial plexus occasionally is injured. This occurrence is somewhat alarming, but it usually recovers with time.

CALLOWAY TEST

Assessment for Dislocation of the Humerus

PROCEDURE

- The test consists of measuring the girth of the shoulder joints bilaterally.
- This test is helpful in the examination of obese patients.
- The examiner loops a flexible tape measure through the axilla (Fig. 4-22).
- The girth is measured at the acromial tip.
- In a positive test, the girth of the affected joint is increased.
- The test is significant for dislocation of the humerus.

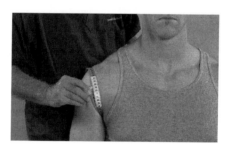

FIG. 4-22

CLINICAL PEARL

Shoulder dislocation results in severe pain. The patient supports the arm with the opposite hand and is hesitant to permit any kind of examination. The lateral outline of the shoulder may be flattened, and if the patient is not too muscular, a small bulge may be seen and felt just below the clavicle. The arm must always be examined for nerve and vessel injury.

CODMAN SIGN
(ALSO KNOWN AS DROP ARM TEST)

Assessment for Tear in the Rotator Cuff Complex

ORTHOPEDIC GAMUT 4-11

CLASSIFICATION OF LONG HEAD OF THE BICEPS INSTABILITY

- Direction of instability
  - Anterior
  - Posterior
  - Anteroposterior
- Extent of instability
  - None
  - Subluxation
  - Dislocation
- Lesion grade
  - 0 (normal)
  - I (minor lesion)
  - II (major lesion)
- Rotator cuff tear or lesion
  - A (intact)
  - B (partial thickness)
  - C (full thickness)

4

PROCEDURE

- The patient's arm is passively abducted.
- The examiner suddenly removes support at some point above 90 degrees, which makes the deltoid contract suddenly (Fig. 4-23).
- If shoulder pain occurs and the patient demonstrates a hunching of the shoulder because rotator cuff function is absent, the sign is present for rotator cuff tear or, more specifically, rupture of the supraspinatus tendon.
- In a modification of Codman sign, the patient's shoulder is abducted to 90 degrees passively.
- The patient tries to lower the arm slowly to the side in the same arc of movement.
- If the patient is unable to return the arm to the side slowly or has severe pain, the test is positive.
- A positive test suggests a tear in the rotator cuff complex.

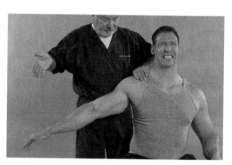

FIG. 4-23

CLINICAL PEARL

The cardinal sign of cuff rupture is persistent weakness. The patient may be conscious of this weakness, but the examiner must often point it out. Sometimes the weakness is easily overlooked. The patient may be able to lift the arm into full abduction or beyond the point of a full-thickness cuff tear. However, if this action is resisted a little, sometimes by as little as the pressure of one finger, even a very strong patient may be unable to abduct or flex the shoulder well.

COSTOCLAVICULAR MANEUVER

Assessment for Thoracic Outlet Syndrome

ORTHOPEDIC GAMUT 4-12

THORACIC OUTLET SYNDROME

Depending on the mechanism and level of compression, several disorders are included under the title of thoracic outlet syndrome:

1. Cervical rib syndrome
2. Scalenus-anticus syndrome
3. Wright hyperabduction syndrome
4. Pectoralis minor syndrome
5. Costoclavicular syndrome

ORTHOPEDIC GAMUT 4-13

SYMPTOMS OF SUBCLAVIAN VENOUS OBSTRUCTION

- Swelling
- Cyanosis
  - Intermittent blueness over the hand, arm, and often the upper chest wall is a common symptom, although this condition is seldom significant enough to be a major complaint.
  - This cyanosis is different than the color changes that are frequently seen in neurogenic TOS and are associated with increased sympathetic activity.
  - The color changes in neurogenic TOS are rubor, pallor, and some cyanosis and are usually limited to the hand.
- Arm pain
- Paresthesia
- Neck pain and occipital headache

PROCEDURE

- The radial pulse is palpated while the patient's shoulders are drawn down and in extension.
- The cervical spine is flexed maximally (Figs. 4-24 and 4-25).
- If the pulses are lost, the test is positive.
- Thoracic outlet syndrome is suggested by a positive test.

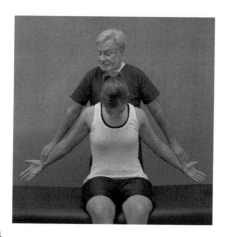

FIG. 4-24

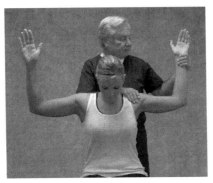

FIG. 4-25 An alternative is to have the patient actively abduct the shoulders and flex the elbows to 90 degrees. The examiner palpates the radial pulse of the affected arm and externally rotates the arm. The test is positive if the pulse disappears.

4

CLINICAL PEARL

Radiating discomfort from neurovascular compression can be associated with sleep or recumbency. This discomfort is a common disturbance that has many descriptive terms applied to it, including *Wartenberg nocturnal dysesthesia, sleep tetany, waking numbness, nocturnal palsy,* and *morning numbness.*

DAWBARN SIGN

Assessment for Subacromial Bursitis

ORTHOPEDIC GAMUT 4-14

BURSAE LOCATIONS

The most commonly present bursae locations are:
1. Subacromial and subdeltoid
2. Between the coracoid and the glenohumeral joint capsule
3. Summit of the acromion
4. Between the infraspinatus and the joint capsule
5. Between the teres major and the long head of the biceps
6. Between the subscapularis and the joint capsule
7. Anterior and posterior to the tendinous insertion of the latissimus dorsi
8. Behind the coracobrachialis muscle

PROCEDURE

- With the patient's arm comfortably at the side, deep palpation of the shoulder by the examiner elicits a well-localized, tender area.
- With the examiner's finger still on the painful spot, the patient's arm is passively abducted by the examiner's other hand.
- The sign is present if the painful spot under the examiner's nonmoving finger disappears as the arm is abducted (Fig. 4-26).
- The sign is significant for subacromial bursitis.

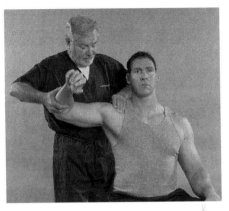

FIG. 4-26

4

CLINICAL PEARL

Subacromial bursitis is not common as a primary condition. The condition may be caused by a direct blow over the shoulder. This blow causes an inflammatory reaction that is aggravated by further motion. Bursitis is usually a secondary reaction. The examiner should search for a primary lesion before beginning treatment.

DUGAS TEST

Assessment for Shoulder Dislocation

ORTHOPEDIC GAMUT 4-15

ANTERIOR SHOULDER DISLOCATION

Radiographic appearances of anterior shoulder dislocation:
1. Bankart lesion, which is an avulsion of a small fragment of the glenoid rim at the site of the triceps insertion
2. Flap fracture, an avulsion of the greater tuberosity
3. Hill-Sachs (hatchet) deformity, an impaction fracture of the posterosuperior surface of the humeral head produced by repetitive traumatization by the inferior glenoid rim after recurrent anterior glenohumeral joint dislocation

---

ORTHOPEDIC GAMUT 4-16

CHRONIC RECURRENT DISLOCATIONS

Four subsets of chronic recurrent dislocations are:
1. Voluntary habitual (emotionally disturbed)
2. Voluntary
3. Not willful (muscular control)
4. Involuntary positional and involuntary unintentional (not demonstrable by patient)

PROCEDURE

- The patient places the hand of the affected shoulder on the opposite shoulder and attempts to touch the chest with the elbow.
- The test is positive if the patient cannot touch the chest wall with the elbow (Fig. 4-27).
- The test is positive in shoulder dislocation.

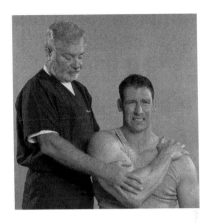

FIG. 4-27

CLINICAL PEARL

In exceptional circumstances, the humeral head can become jammed below the glenoid with the arm pointing directly upward (luxatio erecta), presenting a spectacular appearance sometimes mistaken for hysteria. This condition is a true inferior dislocation. In contrast to anterior dislocation, the humeral head in this situation lies against the vessels and can cause ischemia. The rotator cuff is always damaged.

GEORGE SCREENING PROCEDURE

Assessment for Subclavian Artery Stenosis or Occlusion

ORTHOPEDIC GAMUT 4-17

COMMON PRECIPITATING ACTIVITIES IN PAGET-SCHROETTER SYNDROME OR *EFFORT THROMBOSIS*

- Playing tennis
- Golf
- Baseball
- Throwing a ball
- Rowing a boat
- Swimming
- Gymnastics
- Weightlifting
- Wrestling

ORTHOPEDIC GAMUT 4-18

INDIVIDUALS COMMONLY PREDISPOSED TO PAGET-SCHROETTER SYNDROME OR *EFFORT THROMBOSIS*

- Professional athletes
- Beauticians
- Painters
- Mechanics

PROCEDURE

- With the patient seated, the examiner assesses the patient's blood pressure bilaterally and records it (Fig. 4-28).
- The examiner also assesses the character of the patient's radial pulse bilaterally (Fig. 4-29).
- A difference of 10 mm Hg between the two systolic blood pressure readings and a feeble or absent radial pulse suggest possible subclavian artery stenosis or occlusion on the side of the feeble or absent pulse.
- If the test is negative, the examiner places a stethoscope over the supraclavicular fossa and auscultates the subclavian artery for bruits (Fig. 4-30).
- If bruits are present, subclavian artery stenosis or occlusion is suspected.

4

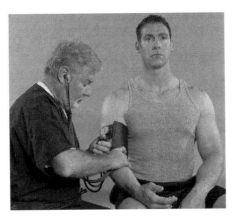

FIG. 4-28

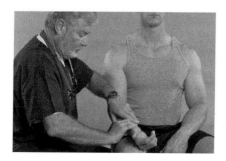

FIG. 4-29

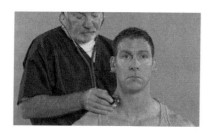

FIG. 4-30

CLINICAL PEARL

The shoulder joint can be linked with the hand in a symptom complex presenting the features of a reflex sympathetic disturbance. The shoulder symptoms may be caused, in part, by the neurovascular upset that develops as a result of sympathetic stimulation. The shoulder complaint is usually secondary to some other factor, but the reflex dystrophy phenomenon has become so predominant that it is mislabeled as the cause when it is actually a result.

HALSTEAD MANEUVER

Assessment for Thoracic Outlet Syndrome

ORTHOPEDIC GAMUT 4-19

SUBTLE SYMPTOMS OF NEUROGENIC THORACIC OUTLET SYNDROME

16 Moderate and mild clinical symptoms and signs suggestive of disputed neurogenic thoracic outlet syndrome:

1. Paresthesias in the whole hand
2. Paresthesias in median digits
3. Paresthesias in ulnar digits
4. Nocturnal paresthesias
5. Diurnal paresthesias
6. Pain in hand
7. Pain in forearm
8. Pain in shoulder
9. Pain in head
10. Pain after pressure of upper trapezius muscle
11. Pain after pressure on Erb point
12. Pain after shoulder mobilization
13. Roos test (3 min)
14. Roos test (paresthesias)
15. Adson maneuver
16. Radial pulse suppression after abduction/external rotation of the shoulder and various positions of the cervical spine

PROCEDURE

- As the radial pulse of the affected arm is palpated, downward traction is applied on the extremity.
- The neck is hyperextended (Fig. 4-31).
- Loss or diminution of the pulse suggests a positive test.
- If the test is negative, it is repeated with the patient rotating the head to the opposite side.
- Thoracic outlet syndrome is suggested by a positive test.

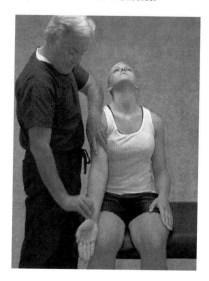

FIG. 4-31

CLINICAL PEARL

Raynaud disease, acroparesthesia, and thromboangiitis obliterans *may be confused* with thoracic outlet compression syndromes, but the former three conditions actually differ profoundly from outlet compression syndromes because Raynaud disease, acroparesthesia, and thromboangiitis obliterans are not accompanied by shoulder discomfort, have no correlation to arm or shoulder movement, and are not affected by body posture.

HAMILTON TEST

Assessment for Dislocation of the Shoulder

ORTHOPEDIC GAMUT 4-20

CAUSES OF NONTRAUMATIC SHOULDER OSTEOARTHRITIS

- Gout
- Septic arthritis
- Rheumatoid arthritis
- Juvenile rheumatoid arthritis
- Alkaptonuria
- Acromegaly
- Epiphyseal dysplasia
- Crystal-induced arthritis
- Apatite deposition disease (Milwaukee shoulder)
- Hemophilia
- Ankylosing spondylitis
- Massive rotator cuff tear
- Steroid-induced avascular necrosis
- Idiopathic avascular necrosis
- Avascular necrosis caused by sickle cell disease
- Lupus erythematosus
- Gaucher disease

ORTHOPEDIC GAMUT 4-21

CAUSES OF POSTTRAUMATIC OSTEOARTHRITIS

- Fracture of the humeral head or glenoid and traumatic dislocation
- Osteoarthritis caused by dislocation is sometime called:
  - Postdislocation osteoarthritis
  - Dislocation arthropathy
  - Dislocation-induced arthropathy

PROCEDURE

- If a straight edge (ruler or yardstick) can rest simultaneously on the acromial tip and the lateral epicondyle of the elbow, the test is positive (Fig. 4-32).
- The positive test is significant for dislocation of the shoulder.

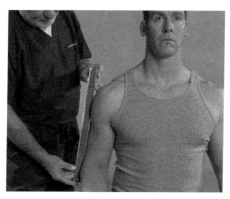

FIG. 4-32

CLINICAL PEARL

Fractures of the humeral head that result in several fragments are usually accompanied by dislocation. Fracture dislocations of the humeral head present several problems: (1) The fragment may obstruct reduction and make open reduction necessary, (2) the reduction will be very unstable, (3) soft-tissue damage and hemorrhage into and around the shoulder lead to joint stiffness, and (4) avascular necrosis of the humeral head can follow fractures through the anatomic neck.

IMPINGEMENT SIGN

Assessment for Overuse Injury to the Supraspinatus or Biceps Tendons

Comment

The terminology for impingement lesions had led to confusion. Many names and causes for this condition have been cited, including *bursitis, tendinitis, acute trauma, overuse, instability, aging, tendon degeneration, vascular deficiencies*, and *mechanical impingement* (Table 4-4). The rotator cuff is the only tendon situated between two bones.

4

TABLE 4-4

CLINICAL PRESENTATIONS OF THE MOST COMMON SHOULDER CONDITIONS

Disorder	Age Group Affected	Key Diagnostic Features
Rotator cuff impingement	Middle-aged	Painful arc within full ROM
Rotator cuff tear	Middle-aged and older adults	Selective weakness of supraspinatus/infraspinatus
Frozen shoulder	Middle-aged	Restriction of passive ROM, external rotation
Calcific tendonitis	Middle-aged	Severe pain; full passive ROM; calcific deposit on radiograph
Acromioclavicular osteoarthosis	Middle-aged and older adults	Pain over joint; radiographic changes
Glenohumeral osteoarthosis	Middle-aged and older adults	Loss of passive ROM; radiographic changes
Shoulder instability	Age <40 years	Recurrent dislocation or subluxation symptoms; clinical signs of instability

ROM, Range of motion.
Adapted from Frost A, Michael Robinson C: The painful shoulder, *Surgery (Oxford)* 24(11):363-367, 2006.

ORTHOPEDIC GAMUT 4-22

IMPINGEMENT SYNDROME

The four stages of impingement syndrome are as follows:

Phase 1: Edema and swelling (correlated with overuse tendonitis from activities requiring repetitive overhead arm action)

Phase 2: Thickening and fibrosis (correlated with incomplete thickness rotator cuff tears)

Phase 3: Comprises complete thickness tearing and bone changes

Phase 4: Cuff tear arthropathy (occurs in a small percentage of neglected cuff tears)

PROCEDURE

- The patient's arm is slightly abducted and moved fully through flexion (Fig. 4-33).
- This move causes a jamming of the greater tuberosity into the anteroinferior acromial surface.
- A positive result is pain in the shoulder.
- A positive test suggests injury to the supraspinatus and sometimes to the biceps tendons.

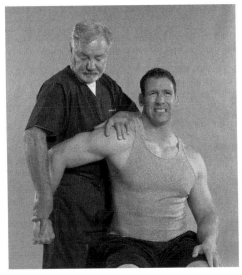

FIG. 4-33 As an alternative, the examiner can internally rotate the affected shoulder. This rotation occurs while the shoulder is abducted to 90 degrees and flexed at the elbow. The arm can also be moved into flexion, which will produce the same jamming effect.

CLINICAL PEARL

The archaic concept of the hunching girdle rhythm as the tell-tale mark of supraspinatus ruptures needs to be discarded. Without resistance, a decrease in the range of motion may not be apparent. Motion must always be assessed against resistance. The presence of consistent weakness helps differentiate a tear from simple chronic tendinitis.

LUDINGTON TEST

Assessment for Rupture of the Long Head of the Biceps Tendon

PROCEDURE

- The patient clasps both hands behind the head.
- The biceps tendons are in resting positions.
- The patient alternately contracts and relaxes the biceps muscles.
- As the patient contracts the muscles, the examiner palpates the biceps tendons (Fig. 4-34).
- The tendon will be felt to contract on the uninvolved side but not on the affected side.
- A positive test result is the loss of tendon contraction.
- A positive test suggests rupture of the long head of the biceps tendon.

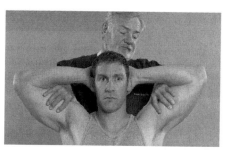

FIG. 4-34

CLINICAL PEARL

A double defect sometimes occurs, with the cuff giving way from the tuberosity on both sides of the tendon. Cuff laxity at this point seriously interferes with biceps function, and the tendon may slip medially over the lesser tuberosity and off the head.

MAZION SHOULDER MANEUVER
(ALSO KNOWN AS SHOULDER ROCK TEST)

Assessment for Significant Pathologic Process of the Shoulder

PROCEDURE

4

- While standing or sitting, the patient places the palm of the affected upper limb over the top of the opposite clavicle.
- From this position, the patient moves the elbow from the chest to the forehead, giving it an inferior to superior rocking motion (Fig. 4-35).
- The maneuver is positive if this action produces or aggravates shoulder or arm pain on the ipsilateral side.
- The pain of any significant pathologic process of the shoulder will be intensified and localized by this maneuver.

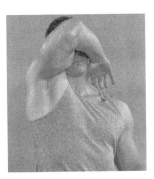

FIG. 4-35

CLINICAL PEARL

Adhesive capsulitis is a common but ill-understood affliction of the glenohumeral joint. Capsulitis is characterized by pain and uniform limitation of all movements but without radiographic change and with a tendency to a slow spontaneous recovery. No evidence of inflammatory or destructive change is seen.

REVERSE BAKODY MANEUVER

Assessment for Cervical Foraminal Compression and Interscalene Compression

---

ORTHOPEDIC GAMUT 4-23

OTHER ANATOMOPATHOLOGIC CAUSES IN NEUROGENIC THORACIC OUTLET SYNDROME

- Anomalous first rib
- Sibson fascia
- Small branches of the subclavian artery or thyrocervical trunk
- Scalene muscles

ORTHOPEDIC GAMUT 4-24

UPPER-EXTREMITY NEUROGENIC SYNDROMES

The important alternative causes of upper-extremity neurogenic syndromes include:
1. Central lesions (tumors involving the spinal cord or its roots)
2. Plexus lesions (tumors at the thoracic inlet, Pancoast tumor)
3. Distal nerve lesions (friction neuritis of the ulnar nerve at the elbow)
4. Pressure on the median nerve in the carpal tunnel

PROCEDURE

- While in the seated position, the patient actively places the palm of the affected extremity on top of the head, raising the elbow to a height approximately level with the head.
- By elevating the arm, interscalene compression increases.
- The sign is present when the radiating pain appears or is worsened with this maneuver (Fig. 4-36).
- The sign helps differentiate between cervical foraminal compression and interscalene compression.

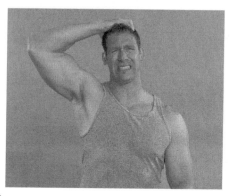

FIG. 4-36

CLINICAL PEARL

Radiographs will show the abnormal rib. If it is small, it is clearly observed in the oblique projections. In cases of suspected vascular obstruction, arteriography is required.

ROOS TEST

Assessment for Thoracic Outlet Syndrome

ORTHOPEDIC GAMUT 4-25

COSTOCLAVICULAR NEUROVASCULAR SPACE

The following actions narrow the costoclavicular neurovascular space:
1. Raising the arm rotates the clavicle posteriorly into the space.
2. Displacing the shoulder posteriorly and interiorly rotates the clavicle posteriorly.
3. Inhaling deeply raises the first rib into the space because the clavicle does not rise with inspiration.

4

PROCEDURE

- While in the seated position, the patient positions both arms at 90 degrees and abducts and externally rotates them.
- The patient repeatedly opens and closes the fists for up to 3 minutes.
- If this maneuver reproduces the usual symptoms of discomfort, the patient probably has thoracic outlet syndrome (Fig. 4-37).

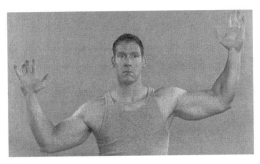

FIG. 4-37

CLINICAL PEARL

Because all of the neurologic, arterial, and venous symptoms are consistently aggravated by both exercise and arm elevation, the most reliable test for the diagnosis of thoracic outlet syndrome is the 3-minute *elevated-arm stress test*.

SHOULDER COMPRESSION TEST

Assessment for Hyperabduction Type of Thoracic Outlet Syndromes

---

ORTHOPEDIC GAMUT 4-26

THORACIC OUTLET

The following signs generally <u>do not</u> implicate the thoracic outlet:
1. Long tract signs such as brisk reflexes or extensor plantar response
2. Loss of tendon reflexes in the arms
3. Horner syndrome
4. Weakness of the upper arm or shoulder

PROCEDURE

- While the patient is seated upright, the examiner palpates the distal apex of the coracoid process and marks it with a flesh pencil.
- With a hypothenar contact, the examiner applies downward pressure over the marked area (Fig. 4-38).
- Production of symptoms that are similar to neurovascular compression of the subclavian artery and brachial plexus constitutes a positive test.
- The test is significant for coracoid pressure syndrome, which is identical to the hyperabduction type of thoracic outlet syndromes.

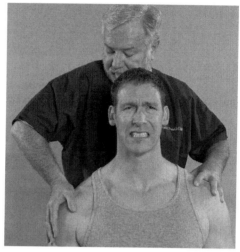

FIG. 4-38

CLINICAL PEARL

The neurovascular bundle may be compressed in the zone distal to the clavicle as the bundle passes beneath the costo-coracoid membrane and pectoralis minor. The pectoralis minor has a particular contribution in this process and is a significant factor in creating the shoulder and radiating symptoms. A patient's degree of skeletal maturation has a great influence on the type of fracture that may result from trauma and the concern physicians have about the sequelae of such injuries. First, the relative softness of the bones of newborns and toddlers increases the likelihood of trauma producing a *greenstick fracture* rather than an ordinary fracture completely separating the two bone fragments. Another crucial consideration in the evaluation of fractures in children is the possible involvement of the epiphyseal plates of the bone in the fracture. If the line of a fracture crosses one of these areas of bone growth, the posthealing alignment of the bone on opposite sides of the plate is disturbed, and the subsequent growth and development of the bone will be asymmetric.

SPEED TEST

Assessment for Bicipital Tendinitis

PROCEDURE

- Shoulder flexion by the patient is restricted.
- The patient further resists forearm supinating and elbow extension.
- A positive test is indicated by increased tenderness in the bicipital groove (Fig. 4-39).
- A positive test suggests bicipital tendinitis.

4

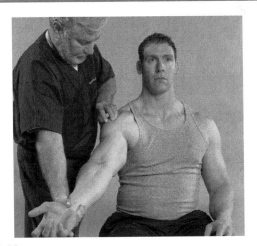

FIG. 4-39

CLINICAL PEARL

Tenosynovitis in the bicipital groove may develop into complete adherence of the tendon, which interdicts any extensive range of motion of the shoulder. The shoulder motion may remain restricted, or the biceps may rupture proximal to the groove.

SUBACROMIAL PUSH-BUTTON SIGN
(ALSO KNOWN AS MAZION CUFF MANEUVER)

Assessment for Rotator Cuff Tear of the Supraspinatus Tendon

Comment

Ruptures of the rotator cuff result from continued deterioration and degeneration (Table 4-5). The tear may be partial or complete.

TABLE 4-5

GOUTALLIER GRADING SYSTEM OF FATTY DEGENERATION OF MUSCLE

Stage	Findings (MRI/CT)
Stage 0	Normal muscle; no fatty streaking
Stage 1	Occasional fatty streaking
Stage 2: fat < 50% of cross	Sectional area (fat < muscle)
Stage 3: fat = 50% of cross	Sectional area (fat = muscle)
Stage 4: fat > 50% of cross	Sectional area (fat > muscle)

CT, Computed tomography; *MRI*, magnetic resonance imaging.

ORTHOPEDIC GAMUT 4-27

ACROMION CHANGES

Three types of acromion changes observed in impingement syndrome:
1. Type 1: flat
2. Type 2: curved
3. Type 3: hooked

PROCEDURE

- The patient is seated with the upper extremities hanging limply at the sides.
- The examiner exerts strong finger or thumb pressure toward the midline at the clavicle, at a point even with the scapular spine (Fig. 4-40).
- The production or increase of shoulder pain indicates a positive test.
- The test is significant for rotator cuff tear of the supraspinatus tendon.

4

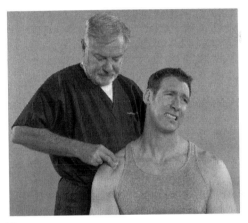

FIG. 4-40

CLINICAL PEARL

Degenerative changes in the supraspinatus tendon may be accompanied by the local deposition of calcium salts. This process may continue without symptoms, although radiographic changes are obvious. However, the calcified material sometimes causes inflammatory changes in the subdeltoid area and results in sudden, severe, and incapacitating pain. When this circumstance occurs, the shoulder is acutely tender and is often swollen and warm to the touch.

SUPRASPINATUS PRESS TEST

Assessment for Tear of the Supraspinatus Tendon or Muscle

ORTHOPEDIC GAMUT 4-28

SUPRASPINATUS SYNDROME

Variations of degeneration that lead to supraspinatus syndrome include the following:

1. In minor tearing of the supraspinatus tendon, tearing or strain of a few degenerate tendon fibers causes an inflammatory reaction with local swelling. Power is not as significantly impaired as it is after a complete tear of the rotator cuff.
2. With supraspinatus tendinitis, an inflammatory reaction is provoked by the degeneration of the tendon fibers.
3. Calcific deposits in the supraspinatus tendon occur when a white, chalky deposit forms within the degenerate tendon and when the lesion is surrounded by an inflammatory reaction. Pain occurs when the calcified material bursts into the surrounding tissue.
4. With subacromial bursitis, the bursal walls are inflamed and thickened by mechanical irritation.
5. With injury to the greater tuberosity, a contusion or undisplaced fracture of the greater tuberosity is a common cause.

PROCEDURE

- The patient abducts the shoulders to 90 degrees.
- The examiner resists the abduction.
- The shoulders are medially rotated and angled 30 degrees forward (the patient's thumbs point to the floor) (Fig. 4-41).
- The examiner again resists abduction.
- If the patient exhibits weakness or experiences pain, the test is positive.
- Weakness and pain indicate a tear of the supraspinatus tendon or muscle.

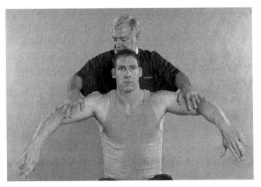

FIG. 4-41

4

CLINICAL PEARL

Painful arc syndrome is sometimes confused with arthritis of the acromioclavicular joint, which also causes pain during a certain phase of the abduction arc. However, with acromioclavicular arthritis, the pain begins later in abduction (not below 90 degrees) and increases, rather than diminishes, as full elevation is achieved.

TRANSVERSE HUMERAL LIGAMENT TEST

Assessment for Torn Transverse Humeral Ligament

ORTHOPEDIC GAMUT 4-29

BICEPS LONG HEAD STRUCTURE

Critical zones in the biceps long head structure:
1. The point where the tendon arches over the humeral head
2. The point where the floor on which the tendon glides changes from bony cortex to articular cartilage

---

PROCEDURE

- The patient's affected shoulder is passively abducted and internally rotated.
- The examiner's fingers are placed on the bicipital groove.
- The patient's shoulder is passively externally rotated (Fig. 4-42).
- If a tendon snap in and out of the groove is felt as the external rotation occurs, the test is positive.
- A positive test suggests a torn transverse humeral ligament.

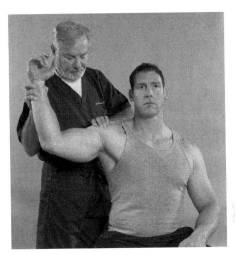

FIG. 4-42

4

CLINICAL PEARL

Conditions involving the bicipital tendon and the bicipital groove are particularly pertinent to athletes because many sports involve the throwing motion of the arm. These athletes include baseball pitchers, football quarterbacks, batters, and tennis players. The throwing motion is especially inhibited by bicipital tendon problems. Recognizing if the defect is an adhesive tenosynovitis, fraying of the tendon, or subluxation or dislocation of the tendon is especially pertinent.

WRIGHT TEST
(ALSO KNOWN AS HYPERABDUCTION MANEUVER)

Assessment for Neurovascular Compromise of the Axillary Artery, as Seen in the Hyperabduction Thoracic Outlet Syndromes

---

ORTHOPEDIC GAMUT 4-30

ELVEY TEST MOVEMENTS

The three superimposed component movements of Elvey test are as follows:
1. Shoulder abduction and lateral rotation and extension behind the coronal plane
2. Forearm supination and elbow extension
3. Wrist and finger extension

PROCEDURE

- Before this test is started, the Allen maneuver at the wrist is performed to establish patency of the radial arteries.
- The patient is seated, with both arms hanging at the sides.
- The examiner palpates the patient's radial pulse.
- Both arms, in turn, are passively abducted to 180 degrees.
- The examiner notes the angle of abduction at which the radial pulse diminishes or disappears on the affected side (Fig. 4-43).
- The examiner compares the results with those on the unaffected side.
- The test is significant for neurovascular compromise of the axillary artery, as seen in hyperabduction thoracic outlet syndromes.
- Many patients have cessation of the radial pulse on abduction without hyperabduction syndrome being present.
- If the nonaffected limb demonstrates radial pulse dampening or cessation at the same approximate degree of abduction as the affected side, the test is not positive for hyperabduction syndrome.

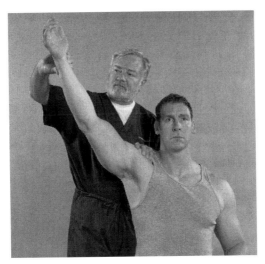

FIG. 4-43

4

CLINICAL PEARL

In most instances of compression hyperabduction of the shoulder, the radial pulse is obliterated; but obliteration of the radial pulse also may occur in the normal extremity. However, a difference is noted. On the affected side, the marginal position is reached sooner than on the normal side. The marginal position is the level of abduction just below that which produces obliteration of the pulse. The patient is often aware of the exact level of abduction at which the symptoms occur.

YERGASON TEST

Assessment for Tenosynovitis or Involvement of the Transverse Humeral Ligament

ORTHOPEDIC GAMUT 4-31

HAWKIN IMPINGEMENT TEST

For the Hawkin impingement test:
- The patient stands while the examiner forward flexes the shoulder to 90 degrees, flexes the elbow to 90 degrees, and forcibly internally rotates the shoulder.
- This movement pushes the supraspinatus tendon against the anterior surface of the coracoacromial ligament.
- Pain indicates a positive test for rotator cuff tendonitis.

ORTHOPEDIC GAMUT 4-32

SUPRASPINATUS TEST: *EMPTY CAN TEST*

In the supraspinatus test:
- The patient's shoulder is abducted to 90 degrees with neutral rotation, and the examiner provides resistance to abduction.
- The shoulder is then medially rotated and angled forward 30 degrees so that the patient's thumb points toward the floor.
- Resistance to abduction is given while the examiner looks for weakness or pain, which reflects a positive result.

ORTHOPEDIC GAMUT 4-33

NEER IMPINGEMENT TEST

- In Neer impingement test, the patient's arm is forcibly elevated through forward flexion by the examiner while the scapula is depressed, causing compression of the greater tuberosity against the anteroinferior acromial surface.
- Discomfort as a result of this maneuver reflects a positive test result.

PROCEDURE

- The patient flexes the elbow.
- The patient attempts to supinate the hand against resistance.
- The patient then resists efforts to extend the elbow (Fig. 4-44).
- If pain over the intertubercular groove develops or is aggravated, the test is positive.
- A positive sign suggests tenosynovitis of the transverse humeral ligament.

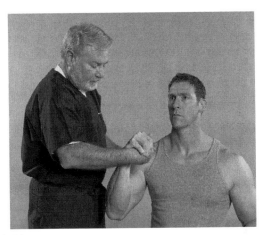

FIG. 4-44

CLINICAL PEARL

The concept that the biceps tendon moves up and down the groove during motion at the glenohumeral joint is questionable. With the bicipital tendon and groove exposed under anesthesia, the biceps tendon remains fixed in the groove during motion. However, the head of the humerus glides up and down the tendon. Contraction of the biceps muscle, by supinating the forearm or flexing the elbow, makes the tendon taut but produces no motion of the tendon in the groove. All movements of the shoulder joint, regardless of the plane in which the arm is elevated, are accompanied by gliding motions of the humerus on the tendon.

CHAPTER FIVE

ELBOW

AXIOMS IN ASSESSING THE ELBOW

- The elbow is a complex hinge joint.
- The elbow is essential to the positioning and full use of the hand.
- Soft-tissue lesions such as lateral epicondylitis and olecranon bursitis occur more often than joint disease.
- Diagnosis of elbow conditions is largely based on pain, location of swelling, presence of point tenderness, and the results of range-of-motion studies.

INTRODUCTION

Although the number of diseases that affect the elbow with any degree of frequency is small, examining the joint often provides clues to diagnosis of specific neuromuscular disease. Pain is the symptom that focuses attention on this joint and prompts the patient to visit the physician. Although it usually reflects a localized process at the elbow, the pain may be referred from the hand and wrist or from the shoulder and neck. Most abnormal actions of the elbow can be compensated by the shoulder; therefore, even moderate compromises of motion, provided they are painless, do not result in disability. Subtle flexion contractures may develop over years without the patient even being aware of the changes or range-of-motion losses. In contrast, significant pain at the elbow incapacitates the entire arm. Sleeves of clothing often cover the elbows; thus, swellings and deformities become cosmetically important only when they are exaggerated. The examiner should note whether swelling is intracapsular or extracapsular, intramuscular or intermuscular. The earliest sign of joint effusion is induration of the capsule around the olecranon or epicondyles. In the flexed position, the hollows of the indurated synovium are totally filled.

When the elbow is extended, the epicondyles and the tip of the olecranon should be at the same level. In normal elbow configuration, when a line is drawn between the epicondyles, the olecranon should bisect and be on the center of the line. When the normal elbow is flexed to an angle of 90 degrees, the tip of the olecranon should be directly below to the line joining the epicondyles. If a line from the

TABLE 5-1

ELBOW JOINT CROSS-REFERENCE TABLE BY SYNDROME PROCEDURE

Elbow	Disease Assessed					
	Lateral Epicondylitis	Radiohumeral Bursitis	Cubital Tunnel Syndrome	Medial Epicondylitis	Neuropathy	Sprain
Test/Sign						
Cozen test	●	●				
Elbow flexion test			●			
Golfer elbow test				●		
Kaplan sign	●					
Ligamentous instability test						●
Mills test	●					
Tinel sign at the elbow					●	

TABLE 5-2

ELBOW JOINT CROSS-REFERENCE TABLE BY SYNDROME

Cubital tunnel syndrome	Elbow flexion test
Lateral epicondylitis	Cozen test
	Kaplan sign
	Mills test
Medial epicondylitis	Golfer elbow test
Neuropathy	Tinel sign at the elbow
Radiohumeral bursitis	Cozen test
Sprain	Ligamentous instability test

olecranon is drawn to each epicondyle, the three prominences and line should form an isosceles triangle.

If the triangle is normal but abnormal in relation to the shaft of the humerus, the patient may have a supracondylar fracture in which the three bony landmarks are displaced posteriorly.

ORTHOPEDIC GAMUT 5-1

ISOSCELES TRIANGLE OF THE ELBOW

If the angles of the isosceles triangle of the elbow are abnormal, the following may exist:
1. Posterior elbow dislocation
2. Fracture of the epicondyle
3. Intracondylar fracture
4. Fracture of the olecranon

The examination of the elbow must be preceded by a precise history to allow emphasis to be placed on particular areas. Complaints usually consist of pain, loss of movement, weakness, clicking, or locking.

ORTHOPEDIC GAMUT 5-2

PRIMARY FUNCTIONS OF THE ELBOW

1. Aids in positioning the hand in appropriate locations
2. Adjusts height and length of the limb
3. Stabilizes the upper extremity for power and fine motor work activities
4. Provides fulcrum for the arm in lifting

ORTHOPEDIC GAMUT 5-3

ELBOW JOINTS

The elbow consists of a complex set of joints that require careful assessment. The articulations of the joint are as follows:
1. Humeroulnar
2. Humeroradial
3. Proximal radioulnar

The patient may complain of sharply localized pain, typical of an extraarticular abnormality, deep joint pain, or the poorly localized pain of ulnar neuropathy with or without typical paresthesia extending to the hand. The functional interplay among the elbow, shoulder, and wrist means that examination of all of these joints may be necessary (Table 5-3). Referred pain in the elbow, especially from the neck or shoulder, is usually diffuse. Examination must include comparison of right and left arms.

TABLE 5-3

FUNCTIONAL ARC MEASUREMENTS FOR SELECTED ACTIVITIES OF DAILY LIVING

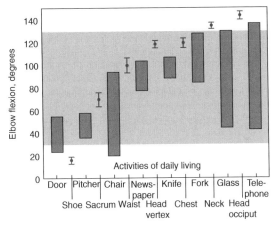

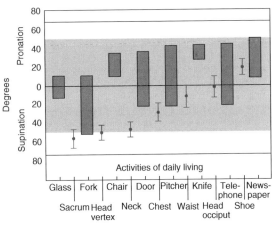

From Kelley WN, et al: *Textbook of rheumatology*, ed 5, Philadelphia, 1997, WB Saunders.

Pain of lateral elbow origin is usually diagnosed as radiohumeral bursitis, epicondylitis, or tennis elbow. All of these problems involve the origin of the wrist extensors (tendinopathy) or, occasionally, radial nerve impingement by musculotendinous structures crossing the elbow joint.

A similar problem may occur on the medial elbow epicondyle because all of the wrist flexors and pronators originate from the medial epicondyle. Affected individuals use flexor-pronator muscle groups repetitively, isometrically or isokinetically. This circumstance is unusual because forceful wrist flexor power is seldom used. Most of powerful hand grasping is accomplished in the dorsiflexed wrist position.

Intraarticular abnormalities such as osteochondritis dissecans of the capitellum result in lateral elbow pain.

Osteochondritis dissecans of the elbow is an idiopathic disorder that affects the capitellum of the humerus, with ensuing avascular necrosis. It is usually seen in the dominant arm of adolescent boys, especially those involved in throwing sports. Panner disease is a condition of unclear origin in which osteochondrosis of the capitellum occurs. It is seen most often in young boys who complain of tenderness and swelling over the lateral aspect of the elbow with limited extension. Direct trauma or inadequate circulation through the elbow joint has been associated with osteochondritis of the capitellum.

ORTHOPEDIC GAMUT 5-4

AVASCULAR NECROSIS OF THE CAPITELLUM

Possible causes of avascular necrosis of the capitellum of the elbow (Panner disease):
1. Bacterial infection
2. Fracture
3. Heredity
4. Vascular insufficiency

An extremely minor fracture of the radial head (chisel fracture) may cause pain that can be confused with tennis elbow. An injury occurring in children and adolescents in whom the medial epicondyle is inflamed with partial separation of the apophysis is *little leaguer's elbow*.

Boxer's elbow (also called *hyperextension overload syndrome* or *olecranon impingement syndrome*) is caused by repetitive valgus extension of the elbow in the boxer's jab or in sports involving throwing. Elbow joint hyperextension injuries usually result from falling on an outstretched arm. The elbow is extended and the forearm supinated.

ORTHOPEDIC GAMUT 5-5

HYPEREXTENSION INJURIES OF THE ELBOW

Structures of the elbow injured with hyperextension forces:
1. Biceps brachii, at its point of insertion on the neck of the radius
2. Brachialis, at its point of insertion on the ulna
3. Brachioradialis
4. Anterior portion of the medial (ulnar) or lateral (radial) collateral ligaments (The medial collateral ligament is injured more often because of the valgus position of the joint.)
5. Elbow capsular and collateral ligament (They can avulse a piece of the condyle, most commonly the medial epicondyle.)

5

Pain in the elbow, particularly extending along the entire arm, in the absence of objective findings at the joint suggests psychogenic origins. Other diseases referring pain to the elbow include myocardial infarction, cervical root lesions, thoracic outlet syndromes, and subdeltoid bursitis. Psychogenic origins are further supported with a history of neurosis, strange behavior, or a bizarre and inconsistent complaint history; diagnostic imaging and laboratory tests are as unimpressive as the physical findings. Carpal tunnel syndrome may cause retrograde radiation of pain to the elbow.

Elbow joint complaints usually consist of pain, loss of movement, weakness, clicking, or locking. The patient may complain of sharply localized pain (typical of an extraarticular abnormality), deep joint pain, or poorly localized pain of ulnar neuropathy with or without typical paresthesias extending to the hand. The functional interplay among the elbow, shoulder, and wrist means that examination of all these joints is necessary. Referred pain in the elbow, especially from the neck or shoulder, is usually diffuse (Table 5-4).

True elbow pain can be related to joint disease; however, it is more commonly caused by lesions of the periarticular tissues. Inflammation of the olecranon bursa *(draftsman's elbow)* may be secondary to several conditions, including repetitive or acute trauma, rheumatoid arthritis, gout, and pseudogout. It is also known as *student's elbow* or *miner's elbow*.

The olecranon bursa is prone to injury by friction or a blow. Additionally, because of its position, swelling occurs easily and is readily visible. It is also a common site involved in crystal arthropathies (gout, or rarely, calcium pyrophosphate arthritis) or in generalized inflammatory arthritis, especially rheumatoid arthritis in which swelling

TABLE 5-4

UPPER EXTREMITY PERIARTICULAR SYNDROME
DIFFERENTIAL DIAGNOSTIC LIST

Region	Periarticular Syndrome	Monarticular Syndrome
Shoulder	Subacromial bursitis Long-head bicipital tendinitis Rotator cuff tear	Pancoast tumor Brachial plexopathy Cervical nerve root injury
Elbow	Olecranon bursitis Epicondylitis	Ulnar nerve entrapment
Wrist	Extensor tendinitis (including de Quervain tenosynovitis) Gonococcal tenosynovitis	Carpal tunnel syndrome
Hand	Palmar fasciitis (Dupuytren contracture)	Ligamentous or capsular injury

Modified from Kelley WN, et al: *Textbook of rheumatology*, ed 5, Philadelphia, 1997, WB Saunders.

of the olecranon bursa may be seen in association with rheumatoid nodules on the ulnar border of the forearm.

Traumatic or repetitive-motion osteochondritis of the radial head occurs in some sports that involve throwing, especially evident in the preadolescent and adolescent athletes. The radioulnar joint is affected by loose bodies and synovial osteochondromatosis. Traumatic partial subluxation of the radial head through the annular ligament occurs in children younger than 8 years.

A *pushed elbow* describes subluxation of the radial head in a proximal direction, which is often seen after a child falls on an outstretched hand. A *pulled elbow* is subluxation of the radial head in a distal direction, which may follow a forceful traction to the forearm.

ESSENTIAL ANATOMY

The elbow acts as a lever system that, along with the other joints, changes the direction of the upper extremity to put the hand in the most effective functional position. The elbow consists of three bones: the distal end of the humerus and the proximal ends of the radius and the ulna. The three articulating surfaces are enclosed in a single synovial cavity. The olecranon bursa is the largest bursa of the elbow, although several smaller bursae are present.

The three major deep nerves of the forearm are the radial, medial, and ulnar nerves. The radial nerve lies anterior to the lateral epicondyle in the arm in its anterior compartment.

Arterial supply to the forearm depends entirely on branches of the brachial artery. The radial artery courses to the lateral side of the forearm and aligns itself with the radius. The ulnar artery is the larger of the two branches of the brachial artery.

ESSENTIAL MOTION ASSESSMENT

Tissue approximation limits elbow flexion to 140 to 150 degrees. Retained flexion motion of 130 degrees or less is impairment in the activities of daily living (Fig. 5-1).

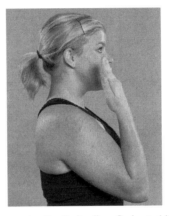

FIG. 5-1 Tissue approximation limits elbow flexion to 140 to 150 degrees.

Elbow extension is 0 degrees. Up to 10 degrees of hyperextension is still within normal limits if the patient has no history of trauma to the joint. The inability to return the elbow to within 10 degrees of the neutral position is impairment in the activities of daily living (Fig. 5-2).

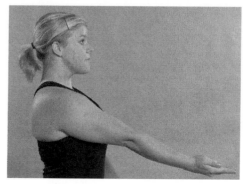

FIG. 5-2 Elbow extension is 0 degrees. Ten degrees of hyperextension is within normal limits if equal bilaterally and in the absence of injury.

Supination of the elbow is limited by tissue stretch to 90 degrees. Retained supination motion of 60 degrees or less is impairment in the activities of daily living (Fig. 5-3).

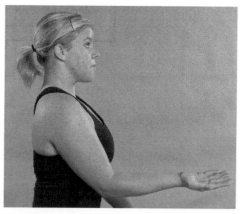

FIG. 5-3 Supination of the elbow is limited, by tissue stretch, to 90 degrees.

Elbow pronation is the same as supination, 80 to 90 degrees. Retained pronation motion of 70 degrees or less is impairment in the activities of daily living (Fig. 5-4).

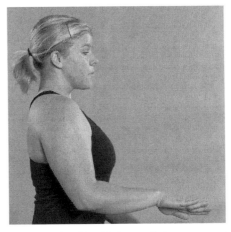

FIG. 5-4 Elbow pronation, 80 to 90 degrees, is the same as supination.

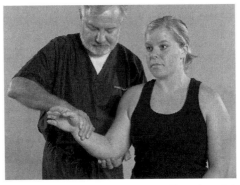

FIG. 5-5 The patient is instructed to flex the elbow through its range of motion against graded resistance applied by the examiner. The examiner's other hand is just proximal to the patient's wrist.

ESSENTIAL MUSCLE FUNCTION ASSESSMENT

The prime movers in flexion of the elbow are the biceps brachii (musculocutaneous nerve, C5, and C6), brachialis (musculocutaneous nerve, C5, and C6), and brachioradialis (radial nerve, C5, and C6) muscles. The flexor muscles of the forearm arising from the medial epicondyle of the humerus are the accessory muscles (Fig. 5-5).

The prime mover in extension of the elbow is the triceps brachii muscle (radial nerve, C7, and C8); the anconeus muscle is an accessory. When the arm is horizontally abducted, the long head of the triceps is shortened over the shoulder joint. When the shoulder is flexed, the long head of the triceps is shortened over the elbow joint and elongated over the shoulder joint (Fig. 5-6).

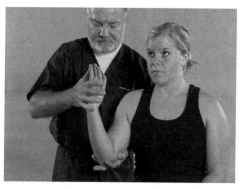

FIG. 5-6 The examiner fixes the patient's arm as described for flexion and instructs the patient to move the elbow through the range of extension motion while providing graded resistance with the other hand just proximal to the patient's wrist.

Although the triceps and anconeus act together in extending the elbow joint, the two muscles can be differentiated. The belly of the anconeus muscle is below the elbow joint and is easily distinguished from the triceps by palpation. Paralysis of the anconeus materially reduces the strength of elbow extension (Fig. 5-7).

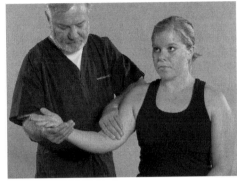

FIG. 5-7 Paralysis of the anconeus materially reduces the strength of elbow extension. The muscle grade of good in-elbow extension strength is actually the result of a normal triceps and a zero anconeus function.

The primary supinators are the biceps brachii and the supinator. The accessory muscle in this movement is the brachioradialis. In addition to its role in supination, the biceps also functions as an elbow flexor. Its total biceps function is well illustrated in the act of twisting a corkscrew into the cork of a bottle and then pulling the cork out of the bottle (Fig. 5-8).

5

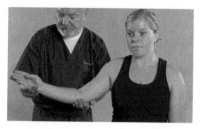

FIG. 5-8 The thenar eminence of the examiner's resisting hand is placed on the dorsal surface of the patient's hand and wrist. The patient begins supination from a position of pronation, and as the arm is moved into supination, the resistance is gradually increased.

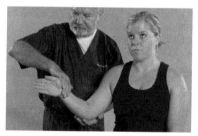

FIG. 5-9 The patient begins forearm pronation from a position of supination. As the patient moves into pronation, the resistance is increased.

The primary pronators are the pronator teres and the pronator quadratus. The accessory muscle in this movement is the flexor carpi radialis. Pronation and supination are complex movements (Fig. 5-9) that occur simultaneously around an axis best described as an imaginary line between the head of the radius proximally and the medial end of the triangular articular disc distally. In the proximal radioulnar joint, the head of the radius can rotate within the perimeter created by the annular ligament.

ESSENTIAL IMAGING

The elbow position of function is 90 degrees of flexion with the forearm midway between supination and pronation. In this position, the olecranon process of the ulna and the medial and lateral epicondyles of the humerus normally form an isosceles triangle when viewed posteriorly; this sign is known as the *triangle sign*. If a fracture, dislocation, or degeneration exists leading to loss of bone or cartilage or both, the distance between the apex and base decreases, and the isosceles triangle no longer exists.

ORTHOPEDIC GAMUT 5-6

THE ELBOW JOINT

Plain-film radiographic films demonstrate that the elbow is a compound joint consisting of:
1. Articulation of the trochlea of the humerus with the trochlear notch of the ulna
2. Articulation of the capitulum of the humerus with the superior surface of the radial head

COZEN TEST

Assessment for Lateral Epicondylitis and Radiohumeral Bursitis

---

ORTHOPEDIC GAMUT 5-7

EXTENSOR-SUPINATOR APONEUROTIC ATTACHMENT

Conditions on the lateral side of the elbow at the extensor-supinator aponeurotic attachment to the lateral epicondyle are:

1. Radioulnar synovitis, marked by development of a pannus of synovium between the radius and ulna
2. Strain in the aponeurosis itself, often directly over the radial head
3. Radiohumeral bursitis

Comment

Because of the proximity of the epicondyle, the radiohumeral joint, and the supinator aponeurosis, diagnosis of exact tissue involvement can be confusing. In many instances, the conditions are caused by the same mechanisms, overuse of the elbow joint (Table 5-5).

TABLE 5-5

CONDITIONS MIMICKING OR CONTRIBUTING TO CHRONIC LATERAL EPICONDYLITIS

Anconeus compartment syndrome
Bursitis
Cervical radiculopathy
Elbow joint components
Hypothyroidism
Lateral epicondyle avulsion
Musculocutaneous nerve entrapment
Non-union of radial neck fracture
Osteoarthritis

TABLE 5-5

CONDITIONS MIMICKING OR CONTRIBUTING TO CHRONIC LATERAL EPICONDYLITIS—cont'd

Posterior interosseous syndrome
Posterolateral rotatory instability of elbow
Radial nerve traction
Radial tunnel syndrome
Rheumatoid arthritis
Strained lateral collateral ligament
Snapping plicae

Adapted from Greenfield C, Webster V: Chronic lateral epicondylitis: survey of current practice in the outpatient departments in Scotland, *Physiotherapy* 88(10):578-594, 2002.

PROCEDURE

- The patient clenches a fist tightly, dorsiflexes it, and maintains a pronated position.
- The examiner, while grasping the patient's lower forearm, applies a flexing force to the dorsiflexion posture of the patient's wrist (Fig. 5-10).
- The test is positive if this action reproduces acute lancinating pain in the region of the lateral epicondyle.
- The test is significant for epicondylitis or radiohumeral bursitis.

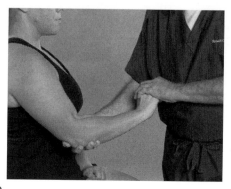

FIG. 5-10

CLINICAL PEARL

Cozen test is the easiest test to perform for lateral epicondy-litis. The patient has often already discovered the pain that accompanies resisted dorsiflexion of the wrist, such as when lifting a gallon of milk. Although the pain of epicondylitis is sometimes exquisite and sharply localized, the condition does not truly differentiate itself from tendinitis or bursitis.

ELBOW FLEXION TEST
(WADSWORTH ELBOW FLEXION TEST)

Assessment for Cubital Tunnel Syndrome and Ulnar Nerve Palsy at the Elbow

ORTHOPEDIC GAMUT 5-8

SITES OF COMPRESSION

Potential sites of compression along the course of the ulnar nerve:
1. The arcade of Struthers
2. The proximal edge of the cubital tunnel retinaculum
3. The cubital tunnel
4. The deep flexor pronator aponeurosis

PROCEDURE

- The patient completely flexes the elbow.
- The elbow is held in the flexed position for up to 5 minutes (Fig. 5-11).
- If tingling or paresthesia occurs in the ulnar distribution of the forearm and hand, the test is positive.
- A positive finding suggests the presence of cubital tunnel syndrome.

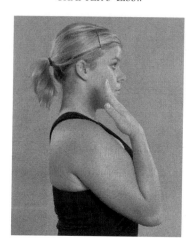

FIG. 5-11

CLINICAL PEARL

This test is not only useful for cubital tunnel syndrome, it may also reveal the mechanism that resulted in injury to the ulnar nerve. The fully flexed elbow is a common posture for the arm during sleep, naturally or chemically induced. Patients may wake up with ulnar palsy symptoms that stem from prolonged neural compression and anoxia.

GOLFER ELBOW TEST

Assessment for Medial Epicondylitis

PROCEDURE

- The patient is seated, the patient's elbow is flexed slightly, and the hand is supinated.
- The patient flexes the wrist against resistance.
- Medial epicondyle pain suggests epicondylitis.
- In more severe medial epicondylitis, the flexor muscle groups are weakened, and the elbow-wrist mechanism can be extended by the examiner (Fig. 5-12).
- Full extension of the elbow-wrist joint localizes the lesion more sharply in medial aponeurosis contractures.

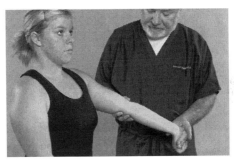

FIG. 5-12

CLINICAL PEARL

This test is a reverse procedure of Cozen test. Cozen test relies on resisted wrist dorsiflexion, but the golfer's elbow test relies on resisted elbow-wrist flexion. The pain associated with medial epicondylitis spreads down the forearm and is often confused with carpal tunnel syndrome symptoms.

KAPLAN SIGN

Assessment for Lateral Epicondylitis

ORTHOPEDIC GAMUT 5-9

IMAGING OF THE ELBOW

Standard plain-film imaging of the elbow involves five views:
1. Anteroposterior
2. Lateral
3. Medial
4. Lateral obliques
5. Axial

ORTHOPEDIC GAMUT 5-10

ELBOW SWELLING

The following are common local swelling locations of the elbow:
1. Olecranon bursa and the radiohumeral bursa
2. Muscle strains or contusions to the tendon, belly, or tenoperiosteal junction
3. Intracapsular effusion

PROCEDURE

- While the patient is seated, the affected upper limb is held straight out with the wrist in slight dorsiflexion.
- Grip strength is assessed with a dynamometer.
- This maneuver is repeated as the examiner firmly encircles the patient's forearm with both hands or with a strap placed approximately 1 to 2 inches below the elbow joint line (Fig. 5-13).
- The sign is present if initial grip strength improves and lateral elbow pain diminishes.

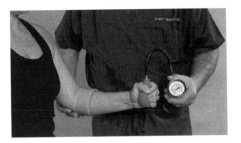

FIG. 5-13

CLINICAL PEARL

Kaplan sign is a good test for discerning the efficacy of tennis-elbow support in the management of a patient's condition. Obviously, if the grip does not improve while the brace is in place, the musculature and epicondylar tissues are not being supported adequately. The condition may be so severe that the use of a brace is not helpful.

LIGAMENTOUS INSTABILITY TEST

Assessment for Medial or Lateral Collateral Ligament Instability at the Elbow

PROCEDURE

- The examiner stabilizes the patient's arm with one hand at the elbow, and the other hand is placed at the wrist.
- The patient's elbow is slightly flexed (20 to 30 degrees), and an adduction (varus) force is applied to test the lateral collateral ligament (Fig. 5-14).
- An abduction (valgus) force is then applied to test the medial collateral ligament (Fig. 5-15).

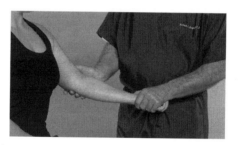

FIG. 5-14

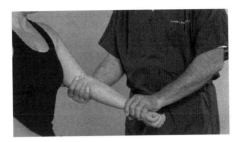

FIG. 5-15

CLINICAL PEARL

Osseous reductions that are felt or heard are not uncommon in elbow ligamentous testing. During this procedure, the radial head may be reduced because of a minor subluxation, or simple adhesion releases may occur. The testing may become the treatment.

MILLS TEST
(ALSO KNOWN AS MILLS MANEUVER)

Assessment for Lateral Epicondylitis

PROCEDURE

- The patient's forearm, fingers, and wrist are passively flexed.
- The forearm is pronated and extended (Fig. 5-16).
- The test is positive if elbow pain increases.
- A positive test indicates lateral epicondylitis (tennis elbow).

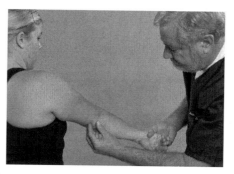

FIG. 5-16

CLINICAL PEARL

Mills test is also a treatment maneuver. One of the principles of management for lateral epicondylitis is the sectioning of the aponeurosis from the epicondyle. In the final maneuvers of Mills test, this separation is accomplished.

TINEL SIGN AT THE ELBOW
(ALSO KNOWN AS FORMICATION SIGN, DISTAL TINGLING ON PERCUSSION [DTP] SIGN, AND HOFFMAN-TINEL SIGN)

Assessment for Ulnar or Radial (Posterior Interosseous) Neuropathy at the Elbow

PROCEDURE

- While the patient is seated, the examiner taps the groove between the olecranon process and the lateral epicondyle with a neurologic reflex hammer (Fig. 5-17).
- The same is repeated for the groove between the olecranon process and the medial epicondyle.
- Hypersensitivity indicates neuritis or neuroma of the respective nerve.

5

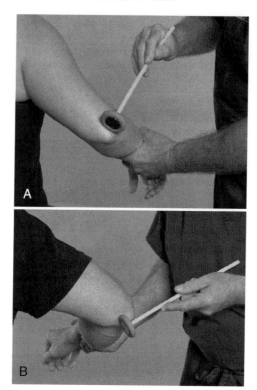

FIG. 5-17

CLINICAL PEARL

An important point to remember is that the tingling elicited by the Tinel sign represents regeneration. Pain and tingling represent injury and degeneration. The more distally the tingling is felt from the site of percussion, the more distally the axons have regenerated.

CHAPTER SIX

FOREARM, WRIST, AND HAND

AXIOMS IN ASSESSING THE FOREARM, WRIST, AND HAND

- Pain in the wrist and hand may have origin in the bones and joints, periarticular soft tissues, nerve roots, peripheral nerves, and vascular structures.
- Pain in the wrist and hand may also be referred from the cervical spine, thoracic outlet, shoulder, or elbow.

INTRODUCTION

Chronic wrist pain has often been called the *lower back pain of hand conditions*. Both areas offer the clinician significant diagnostic and therapeutic challenges. As in the examination of the lower back, a precise evaluation based on thorough knowledge of regional anatomy is essential to successful management (Table 6-1).

The wrist joint is probably the most complicated joint in the body because of its unique arrangement and articulation of the radiocarpal and intercarpal joints. Ligamentous injuries to the carpus can lead to significant and possibly permanent disability. Diagnosis may be difficult with persistent degrees of carpal instability. Definitive treatment modalities have not been perfected. As with most joint injuries, a more thorough understanding of the anatomy and pathogenesis of these injuries is useful (Table 6-2).

Carpal injuries represent a spectrum of bony and ligamentous damage. The names given to the various injuries describe the resultant damage apparent only on radiographs, for example, *lunate dislocation, perilunate dislocation, scaphoid fracture, transscaphoid perilunate fracture-dislocation*, and *transscaphoid transtriquetral perilunate fracture-dislocation*. Each injury is not an entity but part of a continuum.

A stable and pain-free wrist is a prerequisite for normal hand function. In contrast, a painful, unstable, or deformed wrist impairs function. The wrist, a common target of rheumatoid arthritis, is adversely affected by the reaction of synovial tissue on capsuloligamentous structures, articular cartilage, and subchondral bone. The mechanical

TABLE 6-1

FOREARM, WRIST, AND HAND CROSS-REFERENCE TABLE BY ASSESSMENT PROCEDURE

Forearm, Wrist, and Hand

Disease Assessed

Test/Sign	Allen test	Bracelet test	Bunnell-Littler test	Carpal lift sign	Cascade sign
Anterior Interosseous Syndrome					
Carpal Tunnel Syndrome					
Colles Fracture					
Neuroma					
Ulnar Neuropathy					
Aseptic Necrosis					
Tenosynovitis					
Denervation					
Sprain				•	
Carpal Fracture				•	•
Digit Contractures			•		
Rheumatoid Arthritis		•			•
Arterial Stenosis	•				

Test
Dellon moving two-point discrimination test
Finkelstein test
Finsterer sign
Froment paper sign
Interphalangeal neuroma test
Maisonneuve sign
Phalen sign
Pinch grip test
Shrivel test
Test for tight retinacular ligaments
Tinel sign at the wrist
Tourniquet test
Wartenberg sign
Weber two-point discrimination test
Wringing test

6

TABLE 6-2

PRINCIPAL DIFFERENTIAL DIAGNOSIS LIST FOR WRIST PAIN

Radial side	Tenosynovitis (de Quervain disease)
	Osteoarthritis of first carpometacarpal joint
	Scaphotrapeziotrapezoid osteoarthritis
	Scaphoid non-union
	Ganglion
Dorsal, central	Kienböck disease
	Scapholunate dissociation
	Scapholunate advanced collapse (SLAC wrist)
	Intraosseous ganglion
	Ganglion
Ulnar side	Ulnar abutment syndrome
	Ulnar impaction syndrome
	Distal radioulnar joint degenerative arthritis/ instability
	Ulnar head chondromalacia
	Triangular fibrocartilage complex tear
	Extensor carpi ulnaris tendonitis/subluxation
	Lunotriquetral instability
	Pisotriquetral joint disease
	Midcarpal instability

Adapted from Ankarath S: Chronic wrist pain: diagnosis and management, *Curr Orthop* 20(2):141-151, 2006.

TABLE 6-3

FOREARM, WRIST, AND HAND CROSS-REFERENCE TABLE BY SYNDROME OR TISSUE

Anterior interosseous syndrome	Pinch grip test
Arterial stenosis	Allen test
	Tourniquet test
Aseptic necrosis	Finsterer sign
Carpal fracture	Carpal lift sign
	Cascade sign
	Finsterer sign
Carpal tunnel syndrome	Phalen sign
	Tinel sign at the wrist
	Tourniquet test
	Wringing test
Colles fracture	Maisonneuve sign
Denervation	Dellon moving two-point discrimination test
	Shrivel test
	Weber two-point discrimination test

TABLE 6-3

FOREARM, WRIST, AND HAND CROSS-REFERENCE TABLE BY
SYNDROME OR TISSUE—cont'd

Digit contractures	Bunnell-Littler test
	Test for tight retinacular ligaments
Neuroma	Interphalangeal neuroma test
Rheumatoid arthritis	Bracelet test
	Cascade sign
Sprain	Carpal lift sign
Tenosynovitis	Finkelstein test
Ulnar neuropathy	Dellon moving two-point discrimination test
	Froment paper sign
	Tinel sign at the wrist
	Tourniquet test
	Wartenberg sign
	Weber two-point discrimination test

6

ORTHOPEDIC GAMUT 6-1

WRIST CARPAL SYSTEM

The nature of injury of the wrist carpal system is determined by:
1. The type of three-dimensional loading
2. The magnitude and direction of the forces involved
3. The position of the hand at the time of impact
4. The biomechanical properties of the bones and ligaments

---

forces of the different muscle groups acting across the wrist also contribute to deformities.

The initial evaluation of a patient with an injured wrist must be thorough and methodical. In recent years, increased understanding of carpal mechanics and instability patterns, with and without fractures, has increased the importance of accurate examination of the wrist. The diagnosis of *sprained wrist* is not adequate in establishing a proper treatment regimen. By taking a complete history, performing an exact examination, and using appropriate diagnostic aids such as motion views, tomography, bone scans, and arthrography, the clinician can establish an accurate diagnosis of wrist injury. Only after an accurate diagnosis is established can a rational, therapeutic regimen be prepared.

As with any other orthopedic problem, assessment of wrist and hand disorders begins with a complete history (Box 6-1). Painful disorders of the forearm, wrist, and hand can be classified based on the tissue of origin of pain and its distribution.

BOX 6-1

PRÉCIS OF FOREARM WRIST AND HAND DIAGNOSTIC CONSIDERATION

Skin and Subcutaneous Tissue
Forearm
Dorsal hand
Palmar hand
Digits

Bones and Joints
Forearm
Wrist
Hand
Digits:
- Metacarpophalangeal joints
- Interphalangeal joints
- Thumb articulations

Flexor Muscle System
Forearm
Carpal tunnel
Palm and digits

Extensor Muscle System
Forearm
Extensor retinaculum
Dorsal hand
Extensor hood mechanism

Nerves
Superficial nerves
Deep nerves:
- Radial nerve
- Ulnar nerve
- Median nerve

> **BOX 6-1**
>
> PRÉCIS OF FOREARM WRIST AND HAND DIAGNOSTIC
> CONSIDERATION—cont'd
>
> **Vessels**
> Arteries
> Veins
> Lymphatics

ESSENTIAL ANATOMY

The bones of the hand can be divided into four units: a central fixed unit for stability and three mobile units for dexterity and power. The fixed unit is composed of eight carpal bones tightly bound to the second and third metacarpals.

The wrist transmits force between the hand and forearm. Force passes through the capitate bone of the distal carpal row, the scaphoid and lunate bones of the proximal carpal row, and onward proximally to the distal end of the radius. These bones are the ones most likely to be fractured or dislocated in injury of the hand-wrist mechanism. Of the two long bones of the forearm, only the radius has true articulation with the carpal bones. The carpal fractures often involve

> **ORTHOPEDIC GAMUT 6-2**
>
> **MOBILE UNITS OF THE WRIST**
>
> **The three mobile units projecting from the fixed unit of the wrist are:**
> 1. The thumb, for powerful pinch and grasp and fine manipulations
> 2. The index finger, for precise movements alone or with the thumb
> 3. The middle, ring, and little fingers, for power grip

the scaphoid. Scaphoid fractures, with typical tenderness at the anatomic snuffbox, can result in chronic wrist pain because of non-union or collapse of the structure following injury. Wrist radio-carpal trauma can also involve the triangular fibrocartilage complex (Table 6-4).

TABLE 6-4	
TRIANGULAR FIBROCARTILAGE COMPLEX INJURY CLASSIFICATION	
Class I: Traumatic	A. Central perforation
	B. Ulnar avulsion
	a. With distal ulnar fracture
	b. Without distal ulnar fracture
	C. Distal avulsion
	D. Radial avulsion
	a. With sigmoid notch fracture
	b. Without sigmoid notch fracture
Class II: Degenerative (ulnocarpal abutment syndrome)	A. Triangular fibrocartilage complex wear
	B. Triangular fibrocartilage complex wear—with lunate or ulnar chondromalacia
	C. Triangular fibrocartilage complex perforation—with lunate or ulnar chondromalacia
	D. Triangular fibrocartilage complex perforation
	a. With lunate or ulnar chondromalacia
	b. With lunotriquetral ligament perforation
	E. Triangular fibrocartilage complex perforation
	a. With lunate or ulnar chondromalacia
	b. With lunotriquetral ligament perforation
	c. With ulnocarpal arthritis

ORTHOPEDIC GAMUT 6-3

RADIOCARPAL JOINT

The radiocarpal joint consists of the following:
1. The distal surface of the radius
2. The scaphoid and lunate bones
3. The triangular fibrocartilage connecting the medial side of the distal radius with the ulnar styloid process
4. The triquetrum

ESSENTIAL MOTION ASSESSMENT

Movements of the wrist comprise flexion, extension, and ulnar and radial deviation. Flexion-extension movements of the fingers occur at both the metacarpophalangeal (MCP) and the interphalangeal joints (Fig. 6-1).

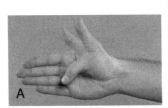
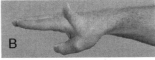
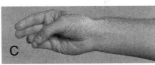

FIG. 6-1 Examples of thumb movements. **A**, Flexion-extension. **B**, Abduction-adduction. **C**, Opposition.

Movements of the thumb are described in terms different from those applied to the other digits because the thumb is positioned in a way that is different from the way the fingers are positioned, and the thumb is capable of unique movements not possible in the other digits.

Opposition is a unique capability, possessed only by the thumb. The goal of opposition is to cause the *pulp* surface (i.e., the rounded eminence directly opposite the nail) of the distal phalanx to face the pulp surfaces of the other digits. This capability is essential to realizing the full range of capabilities for grasping and manipulating objects with the hand.

Creating a cup-shaped recess in the palm of the hand requires movement of the other four digits. This recess allows an object to be cradled in the palm before the fingers are closed over it.

For examination of the wrist-hand range of motion, the middle finger is considered midline (Fig. 6-2). Wrist flexion decreases as the fingers are flexed. Movements of flexion and extension are ultimately limited by muscles and ligaments (Figs. 6-3 and 6-4).

Finger abduction is 20 to 30 degrees at the MCP joints. Finger adduction is 0 degrees at the same joint. The loss of finger abduction or adduction has minimal effect on the activities of daily living.

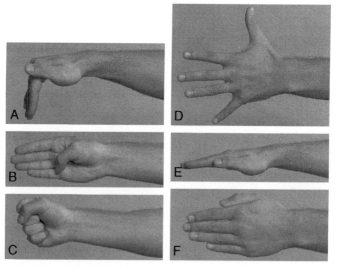

FIG. 6-2 Range of motion of the hand and wrist.

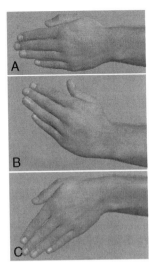

FIG. 6-3 The wrist in a neutral position. Radial deviation of 15 degrees or less and ulnar deviation of 30 degrees or less.

6

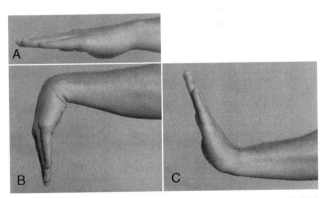

FIG. 6-4 **A**, The wrist in a neutral position. **B**, Wrist flexion. **C**, Wrist extension (dorsiflexion).

Thumb flexion at the carpometacarpal joint is in a range of 45 to 50 degrees. At the MCP joint, the range is 50 to 55 degrees. At the interphalangeal joint, thumb flexion is in a range of 80 to 90 degrees. Extension of the thumb at the interphalangeal joint is 0 to 5 degrees. Thumb abduction is 60 to 70 degrees. Thumb adduction is 30 degrees. Seventy degrees or less of retained flexion of the thumb at the interphalangeal joint and 50 degrees or less retained flexion at the MCP joint are considered impairments of the thumb in the activities of daily living. Zero degrees of extension at the interphalangeal joint is considered the sole impairment of extension for the thumb. Forty degrees or less of radial abduction and 25 degrees or less of adduction are considered impairments of the thumb in the activities of daily living (Fig. 6-5).

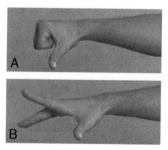

FIG. 6-5 Finger flexion (**A**) at the MCP joints. Extension (**B**) at the MCP joints. Retained active finger flexion of 80 degrees or less at the MCP joint, 90 degrees or less at the proximal interphalangeal joint, and 60 degrees or less at the distal interphalangeal joint serve as an impairment of the fingers in the activities of daily living. Retained active extension of 10 degrees or less at the MCP joint serves as the sole impairment of the fingers in the activities of daily living.

ESSENTIAL MUSCLE FUNCTION ASSESSMENT

ORTHOPEDIC GAMUT 6-4

MUSCLES OF THE HAND

Muscles controlling movements of the hand are divided into two groups:
1. Extrinsic muscles that originate within the arm and forearm
2. Intrinsic muscles, the origins and insertions of which are entirely within the hand (Figs. 6-6 to 6-10)

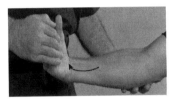

FIG. 6-6 Flexion. The patient flexes the wrist against graded resistance provided by the fingertips of the examiner's other hand placed in the patient's palm.

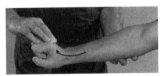

FIG. 6-7 Extension. The patient extends the wrist against graded resistance applied by the examiner's other hand to the dorsal surface of the patient's metacarpals.

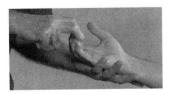

FIG. 6-8 Flexion of the interphalangeal joints of the fingers is accomplished by the long flexor tendons.

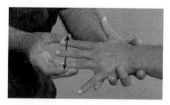

FIG. 6-9 The intrinsic muscles of the hand consist of a central group containing the interossei and lumbricales and the two lateral groups of hypothenar and thenar eminences.

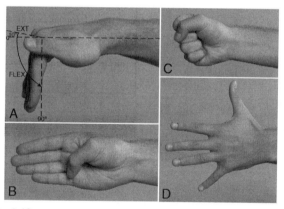

FIG. 6-10 The interosseous and lumbrical muscles are of fundamental importance in the extension of the fingers.

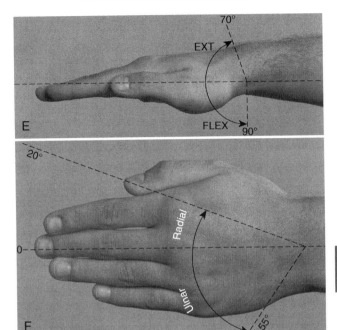

FIG. 6-10, cont'd

ESSENTIAL IMAGING

The importance of routine posteroanterior and lateral radiographs in neutral position of the wrist cannot be overemphasized.

ORTHOPEDIC GAMUT 6-5

SCAPHOLUNATE ADVANCE COLLAPSE (SLAC) WRIST GRADING BASED ON THE EXTENT OF THE DEGENERATIVE CHANGES

Stage 1a: Degenerative changes between the scaphoid and the radial styloid

Stage 1b: Degenerative changes involving the whole of the radio-scaphoid joint

Stage 2: Degenerative arthritis involving the scaphocapitate (midcarpal) joint

---

6

ALLEN TEST

Assessment for Peripheral Vascular Obstruction at the Wrist

ORTHOPEDIC GAMUT 6-6

REFLEX SYMPATHETIC DYSTROPHY– COMPLEX REGIONAL PAIN SYNDROME (RSD-CRPS) LIMB PROTECTION

Three stages of RSD-CRPS limb protection by the patient are:
1. Not allowing palpation or percussion or even light touch of the affected tissue
2. Loss of use, stiffness of soft tissues, loss of joint motion, development of contracture, and atrophy of skin; warmth of hypervascularity turns to coldness; strength and function diminish further
3. Shiny, dry skin; degeneration of muscle tone; further joint stiffness; and both joint and muscle contracture

---

Comment

Diagnosis of reflex sympathetic dystrophy–complex regional pain syndrome (RSD-CRPS) is initially based on clinical symptoms and signs for the upper extremity, which includes painful disuse of the hand and wrist with a high degree of awareness. Supportive laboratory testing includes positive bone scans, hypervascularity (thermography), and positive sweat test with autonomic dysfunction and quantitative sudomotor axon reflex test. Later, osteoporosis can help confirm the diagnosis. The sympathetic dystrophy scale is effective in confirming and rating the severity of this syndrome (Boxes 6-2 and 6-3).

BOX 6-2

PUTATIVE DIAGNOSTIC CRITERIA FOR REFLEX SYMPATHETIC
DYSTROPHY (RSD)–COMPLEX REGIONAL PAIN SYNDROME
(CRPS)

Clinical Symptoms and Signs
Burning pain
Hyperpathia or allodynia
Temperature or color changes
Edema
Hair or nail growth changes

Laboratory Results
Thermometry or thermography
Bone radiograph
Three-phase bone scan
Quantitative sweat test
Response to sympathetic block

Interpretation: If Total of Positive Findings is:
- >6 = probable RSD
- 3–5 = possible RSD
- <3 = unlikely RSD

BOX 6-3

CLASSIFICATION OF COMPLEX REGIONAL PAIN SYNDROME
(CRPS)—MAJOR CATEGORIES

I. Sympathetically maintained pain syndrome (type I and type II)
II. Sympathetically independent pain syndrome (type III)
   A. Category I
- Type I (reflex sympathetic dystrophy) usually follows an initiating noxious event
  - Continuous pain or allodynia and hyperpathia is not limited to the territory of a single peripheral nerve.
  - Disproportionate pain to the inciting event
  - Edema, skin blood flow abnormality
  - Abnormal sudomotor activity
  - Motor dysfunction disproportionate to the inciting event

Continued

BOX 6-3

CLASSIFICATION OF COMPLEX REGIONAL PAIN SYNDROME (CRPS)—MAJOR CATEGORIES—cont'd

- Diagnosis is excluded by the existence of conditions that would otherwise account for the degree of pain and dysfunction.
  - Type II (major causalgia)
    - Major nerve injury, more regionally confined presentation (usually), principally involving the territory of the involved nerve
    - Spontaneous pain or allodynia and hyperpathia is usually limited to the area involved but may spread distally or proximally.
    - Edema, blood flow abnormality
    - Abnormal pseudomotor activity is or has been shown in the region of pain subsequent to the inciting event.
    - Motor dysfunction disproportionate to the inciting event
    - Diagnosis is excluded by conditions that otherwise account for the degree of pain and dysfunction.
  B. Category II
  - Type III CRPS (sympathetically independent pain)
    - Disproportionate pain and sensory change, with motor and tissue change that do not respond to sympathetic block

Adapted from Manning DC: Reflex sympathetic dystrophy, sympathetically maintained pain, and complex regional pain syndrome: diagnoses of inclusion, exclusion, or confusion? *J Hand Ther* 13(4):260-268, 2000.

ORTHOPEDIC GAMUT 6-7

PULSES IN THE WRIST

Pulses are palpated at the wrist in three places:
1. The radial artery lying just medial to the radial styloid process, which passes toward the hand
2. The ulnar artery, which passes just lateral (in the anatomic position) to the pisiform bone
3. The deep radial artery, which crosses the floor of the anatomic snuffbox

PROCEDURE

- The patient is seated and instructed to make a tight fist to express blood from the palm. The examiner uses finger pressure to occlude the radial and ulnar arteries.
- The patient opens and closes the fist to express any remaining blood. The examiner releases the arteries one at a time (Fig. 6-11).
- The sign is negative if the pale skin of the palm flushes immediately after an artery is released.
- The sign is positive if the skin of the palm remains blanched for more than 5 seconds. This test, which should be performed before Wright test, Eden test, and the shoulder hyperabduction maneuver, is significant for revealing vascular occlusion of the artery tested.

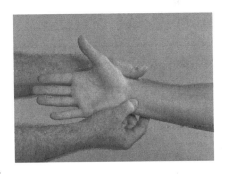

FIG. 6-11

CLINICAL PEARL

This test will often elicit paresthesia when an underlying distal peripheral nerve entrapment syndrome exists (carpal tunnel syndrome). The test is used as an early indicator of other general pathologic conditions only when paresthesia is elicited.

BRACELET TEST

Assessment for Degenerative Changes of the Wrist Articulations (Rheumatoid Arthritis)

ORTHOPEDIC GAMUT 6-8
RHEUMATOID DEFORMITY

Rheumatoid Deformity of the Wrist is Usually Characterized by:
1. Dorsal, distal, and then ulnar displacement of the distal ulna *(caput ulnae syndrome)*
2. Subluxation of the carpus, usually palmarly with supination and radial deviation leading to a zigzag collapse of the wrist and secondary increased ulnar drift
3. Foreshortening and widening of the carpus
4. End-point deformities in which the patient exhibits subluxation, dislocation, or ankylosis of the wrist
5. Digit stance deformities, particularly extension or flexion stance alterations during cascade testing
6. Signs of neurovascular alterations

ORTHOPEDIC GAMUT 6-9

FINDINGS THAT SUGGEST, BUT ARE NOT PATHOGNOMONIC OF, RHEUMATOID ARTHRITIS

- Symmetric swelling of the proximal interphalangeal (PIP) joints
- Boutonnière or swan-neck deformities of several PIP joints
- Swelling or tenderness of the MCP joints
- Ulnar deviation or subluxation of these MCP and PIP joints
- Synovitis of the wrist (especially at the distal ulna)
- Tenderness of the distal ulna
- Swelling of the extensor carpi ulnaris tendon

ORTHOPEDIC GAMUT 6-10

MORE THAN ONE OF THESE MAKES RHEUMATOID ARTHRITIS A LIKELY DIAGNOSIS

- The symptom complex of MCP joint swelling with ulnar deviation of the fingers is present.
- Dorsal interosseous muscle atrophy and extensor swelling at the wrist is virtually pathognomonic of rheumatoid arthritis.
- Caput ulnae syndrome also has a high degree of specificity.
- Subcutaneous nodules in the elbow and forearm may point to early diagnosis of this syndrome.
- The skin is moist, warm, lightly mottled, and thin and may be transparent.
- The erythrocyte sedimentation rate is elevated, but a normal value does not rule out the disease.

6

PROCEDURE

- The examiner gives mild-to-moderate lateral compression of the lower ends of the radius and ulna.
- This compression causes acute forearm, wrist, and hand pain (Fig. 6-12).
- The test is significant for rheumatoid arthritis.

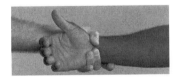

FIG. 6-12

CLINICAL PEARL

The bracelet test can be similar to a manual tourniquet test. The examiner must carefully compress osseous structures and must avoid occluding arterial structures.

BUNNEL-LITTLER TEST

Assessment for Interphalangeal Capsular Contractures

ORTHOPEDIC GAMUT 6-11

Stages of Basal Joint Thumb Arthritis Based on Radiological Appearance

- Stage 1: Articular contours are normal.
  - Patient exhibits slight widening of joint space caused by effusion or ligamentous laxity.
- Stage 2: Slight narrowing of the trapeziometacarpal joint with minimal sclerosis of the subchondral bone.
  - Scaphotrapeziotrapezoid joint is unaffected.
  - Joint debris is less than 2 mm.
- Stage 3: Marked narrowing of the trapeziometacarpal joint.
  - Scaphotrapeziotrapezoid joint are not affected.
  - Joint debris more than 2 mm.
- Stage 4: Identical to stage 3 but with involvement of the scaphotrapeziotrapezoid joint.

PROCEDURE

- The examiner slightly extends the MCP joint while moving the proximal interphalangeal (PIP) joint into flexion.
- A PIP joint that cannot be flexed indicates a tight intrinsic muscle or contracture of the joint capsule, which is a positive finding.
- This joint will not flex fully if the capsule is tight (Fig. 6-13).

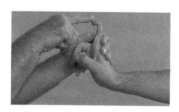

FIG. 6-13

CARPAL LIFT SIGN

Assessment for Carpal Fracture or Sprain

PROCEDURE

- While fixing the other fingers to the examination table, the examiner applies pressure to the dorsum of the digit being examined.
- The patient attempts to lift or extend the finger off the table (Fig. 6-14).
- The sign is present if this action causes pain at the dorsum of the wrist.
- The presence of this sign indicates carpal fracture or sprain.

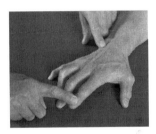

FIG. 6-14

CLINICAL PEARL

Carpal lift is accomplished when the finger is extended against resistance. The earliest sign of carpal fracture or degeneration, before using imaging, is the pain elicited with this test. With a carpal fracture, the carpal lift activity shifts bony fragments and produces the corresponding discomfort.

CASCADE SIGN

Assessment for Internal Derangement of Carpometacarpal Articulations and Internal Derangement of Phalanges

PROCEDURE

- The patient is seated, elbow flexed, and forearm supinated. The patient flexes the fingers at the MCP and PIP joints, as if the hand is gripping a golf club. A complete fist should not be made.
- In the normal hand, the longitudinal axis of the four fingers converges over or near the scaphoid tubercle.
- The sign is present if any of the fingers are askew, which indicates internal derangement of the metacarpals, carpals, or both (Fig. 6-15).

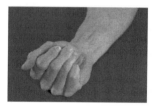

FIG. 6-15

CLINICAL PEARL

A faulty cascade of the fingers, indicating internal derangement of the wrist and hand, is an impediment of the hand grasp in daily activities. Patients usually have adopted accommodating grips. Pain or grip weakness is what precipitates the need for professional care.

DELLON MOVING TWO-POINT DISCRIMINATION TEST

Assessment for Dermatome Sensory Disturbances

ORTHOPEDIC GAMUT 6-12

TWO-POINT DISCRIMINATION

The normal threshold for two-point discrimination distance for the volar surface of the hand varies according to the zone being tested:

1. Between the fingertip and the DIP joint, two-point discrimination is normal from 3 to 5 mm, diminished if 6 to 10 mm, and absent if greater than 10 mm.
2. Between the DIP joint and the PIP joint, normal is 3 to 6 mm, diminished is 7 to 10 mm, and absent is greater than 10 mm.
3. Between the PIP joint and the finger web, normal is 4 to 7 mm, diminished is 9 to 10 mm, and absent is greater than 10 mm.
4. Between the web and the distal palmar crease, normal is 5 to 8 mm, diminished is 9 to 20 mm, and absent is greater than 20 mm.
5. Between the distal crease and the central palm, normal is 6 to 9 mm, diminished is 10 to 20 mm, and absent is greater than 20 mm.
6. At the base of the palm and wrist, normal is 7 to 10 mm, diminished is 11 to 20 mm, and absent is greater than 20 mm.
7. The threshold for the dorsal surface is higher in all zones: normal is 7 to 12 mm, diminished is 13 to 20 mm, and absent is greater than 20 mm.
8. Below the elbow but above the wrist, normal is 40 to 50 mm, diminished is between 55 and 80 mm, and absent is greater than 80 mm.
9. Above the elbow, normal is 65 to 75 mm, diminished is between 80 and 100 mm, and absent is greater than 100 mm.

PROCEDURE

- Two blunt points are moved proximally and distally in the long axis of the digit.
- One or two points of the Boley gauge are randomly used.
- The distance between the two points is decreased until the two points can no longer be distinguished (Fig. 6-16).
- The object is to determine whether the patient can discriminate between being touched with one or two points and the minimal distance at which two points touching the skin are recognized.
- Several areas on the uninvolved hand should be checked because some patients have congenitally abnormal two-point discrimination.

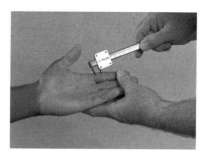

FIG. 6-16

CLINICAL PEARL

A *Janet test* can be performed simultaneously with Dellon test. If the patient's responses are bizarre and do not follow anatomic distributions, psychogenic anesthesia is suspected. The patient is instructed to say *yes* when the stimulus is felt and *no* when the stimulus is not felt. The patient will say *no* if functional anesthesia exists.

FINKELSTEIN TEST

**Assessment for de Quervain Disease
(Hoffman Disease, Tenosynovitis of the Thumb)**

PROCEDURE

- The patient makes a fist with the thumb inside the fingers. The examiner deviates the wrist in an ulnar direction.
- If this action produces pain over the abductor pollicis longus and the extensor pollicis brevis tendons at the wrist, the test is positive (Fig. 6-17).
- Pain indicates tenosynovitis in these two tendons.

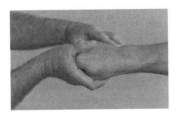

FIG. 6-17

CLINICAL PEARL

Finkelstein test produces an exquisitely painful response when stenosing tenosynovitis is present. Initially, determining the severity of the condition is somewhat easier when the patient actively tucks the thumb in and then deviates the hand and wrist in an ulnar direction. Depending on the response this produces, the passive test can then be performed. The pain elicited by this test is discrete and can be long lasting once excited.

FINSTERER SIGN

Assessment for Lunate Carpal Septic Necrosis

ORTHOPEDIC GAMUT 6-13
KIENBÖCK DISEASE

Kienböck disease staging:

- Stage I: No changes in plain-film radiographs, but magnetic resonance imaging will show decreased signal within the lunate.
- Stage II: Increased density of the lunate in plain-film radiographs. Height of lunate is maintained with no collapse.
- Stage IIIa: Collapse of lunate with loss of carpal height is present, but the scapholunate relationship is maintained.
- Stage IIIb: Collapse of the lunate and loss of carpal height is associated with rotary subluxation of the scaphoid.
- Stage IV: Generalized degenerative arthritis of the carpus associated with fixed rotary subluxation of the scaphoid.

PROCEDURE

- The sign is present when grasping an object hard, clenching the hand, or making a fist fails to show the normal prominence of the third metacarpal on the dorsal surface and when percussion of the third metacarpal elicits tenderness just distal to the center of the wrist joint (Fig. 6-18).
- The test is significant for Kienböck disease (aseptic necrosis of the lunate).

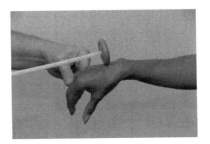

FIG. 6-18

CLINICAL PEARL

For this sign, all the metacarpal heads are percussed. This gross, low-frequency vibration will localize any cortical defect. In addition, an important point to remember is that ganglions are the most common soft tissue swellings of the wrist region. They are usually outpouchings of the capsule from the carpal joints, but they may also arise in relation to the tendons. The most common site of origin is from the scapholunate joint. In nearly every instance, a connection to the underlying joint or tendon sheath exists. Patients often have a painless swelling but, in some cases, may complain only of wrist pain, with no visible swelling. This scenario is particularly likely in early stages when the ganglion is small and not visible.

FROMENT PAPER SIGN ALSO KNOWN AS FROMENT SIGN

Assessment for Ulnar Nerve Palsy

PROCEDURE

- The patient grasps a piece of paper between any two fingers (Fig. 6-19).
- Failure to maintain the grip when the paper is pulled away indicates ulnar nerve paralysis (Fig. 6-20).
- This result indicates a positive test.
- The test indicates ulnar nerve paralysis.

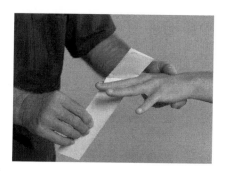

FIG. 6-19

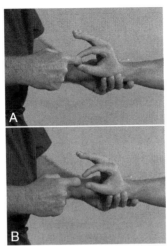

FIG. 6-20 In a modification of the Froment paper test, the patient adducts and flexes the tip of the finger to the tip of the thumb. The examiner tries to pull the digits apart. Failure of the fingers to maintain sufficient strength to resist this motion suggests ulnar nerve paralysis. (Anterior interosseous nerve lesions must be differentiated by electromyogram.)

CLINICAL PEARL

A change from a tip-to-tip pinch grip position to a pulp-to-pulp position is the earliest sign of ulnar entrapment (anterior interosseous nerve lesions must be differentiated). An electromyogram requires more gross muscle deficiency for conclusive findings, and the nerve conduction velocity may be equivocal in the early stages of nerve degeneration.

INTERPHALANGEAL NEUROMA TEST

Assessment for Interdigital Neuroma

PROCEDURE

- Neuromas should be carefully sought out by examination of the area using a slender instrument for palpating, such as the blunt end of a reflex hammer (Fig. 6-21).
- A localized spot in a scar will cause severe pain and is associated with paresthesia.
- The neuroma itself may be felt as a discrete mass.

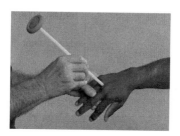

FIG. 6-21

CLINICAL PEARL

Although neuromas in continuity develop more frequently in the lower extremity and near amputations, they do develop elsewhere. Neuromas in continuity are observed at the bifurcation of nerve branches near the base of digits and may result from the chronic mechanical irritation caused by malalignment of the digit structures.

MAISONNEUVE SIGN

Assessment for Colles Fracture

ORTHOPEDIC GAMUT 6-14

COLLES FRACTURE

Poor results from Colles fracture are caused by:
1. Residual dorsal tilt more than 20 degrees (normal, 11 to 12 degrees of volar tilt)
2. Radial inclination more than 10 degrees (normal, 22 to 23 degrees)
3. Articular incongruity more than 2 mm
4. Radial translation more than 2 mm

PROCEDURE

- A positive Maisonneuve sign is characterized by marked hyperextensibility (dorsiflexion) of the hand (Fig. 6-22).
- The sign is present in Colles fracture.

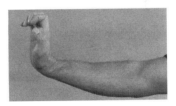

FIG. 6-22

CLINICAL PEARL

Maisonneuve sign remains a finding long after the fracture healing process is completed. A marked hyperextension of the wrist, with or without complaint, warrants imaging.

PHALEN SIGN ALSO KNOWN AS PHALEN SIGN AND PRAYER SIGN

Assessment for Carpal Tunnel Syndrome (Median Nerve Palsy)

PROCEDURE

- The patient's wrists are flexed maximally. The position is held for up to 1 minute as the dorsums are pushed together (Fig. 6-23).
- Tingling sensations that radiate into the thumb, the index finger, and the middle and lateral half of the ring finger are a positive sign.
- A positive sign indicates carpal tunnel syndrome (CTS) caused by median nerve compression (Fig. 6-24).

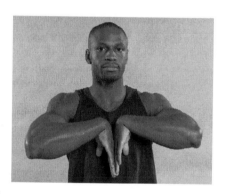

FIG. 6-23

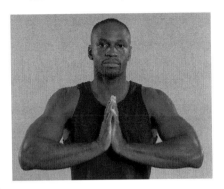

FIG. 6-24

CLINICAL PEARL

Phalen sign duplicates the wrist flexion-extension maneuvers that irritate the median nerve. The presence of Phalen sign is a good indicator that wrist splints will be useful in the management of CTS. As a screening test, a reverse Phalen maneuver can be performed. The patient is asked to press the hands together in the vertical plane and raise the elbows until they are horizontal. Loss of any dorsiflexion should be obvious. The most common cause of lost dorsiflexion is stiffness after a Colles fracture.

6

PINCH GRIP TEST

Assessment for Anterior Interosseous Nerve Syndrome

ORTHOPEDIC GAMUT 6-15

STAGES OF HAND GRASP

Hand grasp consists of three stages:
1. Opening of the hand
2. Closing of the digits to grasp an object
3. Regulating the force of pressure

ORTHOPEDIC GAMUT 6-16

DIVISIONS OF HAND GRASP

Hand grasp is divided into two types:
1. Power
2. Precision

PROCEDURE

- The patient pinches the tips of the index finger and thumb together in tip-to-tip pinch (Fig. 6-25).
- If the patient is unable to pinch tip to tip and has a pulp-to-pulp pinch of the index finger and thumb, the sign for anterior interosseous nerve syndrome is positive (Fig. 6-26).
- This sign may indicate entrapment of the anterior interosseous nerve.

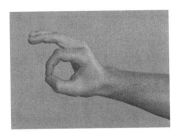

FIG. 6-25

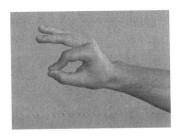

FIG. 6-26

6

CLINICAL PEARL

Even minor irritation of the anterior interosseous nerve produces this sign. The inability to pinch grip tip to tip influences the patient's ability to pick up small objects, which is the dysfunction that usually causes the patient to seek professional care.

SHRIVEL TEST
(ALSO KNOWN AS O'RIAIN SIGN)

Assessment for Peripheral Nerve Denervation

PROCEDURE

- The affected fingers are placed in warm (40° C) water for approximately 30 minutes (Fig. 6-27).
- The fingers are removed from the water and skin wrinkling is observed, especially over the finger pulp.
- Normal fingers wrinkle; denervated fingers do not.
- O'Riain sign is valid only in the first 90 to 120 days after injury, consistent with reactions of degeneration.

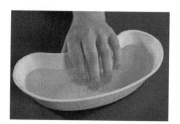

FIG. 6-27

CLINICAL PEARL

Muscle wasting in CTS is a good illustration of the trophic relationship that exists between striated muscle and the nerves that innervate them. When the nerve input to such a muscle is interrupted, the muscle wastes away, loses its strength, and eventually becomes much reduced in size. Even when the nerve-muscle relationship remains intact, if physiologic transmission of impulses is blocked, the muscle similarly wastes away. Smooth muscle is innervated by autonomic nerves, but no such trophic relationship exists in the case of smooth muscle.

TEST FOR TIGHT RETINACULAR LIGAMENTS

Assessment for Fixation of Phalangeal Retinacular Ligaments

ORTHOPEDIC GAMUT 6-17

PROXIMAL INTERPHALANGEAL DISLOCATIONS

Acute dorsal proximal interphalangeal dislocation categories:
I. Hyperextension: joint surfaces in contact
II. Dorsal dislocation: with dorsal dislocation of the middle phalanx on the proximal phalanx (bayonet)
III. Proximal dislocation: fracture of the volar base of the middle phalanx

6

PROCEDURE

- The PIP joint is placed in a neutral position as the distal interphalangeal (DIP) joint is flexed passively (Fig. 6-28).
- If the DIP joint does not flex, the ligaments or capsule are tight or contracted.
- If the PIP joint flexes easily, the retinacular ligaments are tight but the capsule is normal.

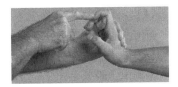

FIG. 6-28

TINEL SIGN AT THE WRIST
(ALSO KNOWN AS FORMICATION SIGN, DISTAL TINGLING ON PERCUSSION [DTP] SIGN, AND HOFFMAN-TINEL SIGN)

Assessment for Peripheral Neuropathy in Median or Ulnar Nerve Distribution

---

ORTHOPEDIC GAMUT 6-18

FIVE PATTERNS OF ULNAR NEUROPATHY DEPENDING ON THE SITE OF THE LESION

- Type I lesion
  - Either outside or just within the proximal end of Guyon canal.
  - Affects the mixed ulnar nerve.
  - All of the hand intrinsic muscles and sensation of the medial 1.5 digits are affected.
  - Dorsal ulnar cutaneous sensory branch distribution is spared.
- Type II lesion
  - Located within Guyon canal and affects only the superficial sensory branch.
  - Creates a pure sensory neuropathy of the medial 1.5 digits.
- Type III lesion
  - Involves the deep motor branch distal to its bifurcation from the superficial sensory nerve but proximal to the motor branch to the hypothenar compartment.
  - Results in a pure motor neuropathy affecting all the hand intrinsics, including the hypothenar muscles.
- Type IV lesion
  - Occurs on the deep motor branch distal to the hypothenar branch; preserves hypothenar function.
  - Affects other ulnar-innervated hand intrinsics.
- Type V lesion
  - Occurs just proximal to the branches supplying the first dorsal interosseous and adductor pollicis muscles; results in decreased activity of these muscle groups only.

PROCEDURE

- The carpal tunnel is percussed at the wrist (Fig. 6-29).
- Tingling in the thumb, index finger, forefinger, and the middle and lateral half of the ring finger is a positive finding.
- Tingling and paresthesia must be felt distal to the point of percussion for a positive finding.
- The test can demonstrate the rate of regeneration of the sensory fibers.
- The most distal point of the abnormal sensation represents the distal limit of nerve regeneration.

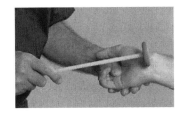

FIG. 6-29

CLINICAL PEARL

Tinel sign is extremely useful in identifying (1) the most proximal point of nerve regeneration or (2) the most distal point of nerve degeneration. These points are one and the same. Tinel sign is most evidenced at the Valleix points (tender points) along the course of the peripheral nerve (as in a neuralgia or neuritis). The examiner also may slide the tip of the index finger across the palm, noting frictional resistance and temperature. Increased thenar resistance from lack of sweating and temperature rise (vasodilation) may occur with median involvement.

TOURNIQUET TEST

Assessment for Neural Irritability as a Result of Posterior Interosseous or Median Nerve Compression

ORTHOPEDIC GAMUT 6-19
TWO TYPES OF POSSIBLE GANGLION CYST
Type I: An expanding cyst in the nerve trunk leaving the epineurium intact
Type II: An expanding cyst that penetrates the epineurium.

Comment

Significant diminution of blood flow to individual digits or to an entire hand results in pale nail beds, slow capillary recovery after skin compression, diminished bleeding after skin puncture, lowering of the skin temperature, and pain of varying intensity. Symptoms and signs of pain, pulselessness, pallor, paresthesia, and paralysis indicate arterial insufficiency or inadequate capillary perfusion (Table 6-5). The coexistence of pallor with cyanosis and rubor is consistent with vasoconstriction and subsequent vasodilation. This sign may occur in the presence of posterior interosseous nerve compression.

TABLE 6-5	
BLOND McINDOE COLD INTOLERANCE SYMPTOM SEVERITY (CISS) QUESTIONNAIRE	
Question	**Score**
1. Which of the following symptoms of cold intolerance do you experience in your injured limb on *exposure to cold?* Please give each symptom a score between 0 and 10, where 0 = no symptoms at all and 10 = the most severe symptoms imaginable.	Not scored
Pain, numbness, stiffness, weakness, aching, swelling, skin color change (white/bluish white/blue)	

TABLE 6-5

BLOND MCINDOE COLD INTOLERANCE SYMPTOM SEVERITY (CISS) QUESTIONNAIRE—cont'd

Question	Score
2. How often do you experience these symptoms? (Please check.)	
Continuously, all the time	10
Several times a day	8
Once a day	6
Once a week	4
Once a month or less	2
3. When you develop cold induced symptoms, on your return to a warm environment are the symptoms relieved? (Please check.)	
Within a few minutes	2
Within 30 minutes	6
After more than 30 minutes	10
4. What do you do to ease or prevent your symptoms occurring? (Please check.)	
Take no special action	0
Keep hand in pocket	2
Wear gloves in cold weather	4
Wear gloves all the time	6
Avoid cold weather, stay indoors	8
Other (please specify)	10
5. How much does cold bother your injured hand in the following situations? (Please score 0–10.)	
Holding a glass of ice water	10
Holding a frozen package from the freezer	10
Washing in cold water	10
When you get out of a hot bath or shower with air at room temperature	10
During cold wintry weather	10
6. Please state how each of the following activities have been affected as a consequence of cold induced symptoms in your injured hand and score each. (Please score 0–4.)	
Domestic chores	0 1 2 3 4
Hobbies and interests	0 1 2 3 4
Dressing and undressing	0 1 2 3 4
Tying your shoelaces	0 1 2 3 4
Your job	0 1 2 3 4

However, the scores given in question #1 do not count; overall, minimal score of 4 and a maximal score of 100. A score of 30 is the cut-off point for abnormal cold intolerance. Numbness is the most frequent cold-induced symptom, present in 80% of the time. Other symptoms of frequency are stiffness (77%), weakness (72%), aching (67%), pain (63%), skin color change (50%) and swelling (33%).

From Irwin MS et al: Cold intolerance following peripheral nerve injury. Natural history and factors predicting severity of symptoms, *J Hand Surg* 22B(3):308-316, 1997.

PROCEDURE

- Application of a pneumatic tourniquet to a normal extremity with pressure elevated to 20 mm Hg above the patient's resting diastolic blood pressure will obliterate arterial inflow and venous outflow; slow motor nerve conduction, decrease sensory conduction, and cause severe pain in the hand and forearm, all of which occur at the site of tourniquet compression.
- Anoxia and nerve compression occur simultaneously, and muscle weakness is evident within 3 to 5 minutes.
- Digital paresthesia occurs, and sensation diminishes gradually to anesthesia in approximately 30 minutes.
- These painful sensations are a combination of muscle and nerve ischemia and nerve compression.
- The appearance of symptoms at less than 20 mm Hg above the patient's resting diastolic blood pressure or sooner than 3 to 5 minutes is a positive test result.
- A positive test indicates neural instability as a result of posterior interosseous nerve or median nerve compression syndromes (Fig. 6-30).

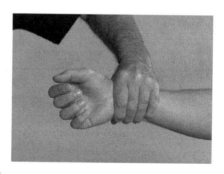

FIG. 6-30

WARTENBERG SIGN

Assessment for Ulnar Palsy

PROCEDURE

- The patient performs a hard grasp strength test with a dynamometer.
- The examiner observes the position and function of the digits in the action.
- If the position of abduction is assumed by the little finger, the sign is present (Fig. 6-31).
- The sign is present in ulnar palsy.

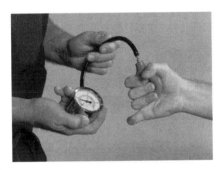

FIG. 6-31

WEBER TWO-POINT DISCRIMINATION TEST

Assessment for Diminished Peripheral Nerve Sensibility

ORTHOPEDIC GAMUT 6-20

TACTILE DISCRIMINATION

Four types of tactile discrimination are:
1. Stereognosis
2. Graphesthesia
3. Extinction
4. Two-point discrimination

ORTHOPEDIC GAMUT 6-21

QUALITIES OF SENSIBILITY

Five elementary qualities of sensibility evoked by stimulation via:
1. Touch-pressure
2. Warmth
3. Coldness
4. Pain
5. Movement and position

ORTHOPEDIC GAMUT 6-22

NEURAL SENSORY UNIT

Factors influencing the neural sensory unit:
1. The diameter of the first-order afferent neuron
2. The properties of the sensory receptors
3. The size and population of the receptive field
4. The threshold for the entire sensory unit

Comment

Ten zones in the hand are tested, six in the territory of the median nerve and four in the territory of the ulnar nerve. The scores are interpreted as suggested by Imai and colleagues (Table 6-6). A score of 6.10 is interpreted as having no sensation.

TABLE 6-6
Imai Classification of Sensory Recovery

Quality of Sensation (Range 1–5)	Filament Marking
1. Normal	2.83
2. Diminished light touch	3.61
3. Diminished protective sensation	4.31
4. Loss of protective sensation	4.56
5. Anesthetic	6.10

From Imai H, Tajima T, Natsuma Y: Interpretation of cutaneous pressure threshold (Semmes-Weinstein monofilament measurement) after median nerve repair and sensory reeducation in the adult, *Microsurgery* 10(2):142-144, 1989.

6

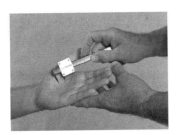

FIG. 6-32

PROCEDURE

- The test should be demonstrated while the patient is watching the procedure. The patient then closes the eyes.
- Several areas on the uninvolved hand are checked because some patients have congenitally abnormal two-point discrimination.
- The testing instrument can be a Boley gauge, a blunt-eye caliper, or an ordinary paper clip.
- Testing is begun distally and proceeds proximally.
- The points of the caliper are set at 10 mm and are brought together progressively as accurate responses are obtained (Fig. 6-32).
- The pressure from the testing instrument should not produce an ischemic area on the skin.
- When two points are applied, they make contact simultaneously.
- The patient indicates immediately if one or two points are felt.
- An interval of 3 to 5 seconds should be allowed between applications of the points.
- A series of one or two points is applied with varied sequence in each finger zone.
- The procedure is performed three times; if the patient does not record two of the three correctly, the result is considered a failure at that test distance.
- If the patient correctly identifies the number of points applied, the testing distance is decreased in varying increments.
- The test has 10 applications of two points and 10 applications of one point at random.
- The total incorrect one-point applications are subtracted from the total of correct two-point applications.
- A score of 5 or more is considered passing.

Abnormal skin texture, such as heavy scales or calluses, has a marked influence on the test results. Testing can be performed in the presence of edema or infection, but the results demonstrate the sensibilities present, which may not reflect the true status of the nerve.

CLINICAL PEARL

As with Dellon moving two-point discrimination test, bizarre responses are reason for suspicion as to the origin of the symptoms. *Janet test* can help identify psychogenic anesthesia.

WRINGING TEST

Assessment for Elbow, Wrist, or Hand Derangement

PROCEDURE

- The patient, using both hands, wrings a towel (Fig. 6-33).
- Paresthesia in the hand indicates CTS.
- Pain elicited at the elbow indicates epicondylitis.
- Wrist discomfort indicates arthropathy or carpal derangement.

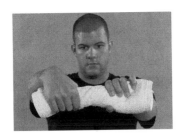

FIG. 6-33

CLINICAL PEARL

The wringing test is useful to determine the area for primary investigation. The patient also may be asked to hold both wrists in a fully flexed position for 1 to 2 minutes. The appearance or exacerbation of paresthesia suggests CTS. This test is the most sensitive clinical test for CTS. Advanced CTS can produce thenar atrophy and distal phalangeal acroasphyxia. The wringing test is particularly useful in eliciting responses in more subtle afflictions of the median nerve.

CHAPTER SEVEN

THORACIC SPINE

AXIOMS IN ASSESSING THE THORACIC SPINE

- The thoracic spine requires evaluation in isolation and in combination with the cervical and lumbar spine.
- Thoracic pain is perplexing and difficult to diagnose.
- The most commonly involved spinal area is the transitional thoracolumbar junction.

INTRODUCTION

Thoracic spinal pain and dysfunction present a particularly challenging clinical dilemma. Thoracic spinal pain may arise from somatic and visceral origins. Pain felt along the thoracic spine may arise from the ribs, the abdomen, or the vertebral column.

The thoracic spine is the part of the vertebral column that is most rigid because of the rib cage. The rib cage, in turn, provides protection for the heart and lungs.

Thoracic pain can occur as a referred visceral symptom, radiating from the chest and abdomen. The pain may also appear as a symptom of musculoskeletal origin. Sudden pain in the thoracic region occurs less often than in the more mobile cervical and lumbar spines.

The structure of the thorax as a whole is such that overall motion of this portion of the spine is limited.

TABLE 7-1

THORACIC SPINE CROSS-REFERENCE TABLE BY ASSESSMENT PROCEDURE

Thoracic Spine

Test/Sign	Disease Assessed											
	Fibrositis	Strain	Fracture	Intercostal Syndrome	Rib Injury	T1–T2 Nerve Root	Myelopathy	Tuberculosis	Sprain	Intervertebral Disc Syndrome	Ankylosing Spondylitis	Scoliosis
Adams positions												●
Amoss sign									●	●	●	
Anghelescu sign								●				
Beevor sign							●					

Continued

7

TABLE 7-1
Thoracic Spine Cross-Reference Table by Assessment Procedure—cont'd

Assessment Procedure	C1	C2	C3	C4	C5	C6	C7	C8	C9
Chest expansion test									•
First thoracic nerve root test						•			
Forestier bowstring sign									•
Passive scapular approximation test						•			
Rib motion test									•
Schepelmann sign				•	•				
Spinal percussion test				•	•	•	•	•	
Sponge test		•	•						
Sternal compression test	•				•				

TABLE 7-2

THORACIC SPINE CROSS-REFERENCE TABLE BY SYNDROME OR TISSUE

Ankylosing spondylitis	Amoss sign
	Chest expansion test
	Forestier bowstring sign
	Rib motion test
Fibrositis	Sponge test
Fracture	Spinal percussion test
Intercostal syndrome	Rib motion test
	Schepelmann sign
Intervertebral disc syndrome	Amoss sign
	Spinal percussion test
Myelopathy	Beevor sign
Rib injury	Rib motion test
	Schepelmann sign
	Sternal compression test
Scoliosis	Adams positions
Sprain	Amoss sign
	Spinal percussion test
Strain	Spinal percussion test
T1–T2 nerve root	First thoracic nerve root test
	Passive scapular approximation test
Tuberculosis	Anghelescu sign

ORTHOPEDIC GAMUT 7-1

THORACIC AREA PAIN

Diagnostic keys for thoracic area pain include the following:
1. Identify postural strain syndromes.
2. Identify radicular syndromes.
3. Always check for myelopathy.

ORTHOPEDIC GAMUT 7-2

MECHANICAL SPINAL SYNDROME CLASSIFICATIONS

1. Posture syndrome. Pain arises as a result of mechanical deformation of normal soft tissues from prolonged end-range loading of periarticular structures.
2. Dysfunction syndrome. Pain occurs as a result of mechanical deformation of structurally impaired tissues (scarred, adhered, or adaptively shortened tissue).
3. Derangement syndrome. Pain occurs as a result of a disturbance in the normal resting position of the affected joint surfaces.
4. Other. Patient exhibits signs and symptoms of other known abnormality (i.e., spinal stenosis, hip disorders, sacroiliac disorders, low back pain in pregnancy, zygapophyseal disorders, spondylolysis and spondylolisthesis, and postsurgical problems).

Adapted from Hefford C: McKenzie classification of mechanical spinal pain: profile of syndromes and directions of preference, *Man Ther* 13(1):75–81, 2008.

ORTHOPEDIC GAMUT 7-3

THORACIC SPINE

Stabilizing influences for the thoracic spine include the following:

- The first element is the vertebral articular process. The interlocking arrangement of the thoracic facets prevents anterior displacement of the vertebra and forms the imbrication of the thoracic spine.
- The second primary stabilizing influence of the thoracic spine is the vertebral body. At the posterior of the vertebral bodies, the height of the body is greater than in the anterior. This circumstance contributes to the thoracic spine kyphosis.
- The third stabilizing influence is the structure of the ribs and their attachments to the spine. The ribs help stiffen the thoracic spine.
- The fourth primary stabilizing influence for the thoracic spine is the structure of the intervertebral disc. The thoracic spine intervertebral discs are more narrow and thin than in the cervical or lumbar spines. They are also less elastic than all the other disc tissues of the spine.

ORTHOPEDIC GAMUT 7-4

THORACOLUMBAR SPINE

To assess range of motion of the thoracolumbar spine, the patient is directed to do the following:

1. Slowly bend forward at the waist and try to touch the toes (while observed for scoliosis) (Figs. 7-1 and 7-2).
2. Bend back as far as possible (hyperextending the spine) (Fig. 7-3).
3. Bend to the right and left side as far as possible (lateral bending with the pelvis stabilized) (Fig. 7-4).
4. Turn to the right and left in a circular motion (with the pelvis stabilized) (Figs. 7-5 and 7-6).

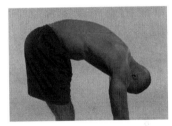

FIG. 7-1 Flexion range of motion in the thoracic spine is 20 to 45 degrees.

7

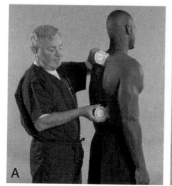
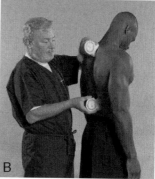

FIG. 7-2 For testing flexion with an inclinometer, the patient is seated or standing. (**A**). The thoracic spine is flexed forward so as not to involve lumbar spine motion (**B**). Both instrument readings are recorded. The T12 value is subtracted from the T1 value to arrive at the thoracic flexion angle.

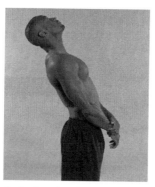

FIG. 7-3 Extension in the thoracic spine is normally 25 to 35 degrees.

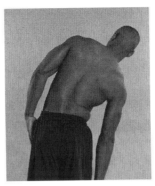

FIG. 7-4 Lateral flexion is approximately 20 to 40 degrees to the right and left.

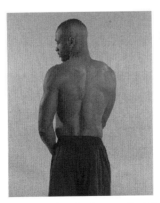

FIG. 7-5 Rotation in the thoracic spine is approximately 35 to 50 degrees.

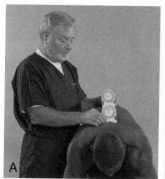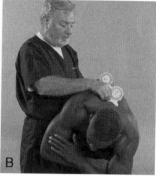

FIG. 7-6 When an inclinometer is used to assess thoracic spinal rotation, the patient is standing. The patient is flexed forward. The T12 measurement is subtracted from the T1 measurement to arrive at the thoracic rotation angle.

ESSENTIAL MUSCLE FUNCTION ASSESSMENT

In addition to te bony and discal stabilizing influences of the thoracic spine are muscles that support the spinal column. The thoracic spinal column serves as the attachment for many of the muscles of the trunk, shoulder, and arm.

During the trunk extension test, the latissimus dorsi, quadratus lumborum, and trapezius assist back extensors. The head and neck extensor muscles and the hip extensors should be tested before the back extensors are tested (Fig. 7-7).

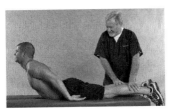

FIG. 7-7 The patient is prone. The patient then attempts trunk extension.

ESSENTIAL IMAGING

Although plain-film radiographs are generally unreliable in the early detection and assessment of osteoporosis, plain-film findings of osteoporosis can be a helpful adjunct to the diagnosis. The trabecular bone becomes sparse, resulting in overall reduction in bone density. Nontraumatic compression deformities are a sure sign that bone density is compromised.

ORTHOPEDIC GAMUT 7-5

VERTEBRAL COMPRESSION DEFORMITIES

Compression deformities of vertebrae may take several shapes:
1. An isolated central end-plate impression may be present.
2. Biconcave end-plate deformities may be present.
3. The segment may lose anterior vertebral body height with maintenance of the end-plate integrity.
4. The segment may demonstrate loss of anterior and posterior vertebral body height.
5. Fractures of the ribs are quite common.

7

ADAMS POSITIONS

Assessment for Pathologic or Structural Scoliosis

Comment

The spinal column centers the mass of the torso and head in a line along the vertical axis that falls through the pelvis. Disturbances of the spine, such as the curvatures associated with scoliosis, may significantly alter the normal balance and coordination of the spine (Table 7-3).

Scoliosis is also classified as either structural or nonstructural. Structural curves are fixed and nonflexible and fail to correct with side bending. Nonstructural curves, on the other hand, are flexible and readily correct with side bending. The Lenke Classification System helps examiners develop a more complete picture of the patient's condition by understanding the scoliosis as multidimensional and considering it from more than one view. The Lenke classification method also gives more detailed shorthand for communicating about scoliosis in professional settings, using a widely understood set of criteria (Table 7-4).

ORTHOPEDIC GAMUT 7-6

SCOLIOSIS

Scoliosis predictive indexing:
1. Curves less than 20 degrees will improve spontaneously more than 50% of the time.
2. No accurate method is available to help predict which curves will improve or worsen.
3. In curves of less than 30 degrees, 20% will progress.
4. Progression is more common in young children, at the beginning of their growth spurt.
5. The larger the curve at detection, the greater the chance of progression.
6. Curves in female patients and double curves in male or female patients are more likely to progress.
7. Scoliosis is more common in female patients than in male patients (idiopathic); 9:1 ratio.

TABLE 7-3

Thoracic Spine Syndromes

	Sprain or Strain	Vertebral Subluxation	Scoliosis	Scheuermann Disease
Physical examination findings	Palpable tenderness over intervertebral joint Supraspinous ligament tenderness Pain on twisting, cervical flexion, or extreme extension Paraspinal myospasm or hypertonicity	Pain over spinous process or supraspinous ligament Flexion or extension fixation; malposition Loss of normal springy end-feel Alteration of normal muscle or joint physiologic response	Structural deformity, such as hip or pelvis unleveling, leg length discrepancy, posterior scapula, high shoulder Muscular asymmetry and unilateral hypertonicity Lateral curvature of spine Chronologic age versus skeletal maturity	Kyphotic deformity of dorsal spine Rigid musculature of thoracic spine Discomfort of back in growing children and adolescents Tight anterior shoulder girdle and thorax
X-ray findings	Usually unremarkable	Normal Need to rule out concomitant mechanical factors that can delay recovery	Lateral deviation of spine (D1 to S1 view)	End-plate irregularity, abnormal vertebral ossification patterns, anterior plate or body deformity, involvement of three or more vertebral bodies More than 40 to 45 degrees of kyphosis

7

Modified from Brier SR: *Primary care orthopedics*, St Louis, 1999, Mosby.

TABLE 7-4

LENKE SCOLIOSIS CLASSIFICATION

Curve Type (1-6)

Lumbar Spine Modifier	Type 1 (Main Thoracic)	Type 2 (Double Thoracic)	Type 3 (Double Major)	Type 4 (Triple Major)	Type 5 (TL/L)	Type 6 (TL/L-MT)
A	1A•	2A•	3A•	4A•		
B	1B•	2B•	3B•	4B•		
C	1C•	2C•	3C•	4C•	5C•	6C•
Possible sagittal structural criteria (To determine specific curve type)	Normal	PT Kyphosis	TL Kyphosis	PT and TL Kyphosis	Normal	TL Kyphosis

•T5-12 sagittal alignment modifier:–, N, or +
−: <10°
N: 10-40°
+: >40°

The Lenke Classification System is simple, accurate, and easy to reproduce and communicate between health care providers. It relies on measurements taken from standard radiographs (X-rays). In this method, the examiner evaluates X-rays of the patient from the front, the side, and in bending positions. Each scoliosis curve is then classified in three steps by the region of the spine, the degree or angle of the curve, and the relationship of the side-to-side curve to the sagittal plane. For example, many scoliosis curves affect the presence or absence of kyphosis, which is the outward or convex curve normally found in the upper back. In addition, each aspect of the curve is evaluated for its relative stiffness or flexibility.

From Dr. Lawrence Lenke, Washington University School of Medicine, St. Louis, Missouri. Available at: www.spinal-deformity-surgeon.com.

PROCEDURE

- If the patient has an S or C scoliosis, the curvature may straighten when the spine flexes forward.
- A curvature that does straighten is a negative sign, indicating evidence of functional scoliosis.
- A positive sign occurs when the scoliosis does not improve after flexing forward.
- A positive sign is evidence of pathologic or structural scoliosis, and it indicates altered morphologic abnormality, pathologic condition, trauma, and subluxation.
- A posterior Adams position requires the examiner to be behind the patient (Fig. 7-8).
- An anterior Adams position requires the examiner to be in front of the patient.

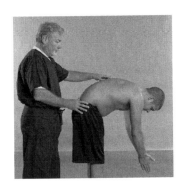

FIG. 7-8

7

CLINICAL PEARL

When the scoliotic curvature disappears in the Adams position, the curves are mild to moderate, or less than 25 degrees. These curves have more of a functional component than a structural component and are amenable to conservative management.

AMOSS SIGN

Assessment for Ankylosing Spondylitis, Severe Sprain, or Intervertebral Disc Syndrome

Comment

Ankylosing spondylitis (AS), an ascending disease, affects the thoracic region after the lumbar. Patients with this condition experience back pain, but the anterolateral chest pain and the limited chest expansion bother them the most. In some patients, these symptoms may occur rather early in the life of the disease, but they usually become bothersome after 6 years of illness. Chest pain, which usually occurs during inspiration, and limited chest expansion are caused primarily by involvement of costovertebral and manubriosternal joints, as well as the costochondral junctions and the clavicular joints. The girdle-like restriction may cause a sense of anxiety and dyspnea, particularly during exertion. However, respiratory problems are surprisingly uncommon, although restricted ventilatory volumes are detected by pulmonary function studies (Table 7-5). Of course, should concomitant disease result in impaired diaphragmatic breathing, a problem is likely to develop.

TABLE 7-5

MODIFIED NEW YORK CRITERIA FOR ANKYLOSING SPONDYLITIS DIAGNOSIS

Clinical criteria	Low back pain and stiffness for more than 3 months that improves with exercise but is not relieved by rest
	Limitation of motion of the lumbar spine both the sagittal and the frontal planes
	Limitation of chest expansion relative to normal values corrected for age and sex
Radiological criterion	Sacroiliitis grade 2 bilaterally or sacroiliitis grade 3–4 unilaterally

Adapted from Moll JMH: New criteria for the diagnosis of ankylosing spondylitis, *Scand J Rheum* 16(suppl 65):12-24, 1987.

PROCEDURE

- The recumbent patient places the hands far behind the body and tries to arise from the supine position to the seated position.
- The patient can also be in a side-lying position.
- The examiner should note the patient's position of comfort and any spinal complaints that the patient presents.
- The patient arises from the side-lying position to a sitting position (Fig. 7-9).
- The sign is present when either action elicits a localized thoracic or thoracolumbar spinal pain.
- The sign suggests ankylosing spondylitis, severe sprain, or intervertebral disc syndrome.

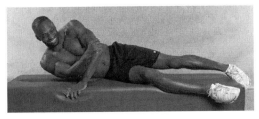

FIG. 7-9

7

CLINICAL PEARL

The patient sometimes defers to a side-lying posture when trying to stand after lying supine. This action represents Amoss sign. Amoss sign may not produce pain, but it reveals stiffness and lack of mobility and is still useful for detecting chronic spondylitis, which, at the least, requires imaging of the thoracolumbar spine.

ANGHELESCU SIGN

Assessment for Tuberculosis of the Vertebrae or Other Destructive Processes of the Spine

ORTHOPEDIC GAMUT 7-7
SIGNS AND SYMPTOMS OF TUBERCULOUS MENINGITIS
• Fever
• Headache
• Meningismus
• Abnormal mental status
• Vomiting
• Malaise-anorexia
• Papilledema
• Cranial-nerve palsies
• Hemiparesis, hemiplegia
• Seizures
• Hydrocephalus (CT scan)

Adapted from Garcia-Monco JC: Central nervous system tuberculosis, *Neurol Clin* 17(4):737-759, 1999.

ORTHOPEDIC GAMUT 7-8

PROBLEMS IN CONFIRMING THE CLINICAL SUSPICION OF TUBERCULOSIS MENINGITIS

- Approximately 45% of patients will have chest radiographic evidence of past or present tuberculosis, and approximately 50% will have a positive tuberculin test.
- Typical routine cerebrospinal fluid (CSF) profile demonstrates a lymphocyte predominant pleocytosis, a raised protein and a low glucose, tuberculous meningitis can be excluded on the absence of these parameters alone.
- The CSF may be acellular in as many as 3% to 6% of human immunodeficiency virus (HIV)-negative patients. The CFS may be acellular in as many as 16% of HIV-positive patients.
- HIV-negative patients may have a neutrophilic predominance in 20% to 25% of HIV-negative patients.
- The protein level may be normal in approximately 6% of HIV patients, the glucose level may be normal in approximately 25% of HIV-negative patients.
- The protein and glucose figures are increased in HIV-positive patients.
- Smears of the CSF, although diagnostic, are positive in only 5% to 20% of cases.
- Culture, though the gold standard, is positive in approximately 40% of cases. Cultures and may take up to 6 weeks to return a positive result.

Adapted from Garcia-Monco JC: Central nervous system tuberculosis, *Neurol Clin* 17(4):737-759, 1999.

PROCEDURE

- Anghelescu sign is used for identifying tuberculosis of the vertebrae or other destructive processes of the spine.
- In the supine position, the patient places weight on the head and heels while lifting the body upward (Fig. 7-10).
- Inability to hyperextend the spine indicates a disease process.

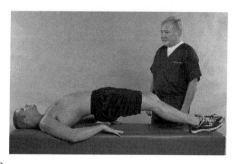

FIG. 7-10

CLINICAL PEARL

When testing for Anghelescu sign, the loss of the ability to achieve a near opisthotonos posture is significant. Although the true opisthotonos posture involves the cervical spine, very few patients normally have enough strength in the neck to accomplish this task.

BEEVOR SIGN

Assessment for Myelopathy Associated with the T10 Spinal Level

---

ORTHOPEDIC GAMUT 7-9

GUILLAIN-BARRÉ SYNDROME DISABILITY SCORE

The Guillain-Barré syndrome (GBS) disability score is a widely accepted scoring system to assess the functional status of patients with GBS in which scores range from 0 (normal) to 6 (dead).

- Poor outcome is a GBS disability score at 6 months of 3 or more, which corresponds with the inability to walk 10 m independently.
- Fairly good outcome is defined as a GBS disability score at 6 months of 2 or less.
- The endpoint is at 6 months because most of the recovery process has occurred by this time in select patients who do recover.
- The GBS index:
  - 0 A healthy state
  - 1 Minor symptoms and capable of running
  - 2 Able to walk 10 m or more without assistance but unable to run
  - 3 Able to walk 10 m across an open space with help
  - 4 Bedridden or chair bound
  - 5 Requiring assisted ventilation for at least part of the day
  - 6 Dead

Adapted from van Koningsveld R et al: A clinical prognostic scoring system for Guillain-Barre syndrome, *Lancet Neurol* 6(7):589–594, 2007.

ORTHOPEDIC GAMUT 7-10

MEDICAL RESEARCH COUNCIL SUM SCORE

1. The Medical Research Council (MRC) sum score is the sum of the scores of six muscle groups, which include shoulder abductors, elbow flexors, wrist extensors, hip flexors, knee extensors, and foot dorsiflexors, bilaterally. Scores range from 60 (normal) to 0 (quadriplegic).
2. The MRC score of an individual muscle group ranges from 0 to 5:
   0 No visible contraction
   1 Visible contraction without movement of the limb
   2 Active movement of the limb, but not against gravity
   3 Active movement against gravity over (almost) the full range
   4 Active movement against gravity and resistance
   5 Normal power

The GBS disability score is probably the easiest to apply in clinical practice, although the MRC sum score might be more accurate. Moreover, a variable measured at 1 week supplies information in an early phase of the disease and therefore might be more helpful in early decision making concerning therapeutic intervention.

Adapted from van Koningsveld R et al: A clinical prognostic scoring system for Guillain-Barre syndrome, *Lancet Neurol* 6(7):589–594, 2007.

PROCEDURE

- Beevor sign, although not an abdominal reflex, is seen during an examination.
- In this test, the recumbent patient lifts the head off the examining table (Fig. 7-11).
- Normally, the upper and lower abdominal muscles contract equally and the umbilicus does not move or drift.
- When the lower abdominal muscles alone are weakened, the umbilicus will be drawn upward by the contraction of the intact upper musculature (Fig. 7-12).
- This effect is associated with a spinal cord lesion at the T10 level.

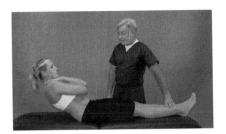

FIG. 7-11

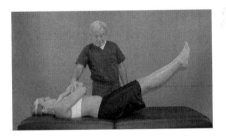

FIG. 7-12

7

CLINICAL PEARL

In the presence of prolonged illness followed by lower extremity paresthesia (regardless of how minor), this test needs to be performed. Beevor sign affords an early, noninvasive indicator of the existence of thoracic spinal cord myelopathy.

CHEST EXPANSION TEST

Assessment for Spinal Ankylosis

PROCEDURE

- The chest diameter is measured at the level of the fourth intercostal space.
- The measurement is taken as the patient exhales maximally.
- A second measurement is made as the patient inhales deeply (Fig. 7-13).
- The normal difference between inspiration and expiration is 5.75 to 7.62 cm (1.5 to 3 inches).

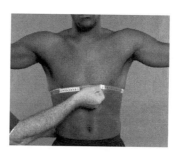

FIG. 7-13

CLINICAL PEARL

Chest expansion measurements are sensitive indicators of early involvement of the costovertebral joints in ankylosing spondylitis. The chest expansion test is often positive before the patient realizes a change in chest comfort.

FIRST THORACIC NERVE ROOT TEST

Assessment for First or Second Thoracic Nerve Root Involvement

---

ORTHOPEDIC GAMUT 7-11

NERVOUS SYSTEM

The four components of the nervous system that refer pain or discomfort follow:
1. The spinal cord
2. The dural sleeve of a nerve root
3. The nerve trunk
4. A peripheral or cutaneous nerve

ORTHOPEDIC GAMUT 7-12

COMMON HISTORICAL AND PHYSICAL FINDINGS IN THORACIC INTERVERTEBRAL DISK HERNIATION

Historical findings
- Pain
- Back pain
- Pain not in back
- Paresthesias
- Numbness
- Tingling
- Weakness
  - Lower extremities
  - Upper extremities
- Bowel/bladder involvement

Physical findings
- Weakness—lower extremities
- Localized spine tenderness
- Sensation abnormalities
- Reflex abnormalities

7

Adapted from Linscott MS, Heyborne R: Thoracic intervertebral disk herniation: a commonly missed diagnosis, *J Emerg Med* 32(3):235-238, 2007.

ORTHOPEDIC GAMUT 7-13

PAIN REFERRAL

Pain referral rules are as follows:

1. Pain refers segmentally. A T5 tissue refers pain to the T5 dermatome. Pain can occupy all or any part of the dermatome. If the patient describes symptoms straddling more than one dermatome or if the pain migrates from one dermatome to another, four possibilities arise: (a) The patient is describing a nonorganic pain; (b) the lesion itself is shifting, which often happens with vertebral element displacements; (c) the lesion is spreading, as in metastasis; or (d) the pain stems from a tissue that cannot refer pain segmentally. An exception of importance is the dura mater, which refers pain extra segmentally.

2. Pain refers distally. The source of symptoms is sought locally or proximally.

3. Referred pain does not cross the midline. A T5 left rib will not cause discomfort on the right side of the body. A pain felt centrally must originate from a central structure. Pain that cannot be accounted for by a unilateral structure must be sought centrally. A pain alternating from one side of the body to the other must have a central source. This central source must be able to shift from one side to the other, such as during an intervertebral disc displacement.

4. The extent of pain reference is controlled. The referred pain is controlled by the size of the dermatome and the position in the dermatome of the tissue lesion. A large dermatome permits greater reference than a small one. A lesion in the proximal part of the dermatome refers pain farther than a lesion in the distal part.

5. The more intense the pain, the more the number of cortical cells that will excited. The spread to adjacent cells in the sensory cortex is interpreted as an enlargement of the painful area.

6. The deeper a soft-tissue lesion lies, the larger the reference to be expected. However, bone lesions produce minimal pain radiation.

PROCEDURE

- Pain from stretching the first thoracic nerve root via the ulnar nerve identifies the T1 or T2 roots.
- Disc lesions at either level are rarities and are not accompanied by easily identifiable neurologic signs.
- If weakness is present, the possibility of serious disease should be considered.
- The affected arm is abducted to 90 degrees. The elbow is flexed with the pronated forearm to 90 degrees.
- The patient places the hand behind the neck (Fig. 7-14).
- The ulnar nerve and the T1 nerve root are stretched.
- A positive test is indicated by scapular pain on the ipsilateral side.

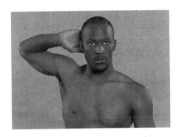

FIG. 7-14

CLINICAL PEARL

The first thoracic nerve root stretch indicates nerve root compression. This stretch can also indicate the existence of an inflammation of the lower two branches of the brachial plexus, a nonvascular thoracic outlet syndrome. This diagnosis is further confirmed by Roos test.

FORESTIER BOWSTRING SIGN

Assessment for Ankylosing Spondylitis

ORTHOPEDIC GAMUT 7-14

THORACIC KYPHOSIS

Patients with thoracic kyphosis are classified into the following two groups:

1. Patients in the first group exhibit a major increase in thoracic kyphosis, with an associated loss of lumbar lordosis and a rigid spine. With sufficient extension of the lumbar spine, compensation can be achieved for the thoracic kyphosis, allowing a horizontal gaze and erect posture.

2. Patients in the second group have thoracic kyphotic deformity but maintain a normal or even increased (compensatory) cervical and lumbar lordosis.

PROCEDURE

- The standing patient performs side bending and reveals ipsilateral tightening and contracture of the paraspinal musculature.
- Normally, the contralateral musculature demonstrates tightening (Fig. 7-15).
- The test is significant for ankylosing spondylitis.

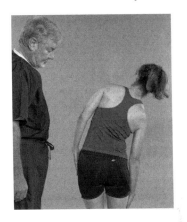

FIG. 7-15

CLINICAL PEARL

Although the presence of Forestier bowstring sign suggests spondylitis, this test also indicates strain and intervertebral disc involvement. Any loss of symmetric motion must be examined further.

7

PASSIVE SCAPULAR APPROXIMATION TEST

Assessment for T1 or T2 Nerve Root Problem

PROCEDURE

- The examiner passively approximates the patient's scapulae.
- Ipsilateral T1 or T2 nerve root problem is indicated by scapular pain (Fig. 7-16).

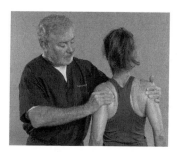

FIG. 7-16

RIB MOTION TEST

Assessment for Hypermobile or Hypomobile Costal Structures

PROCEDURE

- As the supine patient inhales and exhales, the anteroposterior movement of the ribs is palpated (Fig. 7-17).
- Restriction in motion is noted.
- Rib abnormalities during exhalation suggest an elevated rib (lowest rib).
- Rib abnormalities during inhalation suggest a depressed rib (uppermost rib).

7

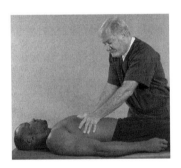

FIG. 7-17

SCHEPELMANN SIGN

Assessment for Costal and Intercostal Tissue Integrity

Comment

Any fixation or aberrant movement of the costovertebral articulations, or ribs, can have an impact on the synovial joints of the dorsal spine. The examiner rarely finds concomitant loss of joint play at the rib angle and corresponding vertebral motor unit. Experts have suggested that the rib cage may act as a splint to the thoracic spine. This splinting effect may prevent stresses placed directly on the midspine. In addition, it may be one of the reasons that thoracic disc herniations are less common. The fully developed ribs protect the underlying thoracic viscera while simultaneously providing attachment sites for a wide variety of muscles (Table 7-6).

TABLE 7-6	
THORACIC CAGE ARCHITECTURE	
Region	**Tissues**
Superiorly	Sternocleidomastoid, sternohyoid, sternothyroid, and anterior, middle, and posterior scalene muscles
Anteriorly	Pectoralis major and minor muscles, mammary glands
Posteriorly	Serratus posterior superior and inferior, and deep back muscles; trapezius, rhomboid minor and major, scapula, and all muscles related to it reset against the thoracic cage
Laterally	Serratus anterior muscles
Inferiorly	Abdominal muscles attaching to thoracic cage (i.e., rectus abdominis, external and internal abdominal oblique, transverses abdominis)

Adapted from Cramer GD, Darby SA: *Basic and clinical anatomy of the spine, spinal cord, and ANS*, St Louis, 1995, Mosby.

PROCEDURE

- Schepelmann sign identifies rib integrity.
- The patient raises the arms while in the seated position and then bends laterally.
- Pain created on the concave side is caused by intercostal neuritis (Fig. 7-18).
- If pain is created on the convex side, the diagnosis is intercostal myofascitis.
- Intercostal myofascitis must be differentiated from the fibrous inflammation of pleurisy.

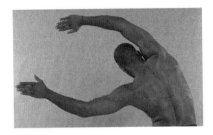

FIG. 7-18

7

CLINICAL PEARL

Schepelmann test provides an efficient method for localizing rib injury. The patient moves actively and can limit the motion according to the pain.

SPINAL PERCUSSION TEST

Assessment for Spinal Osseous and Paraspinal Soft-Tissue Integrity

---

ORTHOPEDIC GAMUT 7-15

MULTIPLE-LEVEL SPINAL FRACTURES

Three patterns of injury in multiple-level spinal fractures are:

Pattern A: The primary lesion occurs between C5 and C7, with secondary injuries at T12 or the lumbar spine

Pattern B: The primary injury occurs at T2 and T4, with secondary injuries in the cervical spine

Pattern C: The primary injury occurs between T12 and L2, with secondary injuries from L4 to L5

ORTHOPEDIC GAMUT 7-16

THORACOLUMBAR FRACTURES

Thoracolumbar fracture classifications (based on three-column concepts) follow:

- Wedge compression fractures cause isolated failure of the anterior column and result from forward flexion.
- In stable burst fractures, the anterior and middle columns fail because of a compressive load.
- In unstable burst fractures, the anterior and middle columns fail in compression, and the posterior column is disrupted.
- Chance fractures are horizontal avulsion injuries of the vertebral bodies caused by flexion about an axis anterior to the anterior longitudinal ligament.
- In flexion distraction injuries, the flexion axis is posterior to the anterior longitudinal ligament. The anterior column fails in compression, and the middle and posterior columns fail in tension.
- Translational injuries are characterized by malalignment of the neural canal, which has been totally disrupted. Usually, all three columns have failed in shear.

PROCEDURE

- While the patient is seated or standing and the thoracic spine is slightly flexed, the examiner percusses the spinous processes and the associated musculature of each of the thoracic vertebrae with a neurologic reflex hammer.
- Evidence of localized pain indicates a possible fractured vertebra.
- Evidence of radicular pain indicates a possible disc lesion.
- Because of the nonspecific nature of this test, other conditions also will elicit a positive pain response.
- If a ligamentous sprain exists, percussion of the spinous processes will elicit pain (Fig. 7-19).
- Percussion of the paraspinal musculature will elicit a positive sign for strain (Fig. 7-20).

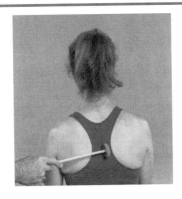

FIG. 7-19

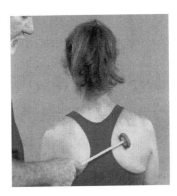

FIG. 7-20

CLINICAL PEARL

When soft-tissue percussion reproduces the complaint, the examiner may expect the same phenomenon from applications of ultrasound to the tissue. The uses of such therapies may be delayed until the soft tissue is no longer reactive to percussion.

SPONGE TEST

**Assessment for Acute Inflammatory
Lesions of the Spine**

ORTHOPEDIC GAMUT 7-17

FIBROMYALGIA TENDER POINT EXAMINATION PROTOCOL

The examiner surveys 18 standard points and three control points. The purpose of the control points is to assess the patient's baseline pain perception.

Palpation technique
- Patient should wear a standard examination gown.
- Survey sites are first located visually and then with light palpation.
- Pressure is applied with the dominant thumb pad perpendicular to each survey site.
- Each site is pressed for a total of 4 seconds only once to prevent sensitization that may occur with repeated palpation.
- The force is increased by 1 kg per second until 4 kg pressure is achieved.
- Whitening of the examiner's nail bed usually occurs when applying 4 kg force.
- Examiners can learn the approximate feel of 4 kg force by using a dolorimeter or by using the thumb to counterbalance the 4-kg weight on a standard scale.

Patient instruction
- "Please say *yes* or *no* if you feel any pain when a specific point is pressed."
- When the patient responds *yes* to indicate pain, the examiner should assess pain severity by asking for a numeric pain intensity rating: on a scale from 0 to 10, where 0 is no pain, and 10 is the worst pain ever experienced.
- By mid test, the patient is reminded of the meaning of the pain intensity range.

Tender point locations for testing
- Seated
  - Mid forehead (control)
  - Occiput: suboccipital muscle insertions
  - Trapezius: midpoint of upper border
  - Supraspinatus: above medial border of scapular spine
  - Gluteal: upper outer quadrant of buttocks
  - Low cervical: anterior aspect of the intertransverse space of C5–C7
  - Second rib: second costochondral junction
  - Lateral epicondyle: 2 cm distal to epicondyle
  - Dorsum right forearm (control): junction of proximal two thirds and distal one third
  - Left thumbnail (control):
- Side lying
  - Greater trochanter: posterior to trochanteric prominences
- Supine, feet slightly apart
  - Knee: medial fat pad proximal to the joint line

Number of positive survey sites: _____	
Sum of survey site scores (SS): _____	
Number of positive control sites: _____	
Sum of control site scores (CS): _____	
FMS Intensity Score (SS/18): _____	
Control Intensity Score (CS/3): _____	
FMS? Widespread pain for more than 3 months: _____ Yes _____ No	
Eleven or more positive survey sites: _____ Yes _____ No	
If answer to both questions is yes, patient fits FMS criteria.	

Adapted from D'Arcy Y, McCarberg BH. New fibromyalgia pain management recommendations, *J Nurs Pract* 1(4):218–225, 2005.

Comment

Common findings on examination include muscle *spasm* or taut bands of muscle, sometimes called nodules by patients; skin sensitivity, in the form of skin roll tenderness of dermatographism; or purplish mottling of the skin, especially of the legs after exposure to the cold. Myofascial pain syndromes also overlap with fibromyalgia (Table 7-7). The relationship of trigger points and tender points is not clear. The location of the trigger point is deep within the muscle belly. Trigger points result in decreased muscle stretch and pain with contraction. A *twitch response* (or jump sign), pathognomonic of an active trigger point, is a visible or palpable contraction of the muscle produced by a rapid snap of the examining finger on the taut band of muscle. A characteristic referred pain pattern is present.

TABLE 7-7

MISDIAGNOSES THAT MAY BE GIVEN TO PATIENTS WHO EVENTUALLY ARE FOUND TO HAVE THE FIBROMYALGIA SYNDROME

Alzheimer disease
Depression
Early spondyloarthropathy
Hypochondriasis
Hypothyroidism
Inflammatory bowel disease
Inflammatory myopathy
Interstitial cystitis
Malingering
Menière–Age disease
Metabolic myopathy
Multiple sclerosis
Neuropathy
Polymyalgia rheumatica
Sciatica
Somatoform pain disorder
Systemic lupus erythematosus/rheumatoid arthritis

From Kelley WN et al: *Textbook of rheumatology*, ed 5, Philadelphia, 1997, WB Saunders.

PROCEDURE

- A hot moist sponge is passed up and down the spine several times (Fig. 7-21).
- If any lesion of the spine is present, pain is felt as the sponge passes over the lesion.
- The test is positive for acute inflammatory lesions of the spine.

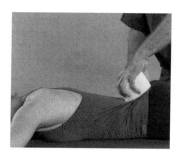

FIG. 7-21

CLINICAL PEARL

As with spinal percussion, the focal areas of tenderness found with the sponge test may be hypersensitive to mechanical stimulation. This sensitivity represents spasmophilia and must be absent before aggressive physical therapy can begin.

STERNAL COMPRESSION TEST

Assessment for Costal Structure Fracture

Comment

Also known as *Tietze syndrome*, costochondritis is an inflammation of the rib cartilage at the costosternal junction. The differential diagnosis includes angina pectoris, intercostal strain and neuralgia, rib subluxation, and, in cases of substantial trauma, rib fracture. The patient with costochondritis complains of point tenderness over one or two rib heads or costal junctions lateral to the sternum (Table 7-8). Symptoms are most commonly localized to the second, third, or fourth costochondral junctions. Abduction of the arm reproduces the patient's pain, which may radiate down the arm. Acute inflammation causes discomfort or pain on deep inspiration as the rib cage expands. Bogginess or swelling over the costal cartilage is possible but does not always occur.

7

TABLE 7-8

THORAX AND RIB SYNDROMES

	Costochondritis (Tietze Syndrome)	Intercostal Strain	Intercostal Neuralgia	Costovertebral Syndrome	Pectoralis Strain
Physical examination findings	Painful arm abduction Palpable tenderness at costosternal junction Commonly at second to fourth rib cartilage Normal results on cardiac examination Exacerbation of pain on stretching of pectoralis muscle	Palpable tenderness at rib interspace Splinting or spasm of affected intercostal muscle Reproduction of pain at deep inspiration with arms overhead	Painful rib interspace Possible strain of intercostal muscle Referral of pain from anterior to posterior or vice versa Exacerbation of pain with deep inspiration or spinal rotation Need to rule out infection (e.g., herpes zoster) and organic disease	Tenderness over rib angle or head Fixation of costovertebral articulation Inferoanterior subluxation of corresponding dorsal vertebral level Muscle guarding, spasm over affected rib cage Palpable spinal rotation or cervicodorsal fixation Referral to anterior thorax possible	Pain on examination at pectoralis muscle, either proximally or distally Swelling or bogginess of muscle belly Discomfort on abduction of arm Ecchymosis at injury site possible Pain reproduced by adduction against resistance Need to rule out costochondral injury, avulsion of pectoralis tendon at proximal humerus
X-ray findings	Usually normal Need to rule out rib fracture in cases of blunt trauma	Not applicable	Only needed for suspected organic disease or rib trauma	Not applicable	Not applicable unless rupture or avulsion is suspected

Adapted from Brier SR: *Primary care orthopedics*, St Louis, 1999, Mosby.

PROCEDURE

- While the patient is in the supine position, the examiner exerts downward pressure on the patient's sternum (Fig. 7-22).
- Localized pain at the lateral border of the ribs indicates a rib fracture.

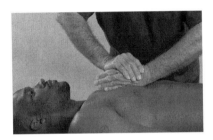

FIG. 7-22

7

CHAPTER EIGHT

LUMBAR SPINE

> **AXIOMS IN ASSESSING THE LUMBAR SPINE**
>
> - Low back pain is common from the second decade of life on.
> - Intervertebral disc disease and disc herniation are most prominent in the third and fourth decades of life.
> - Low back and posterior thigh pain arises from many areas of the spine, including the facet joints, longitudinal ligaments, and the periosteum of the vertebrae.
> - Radicular pain often extends below the knee in the affected dermatome.

INTRODUCTION

As many as 90% of patients with back pain have a mechanical reason for their pain. Mechanical low back pain may be defined as pain secondary to overuse of a normal anatomic structure or pain secondary to trauma or deformity of an anatomic structure. The age of a patient is helpful in determining the potential cause of back pain. In considering spondyloarthropathies, clinical characteristics help in differentiating the diseases belonging in this group (Table 8-3 and Table 8-4). The sex of the patient may also help select potential causes of low back pain. Certain disorders occur more often in men, whereas others are associated more commonly with women. Others occur equally in both sexes (Table 8-5).

Other than the common cold, back pain is the most prevalent human affliction. As stated earlier, most patients have a mechanical cause (muscle strain or annular tear) for their back pain and do not have an underlying, serious, systemic medical illness.

Even if treatment involves only a localized part of the lumbar spine, in each case, the lumbar spine has to be considered as a functional unit consisting of bones, ligaments, intervertebral discs, muscles, and all other soft tissues. Because of their central location, spinal elements represent the focal point for the equilibrium of the body. Because of the many connections and relations, spinal changes influence some

TABLE 8-1

LUMBAR SPINE CROSS-REFERENCE TABLE BY ASSESSMENT PROCEDURE

Disease Assessed

Test/Sign	Lower Extremity Joints	Fracture	Denervation	Myofascitis	Hamstring Spasm	Sacroiliac Lesion	Meningitis	L2–L3–L4	Femoral Nerve	Hip Lesion	Sprain	Spinal Neuropathy	Cord Tumor	Mechanical Lower Back	Subluxation	Dural Adhesions	Intervertebral Foramen Encroachment	Sciatica	Intervertebral Disc Syndrome
Antalgia sign																			●
Bechterew sitting test															●	●	●	●	●
Bilateral leg-lowering test														●			●		●
Bowstring sign												●							
Bragard sign												●	●					●	●
Cox sign																			●

Continued

8

TABLE 8-1

LUMBAR SPINE CROSS-REFERENCE TABLE BY ASSESSMENT PROCEDURE—cont'd

Disease Assessed

Lumbar Spine	Demianoff's sign	Deyerle sign	Double-leg-raise test	Ely sign	Fajersztajn test	Femoral nerve traction test
Lower Extremity Joints						
Fracture						
Denervation						
Myofascitis						
Hamstring Spasm						
Sacroiliac Lesion						
Meningitis						
L2–L3–L4						•
Femoral Nerve					•	•
Hip Lesion					•	
Sprain				•		
Spinal Neuropathy					•	•
Cord Tumor						
Mechanical Lower Back	•		•			
Subluxation						
Dural Adhesions					•	
Intervertebral Foramen Encroachment						
Sciatica		•			•	
Intervertebral Disc Syndrome			•		•	

Test/Sign

Heel/toe walk test

Hyperextension test

Kemp test

Kernig/Brudzinski sign

Lasègue differential sign

Lasègue rebound test

Lasègue sitting test

Lasègue test

Lewin punch test

Lewin snuff test

Lewin standing test

Lewin supine test

Linder sign

Matchstick test

Mennell sign

Milgram test

Continued

8

TABLE 8-1

LUMBAR SPINE CROSS-REFERENCE TABLE BY ASSESSMENT PROCEDURE—cont'd

Disease Assessed	Minor sign	Nachlas test	Neri sign	Prone knee-bending test	Quick test
Lower Extremity Joints					•
Fracture	•				
Denervation					
Myofascitis					
Hamstring Spasm					
Sacroiliac Lesion	•	•	•		
Meningitis					
L2–L3–L4				•	
Femoral Nerve				•	
Hip Lesion					
Sprain					
Spinal Neuropathy					
Cord Tumor					
Mechanical Lower Back		•	•		
Subluxation		•			
Dural Adhesions					
Intervertebral Foramen Encroachment					
Sciatica					
Intervertebral Disc Syndrome	•		•		

Lumbar Spine — Test/Sign

Test									
Schober test			●						
Sicard sign		●							
Sign of the buttock			●						
Skin pinch test			●						
Spinal percussion test			●		●				
Straight-leg-raising test		●		●		●			
Turyn sign									
Vanzetti sign									

8

TABLE 8-2

LUMBAR SPINE CROSS-REFERENCE TABLE BY SYNDROME OR TISSUE

Cord tumor	Bragard sign
	Lasègue test
	Milgram test
	Straight-leg-raising test
Denervation	Matchstick test
	Skin pinch test
Dural adhesions	Bechterew sitting test
	Fajersztajn test
	Lasègue test
	Straight-leg-raising test
Femoral nerve	Ely sign
	Femoral nerve traction test
	Hyperextension test
	Prone knee-bending test
Fracture	Minor sign
	Spinal percussion test
Hamstring spasm	Lewin standing test
Hip lesion	Ely sign
	Sign of the buttock
Intervertebral disc syndrome	Antalgia sign
	Bechterew sitting test
	Bilateral leg-lowering test
	Bragard sign
	Cox sign
	Double-leg-raise test
	Fajersztajn test
	Heel/toe walk test
	Kemp test
	Lasègue rebound test
	Lasègue test
	Lewin punch test
	Lewin snuff test
	Lewin supine test
	Matchstick test
	Milgram test
	Minor sign
	Neri sign
	Skin pinch test
	Spinal percussion test
	Straight-leg-raising test
Intervertebral foramen encroachment	Bechterew sitting test
	Bilateral leg-lowering test
	Lasègue test

TABLE 8-2

LUMBAR SPINE CROSS-REFERENCE TABLE BY SYNDROME OR TISSUE—cont'd

L2–L3–L4	Femoral nerve traction test
	Hyperextension test
	Prone knee-bending test
Lower extremity joints	Quick test
Mechanical lower back	Bilateral leg-lowering test
	Demianoff sign
	Double-leg-raise test
	Kemp test
	Lasègue test
	Nachlas test
	Neri sign
	Schober test
	Sign of the buttock
	Skin pinch test
	Spinal percussion test
Meningitis	Kernig/Brudzinski sign
Myofascitis	Lewin supine test
	Skin pinch test
Sacroiliac lesion	Lasègue test
	Lewin supine test
	Mennell sign
	Minor sign
	Nachlas test
	Neri sign
Sciatica	Bechterew sitting test
	Bragard sign
	Deyerle sign
	Fajersztajn test
	Heel/toe walk test
	Lasègue sitting test
	Lasègue test
	Lewin snuff test
	Lewin standing test
	Lewin supine test
	Sicard sign
	Turyn sign
	Vanzetti sign

8

Continued

TABLE 8-2

LUMBAR SPINE CROSS-REFERENCE TABLE BY SYNDROME OR TISSUE—cont'd

Spinal neuropathy	Bowstring sign
	Bragard sign
	Ely sign
	Femoral nerve traction test
	Heel/toe walk test
	Kemp test
	Lasègue differential sign
	Lasègue sitting test
	Sicard sign
Sprain	Double-leg-raise test
	Spinal percussion test
Subluxation	Bechterew sitting test
	Nachlas test

TABLE 8-3

CLINICAL CHARACTERISTICS OF SPONDYLOARTHROPATHIES

- Typical pattern of peripheral arthritis: predominantly of lower limb, asymmetric
- Tendency to radiographic sacroiliitis
- Absence of rheumatoid factor
- Absence of subcutaneous nodules and other extraarticular features of rheumatoid arthritis
- Overlapping extraarticular features characteristic of the group (e.g., anterior uveitis)
- Significant familial aggregation
- Association with HLA-B27

HLA, Human leukocyte antigen.
Adapted From Kelley WN et al: *Textbook of rheumatology,* ed 5, Philadelphia, 1997, WB Saunders.

TABLE 8-4

DISEASES BELONGING TO THE SPONDYLOARTHROPATHIES

- Ankylosing spondylitis
- Reiter syndrome, reactive arthritis
- Arthropathy of inflammatory bowel disease (Crohn disease, ulcerative colitis)
- Psoriatic arthritis
- Undifferentiated spondyloarthropathies
- Juvenile chronic arthritis: juvenile-onset ankylosing spondylitis

Adapted From Kelley WN et al: *Textbook of rheumatology,* ed 5, Philadelphia, 1997, WB Saunders.

TABLE 8-5

GENDER PREVALENCE IN LOW BACK PAIN

Male predominance	Spondyloarthropathies
	Vertebral osteomyelitis
	Benign and malignant neoplasms
	Paget disease
	Retroperitoneal fibrosis
	Peptic ulcer disease
	Work-related mechanical disorders
Female predominance	Polymyalgia rheumatica
	Fibromyalgia
	Osteoporosis
	Parathyroid disease

Data from Klippel JH, Dieppe PA: *Rheumatology,* vol 1-2, ed 2, London, 1998, Mosby.

8

organs directly, and the functional equilibrium of the spine depends on the efficient performance of other organs.

The spine contributes to many mutual relationships within the total body. With its equilibrium (statics), the spine exerts, influences, and receives forces (dynamics), all of which are interwoven with the far-reaching chain of motion (kinetics). In addition, the spine is able to exercise considerable influence on neighboring structures, as well as on remote organs. This influence is its action on nerves and blood vessels. To a considerable degree, this complicated system depends on the metabolism, the mineral metabolism of the bones, and the nutrition of the bradytrophic ligamentous and disc tissues. Improper function of the endocrine glands also affects the spine.

During fetal development, the spine may be exposed to many influences, such as drug-induced malformations, lack of oxygen, or radiation.

Occupational and daily-living stresses, as well as traumatic influences, may combine to have an unfavorable effect when coupled with the aging process, which has a marked effect on the disc apparatus and the bony substance. More resources for the diagnosis and treatment of spinal diseases are available today than previously.

Degeneration of posture during early years, lack of exercise, physical weakness, and degenerative changes in later life have taken on a serious social significance for the cultures of industrialized nations.

The spine is an intricate and interesting mechanical structure. The spine's functions are mechanical, and it is well suited for serving its basic mechanical roles. The materials used to execute the design are appropriate for enhancing these functions. The spine must transfer loads from the trunk to the pelvis, must allow for physiologic motion, and must protect the spinal cord from damage. When a proper appreciation of normal anatomy and mechanics has been gained, the pathophysiologic features of the diseased or deformed spine become clear.

The lumbar spine is designed to withstand loading and to provide truncal mobility. The primary plane of motion is during flexion-extension, although axial rotation at the L5 level is significant. This rotation in the lower lumbar spine is particularly important, considering that the annulus fails and tears with torsional forces. Coupling in the lumbar spine is the opposite of cervical and thoracic spine coupling. The spinous processes move toward the concavity of the curve in physiologic lateral flexion.

Optimal spinal mobility in relation to age is difficult to pin down. The only generalization that can be made is that spinal mobility is probably greatest during adolescence and early adulthood. This tendency is significant when planning treatment and in determining prognoses.

The anatomic structures of the lumbosacral spine receive specific types of sensory innervation that are associated with distinct qualities of pain (Table 8-6).

TABLE 8-6

SUMMARY OF THE CHARACTERISTICS OF LOW BACK PAIN OF VARIOUS ORIGINS

Source of Pain	Distribution	Nature	Aggravating Factors	Neurologic Changes
Spinal pain	Sclerotomal Local	Sharp Dull	Motion	None
Discogenic pain	Sclerotomal	Deep, aching	Increased intradiscal pressure (e.g., bending, sitting, Valsalva maneuver)	None
Nerve root pain	Radicular	Paresthesias Numbness	Root stretching	Present
Multiple lumbar spinal stenosis pain	Radicular Sclerotomal	Paresthesias Spinal claudication pattern	Lumbar extension Walking	Present
Referred visceral pain	Dermatomal	Deep, aching	Related to affected organ	None

From Kelley WN, et al: *Textbook of rheumatology*, ed 5, Philadelphia, 1997, WB Saunders.

8

ESSENTIAL ANATOMY

The lumbar spine consists of five lumbar vertebrae, numbered L1 to L5, followed by five fused sacral bodies that form the sacrum and the coccyx. The alignment of the lumbar spine generally has a lordotic contour. The normal lordosis is 30 to 50 degrees (apex L3) in a standing person.

ESSENTIAL MOTION ASSESSMENT

Range-of-motion findings are most helpful in pinpointing a vertebral structure that may be compromised in the lumbar spine. Pain at an early point in the extension of the lumbar spine suggests an inflamed posterior joint or pars disease. Painful lumbar flexion in the early-to-middle range connotes a faulty disc mechanism or muscular stain. Because the terminal range of flexion causes the facet joint capsule to stretch, a pain response at this point may indicate a posterior joint sprain.

Patients with acute spasm or significant trauma often have multidirectional complaints and severe limitation of motion in all planes. Therefore, range-of-motion testing may be initially inconclusive as to the severity of the injury.

To assess the contribution made to flexion by the lumbar spine, the examiner should mark the spine at the lumbosacral junction and then 10 cm above and 5 cm below this point. On forward flexion, the distance between the two upper marks should increase by approximately 4 cm, the distance between the lower two remaining unaltered (Figs. 8-1 to 8-4).

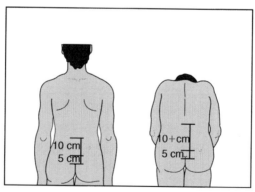

FIG. 8-1

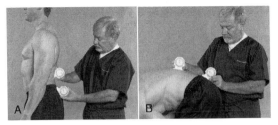

FIG. 8-2 The patient flexes forward, and the angle of both inclinometers is recorded. The sacral inclination is subtracted from the T12 inclination to obtain the lumbar flexion angle.

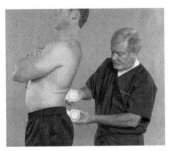

FIG. 8-3 Extension is limited to 35 degrees in the lumbar spine. The patient extends the lumbar spine, and the angles of both instruments are recorded. The sacral inclination angle is subtracted from the T12 inclination angle to obtain the lumbar extension angle.

8

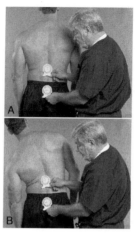

FIG. 8-4 Both instruments are zeroed at the superior aspect of the sacrum, in the coronal plane (**A**). The patient laterally flexes the lumbar spine to one side, and the inclinations of both instruments are recorded (**B**). The sacral angle is subtracted from the T12 angle to obtain the lumbar lateral flexion angle. The procedure is repeated for the range of motion to the opposite side. Lateral flexion of 20 degrees or less to either side is an impairment of the lumbar spine in the activities of daily living.

ESSENTIAL MUSCLE FUNCTION ASSESSMENT

The erector spinae consist of a minor portion (the spinalis) and two major portions (the longissimus and iliocostalis). The spinalis connects spinous processes, and the longissimus and iliocostalis connect homologous portions of the costal and transverse elements of the lumbar, thoracic, and cervical vertebrae and skull.

Useful in screening is muscle testing of the legs, which measures strength on a 5-point scale for extension and flexion (knee), abduction and adduction (hip), and eversion and inversion, as well as dorsiflexion and plantar flexion (foot) (Table 8-7).

TABLE 8-7
LUMBAR RADICULAR SYNDROMES

Disc Level	Any Central Disc Herniation	L5/S1	L4/L5	L3/L4
Nerve root involved	Cauda equina (L4/L5 > L5/S1)	S1	L5	L4
Pain referral pattern	Perineum Low back Buttocks Either or both legs	Unilateral Low back Buttocks Posterior leg	Unilateral Low back Buttocks Lateral leg and thigh	Unilateral Low back Buttocks Posterolateral leg
Motor deficit	Unilateral or bilateral leg weakness	Unilateral weakness; plantar flexion of foot; difficulty with toe walking	Unilateral weakness; dorsiflexion of foot; difficulty with heel walking	Unilateral quadriceps weakness
Sensory deficit	Perineum/buttocks, low back, thighs, legs, feet	Lateral foot, posterolateral calf	Lateral calf; between the first and second toes	Knee distal, anterior thigh
Reflexes compromised	Ankle jerk	Ankle jerk	0	Knee jerk

From Demeter SL, Andersson GBJ, Smith GM: *Disability evaluation*. St Louis, 1996, Mosby.

8

ORTHOPEDIC GAMUT 8-1

LOWER EXTREMITY MUSCULATURE

Sequential innervation lower extremity musculature:

1. L2 and L3 supply hip flexion
2. L4 and L5 hip extension
3. L3 and L4 supply knee extension
4. L5 and S1 knee flexion
5. L4 and L5 supply ankle dorsiflexion
6. S1 and S2 ankle plantar flexion
7. L4 supplies ankle inversion
8. L5 and S1 supply ankle eversion

For patients in whom the objective findings do not match the subjective complaints, close observation helps identify the inconsistencies (Table 8-8). A finding of three or more of the five signs of the Waddell index is clinically significant. Isolated positive signs are ignored.

TABLE 8-8

NONORGANIC PHYSICAL SIGNS INDICATING
ILLNESS BEHAVIOR

	Physical Disease/ Normal Illness Behavior	**Abnormal Illness Behavior**
Symptoms		
Pain	Anatomic distribution	Whole leg pain Tailbone pain
Numbness	Dermatomal	Whole leg numbness
Weakness	Myotomal	Whole leg giving way
Time pattern	Varies with time and activity	Never free of pain
Response to treatment	Variable benefit	Intolerance of treatments Emergency admissions to hospital

TABLE 8-8

NONORGANIC PHYSICAL SIGNS INDICATING
ILLNESS BEHAVIOR—cont'd

	Physical Disease/ Normal Illness Behavior	Abnormal Illness Behavior
Signs		
Tenderness	Anatomic distribution	Superficial Widespread nonanatomic
Axial loading	No lumbar pain	Lumbar pain
Simulated rotation	No lumbar pain	Lumbar pain
Straight leg raising	Limited on distraction	Improves with distraction
Sensory	Dermatomal	Regional
Motor	Myotomal	Regional, jerky, giving way

From Demeter SL, Andersson GBJ, Smith GM: *Disability evaluation,* St Louis, 1996, Mosby.

The iliacus arises from the iliac fossa and joins the psoas under the inguinal ligament. The iliacus then crosses the hip joint capsule and inserts into the lesser trochanter of the femur. These muscles flex the lumbar spine and bend it toward the same side. The quadratus lumborum, which lies lateral to the vertebral column, arises from the posterior part of the iliac crest and iliolumbar ligament and inserts into the twelfth rib and the tips of the transverse processes of the upper four lumbar vertebrae. This muscle fixes the diaphragm during inspiration and bends the trunk toward the same side when it acts alone (Figs. 8-5 to 8-7).

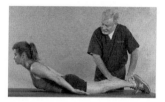

FIG. 8-5 The patient is lying prone on the examination table. The patient then extends the trunk.

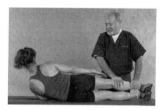

FIG. 8-6 Lateral flexion of the trunk requires a combination of lateral flexion and hip abduction. The patient is side lying, with the head, upper trunk, pelvis, and lower extremities in a straight line. During the test, the patient laterally flexes the trunk away from the examination table.

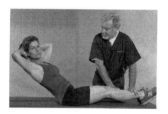

FIG. 8-7 Raising the trunk obliquely forward combines trunk flexion and rotation. The patient is supine on the examination table, and the legs are supported by the examiner.

ESSENTIAL IMAGING

A variety of radiographic views can be taken when the lumbosacral region is evaluated. The standard views consist of the anteroposterior (AP), lateral, oblique, and either a frontal or a lateral lumbosacral spot.

ANTALGIA SIGN

Assessment for Posterolateral, Posteromedial, and Posterocentral Intervertebral Disc Protrusion

Comment

Two major types of low back abnormalities center on the intervertebral disc: acute impairment from herniated discs and chronic impairment from degenerative disc disease (Table 8-9).

TABLE 8-9

LUMBAR DISC SYNDROMES

	Lumbar Herniated Nucleus Pulposus	Degenerative Disc Disease

Physical examination findings	Back or leg pain
	Sciatic nerve tension signs:
	    Positive straight leg raise less than 60 degrees
	    Positive Bragard sign
	    Positive bowstring sign
	    Positive Bechterew test
	    Painful arc of lumbar flexion, extension, or both
	True nerve root signs:
	    Radiculopathy
	    Motor or sensory deficit
	    Paresthesias
	    Diminished or absent deep-tendon reflexes
	    Possible antalgia, muscle spasm, instability
		Morning stiffness
		Lumbopelvic hypomobility
		Pain in lumbar flexion
		History consistent with spinal degeneration

X-ray findings	Need to rule out organic abnormality Hypolordosis secondary to muscle spasm Possible loss of intervertebral disc height Possible diagnosis of degenerative arthritis	Radiologic signs in acute exacerbation Spur formation Loss of intervertebral disc height Discogenic spondylosis Compatible findings on CT or MRI scans

CT, Computed tomography; *MRI,* magnetic resonance imaging.
Adapted from Brier SR: *Primary care orthopedics,* St Louis, 1999, Mosby.

ORTHOPEDIC GAMUT 8-2

DISC INJURIES

Definitions of disc injuries are as follows:

1. *Disc protrusion* is present when nuclear material does not extend beyond the annulus in a contained herniated nucleus pulposus.

2. *Disc extrusion* is a focal herniation contained by the posterior longitudinal ligament that extends into the spinal canal.

3. *Sequestered disc* is a free fragment that has broken off or through the annular peripheral fibers in the vertebral canal (prolapsed).

A disc may protrude lateral to a nerve root, medial to a nerve root, under a nerve root, or central to the nerve root.

PROCEDURE

- When the disc protrudes lateral to the nerve root, the patient assumes an antalgic lean away from the side of the disc lesion or pain (Fig. 8-8).
- When the disc protrudes medial to the nerve root, the patient assumes an antalgic lean into the side of the disc lesion or pain (Fig. 8-9).
- With a central disc lesion, the patient assumes a flexed posture of the lumbar spine, with or without leaning to either side (Fig. 8-10).
- With protrusion under the nerve root, the patient may not lean at all.

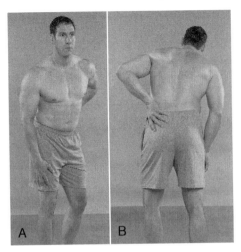

FIG. 8-8

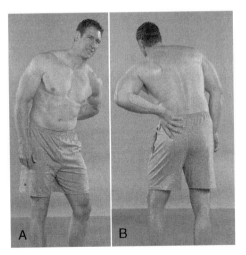

FIG. 8-9

8

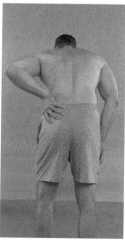

FIG. 8-10 With a central disc lesion, the patient assumes a flexed posture of the lumbar spine, with or without leaning to either side.

CLINICAL PEARL

If the antalgia is not readily apparent in a static posture, it will appear with forward flexion of the trunk. If a disc protrusion exists, even in the mildest degree, trunk flexion exerts enough pressure to irritate the inflamed muscle or to stretch neural structures over the bulging disc. The antalgia is manifested at this point. Patients with lower back pain might stiffen the trunk and pelvis and hyperextend the knees in an effort to decrease the number of degrees of freedom.

BECHTEREW SITTING TEST

Assessment for Sciatica, Intervertebral Disc Lesion, Vertebral Exostoses, Dural Sleeve Adhesions, Muscular Spasm, or Vertebral Subluxation

PROCEDURE

- While in a seated position, the patient attempts to extend each leg, one at a time.
- The examiner restricts the patient's attempts at hip flexion with downward pressure on the thigh (Fig. 8-11).
- This extension is followed by an attempt to extend both legs.
- The test is positive if backache or sciatic pain is increased or if the maneuver is impossible.
- In disc involvement, extending both legs will usually increase the spinal and sciatic discomfort.
- A positive test indicates sciatica, a disc lesion, exostoses, adhesions, spasm, or subluxation.

8

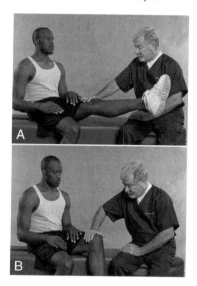

FIG. 8-11

CLINICAL PEARL

Simple flattening or even reversing the lumbar curve is often not associated with radicular pain. The pain is localized in the lower lumbar spine, and any movement of the spine accentuates the pain. In these instances, the prime pathologic feature is sprain of an intervertebral joint rather than root irritation.

BILATERAL LEG-LOWERING TEST

Assessment for Mechanical Lumbosacral Lesion, Intervertebral Disc Lesion, or Vertebral Exostoses

PROCEDURE

- The patient lowers the straightened legs from a 90-degree angle to a 45-degree angle (Fig. 8-12).
- The test is positive if the legs drop or if the move produces pain.
- A positive test indicates lumbosacral involvement, disc lesions, or exostoses.

8

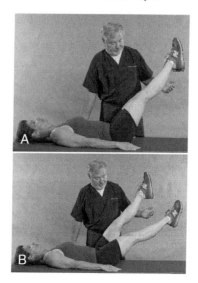

FIG. 8-12

BOWSTRING SIGN

Assessment for Lumbar Nerve Root Compression

ORTHOPEDIC GAMUT 8-3

LUMBOSACRAL NERVE ROOTS

After leaving the dural sac, the lumbosacral nerve roots run caudally and laterally in the direction of departure from the spinal canal:

1. The fourth lumbar root (L4) leaves the dural sac slightly caudal of the intervertebral disc between the third and fourth lumbar vertebrae (third lumbar disc).
2. The fifth lumbar root (L5) leaves the dural sac near the level of the fourth lumbar disc.
3. The first sacral root (S1) leaves the dural sac medial of S1 and slightly below the level of the L5 disc.

ORTHOPEDIC GAMUT 8-4

WALLERIAN DEGENERATION SEQUENCE

8

- When axonal continuity is disrupted by mechanical compression or nerve trunk ischemia:
  - Axons distal to the stump divide finely and begin to degenerate.
  - At the same time, the myelin sheaths that have lost axons begin to break down.
- Wallerian degeneration occurs peripheral to the site of compression in the anterior root and central to this site (i.e., toward the spinal cord) in the posterior root when the cauda equina or nerve root is compressed by a herniated intervertebral disc or spinal canal stenosis.
- Nerve roots have a regenerative capacity similar to that of peripheral nerves.
- While regeneration of the anterior root approximates that of peripheral nerves, recovery of sensation presents problems in the posterior root because degeneration extends into the spinal cord.

PROCEDURE

- With the patient in the supine position, the examiner moves the patient's leg until it is above the examiner's shoulder.
- At this point, firm pressure should be exerted on the hamstring muscles (Fig. 8-13).
- If pain is not elicited, pressure is applied to the popliteal fossa.
- Pain in the lumbar region or radiculopathy is a positive sign for nerve root compression.

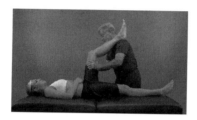

FIG. 8-13

CLINICAL PEARL

Nerve roots must change their lengths depending on the degree of flexion, extension, lateral flexion, and rotation of the lumbar spine. Lumbar nerve roots that are limited in motion by fibrosis of either intraspinal or extraspinal origin will create traction on the nerve root complex, causing ischemia and secondary neural dysfunction.

BRAGARD SIGN

Assessment for Sciatic Neuritis, Spinal Cord Tumor, Intervertebral Disc Lesions, and Spinal Nerve Irritation

PROCEDURE

- If the Lasègue test or the straight-leg-raising test is positive, the leg is lowered below the point of discomfort, and the foot is sharply dorsiflexed (Fig. 8-14).
- The sign is present if pain is increased.
- The presence of the sign is a finding associated with sciatic neuritis, spinal cord tumors, intervertebral disc lesions, and spinal nerve irritations.

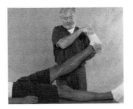

FIG. 8-14

8

CLINICAL PEARL

Either the *Bragard sign* or the *Hyndman sign* (for neck flexion movement) must be accomplished as a finishing maneuver in any positive straight-leg-raising test. Pain that increases during neck flexion, ankle dorsiflexion, or both indicates an inflamed nerve root. Pain that does not increase with these maneuvers may indicate a problem in the hamstring area or in the lumbosacral or sacroiliac joints.

COX SIGN

Assessment for Prolapse of Intervertebral Disc Nucleus

Comment

Several maneuvers tighten the sciatic nerve and compress an inflamed nerve root against a herniated lumbar disc. With the straight-leg-raising tests, the L5 and S1 nerve roots move several millimeters at the level of the foramen. The L4 nerve root moves a smaller distance, and the proximal roots show little motion. The straight-leg-raising tests are most important and valuable for detecting lesions of the L5 and S1 nerve roots. Young patients with herniated discs have marked propensities for positive straight-leg-raising tests. Although the test itself is not pathognomonic, a negative test rules out the possibility of a herniated disc. After age 30, a negative straight-leg-raising test no longer precludes this diagnosis. Lumbosacral transitional vertebrae complicate this further (Table 8-10).

TABLE 8-10

Castellvi Classification of Lumbosacral Transitional Vertebra

- Type I: dysplastic transverse process
  - Type Ia (unilateral) height >19mm
  - Type Ib (bilateral) height >19 mm
  - Type I is not considered a true lumbosacral transitional vertebra because no articulation with the sacrum is present
- Type II: incomplete lumbarization/sacralization
  - Type IIa enlarged transverse process with unilateral pseudoarthrosis with the adjacent sacral ala
  - Type IIb enlarged transverse process with bilateral pseudoarthrosis with the adjacent sacral ala
- Type III: complete lumbarization/sacralization
  - Type IIIa enlarged transverse process that has unilateral complete fusion with the adjacent sacral ala
  - Type IIIb enlarged transverse process that has bilateral complete fusion with the adjacent sacral ala
- Type IV: mixed (type IIa on one side and type IIIa on the other)

PROCEDURE

- Cox sign occurs during straight leg raising when the pelvis rises from the table instead of the hip flexing (Fig. 8-15).
- Cox sign is present when patients have a prolapse of the nucleus into the intervertebral foramen.

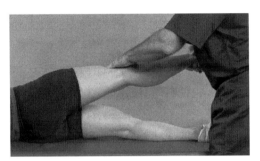

FIG. 8-15

CLINICAL PEARL

Cox sign is a consistent finding associated with disc prolapse. The sign is often overlooked in the patient's pain presentation. A false-negative test result may occur if the examiner does not observe the movements of the buttocks on the affected side. The sign is present the moment hip flexion motion is locked and the buttock rises from the examination table.

DEMIANOFF SIGN

Assessment for Spasm of the Sacrolumbalis (Iliocostalis Lumborum) Musculature

---

ORTHOPEDIC GAMUT 8-5

COMMON INFECTIVE ORGANISMS IN DISCITIS

- *Neisseria gonorrhoeae*
- *Neisseria meningitidis*
- *Listeria monocytogenes*
- *Mycoplasma*
- *Ureaplasma urealyticum*

ORTHOPEDIC GAMUT 8-6

DISC SPACE INFECTION

The radiographic evidence of established disc space infection includes:

1. Symmetric destruction of adjacent end-plate surfaces of two vertebrae
2. Loss of disc height
3. Reactive new bone formation
4. Sclerosis of bone end-plates, with or without evidence of bone destruction or bone formation
5. Soft-tissue abscesses
6. Kyphosis or subluxation after previous significant bone destruction

PROCEDURE

- While the patient is in the supine position, the examiner performs a straight-leg-raising test with either leg.
- The sign is present when this action produces a pain in the lumbar region.
- This pain prevents the patient from raising the leg high enough to form an angle between the examination table and the leg of 15 degrees or more (Fig. 8-16).
- The sign differentiates pain that originates in the sacrolumbalis muscles from lumbar pain of any other origin.
- A positive test demonstrates that the pain is caused by the stretching of the sacrolumbalis (iliocostalis lumborum).

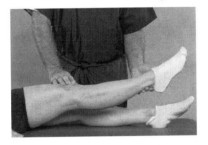

FIG. 8-16

8

CLINICAL PEARL

Demianoff sign is clearly separate from Cox sign. Demianoff sign involves production of lower back pain, which prevents further raising of the leg. Sciatica is absent. Cox sign is present when the pelvis is locked, which prevents further elevation of the leg because of increasing sciatica.

DEYERLE SIGN

Assessment for Sciatic Nerve Irritation

Comment

Occasionally, L4 lesions may also cause similar symptoms and signs. The phase of degeneration or spondylosis often determines the level of intervention (Table 8-11).

TABLE 8-11

Overview of Scheme of Treatment Relative to the Phase of Spondylosis

Phase	Lesion	Treatment
Dysfunction	Facet joint	Mobilization, manipulation, injection
	Sacroiliac joint	
	Myofascial syndromes	Mobilization, manipulation, injection
	Disc herniation	Contract stretching, injection
		Epidural injection, discectomy
Unstable	Disc herniation	Epidural injection, discectomy
	Segmental instability	Injection, fusion
	Lateral stenosis	Nerve root block, decompression, fusion
	Central stenosis	
	Degenerative olisthesis	Epidural injection, decompression, fusion
	Isthmic olisthesis	Epidural injection, decompression, fusion
		Epidural injection, decompression, fusion
Stabilization	Disc herniation	Epidural injection, discectomy
	Lateral stenosis	Nerve root block, decompression
	Central stenosis	Epidural injection, decompression
	Degenerative olisthesis	Epidural injection, decompression, rarely fusion
	Isthmic olisthesis	Epidural injection, decompression, rarely fusion

From Kirkaldy WH: *Managing low back pain*, ed 4, Philadelphia 1999, Churchill Livingstone.

PROCEDURE

- While the patient is seated, the affected leg is passively extended at the knee until pain is reproduced.
- The knee is then slightly flexed while strong pressure is applied by the examiner into the popliteal fossa (Fig. 8-17).
- The sign is present if this pressure increases radicular symptoms.
- The sign demonstrates irritation of the sciatic nerve above the knee.
- This irritation is caused by stretching the nerve over an abnormal mechanical obstruction.

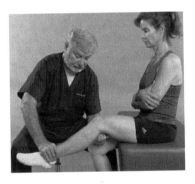

FIG. 8-17

8

CLINICAL PEARL

Deyerle sign is a variation of the Lasègue sitting test. The sign demonstrates the effects of inflammation or partial denervation (neural compression) in the sciatic distribution. The pain response may be caused by myalgic hyperalgesia as a response to denervation hypersensitivity.

DOUBLE-LEG-RAISE TEST

ALSO KNOWN AS BILATERAL STRAIGHT-LEG-RAISING TEST

Assessment for Lumbosacral Joint Involvement

PROCEDURE

- While the patient is supine, the examiner performs a straight-leg-raising test on each of the patient's lower extremities, noting the angle at which the pain is produced.
- Next, both lower limbs are raised together.
- If pain is produced at an earlier angle by raising both legs together, the test is positive (Fig. 8-18).
- In the presence of disc disease with resulting vertebral instability, the double-leg-raising movement will cause pain in the lumbar area.
- The test is specific and highly accurate for lumbosacral joint involvement.

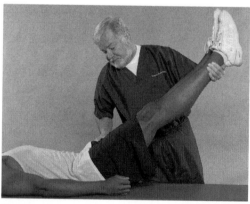

FIG. 8-18

CLINICAL PEARL

Atypical cases of disc prolapse are common. A definite history of injury or strain is often lacking. The pain may begin gradually rather than suddenly, and the symptoms may be confined to the back and never radiate down the leg. On the other hand, the pain is sometimes felt predominantly in the limb and is scarcely perceptible in the back.

8

ELY SIGN

ELY HEEL-TO-BUTTOCK TEST

Assessment for Lumbar Radicular or Femoral Nerve Inflammation

Comment

The size of the lumbar vertebral canal ranges from 12 to 20 mm in its AP dimension at the mid sagittal plane and 18 to 27 mm in its transverse diameter. Stenosis has been defined as a narrowing below the lowest value of the range of normal (Table 8-12).

TABLE 8-12

DIMENSIONS OF THE LUMBAR VERTEBRAL FORAMINA (VERTEBRAL CANAL)*

Dimension	Size (Range)[†]
Anteroposterior (in midsagittal plane)	12–20 mm
Transverse (interpedicular distance)	18–27 mm

*Dimensions below the lowest value indicate spinal (vertebral) canal stenosis.

[‡] A typical vertebral foramen is rather triangular (trefoil) in shape. However, the upper lumbar vertebral foramina are more rounded than the lower lumbar foramina. L1 is the most rounded, and each succeeding lumbar vertebra becomes increasingly triangular, with L5 most dramatically trefoil of all. From Dommisse GF, Louw JA: Anatomy of the lumbar spine. In Floman Y, editor: *Disorders of the lumbar spine*, Rockville, Md, and Tel Aviv, Israel, 1990, Aspen and Freund Publishing House.

[†] Dimensions of lumbar vertebral foramina are usually smaller than those of the cervical region but larger than those of the thoracic region. From Cramer GD, Darby SA: *Basic and clinical anatomy of the spine, spinal cord, and ANS,* St Louis, 1995, Mosby.

ORTHOPEDIC GAMUT 8-7

MODIFIED ARNOLD INTERNATIONAL CLASSIFICATION OF LUMBAR SPINAL STENOSIS AND NERVE ROOT ENTRAPMENT SYNDROMES

- Congenital stenosis
  - Idiopathic
  - Achondroplastic
- Acquired stenosis
  - Degenerative
  - Combined
  - Spondylolisthetic, spondylolytic
  - Iatrogenic
  - Posttraumatic
  - Paget disease
  - Fluorosis
- Degenerative lumbar spinal stenosis with scoliosis

ORTHOPEDIC GAMUT 8-8

8

COMPLEX REGIONAL PAIN SYNDROME DIAGNOSTIC CRITERIA (INTERNATIONAL ASSOCIATION FOR THE STUDY OF PAIN)

1. Complex regional pain syndrome type I (CRPS-I) is a syndrome that develops after an initiating noxious event.
2. Spontaneous pain or allodynia/hyperalgesia occurs, is not limited to the territory of a single peripheral nerve, and is disproportionate to the inciting event.
3. Evidence exists or has existed of edema, skin blood flow abnormality, or abnormal sudomotor activity in the region of the pain since the inciting event.
4. This diagnosis is excluded by the existence of conditions that would otherwise account for the degree of pain and dysfunction.
5. For the diagnosis of CRPS-I, criteria 2 through 4 must be fulfilled.

PROCEDURE

- The patient is prone, with the toes hanging over the edge of the table and legs relaxed.
- One or the other heel is approximated to the opposite buttock (Fig. 8-19).
- After flexion of the knee, the thigh is hyperextended.
- With any significant hip lesion, performing this test will normally be impossible.
- With irritation of the iliopsoas muscle or its sheath, extending the thigh to any normal degree will be impossible.
- This test will aggravate inflammation of the lumbar nerve roots and will be accompanied by production of femoral radicular pain.
- The test will also stretch lumbar nerve root adhesions, which will be accompanied by upper lumbar discomfort.

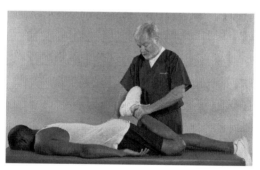

FIG. 8-19

CLINICAL PEARL

In the uncommon cases of high lumbar and mid lumbar disc prolapse, the pain radiates toward the groin and front of the thigh rather than to the back of the thigh and leg.

FAJERSZTAJN TEST

ALSO KNOWN AS WELL-LEG-RAISING TEST OF FAJERSZTAJN, PROSTRATE LEG-RAISING TEST, SCIATIC PHENOMENON, AND CROSS-OVER SIGN

Assessment for Lumbar Nerve Root Lesion Caused by Intervertebral Disc Syndrome or Dural Sleeve Adhesion

---

ORTHOPEDIC GAMUT 8-9

LUMBAR CENTRAL CANAL STENOSIS

Structural causes for lumbar central canal stenosis are as follows:

1. *Osseous:* inferior facet arthrosis
2. *Discogenic:* central disc herniation
3. *Ligamentous:* ligamentum flavum buckling in degenerative spinal disease

---

8

PROCEDURE

- Straight-leg-raising and dorsiflexion of the foot are performed on the asymptomatic side of a sciatic patient (Fig. 8-20).
- When this test causes pain on the symptomatic side, Fajersztajn sign is present.
- The sign indicates sciatic nerve root involvement, such as a disc syndrome or dural root sleeve adhesions.

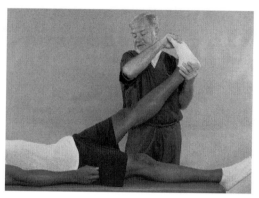

FIG. 8-20

CLINICAL PEARL

Several factors my produce pain in the back or lower extremities. Some of these causes are (1) tumors of the spinal cord or cauda equina, (2) tumors of the spinal column, (3) tuberculosis of the spine, (4) osteoarthritis, (5) tumors of the ilium or sacrum, (6) spondylolisthesis, (7) prolapsed intervertebral disc, (8) ankylosing spondylitis, (9) vascular occlusion, (10) intrapelvic mass, and (11) arthritis of the hip. All of these possible causes must be considered in differential diagnosis.

FEMORAL NERVE TRACTION TEST

Assessment for Mid Lumbar Nerve Root Involvement (L2, L3, and L4)

Comment

A large, midline disc herniation can compress several nerve roots of the cauda equina and can mimic an intraspinal tumor. Usually, lower back and perineal symptoms predominate, with radicular symptoms being masked. Difficulty with urination, such as frequency or overflow incontinence, may develop early. In men, a recent history of sexual impotence may be elicited. The patients experience pain down the posterior thighs to the soles of the feet accompanied by weakness of the legs and feet. L2, L3, and L4 radiculopathies are less common than the L5 and S1 radiculopathies, probably because of their relatively short course within the cauda equina, which makes them less susceptible to compression (Table 8-13).

TABLE 8-13

DIFFERENTIAL ELECTRODIAGNOSIS OF UPPER LUMBAR RADICULOPATHY

	Femoral Neuropathy	Lumbar Plexopathy	Lumbar Radiculopathy
Thigh adductors	Normal	Denervation	Denervation
Tibialis anterior	Normal	Denervation*	Denervation*
Saphenous SNAP[†]	Low or absent[‡]	Low or absent[‡]	Normal
Paraspinal fibrillations	Absent	Absent	Usually present

SNAP, Sensory nerve action potential.

*Abnormal in L4 radiculopathy/plexopathy only.

[†]May be technically difficult, particularly in the elderly patients or if leg edema is present.

[‡]Normal in purely demyelinating lesions.

From Katirji B: *Electromyography in clinical practice: a case study approach,* St Louis, 1998, Mosby.

8

ORTHOPEDIC GAMUT 8-10

UPPER LUMBAR RADICULOPATHY

The electrophysiologic confirmation of an upper lumbar radiculopathy is challenging for the following reasons:

1. The exact compressed root is difficult to identify among upper lumbar roots because of the limited number of muscles innervated by the roots.
2. The myotomal representation of these roots occurs in proximally situated muscles, mostly above the knee (except for the tibialis anterior).
3. A lack of available sensory nerve action potential exists for confirming that the upper lumbar lesion is preganglionic.

PROCEDURE

- The side-lying patient slightly flexes the hip and knee on the unaffected side.
- With neck slightly flexed, the patient's back is straight (not hyperextended).
- The affected limb is extended at the hip 15 degrees.
- The affected knee is flexed, stretching the femoral nerve (Fig. 8-21).
- If the test is positive, pain radiates into the anterior thigh.

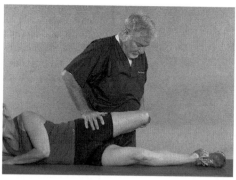

FIG. 8-21

CLINICAL PEARL

Upper lumbar disc disturbances may cause weakness of the quadriceps muscle and a diminished or absent patellar reflex. The straight-leg-raising tests and signs may be negative. Pinwheel examination usually reveals hyperesthesia or hypoesthesia of the L4 dermatome.

8

HEEL/TOE WALK TEST

Assessment for L5 or S1 Nerve Root Motor Deficiency

Comment

Muscle weakness, atrophy, or the inability to perform functional testing maneuvers all suggest the presence of nerve root compression that is more significant than the alteration of sensation (Table 8-14).

TABLE 8-14

SPECIFIC DORSOLUMBAR RADICULOPATHY PATTERNS

Nerve	HNP	Foramen	Muscle	Reflex	Sensation
T10					Umbilicus
T12					Pubis
L1	T12–L1	L1–L2			Upper anterior thigh
L2	L1–L2	L2–L3			Mid anterior thigh
L3	L2–L3	L3–L4	Quadriceps femoris		Lower anterior thigh
L4	L3–L4	L4–L5	Quadriceps femoris Anterior tibial	Patella	Anterior thigh Medial leg Foot (occasionally)
L5	L4–L5	L5–S1	Anterior tibial EHL	Posterior tibial	Lateral leg Dorsum of foot Big toe
S1	L5–S1	Heel raise Peroneal		Achilles tendon	Posterior leg Sole of foot Lateral foot Little toe

EHL, Extensor hallicis longus; *HNP*, herniated nucleus pulposus.
Adapted from Brier SR: *Primary care orthopedics*, St Louis, 1999, Mosby.

> ### ORTHOPEDIC GAMUT 8-11
>
> ### ANATOMIC RELATIONS BETWEEN THE SCIATIC NERVE AND THE PIRIFORMIS MUSCLE
>
> - Both peroneal and tibial components of sciatic nerve pass inferior to the piriformis muscle.
> - Tibial component of the sciatic nerve passes inferior to the piriformis muscle; the common peroneal nerve passes through the muscle.

When the leg is shaken, such as during the test for alternating motion rate, the foot will be unstable and flop about. The foot is less floppy with central disorders (upper motor neuron lesions) and may be fixed in plantar flexion. When dorsiflexion of the ankles and toes is weak, the toes of the spastic leg are dragged during walking. Before the examiner concludes that weakness of dorsiflexion is present, the foot should be passively dorsiflexed to be certain that previous weakness, now healed, did not permanently shorten the gastrocnemius. Not unusual is for patients with severe L5 radiculopathy, in whom significant motor axon loss has occurred, to have foot drop (Table 8-15).

8

TABLE 8-15

ELECTROPHYSIOLOGIC DIFFERENCES BETWEEN
L5 RADICULOPATHY AND PERONEAL NEUROPATHY

	L5 Radiculopathy	Peroneal Neuropathy
Nerve Conduction Studies		
Peroneal CMAP, recording extensor digitorum brevis	Normal or low amplitude	Conduction block at fibular head, low amplitude, or both
Peroneal CMAP, recording tibialis anterior	Normal or low amplitude	Conduction block at fibular head, low amplitude, or both
Superficial peroneal SNAP	Normal	Low or absent; normal in deep peroneal or purely demyelinating lesions

Continued

TABLE 8-15

ELECTROPHYSIOLOGIC DIFFERENCES BETWEEN
L5 RADICULOPATHY AND PERONEAL NEUROPATHY—cont'd

	L5 Radiculopathy	Peroneal Neuropathy
Needle EMG		
Tibialis anterior	Abnormal	Abnormal
Extensor digitorum brevis	Abnormal	Abnormal
Extensor hallucis	Abnormal	Abnormal
Peroneus longus	Abnormal	Abnormal; normal in selective deep peroneal lesions
Tibialis posterior	Abnormal	Normal
Flexor digitorum longus	Abnormal	Normal
Gluteus medius	May be normal	Normal
Tensor fasciae latae	May be normal	Normal
Lumbar paraspinals	May be normal	Normal

CMAP, Compound muscle action potential; EMG, electromyography; SNAP, sensory nerve action potential.

From Katirji B: *Electromyography in clinical practice: a case study approach,* St Louis, 1998, Mosby.

PROCEDURE

- The examiner observes the patient walking on the toes, which requires each foot, one at a time, to support the patient's body weight completely (Fig. 8-22).
- If weakness exists, the heel will drop while the patient is walking.
- The contours of the musculature may demonstrate atrophy or hypertrophy.
- Having the patient walk on the heels is an especially valuable screening test because many muscular and neural disorders result in weakened dorsiflexion of the ankles and toes (Fig. 8-23).
- The patient may need help maintaining balance during this maneuver.
- The normal patient can hold the foot and toes anteriorly off the floor while strongly dorsiflexing the great toe during walking on the heels.
- If the patient can perform this maneuver, foot drop does not exist.

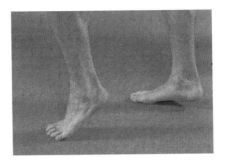

FIG. 8-22

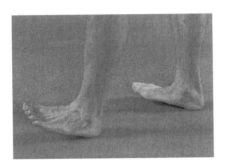

FIG. 8-23

8

CLINICAL PEARL

The inability to walk on the toes indicates an L5–S1 disc problem based on weakness of the calf muscles supplied by the tibial nerve. The inability to walk on the heels indicates an L4–L5 disc problem based on weakness of the anterior leg muscles supplied by the common peroneal nerve.

HYPEREXTENSION TEST

Assessment for L3 and L4 Nerve Root Inflammation

ORTHOPEDIC GAMUT 8-12

MODIFIED WILTSE CLASSIFICATION OF LUMBAR SPONDYLOLISTHESIS ETIOLOGY

- Type 1, dysplastic (congenital) spondylolisthesis (congenital dysplasia of articular processes)
  - Type 1a. The articular processes of L5 and S1 are dysplastic, having a horizontal rather than coronal orientation.
  - Type 1b. The orientation of the facet joints is sagittal and the facets are malformed, allowing spondylolisthesis to occur typically in adult life.
  - Type 1c includes other congenital malformations of the lumbar spine that permit spondylolisthesis.
- Type 2, isthmic (lytic) spondylolisthesis (This type occurs in the presence of bilateral pars defects, which can result from a variety of causes.)
  - Type 2a. Lytic defects arise in the pars because of congenital weakness in the bone or repeated mechanical strain or both.
  - Type 2b. The elongated pars is a true stress fracture of the pars.
  - Type 2c. The pars fractures under acute trauma in cases that show complex fractures of the spine. Acute isolated pars fracture is exceedingly rare.
- Type 3, degenerative spondylolisthesis (This type is the most common cause of lumbar spondylolisthesis in patients older than 50 years. The neural arch is intact and the slip occurs because of degenerative changes in the facet joints with associated disc degeneration.)
- Type 4, traumatic spondylolisthesis (This type is rare and results from fractures or dislocations involving any part of the neural arch except the pars interarticularis, for example, the pedicle or the facet joints. It is almost always secondary to severe trauma.)

ORTHOPEDIC GAMUT 8-12

MODIFIED WILTSE CLASSIFICATION OF LUMBAR SPONDYLOLISTHESIS ETIOLOGY—cont'd

- Type 5, pathological spondylolisthesis (This type can be divided into two types.)
  - Type 5a can occur when a generalized bone disease weakens the spine (i.e., Paget disease, osteoporosis, osteogenesis imperfecta, achondroplasia, arthrogryposis, osteopetrosis).
  - Type 5b can occur when a focal disease process weakens the pars interarticularis, resulting in pathologic fracture and spondylolisthesis (i.e., syphilis, tuberculosis, neoplastic processes).
- Type 6, iatrogenic spondylolisthesis (This type can follow spinal decompression performed for spinal stenosis, laminectomy for disc removal, or any other spine surgery in which decompressing the spinal canal is necessary.)

PROCEDURE

- The patient is prone, and the legs are fully extended.
- The examiner anchors the patient's lumbosacral spine with one hand.
- With the other hand, the examiner slowly extends the hip of the patient's affected leg (Fig. 8-24).
- The test is positive if the patient experiences radiating pain in the anterior thigh.
- A positive test indicates inflammation of the L3 and L4 nerve roots.

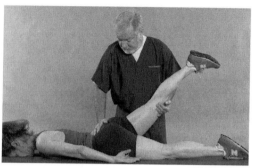

FIG. 8-24

CLINICAL PEARL

Five criteria have been established for diagnosis of sciatica caused by a herniated intervertebral disc. (1) Leg pain is the dominant symptom when compared with back pain, and it affects only one leg and follows a typical sciatic or femoral nerve distribution. (2) Paresthesia is localized to a dermatomal distribution. (3) Straight leg raising is reduced to 50% of what is considered normal, and pain is elicited in the symptomatic leg when the unaffected leg is elevated. This pain radiates proximally or distally with digital pressure on the tibial nerve in the popliteal fossa. (4) Two of four neurologic signs (atrophy, motor weakness, diminished sensory appreciation, and diminution of reflex activity) are present. (5) A contrast study or other diagnostic imaging is positive and corresponds to the clinical level.

KEMP TEST

Assessment for Intervertebral Nerve Root Encroachment, Muscular Strain, Ligamentous Sprain, or Pericapsular Inflammation

---

ORTHOPEDIC GAMUT 8-13

MECHANISMS OF LUMBAR FACET PAIN

1. The facet joint can carry a significant amount of the total compressive load on the spine when the human spine is hyperextended.
2. Extensive stretch of the human facet joint capsule occurs when the spine is in the physiologic range of extreme extension.
3. An extensive distribution of small nerve fibers and free and encapsulated nerve endings exists in the lumbar facet joint capsule, including nerves containing substance P, a putative neuromodulator of pain.
4. Low- and high-threshold mechanoreceptors fire when the facet joint capsule is stretched or is subject to localized compressive forces.
5. Sensitization and excitation of nerves in facet joint and surrounding muscle occur when the joint is inflamed or exposed to certain chemicals that are released during injury and inflammation.
6. Marked reduction in nerve activity occurs in facet tissue injected with hydrocortisone and lidocaine.

8

ORTHOPEDIC GAMUT 8-14

DISC PROLAPSE

Disc prolapse usually follows lifting or twisting while the trunk is in flexion:

1. During the first stage, trunk flexion flattens the discs anteriorly and opens out the intervertebral space posteriorly.
2. During the second stage, as soon as the weight is lifted, the increased axial compression force crushes the whole disc and violently drives the nuclear substance posteriorly until it reaches the deep surface of the posterior longitudinal ligament.
3. During the third stage, when the trunk is nearly straight, the path taken by the herniating mass is closed by the pressure of the vertebral plateaus, and a hernia remains trapped under the posterior longitudinal ligament.

PROCEDURE

- While in a seated position, the patient is supported by the examiner, who reaches around the patient's shoulders and upper chest from behind.
- The patient is directed to lean forward to one side and then around until the patient is eventually bending obliquely backward (Fig. 8-25).
- The maneuver is similar to that used for cervical compression.
- If this compression causes or aggravates a pattern of radicular pain in the thigh and leg, the sign is positive and indicates nerve root compression.
- Local back pain should be noted, but it does not constitute a positive test.
- However, local back pain may indicate a strain or sprain and thus be present when the patient leans obliquely forward or at any point in motion.
- Because elderly adults are less prone to an actual herniation of a disc because of lessened elasticity involved in the aging process, other reasons for nerve root compression are usually the cause.
- Degenerative joint disease, exostoses, inflammatory or fibrotic residues, narrowing from disc degeneration, and tumors must all be considered.
- This test must elicit a more positive finding when the patient is standing than when sitting (Fig. 8-26).

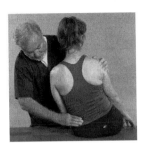

FIG. 8-25

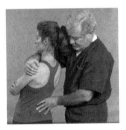

FIG. 8-26

8

CLINICAL PEARL

Kemp test can be performed when the patient is either standing or sitting. Sitting increases intradiscal pressure and therefore maximizes stress on the disc. Standing increases weight bearing and maximizes stress to the facets. The test should be performed in both positions.

KERNIG/BRUDZINSKI SIGN

Assessment for Meningeal Irritation or Inflammation

ORTHOPEDIC GAMUT 8-15

MENINGEAL PATHOGENS AND ASSOCIATED OR PREDISPOSING CONDITIONS*

Organism	Associated Factors/Condition
Streptococcus pneumoniae	Pneumonia
	Otitis media
	Acute sinusitis
	Diabetes
	Splenectomy
	Hypogammaglobulinemia
	Head trauma
	CSF rhinorrhea
	Neonates, elderly adults
	Alcoholism, cirrhosis, peritonitis
Neisseria meningitidis	College dormitory living
	Exposure in an endemic area
	Complement deficiencies
	Splenectomy
	Hypogammaglobulinemia
Listeria monocytogenes	Immunosuppressive therapy
	Organ transplantation
	Pregnancy
	Diabetes
	Alcoholism
	Neonates, elderly adults
Enteric gram-negative bacilli	Diabetes
	Cirrhosis, alcoholism
	Craniotomy
	Head trauma

CSF, Cerebral spinal fluid.

*Adapted from Roos KL: Bacterial meningitis, *Curr Treat Options Neurol* 1(2): 147-156, 1999.

ORTHOPEDIC GAMUT 8-15

MENINGEAL PATHOGENS AND ASSOCIATED OR PREDISPOSING CONDITIONS*—cont'd

Organism	Associated Factors/Condition
Staphylococcus	CSF shunt Ommaya reservoir Lumbar puncture Infective endocarditis Parameningeal infection (empyema, epidural abscess, osteomyelitis)
Streptococcus agalactiae	Neonates, elderly adults Diabetes Alcoholism Acquired immunodeficiency syndrome
Haemophilus influenzae type b	Age over 60 Otitis media Sinusitis CSF leak Immunodeficiency Diabetes Alcoholism

8

PROCEDURE

- For the Brudzinski part of the sign, the patient is in the supine position, and the examiner passively flexes the patient's head.
- The sign is present if flexion of both knees occurs (Fig. 8-27).
- The sign is often accompanied by flexion of both hips and is present with meningitis.
- For the Kernig part of the sign, the patient is supine.
- The examiner flexes the patient's hip and knee of either leg to 90 degrees.
- The examiner attempts to completely extend the patient's leg (Fig. 8-28).
- If this maneuver causes pain, the sign is present.
- The sign is often accompanied by involuntary flexion of the opposite knee and hip and is present in meningitis.

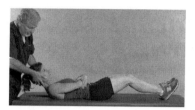

FIG. 8-27

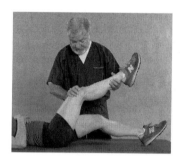

FIG. 8-28

CLINICAL PEARL

After myelographic examination, a percentage of patients experience general malaise, headache, nausea, pain, and stiffness for a week or longer, and the symptoms are strikingly aggravated by the erect position or activity. These conditions may be signs of arachnoiditis. Subarachnoid fibrosis typically affects the lowermost segment of the thecal sac. This whole process represents meningismus or the apparent irritation of the spinal cord in which the symptoms simulate meningitis. However, no actual infectious agent—such as bacteria, fungi, or viruses—can be found.

LASÈGUE DIFFERENTIAL SIGN

Assessment for Intervertebral Radiculopathy *Versus* Hip Joint Disease

Comment

Examination often reveals restriction of low back motion. Bending toward the affected side typically exacerbates the pain. Variable degrees of local tenderness and muscle guarding are present. In an attempt to relieve tension on the nerve root, the patient may list or bend away from the painful side and stand with the affected hip and knee slightly flexed. A characteristic clinical picture may be present, depending on the level of nerve root involvement (Table 8-16).

ORTHOPEDIC GAMUT 8-16

MODIFIED ALTMAN CLASSIFICATION OF HIP OSTEOARTHRITIS

8

Different classification systems have been described using as criteria the direction of migration of the femoral head and the evolution of the destructive changes within the joint. The two main types of head migration are as follows:

- The superior migration (or eccentric) may be superolateral or superomedial. The differential diagnosis of the superior migration pattern of the hip includes the calcium pyrophosphate dihydrate crystal deposition disease and the osteonecrosis, both of which might be complicated by secondary degenerative changes.
- The medial migration (concentric) is also known as axial or global. The concentric loss of articular cartilage poses diagnostic difficulties because it should be differentiated from infectious arthritis and rheumatoid arthritis.

TABLE 8-16

LUMBAR DISC SYNDROME PATTERNS

Level	Pain	Sensory	Motor Weakness Atrophy	Reflex
L3–L4 (L4 root)	Low back, posterolateral aspect of thigh, across patella, anteromedial aspect of leg	Anterior aspect of knee, anteromedial aspect of leg	Quadriceps (knee extension)	Knee jerk
L4–L5 (L5 root)	Lateral, posterolateral aspect of thigh, leg	Lateral aspect of leg, dorsum of foot, first web space, great toe	Great toe extension, ankle dorsiflexion, heel walking difficult (foot drop may occur)	Minor (posterior tibial jerk depressed)
L5–S1 (S1 root)	Posterolateral aspect of thigh, leg, heel	Posterior aspect of calf, heel, lateral aspect of foot (three toes)	Calf, plantar flexion of foot, great toe; toe walking weak	Ankle jerk
Cauda equina syndrome (massive midline protrusion)	Low back, thigh, legs; often bilateral	Thighs, legs, feet, perineum; often bilateral	Variable; may be bowel, bladder incontinence	Ankle jerk (may be bilateral)

Adapted from Mercier LR, Pettid FJ: *Practical orthopedics*, ed 4, St Louis, 1995, Mosby.

PROCEDURE

- If the examiner flexes the hip of a patient with sciatica while the knee is extended and this movement elicits pain but flexing the thigh on the pelvis while the knee is flexed produces no sciatic pain, the sign is present (Fig. 8-29).
- This sign rules out hip joint disease.

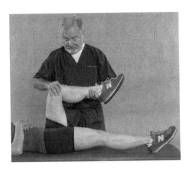

FIG. 8-29

8

CLINICAL PEARL

Lasègue described how painful sciatica is for patients when the sciatic nerve is stretched by extending the knee while the hip is flexed. He also described the pain relief that occurs when the knee was then flexed. This reaction is the classic leg-raising sign. Variations of this sign, with interpretations of its meaning, lend much more knowledge to the examining physician than merely noting at what degree of leg raise the patient experiences either back pain, leg pain, or both.

LASÈGUE REBOUND TEST

Assessment for Intervertebral Nerve Root Lesion, Piriformis Muscular Spasm, Ischiotrochanteric Groove Adhesion, or Intervertebral Disc Syndrome

---

ORTHOPEDIC GAMUT 8-17

CAUSES AND PREDILECTION FOR PIRIFORMIS SYNDROME

- The female-to-male predominance is 6:1.
- The most common cause of piriformis syndrome is trauma to the pelvis or buttock (50%).
- However, the trauma is usually not dramatic and may occur several months before initial symptoms.
- Prolonged sitting, although uncommon, has been recognized as a cause of piriformis syndrome.

ORTHOPEDIC GAMUT 8-18

DISC HERNIATION VERSUS OTHER CAUSES OF BACK PAIN

The following elements apply when early disc herniation is difficult to differentiate from other causes of back pain:

1. Plain-film roentgenograms are indicated within 2 to 4 weeks of onset.
2. Electromyography, computed tomography (CT), magnetic resonance imaging (MRI), or myelography confirm the diagnosis.
3. Electromyography (EMG), CT, and MRI are not usually indicated for at least 4 to 6 weeks from onset.
4. EMG, CT (if surgical intervention is being contemplated), or MRI is indicated if other more serious spinal disease is suspected.
5. Discography is considered to be of only limited value.

PROCEDURE

- To continue a differential after the straight-leg-raising test, the examiner fixes the patient's pelvis on the same side by pressing heavily with a hand on the region of the ipsilateral anterosuperior iliac spine and repeats this straight-leg-raising test.
- Any undue pain experienced by the patient is associated with sciatic involvement resulting from a nerve root disorder, piriform spasm, or ischiotrochanteric groove adhesions.
- Differentiation of piriformis spasm from other causes can be accomplished by reproducing the pain during internal rotation of the femur when it is at a lower level than the original point of pain.
- After a positive Lasègue test, the examiner may permit the leg to drop to the examination table without warning the patient (Fig. 8-30).
- If this Lasègue rebound test causes a marked increase in the back pain, sciatic neuralgia, and muscle spasm, then disc involvement is suspected.

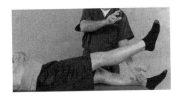

FIG. 8-30

8

CLINICAL PEARL

The relationship of the lumbar roots and the lumbar discs is of major clinical importance. A massive posterior extrusion of one of the lumbar discs may severely injure the cauda equina (both intrathecal and extrathecal roots). Although these lesions are rare, they do occur. In these instances, the size and shape of the spinal canal and the size of the extruded mass are major factors in the severity of the clinical syndrome.

LASÈGUE SITTING TEST

Assessment for Sciatic Nerve Inflammation

ORTHOPEDIC GAMUT 8-19

ETIOLOGY OF NEUROGENIC CLAUDICATION PAIN

- Direct compressive forces on the nerves, particularly in the lateral recesses and foramina of the lumbar spinal canal, where the nerves exit
- Compromised blood supply to the nerve root as a result of the compression, leading to nerve pain similar to the muscular pain of vascular claudication
- Lack of nerve root nutrition resulting from stenosis-induced stagnation of cerebrospinal fluid

---

ORTHOPEDIC GAMUT 8-20

LUMBAR CANAL STENOSIS

Electromyographic (EMG) findings in lumbar canal stenosis include the following:

1. An entirely normal EMG
2. Absent H-reflex only, unilaterally or bilaterally
3. Denervation in a single root distribution (single radiculopathy), unilaterally or bilaterally and asymmetrically
4. Occurrence of bilateral and asymmetric lumbosacral radiculopathies, affecting the L5, S1, and S2 roots (the most common EMG finding associated with lumbar canal stenosis) (Table 8-17)

ORTHOPEDIC GAMUT 8-21

LUMBOSACRAL RADICULOPATHY

Electromyographic (EMG) limitations in lumbosacral radiculopathy are as follows:

1. If the dorsal root is the only root compressed, and if the ventral root is normal, then the EMG examination is normal. This scenario occurs in a significant number of patients whose symptoms are limited to pain or paresthesia or both. Thus, a normal EMG does not exclude root compression.

2. Fibrillation potentials can be absent from the paraspinal muscles, particularly in chronic radiculopathies. This circumstance is likely caused by reinnervation. In contrast, fibrillation potentials can be present in the paraspinal muscles after lumbar laminectomy because of denervation during surgical exposure.

3. The lower-extremity sensory nerve action potentials (SNAPs) often are unevocable bilaterally in elderly patients. When this circumstance occurs, differentiating a preganglionic lesion (i.e., lumbosacral radiculopathy) from a postganglionic lesion (i.e., lumbosacral plexopathy) is often difficult unless fibrillation potentials are evident in the paraspinal muscles.

4. No SNAPs have been devised to assess the L2 or L3 fibers up to the dorsal root ganglion, and the saphenous SNAP is not technically reliable (especially in elderly and obese patients) to assess the L4 fibers. Thus, separating an upper lumbar radiculopathy (especially L2 and L3) from lumbar plexopathy is often difficult unless fibrillations are present in the paraspinal muscles.

8

ORTHOPEDIC GAMUT 8-22

DISTINGUISHING FEATURES OF RESTLESS LEGS SYNDROME

- Onset at rest, restless leg syndrome is unrelated to body position or other activity and occurs when resting or lying down.
- The patient has an internal urge to move a body part, usually the limbs (not a spontaneous general body movement).
- Focal akathisia is relieved immediately (at least partially) by movement of the affected limb.
- Relief with movement persists as long as the limb is being moved.
- Symptoms may reoccur as soon as movement ceases.
- Usually a time of day exists when symptoms are not present or are less severe, typically a circadian pattern when symptoms appear at the end of the day or at bedtime.
- No signs of disease are found in the affected limbs.

ORTHOPEDIC GAMUT 8-23

DIFFERENTIAL DIAGNOSIS FOR RESTLESS LEGS SYNDROME*

- Neuropathic pain syndromes
- Peripheral neuropathy
- Arthritis
- Nocturnal leg cramps
- Restless insomnia
- Painful legs and moving toes
- Vascular insufficiencies
- Drug-induced akathisia

*Adapted from Allen RP, Earley CJ: Restless legs syndrome: a review of clinical and pathophysiologic features, *J Clin Neurophysiol* 18(2):128-147, 2001.

ORTHOPEDIC GAMUT 8-24

DIAGNOSTIC CRITERIA OF RESTLESS LEGS SYNDROME*

Essential criteria:
1. Urge to move legs is usually accompanied or caused by uncomfortable or unpleasant sensations in the legs.
2. Urge to move or unpleasant sensation begins or worsens during periods of rest or inactivity.
3. Urge to move or unpleasant sensation is partially or totally relieved by movement as long as activity continues.
4. Urge to move or unpleasant sensation is worse in the evening or at night than during the day, or the urge occurs only during the evening or at night.

Supportive clinical features:
1. Positive family history
2. Response to dopaminergic therapy (>90%)
3. Periodic limb movements (during wakefulness or sleep)

Associated features:
1. Natural clinical course
2. Sleep disturbance
3. Medical or physical evaluation is generally normal

*Adapted from Allen RP, Earley CJ: Restless legs syndrome: a review of clinical and pathophysiologic features, *J Clin Neurophysiol* 18(2):128-147, 2001.

8

TABLE 8-17

Electrophysiologic Differentiation of Chronic S1/S2 Radiculopathy

	Chronic S1/S2 Radiculopathy	Tarsal Tunnel Syndrome	Peripheral Polyneuropathy
Nerve Conduction Studies			
Sural sensory study*	Normal	Normal	Usually abnormal
Peroneal motor study	Normal or low amplitude	Normal	Low amplitude or slow latency or both
Tibial motor study	Normal or low amplitude	Low amplitude or slow latency or both	Low amplitude or slow latency or both
Motor conduction velocities	Normal or slowed	Normal	Slowed
Plantar studies*	Normal	Slow latencies or absent	Slow latencies or absent
H-reflex*	Abnormal	Normal	Abnormal
Upper extremity conductions	Normal	Normal	Can be abnormal
Needle EMG			
AH/ADQP	Denervated	Denervated	Denervated
EDB†	Denervated	Normal	Denervated
Medial gastrocnemius	Denervated	Normal	Denervated
Tibialis anterior	Normal	Normal	Denervated
Paraspinal muscles	Normal or fibs	Normal	Normal or fibrillations
Symmetry of findings (when bilateral)	Asymmetric	Asymmetric	Symmetric

ADQP, Abductor digiti quinti pedis; *AH*, abductor hallucis; *EDB*, extensor digitorum brevis; *EMG*, electromyography.

*Commonly absent in asymptomatic elderly subjects.

†May be denervated, selectively, in healthy subjects.

From Katirji B: *Electromyography in clinical practice: a case study approach*, St Louis, 1998, Mosby.

PROCEDURE

- The patient is seated upright on the edge of a table with the legs dangling.
- The examiner faces the patient and extends the patient's leg at the knee.
- The lower extremity from the hip to the foot is made parallel with the floor (Fig. 8-31).
- When radiculoneuropathy is not present, the patient should not experience discomfort from this action.
- Initially, the significance of the test is the same as the Lasègue test.
- However, the modification of performing the straight leg raise while the patient is in the seated position provides several advantages.
- In the supine position, straight leg raising may be difficult because the patient may squirm and shift the pelvis, making the leg abduct and rotate.
- The apprehensive patient may attempt to ward off anticipated pain and make the test positive sooner than is warranted.
- When the test is performed in the seated position, the patient faces the examiner, feels more secure and at ease, and is less likely to even know the part is being tested.
- The test has excellent, objective values when the examiner is able to determine immediately the slightest attempt on the part of the patient to withdraw by leaning back from the induced pain.

8

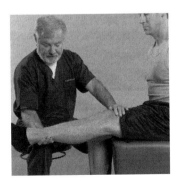

FIG. 8-31

CLINICAL PEARL

By raising the patient's foot, the examiner has performed a modified straight-leg-raising test. Because the thigh is already flexed to 90 degrees in this position, straightening the knee to the horizontal places stretching forces on the nerve roots. The results of this seated tension should correspond to the results obtained from the tests performed in the supine position.

LASÈGUE TEST

ALSO KNOWN AS LASÈGUE SIGN

Assessment for Sciatica Resulting from Lumbosacral or Sacroiliac Lesions, Lumbar Subluxation Syndrome, Intervertebral Disc Lesion, Spondylolisthesis, Dural Sleeve Adhesions, or Intervertebral Foramen Occlusion (Encroachment)

ORTHOPEDIC GAMUT 8-25

LASÈGUE TEST

Interpretations of the Lasègue test:

1. When the patient is supine and the lower limbs are resting on the examination table, the sciatic nerve and its roots are under no tension.
2. When the lower limb is raised while the knees are flexed, the sciatic nerve and its roots are still under no tension.
3. If the knee is extended while the leg is elevated, the sciatic nerve, which must cover a longer distance, is subjected to increasing tension. In the normal patient, the nerve roots slide freely through the intervertebral foramen, and no pain results. When the lower limb is nearly vertical for people with diminished flexibility, pain is felt on the posterior aspect of the thigh as a result of stretching the hamstrings. However, this pain does not constitute a positive Lasègue sign.
4. When one nerve root is trapped in the foramen or when the root must cover a longer distance because of a prolapsed disc, any stretching of the nerve will become painful with moderate elevation of the lower limb. This result constitutes a positive Lasègue sign, which is evident before 60 degrees of flexion is attained. Pain may be elicited at 10, 15, or 20 degrees of flexion, which allows a rough quantification of the severity of the lesion.

8

ORTHOPEDIC GAMUT 8-26

PRECAUTIONS FOR LASÈGUE TEST

Two precautions to observe in performing Lasègue test:
1. The examiner must always elicit the Lasègue sign cautiously and stop when the patient feels pain.
2. The examiner must never attempt to elicit the Lasègue sign when the patient is under general anesthesia because the protective pain reflex is absent. The reflex can occur when the patient is being placed prone on an operating table and the hips are allowed to flex while the knees are extended. Hip flexion must always be associated with knee flexion, which relaxes the sciatic nerve and the trapped root.

PROCEDURE

- The patient lies supine with legs extended.
- The examiner places one hand under the ankle of the patient's affected leg and the other hand on the knee and flexes the thigh on the pelvis while the knee is flexed.
- The examiner then slowly extends the patient's knee while the leg is elevated (Fig. 8-32).
- If this maneuver is markedly limited because of pain, the test is positive and suggests sciatica from lumbosacral or sacroiliac lesions, subluxation syndrome, disc lesions, spondylolisthesis, adhesions, or intervertebral foramen occlusion.

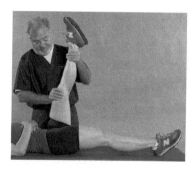

FIG. 8-32

CLINICAL PEARL

Whenever the presence of the Lasègue sign is questionable, the examiner should combine this test with flexion of the cervical spine *(Lindner sign)*. This combination places the greatest pull and stretch on the nerve roots behind the intervertebral discs and often elicits pain.

8

LEWIN PUNCH TEST

Assessment for Generalized Spinal Lesion or Intervertebral Disc Protrusion

PROCEDURE

- Punching the buttock produces a referred pain in the back.
- While the patient is standing, the examiner percusses (punches) the side of the patient's buttock with the lesion (Fig. 8-33).
- If this percussion (punch) elicits pain, the test is positive.
- Punching the opposite buttock should not elicit pain.
- The test is significant for a spinal lesion, usually involving a protruded disc.

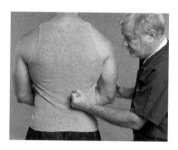

FIG. 8-33

CLINICAL PEARL

In some instances of an acute attack, even light fist percussion over the lumbar spine in the midline will produce such severe accentuation of the local and radiating pain that the patient's knees may buckle. Some evidence of a vasovagal response may be found. In patients with spondylolysis or spondylolisthesis, hamstring tightness and the classic Phalen-Dickson sign—a knee-flexed, hip-flexed gait—may be demonstrated, regardless of degree of slippage. The mechanism for hamstring tightness is unclear, but it may be caused by nerve root irritation from the instability. For higher degrees of slip, the sacrum becomes more vertical so that the pelvis is more flexed and the hips cannot hyperextend enough to maintain upright posture. Therefore, the patient must flex the knees to stand upright.

8

LEWIN SNUFF TEST

Assessment for Intervertebral Disc Rupture or Space-Occupying Mass

PROCEDURE

- An aromatic substance is introduced, and the patient is instructed to sniff it up the nostril so as to induce sneezing.
- The test is positive when sneezing elicits an exacerbation of well-localized spinal and radicular pain (Fig. 8-34).
- The test is significant for intervertebral disc rupture.

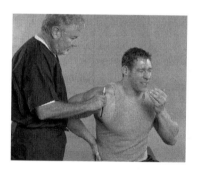

FIG. 8-34

CLINICAL PEARL

The sneeze produces a sudden Valsalva maneuver. If the examiner assumes that motion of an irritated nerve root over a disc bulge is one of the causes of pain, any production of a Valsalva effect abruptly increases the patient's pain as the defect appears and disappears and thereby moves the nerve root over the disc.

LEWIN STANDING TEST

Assessment for Unilateral or Bilateral Hamstring Spasm

PROCEDURE

- The patient is standing.
- From behind, the examiner stabilizes the patient's pelvis with one hand while sharply pulling the knee on that side into extension (Fig. 8-35).
- The examiner then repeats this move on the opposite side and braces a shoulder against the patient's sacrum and sharply pulls both of the patient's knees into extension.
- The test is positive when pulling one or both knees into extension elicits pain that is followed by one or both knees snapping back into flexion.
- This positive finding represents unilateral or bilateral hamstring spasm.

8

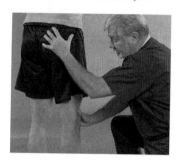

FIG. 8-35

CLINICAL PEARL

Tight or contracted hamstrings pull eccentrically on the pelvis. The patient with suspected tight hamstring disorder can be examined in the supine position. Keeping the hips and buttocks in contact with the table, straight leg raising is performed bilaterally. The comparison will indicate any hamstring contracture or tightness.

LEWIN SUPINE TEST

Assessment for Lumbar Arthritis, Lumbar Fibrosis, Spondylosis, Sacroiliac or Lumbosacral Arthrosis, or Sciatica

Comment

With lumbar spondylosis accompanied by a stenotic lumbar spinal canal, the physical examination is unrevealing despite intermittent symptoms that are often severe. Flexion and straight leg raising are often performed without difficulty. Severe pain during lumbar extension may be the only positive result. Rheumatoid arthritis must be included in the differential diagnoses (Tables 8-18 and 8-19).

ORTHOPEDIC GAMUT 8-27

DISC DEGENERATION

Observations in disc degeneration:
1. Disc degeneration may occur and may remain asymptomatic.
2. Disc degeneration may be associated with changes within the disc itself, which may produce pain.
3. Disc degeneration may give rise to mechanical instability that renders the spine vulnerable to trauma.

8

TABLE 8-18

LARSEN AND THE MODIFIED LARSEN RHEUMATOID ARTHRITIS GRADING SYSTEM

	Larsen Systems	Modified Larsen System Erosions		Joint Space Narrowing (JSN)
Grade 0	Intact bony outlines and normal joint space	Definitely no erosions	and/or	Definitely no JSN
		"There is no doubt that there is no damage at all"		"There is no doubt that there is no damage at all"
Grade 1	Erosion less than 1 mm in diameter or joint space narrowing	Possible erosions	and/or	Possible JSN
		"I am not sure whether what I am seeing is an erosion, and I could not assign this finding to either grade 0 or grade 2"		"I am not sure whether JSN is present, even if I compare with neighboring joints, and I could not assign this finding to either grade 0 or grade 2"
Grade 2	One or several small erosions	Definite, but moderate, erosions	and/or	Define, but moderate, JSN
		"I am sure that some damage is present, but I had to look extensively to come to this conclusion; it is definitely not striking"		"I am sure that some damage is present, but I had to look extensively to come to this conclusion; it is definitely not striking"
		Striking erosions, bony outlines at joint line more than 50% preserved		Striking JSN, but both subchondral bony outlines still separated
Grade 3	Marked erosions	"Damage is gross, visible at first glance. Definitely more than what grade 2 would be, but the joint line is intact"		"Damage is gross, visible at first glance, even from some distance. Definitely more than what grade 2 would be"

Grade 4	Severe erosions: there is usually no joint space left: the original bony outlines have been partly preserved	Severe erosions, bony outlines at joint line less than 50% preserved	and/or	Complete JSN, subchondral bony outlines in contact
		The joint appears completely destroyed, but a portion of the joint line is still intact		
Grade 5	Mutilating changes: the bony outlines have been completely destroyed	Complete disorganization of the joint, bony outlines destroyed	and/or	Complete disorganization of the joint, bony outlines destroyed

The following joints are graded: five metacarpophalangeal joints, the interphalangeal joint of the thumb, four proximal interphalangeal joints, and four quadrants of the wrist on both sides, to give a total of 28 joints or sectors.

Either erosions or joint space narrowing must be present to assign to more than grade 1. If both are present, the worse finding is taken into account. Any amount of erosion or JSN associated with dislocation of the joint = grade 5.

Adapted from Zangger P et al: Assessing damage in individual joints in rheumatoid arthritis: a new method based on the Larsen system, *Joint Bone Spine* 71(5):389-396, 2004.

TABLE 8-19

LUMBAR SPINAL RHEUMATOID ARTHRITIS LESION GRADES

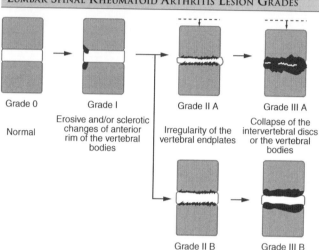

Grade 0	Grade I	Grade II A	Grade III A
Normal	Erosive and/or sclerotic changes of anterior rim of the vertebral bodies	Irregularity of the vertebral endplates	Collapse of the intervertebral discs or the vertebral bodies

Grade II B   Grade III B

Grades II and III are further divided into two types. Type A includes grade IIA (presence of disc narrowing) and grade IIIA (disc space collapsed and vertebral bodies fused), and type B includes grade IIB (absence of disc narrowing) and grade IIIB (vertebral body collapsed but intervertebral disc remains or appears ballooned).

From Sakai T et al: Radiological features of lumbar spinal lesions in patients with rheumatoid arthritis with special reference to the changes around intervertebral discs, *Spine J* 8(4): 605–611, 2008.

PROCEDURE

- While the patient is supine, the examiner supports the patient's legs on the table.
- The patient is directed to sit up without using the hands (Fig. 8-36).
- The test is positive if the patient is unable to perform this action.
- A positive test is often associated with lumbar arthritis, lumbar fibrosis, degenerative disc thinning with protrusion, sacroiliac or lumbosacral arthritis, and sciatica.
- The patient is often able to localize the site of the complaint.

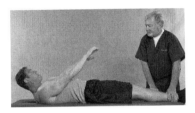

FIG. 8-36

8

CLINICAL PEARL

The security and comfort of the back depend not only on the lumbar muscles and ligaments, but also on the strength of the abdominal wall and prevertebral muscles. The abdomen should be palpated to determine whether divarication of the rectus abdominis muscle is present. The clinical test for diagnosis of rectus divarication involves instructing the supine patient to raise the head from the examination table. The examining hand can easily feel the gap between the contracted pillars of the rectus, and the fingers will sink into the soft abdominal wall. The width of the gap may vary from 1 cm to a hand's breadth.

LINDNER SIGN

**Assessment for Lumbar Nerve Root
Irritation or Inflammation**

ORTHOPEDIC GAMUT 8-28

UNILATERAL DISC HERNIATION BETWEEN L3 AND L4

Unilateral disc herniation between L3 and L4 usually compresses the fourth lumbar root as it crosses the disc before exiting at the L4 intervertebral foramen with the following results:

1. Pain may be localized around the medial side of the leg.
2. Numbness may be present over the anteromedial aspect of the leg.
3. The quadriceps and hip adductor group, both innervated from L2, L3 and L4, may be weak and, in extended ruptures, atrophic.
4. Reflex testing may reveal a diminished or absent patellar tendon reflex (L2, L3, and L4) or tibialis anterior tendon reflex (L4).
5. Sensory testing may show diminished sensibility over the L4 dermatome, the isolated portion of which is the medial leg, and the autonomous zone, which is at the level of the medial malleolus.

ORTHOPEDIC GAMUT 8-29

UNILATERAL DISC HERNIATION BETWEEN L4 AND L5

Unilateral disc herniation between L4 and L5 results in compression of the fifth lumbar root with the following results:
1. Fifth lumbar root radiculopathy should produce pain in the dermatomal pattern.
2. Numbness, when present, follows the L5 dermatome along the anterolateral aspect of the leg and the dorsum of the foot, including the great toe.
3. The autonomous zone for this nerve is the first web of the foot and the dorsum of the third toe. Weakness may involve the extensor hallucis longus (L5), gluteus medius (L5), or extensor digitorum longus and brevis (L5).
4. Reflex change is not usually found.
5. A diminished tibialis posterior reflex is possible but difficult to elicit.

ORTHOPEDIC GAMUT 8-30

UNILATERAL DISC HERNIATION BETWEEN L5 AND S1

8

In a unilateral disc herniation between L5 and S1, the findings of an S1 radiculopathy are noted as follows:
1. Pain and numbness involve the dermatome of S1.
2. The S1 dermatome includes the lateral malleolus and the lateral and plantar surface of the foot, occasionally including the heel.
3. Numbness is present over the lateral aspect of the leg and, more important, over the lateral aspect of the foot, including the lateral three toes.
4. The autonomous zone for this root is the dorsum of the fifth toe.
5. Weakness may be demonstrated in the peroneus longus and brevis (S1), gastrocnemius-soleus (S1), or gluteus maximus (S1).
6. In general, weakness is not a usual finding in S1 radiculopathy.
7. Occasionally, mild weakness may be demonstrated by asymmetrical fatigue with exercise of these motor groups.
8. The ankle jerk usually is reduced or absent.

PROCEDURE

- Passive flexion of the patient's head onto the chest can be accomplished in a supine, seated, or standing position (Fig. 8-37).
- If pain occurs in the lumbar spine and along the sciatic nerve distribution, the test is positive and, according to Lindner, is an indication of root sciatica (Fig. 8-38).

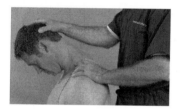

FIG. 8-37

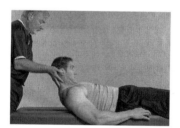

FIG. 8-38

CLINICAL PEARL

Flexion of the head to the chest increases the traction of the nerve root against the disc bulge. When the disc is a contained disc, in which the annulus is not ruptured, the flexion or maintenance of a flexed position of the trunk obliterates the disc bulge. Motion of an irritated nerve root over a bulging disc is often the source of the patient's back and leg pain. Relief of pain with trunk flexion occurs only because the disc bulge has disappeared.

MATCHSTICK TEST

Assessment for Denervation Hypersensitivity

Comment

Many cases of acute low back pain that are not correctly identified evolve into a chronic spinal problem with significant disability at the muscular level (Table 8-20). Patients with muscular dysfunction of the lumbar spine can have varying types of clinical findings and case histories.

TABLE 8-20

SITES OF LUMBOPELVIC SOFT-TISSUE SYNDROMES/ MYOFASCIAL TRIGGER POINTS

Diagnosis	Site of Complaint
Quadratus lumborum syndrome	Gluteal region, anterior iliac spine, greater trochanter of femur
Gluteus maximus or medius syndrome	Sacral and gluteal region, lateral hip
Gluteus minimus syndrome	Lateral hip, thigh, and calf
Chronic lumbar strain (spinal erector muscles)	Laterally to ribs, caudally toward lumbosacral junction
Piriformis syndrome	Sacroiliac region; posterior hip, thigh, calf; possibly sole of foot

Adapted from Brier SR: *Primary care orthopedics*, St Louis, 1999, Mosby.

8

ORTHOPEDIC GAMUT 8-31

MUSCLE SYNDROMES OF THE LUMBOPELVIC SPINE

Common findings in muscle syndromes of the lumbopelvic spine are as follows:

1. Hip inflexibility, especially hamstring and psoas insufficiency
2. Weakness of the hip and spine extensor mechanism
3. Intersegmental lumbosacral fixation
4. Myofascial trigger points in the spinal erector, quadratus lumborum, gluteal musculature, and psoas muscles
5. Referred zones of pain to the hip, buttocks, thigh, and lateral lower leg
6. Severe tightness of the outward rotators of the hip
7. Muscle hypertonicity
8. Palpable tenderness with pressure or stretch
9. Taut, tender, or ropelike muscle fibers

ORTHOPEDIC GAMUT 8-32

MIXED MOTOR PERIPHERAL NERVE LESION

Effects of a mixed motor (motor, sensory, and sympathetic) peripheral nerve lesion:

1. Flaccid paralysis (motor)
2. Loss of reflexes (motor)
3. Muscle wasting and atrophy (motor)
4. Loss of sensation (sensory)
5. Trophic changes in the skin (sensory), loss of secretions from sweat glands (sympathetic)
6. Loss of pilomotor response (sympathetic)

PROCEDURE

- Trophedema is nonpitting to digital pressure. However, when a blunt instrument, such as the end of a matchstick or cotton-tip applicator is used, the indentation produced is clear cut and persists for several minutes, which is distinctly longer than such an indentation would persist in normal skin (Fig. 8-39).
- The matchstick test may be positive and yield deep indentations over an extensive area (commonly over the lower back and hamstrings), or, in mild cases, the test may yield only slight indentations of skin overlying a tender motor point or the neurovascular hilus.

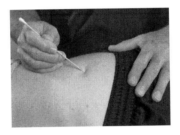

FIG. 8-39

8

CLINICAL PEARL

Complex regional pain syndrome (CRPS) can occur in any disease that produces pain. This type of dystrophy is a likely secondary condition after 4 months of unrelenting pain from the primary disorder. The earliest sign, other than the symptoms of burning or stinging pain, is localized trophedema. The matchstick test can be applied to any cutaneous area of pain because the test is sensitive to the earliest changes in fluid management in the skin by the sympathetically operated cutaneous vascularity. The result of this test becomes the earliest warning sign of the advancing CRPS type I. An intervertebral disc syndrome with protracted nerve root compression is a common onset mechanism.

MENNELL SIGN

Assessment for Pathologic Involvement of the Sacroiliac Joint Structures

---

ORTHOPEDIC GAMUT 8-33
SACROILIAC PAIN

The radicular component of sacroiliac pain is referred pain similar to pain associated with:
1. The painful tendon attachment
2. Periosteal pain
3. The deep aching associated with compression of a small blood vessel
4. The irritation of a sensory nerve penetrating the fascia
5. Straight leg raising that may be uncomfortable but not radicular

---

ORTHOPEDIC GAMUT 8-34
LUMBOPELVIC TENDERNESS

Common areas of palpable lumbopelvic tenderness:
1. Medial to the posterior-superior iliac spine is the most superficial posterior ligament of the sacroiliac joint. Tenderness here suggests a pathologic condition involving the sacroiliac joint.
2. Lateral to the posterior-superior iliac spine is the puny part of the gluteal muscle origin that may be torn by minor trauma. Tenderness here suggests a pathologic condition resulting from a muscle tear.
3. Above the posterior-superior iliac spine is where the sacrospinalis muscle joins its tendon. Muscle fiber tears frequently occur at this junction during minor lifting trauma.
4. Above and medial to the posterior-superior iliac spine is the area over the interlaminar facet joint, where tenderness may be felt if dysfunction is present.
5. Medial and inferior to the posterior-superior iliac spine is the area where local tenderness may be felt from a pathologic condition involving a disc.

ORTHOPEDIC GAMUT 8-34

LUMBOPELVIC TENDERNESS—cont'd

6. Tenderness lateral to the ischial tuberosity, where the sciatic trunk emerges from beneath the piriformis muscle, suggests either tightness of the muscle or a pathologic condition of a radicular origin.
7. Tenderness elicited by deeply rolling with the fingers over the sciatic trunk in the back of the thigh indicates neuritis.

PROCEDURE

- The examiner places a thumb over the posterior-superior iliac spine (PSIS), exerts pressure, slides the thumb outward, and then slides it inward (Fig. 8-40).
- The sign is positive if tenderness is increased.
- This result is significant if, when sliding outward, sensitive deposits in structures on the gluteal aspect of the PSIS are noted.
- If, when sliding inward, tenderness is increased, this is a significant result for strain of the superior sacroiliac ligaments.
- Confirmation can be made if tenderness is increased when the examiner posteriorly pulls the anterior-superior iliac spine while standing behind the patient or when the examiner pulls the PSIS forward while standing in front of the patient.
- This test is helpful in determining that tenderness is caused by strained superior sacroiliac ligaments.
- A positive result indicates deposits in the structure or adjacent to the structure of the sacroiliac joint.
- These deposits are the result of ligamentous strain or sprain.

8

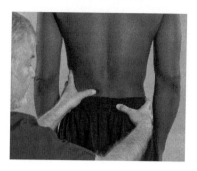

FIG. 8-40

CLINICAL PEARL

This method of tissue examination provides pertinent information, providing the results are accurately interpreted. Palpation of the lumbosacral region, with the patient in either the erect or the prone position, may evoke tender areas in the midline, at the level of the disc lesion, and in the paravertebral area on the side of the nuclear extrusion. The ability to elicit tenderness along the iliac crest or even over the posterior aspect of the sacroiliac joint on the side of an irritated nerve root is not uncommon.

MILGRAM TEST

Assessment for Intervertebral Disc Syndrome or Space-Occupying Mass

ORTHOPEDIC GAMUT 8-35

DISORDERS MIMICKING DISC DISEASE

Common disorders that mimic intervertebral disc disease:
1. Ankylosing spondylitis
2. Multiple myeloma
3. Vascular insufficiency
4. Arthritis of the hip
5. Osteoporosis with stress fractures
6. Extradural tumors
7. Peripheral neuropathy
8. Myofascial trigger points and herpes zoster

ORTHOPEDIC GAMUT 8-36

OTHER CAUSES OF SCIATICA

Causes of sciatica not related to disc herniated nucleus pulposus:
1. Synovial cysts
2. Rupture of the medial head of the gastrocnemius
3. Sacroiliac joint dysfunction
4. Lesions in the sacrum and pelvis
5. Fracture of the ischial tuberosity

8

ORTHOPEDIC GAMUT 8-37

ACTIVE STRAIGHT-LEG-RAISING TEST

- The active straight-leg-raising (ASLR) test is a check for over-loading of ligaments of the pelvic ring or lumbopelvic junction or both.
- In this test, performed in supine position, a subject raises one leg, with the knee extended, 20 cm above the examination surface.
- The test is scored, only by the patient, rating the impairment on a 6-point Likert scale.
- The ASLR test is a valid and reliable test to discriminate between patients with pregnancy-related low back pain and healthy subjects and to test the severity of pregnancy-related low back pain.
- However, objective measurements are lacking.

PROCEDURE

- The patient is lying supine with both lower limbs straight out and is directed to raise the limbs until the heels are 6 inches off the table.
- The patient holds the position for as long as possible.
- The test is positive if the patient experiences lower back pain (Fig. 8-41).
- Because this maneuver increases the subarachnoid pressure, if the patient can hold the position for 30 seconds without pain, a pathologic condition of intrathecal origin can be ruled out.
- If the test is positive, the patient may have a pathologic condition, such as a herniated disc, in or outside the spinal cord sheath.

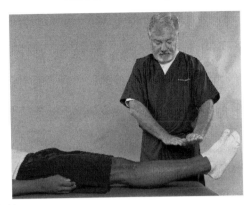

FIG. 8-41

CLINICAL PEARL

This test increases thecal pressure. The ability to hold this position for any time rules out a pathologic condition of thecal origin.

8

MINOR SIGN

**Assessment for Sacroiliac Lesions, Lumbosacral
Strains and Sprains, Lumbopelvic Fractures,
Intervertebral Disc Syndrome, Muscular Dystrophy,
and Dystonia**

PROCEDURE

- Sciatic radiculitis is suggested by how a patient with this condition
  rises from a seated position.
- The patient supports the body with the uninvolved side by balanc-
  ing on the healthy leg, placing one hand on the back, and flexing
  the knee and hip of the affected limb (Fig. 8-42).
- The sign is often present with sacroiliac lesions, lumbosacral
  strains and sprains, fractures, disc syndromes, dystrophies, and
  myotonia.

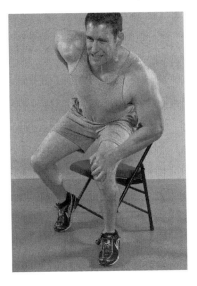

FIG. 8-42

CLINICAL PEARL

With lumbar disc lesions, all movements of the spine—extension, flexion, lateral flexion, and rotation—are affected. With an acute lesion, extension and flexion are seriously restricted, but lateral flexion and rotation are free. The degree of restriction is governed by the phase and severity of the local pathologic process. During an acute attack, the striking feature of the spine is the complete loss of its inherent flexibility. The patient avoids motion in any direction.

NACHLAS TEST

Assessment for Sacroiliac or Lumbosacral Disorder

Comment

A most comprehensive low back differential diagnosis system based on symptoms is that developed by the Quebec Task Force (Table 8-21).

ORTHOPEDIC GAMUT 8-38

DIFFERENTIAL RED FLAGS IN LOW BACK PAIN

- Advanced age
- Bowel or bladder incontinence retention
- Constant progressive pain at night
- Intravenous drug use
- Prior cancer
- Trauma
- Fever
- Prolonged systemic steroid use
- Saddle anesthesia
- Systemic illness or infection
- Unexplained weight loss

TABLE 8-21

DURATION OF SYMPTOMS AND WORKING STATUS CLASSIFICATION OF LOW BACK PAIN DISORDERS

Classification	Symptoms	Duration of Symptoms from Onset	Working Status at Time of Evaluation
1	Pain without radiation	a (<7 days)	W (working)
2	Pain + radiation to extremity, proximally	b (7 days–7 wks)	I (idle)
3	Pain + radiation to extremity, distally	c (>7 wks)	
4	Pain + radiation to upper/lower limb neurologic signs		
5	Presumptive compression of a spinal nerve root on a simple roentgenogram (i.e., spinal instability or fracture)		
6	Compression of a spinal nerve root confirmed by Specific imaging techniques (i.e., computerized) Other diagnostic techniques (i.e., electromyography, venography)		
7	Spinal stenosis		
8	Postsurgical status, 1-6 mos after intervention		
9	Postsurgical status, >6 mos after intervention		
	9.1 Asymptomatic		
	9.2 Symptomatic		
10	Chronic pain syndrome		W (working)
11	Other diagnoses		I (idle)

Adapted from Pope MH et al: *Occupational low back pain assessment, treatment and prevention,* St Louis, 1991. Mosby.

8

PROCEDURE

- To eliminate lumbosacral muscular influence in this test, the patient is placed prone and relaxed on a rigid table.
- Pain in the lower back and lower extremity is noted during passive flexion of the knee.
- The test is positive if pain is noted in the sacroiliac area or lumbosacral area or if the pain radiates down the thigh or leg (Fig. 8-43).
- A positive test indicates a sacroiliac or lumbosacral disorder.

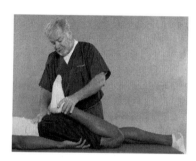

FIG. 8-43

CLINICAL PEARL

Intermittent prolapse of nuclear material is called a *concealed disc* or *occult disc*. Degenerated nuclear material still within the confines of the annulus, which may be weakened by degenerative process but remains intact, may bulge beyond its normal limits when the spine is subjected to certain stresses. Depending on the stresses, the prolapse appears and then disappears. Extension and hyperextension of the spine favor the prolapse, which can produce a defect in the anterior aspect of a myelographic column of dye. When the spine is relieved of stress, such as when the patient is relaxed and lying in the prone position, the defect disappears.

NERI SIGN

Assessment for Lower Intervertebral Disc Syndrome, Lumbosacral and Sacroiliac Strain, or Lumbopelvic Subluxation

---

ORTHOPEDIC GAMUT 8-39

ALTERATIONS IN SPINAL BALANCE AND CURVATURE

Alterations of spinal balance and curvature are implicated in the development of a variety of spinal disorders:

- Acute and chronic low back pain
- Disc degeneration
- Spondylosis
- Ossification of spinal ligaments
- Adolescent idiopathic scoliosis
- Scheuermann kyphosis
- Impaired ribcage expansion
- Early osteoarthritis and disc degeneration
- Osteoporosis and vertebral compression fractures
- Spondylolisthesis

8

ORTHOPEDIC GAMUT 8-40

LUMBAR NERVE ROOT ANOMALIES

- Type I
  - Intradural anastomosis between rootlets at different levels
- Type II
  - Anomalous origin of the nerve roots separated into four subtypes:
    - Cranial origin
    - Caudal origin
    - Combination of cranial and caudal origin
    - Conjoined nerve roots
- Type III
  - Extradural anastomosis between roots
- Type IV
  - Extradural division of the nerve root

PROCEDURE

- While in a standing posture, the patient is directed to bow forward.
- The sign is present when the patient flexes the knee on the affected side (Fig. 8-44).
- The trunk flexion action causes pain in the leg.
- This pain is a common sign with lower disc problems, as well as lumbosacral and sacroiliac strain subluxations.

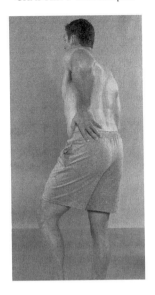

FIG. 8-44

CLINICAL PEARL

Muscle tenderness may be associated with nerve root irritation. With an acute attack, tenderness of the buttock, thigh, and calf on the affected side is often demonstrable. When pain is localized to a specific area along the course of the sciatic nerve, thorough regional examination is essential for ruling out local lesions, such as an abscess, neurofibroma, glomus tumor, lipoma, or sterile abscess, that irritate the sciatic nerve.

PRONE KNEE-BENDING TEST

Assessment for L2 or L3 Nerve Root Lesion, Femoral Nerve Inflammation, or Quadriceps Muscular Strain

ORTHOPEDIC GAMUT 8-41

FRANK DEGENERATION OF THE FACETS

Frank degeneration of the facets may be associated with the following three clinically important conditions:
1. Degeneration of the facets is part of the overall process of spinal degeneration and significantly contributes to pain in patients with multilevel spinal osteoarthritis.
2. Degeneration of the facets, with associated development of osteophytes projecting into the lateral recess and central spinal canal, is a significant part of degenerative spinal stenosis.
3. Degeneration of the facets is sometimes associated with a ventrally projecting synovial cyst, which impinges on the nerve root and thus is part of the differential diagnosis of sciatica.

ORTHOPEDIC GAMUT 8-42

CAUSES OF MERALGIA PARESTHETICA (LATERAL FEMORAL NERVE COMPRESSION)

A variety of causes for meralgia paresthetica exists (most common in bold type):

- Abdominal distention
- Cholecystectomy
- Direct trauma
  - **Iatrogenic complications after thoracoabdominal surgery**
  - Idiopathic causes
  - **Iliac bone graft harvesting**
  - Laparoscopic inguinal hernia repair
  - Limb length discrepancy
  - Metastatic carcinoma in the iliac crest
  - Myomectomy
  - Neuropathy involving the lateral cutaneous nerve
  - Neuropathy of diabetes mellitus and thyroid diseases
  - Obesity and pregnancy
  - Rare complication of heart operations
  - Retroperitoneal tumors
  - Seat belt injury
  - **Tight clothing**

PROCEDURE

- The patient is prone as the knees are passively flexed so that the heels touch the buttocks.
- An L2 or L3 nerve root lesion is indicated by unilateral lumbar pain (Fig. 8-45).
- The test stretches the femoral nerve.

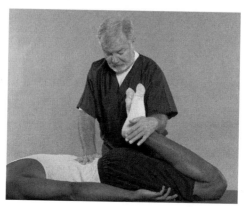

FIG. 8-45

CLINICAL PEARL

Prone knee flexion can provide provocative testing for lumbar disc protrusion. The pathophysiologic aspect of this test depends on compression of spinal nerves during hyperextension of the lumbar spine. The compression intensifies intervertebral disc protrusion into the spinal canal. The lumbar intervertebral foramina are narrowed, and the spinal canal cross-sectional area is decreased by lumbar extension. The presence of a protruded disc that has not produced other physical findings may be detected by this test.

QUICK TEST

Assessment for Lower Back or Lower Extremity Screening

ORTHOPEDIC GAMUT 8-43

LOW BACK PAIN

Considering low back pain under three headings is helpful:
1. Back pain may be associated with a spinal pathologic process, such as vertebral infections, tumors, ankylosing spondylitis, polyarthritis, Paget disease, and primary neurologic disease.
2. Back pain may be associated with nerve root pain. The most common causes are intervertebral disc prolapse and compression of nerve roots within the neural canals.
3. Back pain may be caused by disturbance of the mechanics of the spine (mechanical back pain). This group is the largest group of conditions that cause back pain.

8

PROCEDURE

- The Quick test is accomplished with the patient standing.
- The patient squats down and stands again (Fig. 8-46).
- This action will help the examiner quickly assess the integrity of the ankles, knees, and hips.
- If the patient can fully squat without any symptoms, these joints are free of disease related to the pain complaint.

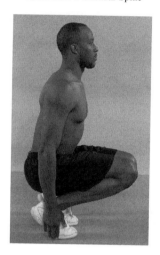

FIG. 8-46

SCHOBER TEST

Assessment for Lumbar Spine Motion

PROCEDURE

- Schober test is used to assess lumbar spine flexion.
- A point is marked at the spinous process level of S2. Points 0.5 cm below S2 and 10 cm above the S2 level are marked.
- The distance between the two S2 reference points is measured.
- The patient flexes forward. The distance between the S2 reference points is remeasured.
- The difference between the two measurements indicates the amount of lumbar flexion.
- Normally, the S2 reference points should separate at least 5 to 8 cm (Fig. 8-47).

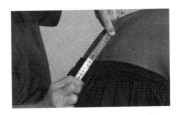

FIG. 8-47

CLINICAL PEARL

For a modification of this test, the patient is placed in a maximal flexion position (seated or standing), and starting from the upper sacral spinous prominence, three 10-cm segments are marked up the spine. The distances between the marks are then remeasured while the patient is erect. The lowest segment should shorten by at least 50%, the middle should shorten by 40%, and the upper should shorten by 30%. The shortening effect will be greater in tall subjects.

SICARD SIGN

Assessment for Sciatic Radiculopathy

Comment

Once a fragment transgresses the peridural membrane, epidural fat and the epidural venous plexus, the nerve root itself presumably acts as an impediment to further posterior migration.

ORTHOPEDIC GAMUT 8-44

LOCATION OF LESION WITHIN AN INTERVERTEBRAL DISC

Standardization of the nomenclature used in reporting the location of disc lesions in the lumbar spine (Whiltse system). In the Whiltse system, areas in the axial plane (medial to lateral), are called _zones_, and in the craniocaudal direction, they are called _levels_.

- Zones are:
  - The central canal zone
  - The subarticular zone
  - The foraminal zone
  - The extraforaminal zone
- In the caudocranial direction, levels from above downward are:
  - The supra pedicle level
  - The pedicle level
  - The infra pedicle level
  - The disc level

ORTHOPEDIC GAMUT 8-45

DISC FRAGMENT MIGRATION

- When a fragment ruptures the posterior longitudinal ligament and enters the anterior extradural space as a distinct entity, it migrates in 35% to 72% of cases.
- Subligamentous herniations (contained) and noncontained herniations, which rupture the posterior longitudinal ligament, can migrate away from the interspace.
- Lateral migration (e.g., from the subarticular zone to the foraminal zone) at the level of the interspace is probably the most common pattern.
- Rostral and caudal migration (e.g., from disc level to pedicle level) together are the most clinically important modes of migration because they may result in retained fragments.
- Migration of disc material posterior to the dura is an uncommon condition.

PROCEDURE

- While the patient is supine, the extended leg is raised to a point just short of that which produces pain.
- When the sign is present, dorsiflexion of the great toe reproduces sciatic pain (Fig. 8-48).
- The test is significant for sciatic radiculopathy.

8

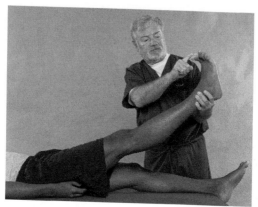

FIG. 8-48

CLINICAL PEARL

The second, third, and fourth nerve roots do not have an increase in tension during straight leg raising, but they do undergo an increase in tension during the femoral stretch tests.

SIGN OF THE BUTTOCK

Assessment for Gluteal Bursitis, Tumor, or Abscess

ORTHOPEDIC GAMUT 8-46

BENIGN SOFT-TISSUE TUMORS

- Vascular
    - Venous malformation
    - Arteriovenous malformation
    - Glomus tumor
- Lipomatous
    - Lipoma
    - Hibernoma
    - Chondroid lipoma
    - Fibrolipoma
    - Atypical lipoma
    - Lipoma arborescens
    - Lipoblastoma
    - Myelolipoma
    - Myolipoma
    - Angiolipoma
- Fibrous
    - Fibromatosis
    - Elastofibroma
    - Fibroma of tendon sheath
    - Solitary fibrous tumor
    - Calcifying aponeurotic fibroma
    - Infantile myofibroma
    - Reactive fibroblastic tumor
- Neurogenic
    - Schwannoma
    - Neurofibroma
    - Neuroma
- Myxomas
- Chondral
    - Soft-tissue chondroma
- Synovial
    - Giant cell tumor of tendon sheath

8

PROCEDURE

- A passive unilateral straight-leg-raising test is performed on a supine patient.
- When unilateral restriction is encountered, the knee is flexed to determine if hip flexion increases (Fig. 8-49).
- If the lumbar spine is the source of complaint, hip flexion will increase.
- A positive sign of the buttock occurs when hip flexion does not increase with knee flexion.
- The sign is present in bursitis, tumor, or abscess.

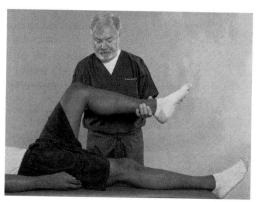

FIG. 8-49

CLINICAL PEARL

Trochanteric bursitis causes localized pain and tenderness over the trochanter and occasionally causes pain that radiates down the lateral thigh. The pain is particularly strong when lying on the affected side. Pain from ischiogluteal bursitis is felt posteriorly and is particularly exacerbated by sitting.

SKIN PINCH TEST

Assessment for Fibrositic Infiltration

ORTHOPEDIC GAMUT 8-47

CAUDA EQUINA SYNDROME

The clinical characteristics of cauda equina syndrome (CES triad of signs) include the following:
1. Anesthesia in the distribution of the S2–S4 nerve roots, which supply the perineum in the distribution of a person sitting on a saddle, leading to the term saddle anesthesia
2. Disturbance of bladder and bowel control with urinary incontinence or retention and fecal incontinence (Any urinary disturbance in a patient with back pain constitutes an emergency and requires urgent investigation.)
3. Lower extremity weakness

ORTHOPEDIC GAMUT 8-48

CAUDA EQUINA SYNDROME DIAGNOSTIC ESSENTIALS

- Presentation: low back pain, radicular symptoms, lower-extremity paresthesias, lower-extremity weakness, urinary or fecal retention, incontinence, gait abnormalities, and frequent falls
- Examination
  - Leg weakness
  - Decreased or absent deep-tendon reflexes
  - Saddle anesthesia
  - Decreased or absent sphincter tone
- Tests
  - Positive straight-leg-raising
  - Abnormal sphincter tone
  - Postvoid residual above 100–200 mL
  - Obtain urgent whole spine magnetic resonance imaging

8

PROCEDURE

- The skin pinch test involves smoothly rolling the skin over the spinous process of the vertebrae by using the forefingers over the advancing thumbs (Fig. 8-50).
- The skin is picked up before rolling it.
- Skin rolling is then performed over each side of the back.
- Fibrositic infiltration and trigger points are demonstrated by tightness and acute tenderness.
- The patient will experience tightness and tenderness maximally over the level at which a pathologic bone condition exists or over the vertebra above the level at which a pathologic joint or disc condition exists.

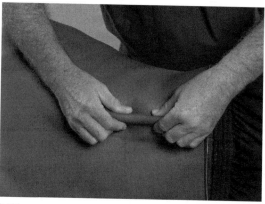

FIG. 8-50

CLINICAL PEARL

Trophedematous subcutaneous tissue has a boggy, inelastic texture when rolled between the thumb and finger. This type of tissue is distinguishable from subcutaneous fat. When a patch of skin and subcutaneous tissue a centimeter in diameter is gently squeezed together, instead of immediately forming a fold of flesh, trophedematous tissue does not budge, or it finally yields altogether, with a sudden expanding movement similar to that of inflating a rubber dinghy or air mattress.

SPINAL PERCUSSION TEST

Assessment for Osseous or Soft-Tissue Injury in the Lumbar Spine

---

ORTHOPEDIC GAMUT 8-49

SPINAL TRAUMA MECHANISMS

Spinal trauma mechanisms:
1. Hyperextension
2. Flexion
3. Flexion combined with rotation
4. Axial displacement (compression)

ORTHOPEDIC GAMUT 8-50

OSTEOPOROTIC COMPRESSION FRACTURE CLASSIFICATION

- Type I compression fracture involving the anterior column only
  - Type Ia is a compression fracture with union.
  - Type Ib is a compression fracture with non-union.
- Type II fracture involving both the anterior and middle column
  - Type IIa is a compression fracture with union.
  - Type IIb is a compression fracture with non-union.
- Type II compression fractures have a higher incidence of non-union than type I.
- In both type I and II non-union groups, fractures achieve greater increase in vertebral body height after vertebroplasty than both type I and type II union group fractures.
- In both non-union groups, fractures achieve a greater reduction of kyphotic angle postvertebroplasty than type I and II union group fractures.

8

ORTHOPEDIC GAMUT 8-51

ANTERIOR VERTEBRAL COMPRESSION FRACTURES

Roentgenographic findings in anterior vertebral compression fractures:

1. Buckling of the anterior vertebral body cortex
2. Wedge deformity of the fractured vertebral body, with loss of the vertebral body height anteriorly compared with its posterior height
3. Possibility of some focal increase in kyphosis
4. A zone of condensation caused by compaction of the trabecular elements of the spongiosa, appearing as a band of increased osseous density through the medullary bone beneath the affected end-plate
5. Vertebral end-plate fractures occur more frequently in the lower thoracic and upper lumbar spines.
6. Vertebral body compression fractures may be suspected when a *frog-face* sign is exhibited on the anteroposterior study.
7. Paraspinal soft-tissue injury is often observed with spinal compression fractures.

ORTHOPEDIC GAMUT 8-52

SPINAL FRACTURES

Other forms of spinal fractures may include the following:

1. Lateral body compression-type fractures
2. Pillar fractures
3. Lamina-pedicle fractures
4. Transverse process fractures

ORTHOPEDIC GAMUT 8-53
INTRA DISCAL PRESSURE

Compressive forces that influencing intra discal pressure:

1. *Standing:* Disc pressure is equal to 100% of body weight.
2. *Supine:* Disc pressure is less than 25% of body weight.
3. *Side lying:* Disc pressure is less than 75% of body weight.
4. *Standing and bending forward:* Disc pressure is approximately 150% of body weight.
5. *Supine with both knees flexed:* Disc pressure is less than 35% of body weight.
6. *Seated in a flexed position:* Disc pressure is approximately 85% of body weight.
7. *Bending forward in a flexed posture and lifting:* Disc pressure is approaching 275% of body weight.

PROCEDURE

- While the patient is standing and the trunk is slightly flexed, the examiner uses a neurologic hammer to percuss the spinous processes and the associated musculature of each of the lumbar vertebrae (Fig. 8-51).
- Evidence of localized pain indicates a possible vertebra fracture.
- Evidence of radicular pain indicates a possible disc lesion.
- Because of the nonspecific nature of this test, other conditions will also elicit a positive pain response.
- For example, a ligamentous sprain will cause pain when the spinous processes are percussed.
- Percussing the paraspinal musculature will elicit a positive sign for muscular strain (Figs. 8-52 and 8-53).

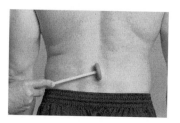

FIG. 8-51

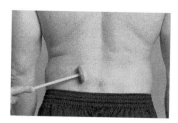

FIG. 8-52

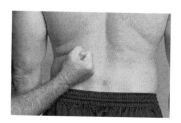

FIG. 8-53

CLINICAL PEARL

When soft-tissue percussion reproduces the complaint, the examiner may expect the same phenomenon from the use of ultrasound on the tissue. The uses of such therapies may be delayed until the soft tissue is no longer reactive to percussion.

STRAIGHT-LEG-RAISING TEST

Assessment for Space-Occupying Mass in the Path of a Nerve Root, Sacroiliac Inflammation, and Lumbosacral Involvement

ORTHOPEDIC GAMUT 8-54

UNILATERAL STRAIGHT LEG RAISING

The following are dynamics of unilateral straight leg raising:

1. The slack in sciatic arborization is taken up from 0 to 35 degrees. No dural movement is observed.

2. When approaching 35 degrees, tension is applied to the sciatic nerve roots.

3. In the range of 35 to 70 degrees, the sciatic nerve roots tense over the intervertebral disc. The rate of nerve root deformation diminishes as the angle increases.

4. Above 60 to 70 degrees, practically no further deformation of the root occurs during further straight leg raising, and the pain probably originates in the joint.

8

PROCEDURE

- The patient lies supine with the legs extended.
- The examiner places one hand under the heel of the patient's affected leg and the other hand on the knee.
- With the limb extended, the examiner flexes the patient's thigh on the pelvis.
- If this maneuver is markedly limited because of pain, the test is positive and may suggest sciatica from lumbosacral or sacroiliac lesions, subluxation syndrome, disc lesions, spondylolisthesis, adhesions, or intervertebral foramen occlusion.
- The exacerbation of pain by raising the extended leg is further evidence of the effects of traction on a sensitized nerve root (Fig. 8-54).
- Normally, the leg can be raised 15 to 30 degrees before the nerve root is tractioned through the intervertebral foramen.
- Pain, duplicating sciatica, that is elicited by this maneuver indicates a space-occupying lesion—such as lumbar disc protrusion, tumor, adhesions, edema, and tissue inflammation—at the nerve root level.

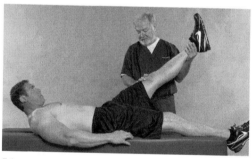

FIG. 8-54

CLINICAL PEARL

As many authors have pointed out, the nerve roots have a narrow range of movement for stretching. Most authors also conclude that the nerve roots in normal conditions are not stretched by the straight-leg-raising test until 35 to 70 degrees of angulation have been reached. However, if the nerve exists with a space-occupying mass (protrusion of disc material) that deflects the nerve's normal pathway, the amount of allowable stretch is already used up by the mass. In this case, the positive sign, pain radiating down the sciatic distribution, occurs at a much lower angulation. This pain has been misconstrued by many researchers to indicate the involvement of the sacroiliac joint instead of the sensitive finding that a nerve root compression syndrome exists. Sciatica that is in the leg and produced from 0 to 30 degrees is caused by nerve root compression. Sciatica that is in the leg and produced from 30 to 60 degrees is probably caused by sacroiliac joint disease. Sciatica that is in the leg and produced above 60 degrees is probably caused by lumbosacral disease.

A cardinal point is that most, if not all, ranges of movement given for the sciatic nerve roots are based on the absence of a space-occupying mass. The angles change dramatically in the presence of disease. This change is the basis of the Cox sign, which reveals the diseased or compressed nerve root, and Demianoff sign, which reveals the normal nerve root but diseased sacroiliac or lumbosacral musculature.

8

TURYN SIGN

Assessment for Sciatic Radiculopathy

ORTHOPEDIC GAMUT 8-55

LUMBAR DISC DISEASE CLASSIFICATION

Variation of the lumbar disc disease classification model is as follows:

- Disc protrusion
  - Type I: peripheral annular bulge
  - Type II: localized annular bulge
- Disc herniation
  - Type I: prolapsed intervertebral disc
  - Type II: extruded intervertebral disc
  - Type III: sequestered intervertebral disc

ORTHOPEDIC GAMUT 8-56

CATEGORIES OF LOW BACK PAIN

1. *Viscerogenic pain:* Pain that originates from the kidneys, sacro-iliac, pelvic lesions, and retroperitoneal tumors. This type of pain is neither aggravated by activity nor relieved by rest.
2. *Neurogenic pain:* Pain commonly caused by neurofibromas, cysts, and tumors of the nerve roots in the lumbar spine.
3. *Vascular pain:* Pain characterized by intermittent claudication from aneurysms and peripheral vascular disease.
4. *Spondylogenic pain:* Pain directly related to the pain originating from soft tissues of the spine and sacroiliac joint.
5. *Psychogenic pain:* Pain that is quite uncommon and ascribed to nonorganic causes.

XORTHOPEDIC GAMUT 8-57

SPINAL EPIDURAL HEMATOMA

Spinal epidural hematoma (SEH) is a rare disease and remains a challenge for clinical diagnosis. Traumatic SEH is less common than spontaneous lesion, and incidence is estimated at less than 1% to 1.7% of all spinal injuries. Traumatic causes include:

- Vertebral fractures
- Obstetrical birth trauma
- Lumbar punctures
- Postsurgical bleeding
- Epidural anesthesia
- Missile injuries

ORTHOPEDIC GAMUT 8-58

RISK FACTORS FOR SPINAL EPIDURAL HEMATOMA

- Cervical spondylosis
- Rheumatoid arthritis
- Paget disease
- Ankylosing spondylitis

8

ORTHOPEDIC GAMUT 8-59

SCIATICA

Origins of sciatica:
1. Prolapsed intervertebral disc pressure, infection, and traumatic sciatic neuritis, perineural fibrositis, infections, and tumors of the spinal cord
2. Lumbosacral and sacroiliac sprain and strain, degenerating intervertebral discs, fibrositis, osteomyelitis, hip joint disease, and secondary carcinomatous deposits in bone
3. Nephrolithiasis, prostatic, renal, and anal disease
4. Toxic and metabolic disorders, conversion hysteria, and arterial insufficiency

PROCEDURE

- When the patient is in the supine position with both lower limbs resting straight out on the table, dorsiflexion of the great toe elicits pain in the gluteal region (Fig. 8-55).
- The sign is significant for sciatic radiculopathy.

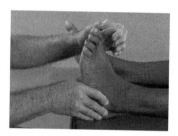

FIG. 8-55

CLINICAL PEARL

A straight-leg-raising test that is positive under 30 degrees reveals a large disc protrusion. The nerve root is stretched long before it would normally be. The straight-leg-raising test is most useful for identifying L5–S1 disc lesions because the pressures on the nerve root are highest at this level. During straight leg raising, L4–L5 is not as apt to give as much pain as the L5–S1 because the pressure between the disc and the nerve root at L4–L5 is one half that at L5–S1. Therefore the L5–S1 disc lesion gives more pain in the lower back and leg than does the L4–L5 disc lesion. No movement on the nerve root occurs until straight leg raising reaches 30 degrees. No movement on L4 occurs during a straight-leg-raising test. From this circumstance, the presence of a Turyn sign indicates a large disc protrusion at the level of the L5–S1 nerve root.

VANZETTI SIGN

Assessment for Sciatic Scoliosis

ORTHOPEDIC GAMUT 8-60

DEGENERATIVE LUMBAR SCOLIOSIS CLASSIFICATION

- Type I: minimal or no lumbar vertebral rotation
  - Type IA: back pain without radicular symptoms is present.
  - Type IB: sciatic pain (from the lumbosacral hemi curve) back pain may or may not be present.
  - Type IC: femoral pain (from the major curve) back pain may or may not be present.
- Type II: rotatory olisthesis (intersegmental rotation and translation)
  - Type IIA: back pain without radicular symptoms is present.
  - Type IIB: sciatic pain (from the lumbosacral hemi curve) back pain may or may not be present.
  - Type IIC: femoral pain (from the major curve) back pain may or may not be present.
- Type III: rotatory olisthesis and structural coronal
  - More than 4 cm distance from C7 plumb line *or*
  - Positive sagittal imbalance (>2 cm from anterior sacral corner)
  - Type IIIA: back pain without radicular symptoms is present.
  - Type IIIB: sciatic pain (from the lumbosacral hemi curve) back pain may or may not be present.
  - Type IIIC: femoral pain (from the major curve) back pain may or may not be present.

8

ORTHOPEDIC GAMUT 8-61

SCOLIOSIS

In scoliosis, the deformity is usually one of the following:
1. Compensatory, resulting from tilting of the pelvis from real or apparent shortening of one leg
2. Sciatic, resulting from a unilateral protective muscle spasm, especially accompanying a prolapsed intervertebral disc

PROCEDURE

- With sciatica, the pelvis is always horizontal even though scoliosis exists (Fig. 8-56).
- When scoliosis is present with other spinal lesions, the pelvis will be tilted.

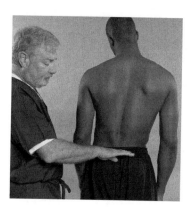

FIG. 8-56

CLINICAL PEARL

Vanzetti sign allows quick observation of the patient to determine the source of the patient's antalgia before performing the more aggressive assessments of the lumbosacral spine.

CHAPTER NINE

PELVIS AND SACROILIAC JOINT

AXIOMS IN ASSESSING THE PELVIS AND THE SACROILIAC JOINTS

- The primary function of the pelvis, including the bones, joints, ligaments, and muscles, is mechanical transfer of weight.
- A secondary function of the bony pelvis is protection of viscera.

INTRODUCTION

The pelvis is a uniquely devised mechanism designed to transfer the body weight from the single weight-bearing axis of the trunk to the bipolar weight bearing of the lower extremities. The spine attaches to the pelvis by a single connection to the sacrum. Weight transfers through the bony ring of the pelvis from the spinal column to the two lower extremities. Enclosed within the pelvis are the bladder, the female genitalia, the rectum, and the great vessels and nerves that extend to the lower extremities.

Narrow, closely fitted, irregularly shaped, and cartilage-covered surfaces of the posterior and internal ilium and the lateral border of the sacrum form the sacroiliac articulation. The lumbosacral trunk lies anteriorly in direct relationship to the sacroiliac articulation. An inflammatory neuritis is a common accompaniment of sacroiliac arthritis. The anterior ligaments are thin and easily distended by intraarticular swelling.

The upper two thirds of the joint are covered posteriorly by the posterior end of the ilium. The lower third of the joint is covered by the sacroiliac ligaments but can often be palpated in thin individuals.

The conditions that affect the sacroiliac joints are those that involve any joint. The sacroiliac articulation is a favored site for tuberculous infection and is often the starting point for ankylosing spondylitis. Degenerative arthritic changes are often significant at this joint.

TABLE 9-1

PELVIS AND SACROILIAC CROSS-REFERENCE TABLE BY ASSESSMENT PROCEDURE

Pelvis

Test/Sign	Disease Assessed					
	Sacroiliac Abnormality	Lumbosacral Syndrome	Sprain	Subluxation	Fracture	Pyogenic Sacroiliitis
Anterior innominate test	●					
Belt test	●	●				
Erichsen sign	●					
Gaenslen test	●	●				
Gapping test	●		●			
Goldthwait sign	●	●				
Hibbs test	●		●	●		

Test					
Iliac compression test					●
Knee-to-shoulder test	●	●	●		●
Laguerre test		●	●		●
Lewin-Gaenslen test		●	●		●
Piedallu sign		●	●		●
Sacral apex test		●	●		●
Sacroiliac resisted-abduction test		●	●		
Smith-Petersen test				●	●
Squish test			●		
Yeoman test		●	●		●

TABLE 9-2

Pelvis and Sacroiliac Joint Cross-Reference Table by Syndrome or Tissue

Fracture	Iliac compression test
Lumbosacral syndrome	Belt test
	Gaenslen test
	Smith-Petersen test
Pyogenic sacroiliitis	Knee-to-shoulder test
Sacroiliac disease	Anterior innominate test
	Belt test
	Erichsen sign
	Gaenslen test
	Gapping test
	Goldthwait sign
	Hibbs test
	Iliac compression test
	Knee-to-shoulder test
	Laguerre test
	Lewin-Gaenslen test
	Piedallu sign
	Sacral apex test
	Smith-Petersen test
	Yeoman test
Sprain	Gapping test
	Hibbs test
	Iliac compression test
	Knee-to-shoulder test
	Laguerre test
	Lewin-Gaenslen test
	Piedallu sign
	Sacral apex test
	Sacroiliac resisted-abduction test
	Squish test
	Yeoman test
Subluxation	Hibbs test
	Iliac compression test
	Knee-to-shoulder test
	Laguerre test
	Lewin-Gaenslen test
	Piedallu sign
	Sacral apex test
	Sacroiliac resisted-abduction test
	Yeoman test

The stability of the sacroiliac joint lies in the nature of its articular surfaces and ligaments. Cardinal in this role are the dense, interosseous ligaments lying dorsal to the joint and the ventral sacroiliac ligament covering its anterior aspect.

In ankylosing spondylitis, the patient complains of spinal pain and stiffness. The sacroiliac joints are affected initially; increasing loss of spinal mobility can lead to loss of the lumbar lordosis.

A common tender fatty nodule in the sacroiliac area is sometimes called the **episacroiliac lipoma** or *back mouse*. In this instance, fatty tissue herniates through the normal deep fascia and become edematous and a source of pain. Clinically, the patient complains of pain in the tender nodules that are palpable and often bilateral. The mass is usually palpable as a mobile soft tumor that slips beneath the examining finger. Such a lipoma mass must be differentiated from the peripelvic serosanguineous cyst.

ESSENTIAL ANATOMY

The two innominate bones (or *hip* bones), the sacrum, and the coccyx make up the pelvis. The innominate bone consists of the ilium, ischium, and pubis.

ORTHOPEDIC GAMUT 9-1
INNOMINATE BONE

Exterior surfaces of the innominate bones:
1. An upper area, the lateral surface of the ilium
2. A central depressed socket, the acetabulum
3. A lower region, in which curved rami of the pubis and ischium form the obturator foramen

---

ORTHOPEDIC GAMUT 9-2
SUPERIOR HALF OF THE PELVIS

Interior surfaces of the superior half of the pelvis include:
1. Superiorly, the iliac fossa, a shallow depression in the ilium
2. A posterior roughened articular surface
3. Inferiorly, the medial surface of obturator foramen

9

The lumbosacral plexus takes shape on the medial surface of the levator ani muscle (Table 9-3).

TABLE 9-3
SACRAL PLEXUS

Anterior Divisions	Posterior Divisions
Nerve to quadratus femoris/ inferior gemellus	Nerve to piriformis
Nerve to obturator internus/ superior gemellus	Superior gluteal nerve
Posterior femoral cutaneous nerve*	Inferior gluteal nerve
Tibial nerve	Posterior femoral cutaneous nerve*
Pudendal nerve	Common peroneal nerve
Pelvic splanchnic nerves	Perforating cutaneous nerve
Nerve to levator ani/coccygeus	

*Both divisions contribute to this nerve.
Adapted from Mathers LH et al: *Clinical anatomy principles,* St Louis, 1996, Mosby.

ESSENTIAL MOTION ASSESSMENT

Although firmly constrained by its ligaments, the sacroiliac joint exhibits movements that are small in magnitude and complex in nature. The amplitude of nutation of the sacrum is normally not more than 2 mm or 2 degrees.

ESSENTIAL MUSCLE FUNCTION ASSESSMENT

The gluteal and erector muscles aid in stabilizing the spine and provide extension. To evaluate functional strength in spinal extension, the examiner places the patient in a prone position. The patient raises one arm out straight in front and simultaneously lifts the leg on the opposite side out straight. The patient holds this position for 5 to 10 seconds, and the examiner notes any fatigue or inability to gain a healthy contraction, especially on the side of the leg lift. This side activates the hip and spinal extensor mass. The patient repeats the exercise on the opposite side, and the examiner compares the observations.

ORTHOPEDIC GAMUT 9-3

LUMBOPELVIC FLEXIBILITY TESTING PROCEDURES

1. *Spinal erector muscles:* With the patient in the supine position, the examiner gently bends the patient's knee to the chest.

2. *Hip flexor muscles:* With the patient prone, the examiner places the patient's affected hip into extension and then abducts the thigh.

3. *Hamstring muscles:* Placing the patient supine and keeping the patient's hips and buttocks down to the table, the examiner performs a straight leg raise with the patient's knee held in extension.

4. *Gluteal muscles:* The patient should be supine and placed in hip flexion with a bent knee. The lower leg can be internally rotated with thigh adduction to facilitate a stretch of the rotator muscles of the hip, such as the gluteus medius and piriformis.

5. *Quadriceps muscles:* With the patient prone and the examiner's inferior hand on the patient's affected knee, the examiner uses the shoulder to move the patient's lower leg gently toward the ipsilateral buttock to induce knee flexion.

ESSENTIAL IMAGING

The pelvis can be well visualized by a routine anteroposterior (AP) roentgenogram. In addition, the sacrum and coccyx may be studied by lateral views and AP views angled 15 degrees cephalad and caudad.

Radiographic evaluation can play an important role in ruling out an inflammatory arthritis. Conditions such as ankylosing spondylitis can have a clinical presentation similar to other spondyloarthropathies, with referral of pain into the hip and gluteal regions. After pregnancy, conditions such as osteitis condensans ilii can also be identified with plain films. In this case, the soft-tissue findings cannot be evaluated with plain films.

ANTERIOR INNOMINATE TEST

ALSO KNOWN AS MAZION PELVIC MANEUVER

Assessment for Unilateral Forward Displacement of the Ilia on the Sacrum

Comment

Many cases of acute low back pain that are not correctly identified evolve into a chronic spinal problem with significant disability at the muscular level (Table 9-4). Muscular fixation alone can be the cause of spinal joint dysfunction.

TABLE 9-4

LUMBOPELVIC SYNDROMES

Diagnosis	Site of Complaint
Quadratus lumborum syndrome	Gluteal region, anterior iliac spine, greater trochanter of femur
Gluteus maximus or medius syndrome	Sacral and gluteal region, lateral hip
Gluteus minimus syndrome	Lateral hip, thigh, and calf
Chronic lumbar strain (spinal erector muscles)	Laterally to ribs, caudally toward lumbosacral junction
Piriformis syndrome	Sacroiliac region; posterior hip, thigh, calf; possibly sole of foot

Adapted from Brier SR: *Primary care orthopedics*, St Louis, 1999, Mosby.

ORTHOPEDIC GAMUT 9-4

LUMBOPELVIC MUSCLES

Results of lumbopelvic muscle contractures:
1. Contracture of lumbodorsal fascia
2. Anterior pelvic tilt
3. Inappropriate transfer of loads to the lumbar spine
4. Difficulty in attaining the proper biomechanical posture for lifting

ORTHOPEDIC GAMUT 9-5

LUMBOPELVIC SPINE MUSCULAR SYNDROMES

Clinical findings of lumbopelvic spine muscular syndromes:
1. Hip inflexibility
2. Weakness of the hip and spine extensor mechanism
3. Intersegmental lumbosacral fixation
4. Myofascial trigger points in the spinal erector, quadratus lumborum, gluteal musculature, and psoas muscles
5. Referred zones of pain to the hip, buttocks, thigh, and lateral lower leg
6. Severe tightness of the outward rotators of the hip
7. Muscle hypertonicity
8. Palpable tenderness with pressure or stretch
9. Taut, tender, or ropelike muscle fibers

PROCEDURE

- The patient with lower trunk pain is in the standing position and is instructed to place the lower extremity that is opposite the painful side approximately 2 or 3 feet in front of the foot of the other extremity.
- This position is such that the patient appears to be taking a big step forward.
- The patient then bends the upper trunk acutely over the forward extremity so as to put all the weight on the front leg.
- The patient flexes to the point at which the heel of the back foot rises from the floor (Fig. 9-1).
- The production or aggravation of lower trunk pain on the side of the posterior leg indicates a positive test.
- A positive test indicates unilateral forward displacement of the ilia (anterior innominate) in relation to the sacrum.

9

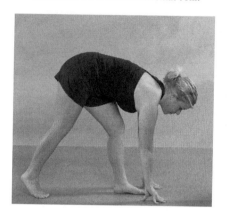

FIG. 9-1

CLINICAL PEARL

The sacroiliac joint, most inaccessible to palpation, is difficult to assess clinically. Only florid inflammation or damage to the fibrous portion is likely to result in local posterior tenderness. This tenderness is probably ligamentous.

BELT TEST

SUPPORTED ADAMS TEST

Assessment for Sprain of the Sacroiliac Ligaments or Lumbosacral Capsular Sprain

PROCEDURE

- The patient with lower back symptoms is in the standing position.
- The patient flexes the dorsolumbar spine while the examiner notes the amount of movement necessary to aggravate the pain.
- While positioned behind the patient, the examiner grasps the patient's iliac crests and braces a hip against the patient's sacrum.
- The patient flexes the spine again as the examiner immobilizes the patient's pelvis (Fig. 9-2).
- If the lesion is of a pelvic nature, flexing the spine with the pelvis immobilized will not reproduce the discomfort.
- If the lesion is of a spinal nature, the pain will be aggravated in both instances.

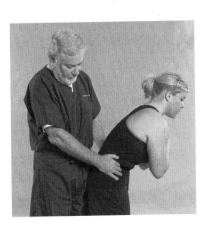

FIG. 9-2

CLINICAL PEARL

Because of the stabilizing effect of the very strong ligamentous structures, sprain of the sacroiliac ligaments accompanies sacroiliac subluxation and is a subluxation sprain. Posterior subluxation results from a flexion-type injury, which occurs with activities such as lifting or pushing. Anterior subluxation results from extension-type injuries, which occur when falling forward or extending the leg.

ERICHSEN SIGN

Assessment for Sacroiliac Disease *versus* Pathologic Conditions Involving the Hip Joint

ORTHOPEDIC GAMUT 9-6

ACETABULAR FRACTURES

In general, acetabular fractures involve one or more of the following:
1. The posterior rim
2. The posterior column
3. The anterior column
4. The quadrilateral plate

PROCEDURE

- While the patient is prone, the examiner places the hands over the dorsum of the ilia and proceeds to give a forceful, sharp, bilateral thrust toward the midline (Fig. 9-3).
- The sign is present when this procedure produces pain over the sacroiliac area.
- Pain is felt in sacroiliac joint disease but not in hip joint disease.

9

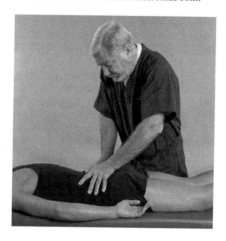

FIG. 9-3

CLINICAL PEARL

Patients who possess an anomalous relation of the piriformis muscle to the sciatic nerve are particularly susceptible to developing symptoms of sciatic neuritis when the muscle is hypertonic or spastic. Approximately 10% of the population possesses such an anomaly. A reflex spasm of this muscle may occur because of intraarticular sacroiliac subluxation and sacroiliac irritation. Such a spasm is probably the cause of a positive Lasègue test, which is positive in the range of 20 to 45 degrees.

Cross-legged sitting results in a relative elongation of the piriformis muscle of 11.7% compared with normal sitting and even 21.4% compared with standing. Application of piriformis muscle force results in inward deformation of the pelvic ring and compression of the sacroiliac joints and the dorsal side of the pubic symphysis.

GAENSLEN TEST

Assessment for Sacroiliac Disease

ORTHOPEDIC GAMUT 9-7

PELVIC RING

Five distinct different types of joints of the pelvic ring:
1. The lumbosacral zygapophyseal joints
2. The anterior lumbosacral
3. Coxal (hip)
4. Sacroiliac joint
5. Symphysis pubis

ORTHOPEDIC GAMUT 9-8

SACROILIAC JOINTS

Sacroiliac joint movement contributions:
1. Locomotion
2. Spinal and thigh movement
3. Changes of position (e.g., from lying to standing, standing to sitting)

9

PROCEDURE

- The patient is lying supine.
- The examiner acutely flexes the knee and thigh of the patient's unaffected leg to the abdomen.
- This move brings the lumbar spine firmly into contact with the table and fixes both the pelvis and the lumbar spine.
- With the examiner standing at a right angle to the patient, the patient is brought well to the side of the table, and the examiner slowly hyperextends the patient's affected thigh (Fig. 9-4).
- This hyperextension is accomplished by gradually increasing the pressure of one hand on top of the knee while the examiner's other hand is on the flexed knee.

- The hyperextension of the affected hip exerts a rotating force on the corresponding half of the pelvis.
- The pull is made on the ilium, through the Y-ligament, and the muscles attached to the anterior iliac spine.
- The test is positive if pain is felt in the sacroiliac area or referred down the thigh.
- The test is performed bilaterally.
- If the test is negative, a lumbosacral lesion is suspected.
- The test is usually contraindicated in older patients.

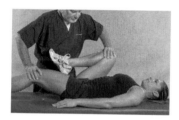

FIG. 9-4

CLINICAL PEARL

Sacroiliac joint involvement produces local pain over the joint, or pain that is referred to (1) the groin on the same side, (2) the posterior thigh on the same side, and (3) down the leg, which is less often. Pain is often increased by lying on the affected side.

GAPPING TEST

Sacroiliac Stretch Test

Assessment for Sprain of the Anterior Sacroiliac Ligaments

ORTHOPEDIC GAMUT 9-9

OSTEITIS PUBIS

Primary clinical types of osteitis pubis:
1. Noninfectious osteitis pubis, associated with urologic procedures, gynecologic procedures, and pregnancy
2. Infectious osteitis pubis, associated with local or distant infection loci
3. Athletic or mechanical trauma osteitis pubis
4. Degenerative or rheumatologic osteitis pubis

PROCEDURE

- The patient lies supine, and the examiner places both hands on the patient's anterosuperior spine of each ilium and presses laterally downward.
- Crossing the arms increases the lateral component of the strain on the ligaments (Fig. 9-5).
- The pelvis must not be allowed to rock because the lumbar spine then moves.
- The examiner's hands can cause anterior iliac spine discomfort as a result of compression of the skin against the osseous structures.
- The expected finding is not local pain but rather aggravation of the gluteal symptoms.
- The response to the test is positive only if unilateral gluteal or posterior crural pain is elicited.
- The test is significant for anterior sacroiliac ligament sprain.

9

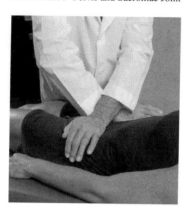

FIG. 9-5

CLINICAL PEARL

Stretching the anterior ligaments in the manner described is the most delicate test for the sacroiliac joint. Patients recovering from a sacroiliac injury may say that all pain ceased some days before. Patients walk and bend painlessly; yet for 7 to 10 days after subjective recovery, the straining of the joint that occurs in the gapping test still evokes discomfort. This test clearly applies more stress to sacroiliac ligaments than ordinary daily activities. If a patient has symptoms referable to the sacroiliac joint, this maneuver will elicit them.

GOLDTHWAIT SIGN

Assessment for Sacroiliac Joint Sprain Versus a Lumbosacral Spine Abnormality

PROCEDURE

- The patient is supine.
- The patient's affected leg is raised slowly while one of the examiner's hands is under the lumbar portion of the patient's spine.
- If pain is brought on before the lumbar spine begins to move, a sacroiliac lesion is probably present.
- The lesion may be caused by arthritis or by a sprain of the ligaments that involve the sacroiliac joint (Fig. 9-6).
- If pain does not come on until after the lumbar spine begins to move, the disorder is more likely to have its origin in the lumbosacral area or, less commonly, in the sacroiliac area.
- The test is repeated with the unaffected limb.
- A positive sign of a lumbosacral lesion is elicited if pain occurs at approximately the same height as it did with the affected limb.
- If the unaffected leg can be raised higher than the affected leg, it signifies sacroiliac involvement of the affected side.

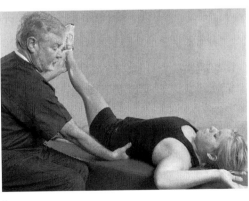

FIG. 9-6

CLINICAL PEARL

This test is similar to the Lasègue test, the straight-leg-raising test, and Smith-Petersen test. All of these tests have in common the use of the affected leg as a lever to stretch the suspect tissue, whether neural or ligamentous. The key to differentiation is the determination of the moment of L5–S1 separation, reflecting lumbosacral movement.

HIBBS TEST

Assessment for Sacroiliac Disease

Comment
Evaluation of the SI-joint is challenging. First, the SI-joint is subject to a wide range of normal anatomic variation. Second, its unusual location and its oblique position make direct palpation almost impossible.

PROCEDURE

- While the patient is in the prone position, the examiner stabilizes the patient's pelvis on the nearest side by placing one hand firmly on the dorsum of the iliac bone.
- With the other hand around the patient's ankle, the opposite knee is flexed to a right angle.
- The knee is flexed to its maximum without elevating the thigh from the examination table.
- From this position, the examiner slowly pushes the patient's leg laterally, causing strong internal rotation of the femoral head (Fig. 9-7).
- The test is performed bilaterally.
- The production of pelvic pain is a positive finding.
- The test is significant for a sacroiliac lesion.
- In the absence of hip involvement, stress is transmitted through the hip joints into the sacroiliac mechanism, producing pain.

9

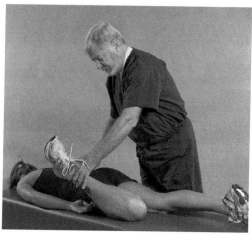

FIG. 9-7

CLINICAL PEARL

Tuberculosis is now rare in developed countries but remains a scourge elsewhere. Complications may be serious because of the formation of sinuses. These sinuses may become secondarily infected and may cause paraplegia (Pott paraplegia) because of (1) pus and intracellular pressure, (2) mechanical injury to the nervous system (cord) caused by bony pressure, or (3) vascular embarrassment of the nervous system where it crosses the bony infection. Hibbs test is not specific for tuberculosis of the sacroiliac joint but is correlated with other systemic findings that may suggest the existence of this type of tuberculosis. At the least, Hibbs test reveals mechanical dysfunction of the sacroiliac joint.

ILIAC COMPRESSION TEST

COMPRESSION OF THE ILIAC CRESTS

Assessment for Sacroiliac Lesions, Sprain, Inflammation, Subluxation, and Fracture

PROCEDURE

- The patient is in a side-lying position.
- The examiner compresses the patient's superior ilium toward the floor (Fig. 9-8).
- Forward rolling motion of the sacrum occurs.
- Increased pressure in the sacroiliac joint suggests a sacroiliac lesion.
- This pressure may also indicate a sprain of the posterior sacroiliac ligaments.
- A positive finding is significant for sacroiliac lesions.

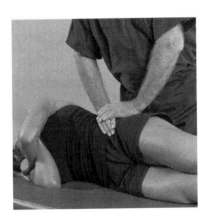

FIG. 9-8

9

CLINICAL PEARL

Fractures of the pelvis are serious in and of themselves and may result in long-term disability. However, even more important is that these fractures are often complicated by damage to the soft tissues, urethra, bladder, bowel, blood vessels, and nerves. These complications can be fatal. Genitourinary complications occur in approximately 20% of pelvic fractures, and the overall mortality is 5%.

KNEE-TO-SHOULDER TEST

Assessment for Sacroiliac Mechanical Dysfunction and Pyogenic Sacroiliitis *(Correlated with Systemic Findings)*

ORTHOPEDIC GAMUT 9-10

PATIENT GROUPS SUSCEPTIBLE TO PYOGENIC INFECTION OF THE SACROILIAC JOINT

1. Children
2. Parenteral drug users
3. Immunosuppressed patients
4. Patients with endocarditis
5. Patients with pelvic inflammatory disease
6. Patients with gynecologic infections
7. Following uncomplicated pregnancy and labor
8. Patients with sickle cell disease (secondary salmonella) infection
9. Trauma*

---

*Estimated 10% of cases have a history of pelvic trauma.

PROCEDURE

- The patient is supine. The patient's knee and hip are flexed, and the hip is adducted.
- This position rocks the sacroiliac joint.
- The knee is approximated to patient's opposite shoulder (Fig. 9-9).
- A positive test is indicated by pain in the ipsilateral sacroiliac joint.
- A positive test indicates sacroiliac mechanical dysfunction, which may include pyogenic sacroiliitis when correlated with other system findings.

9

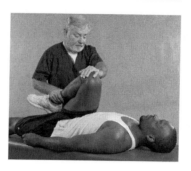

FIG. 9-9

CLINICAL PEARL

With acute sacroiliac pyogenic infections, the onset is usually rapid and very painful. Swelling is intense, and tenderness is widespread. The patient resists movement and experiences pyrexia and general malaise. Pyogenic infections occurring in patients with rheumatoid arthritis often have a much slower onset. Although the sacroiliac joint is swollen, other inflammatory changes are often suppressed, especially if the patient is receiving steroids. In the early stages, both modes of onset will mimic simple mechanical injury of the sacroiliac joint.

LAGUERRE TEST

Assessment for a Sacroiliac Intraarticular Abnormality

PROCEDURE

- The patient is in a supine position.
- The patient's involved hip is flexed, abducted, and laterally rotated (Fig. 9-10).
- An overpressure at the end of the range of motion is applied.
- The opposite anterior-superior iliac spine is stabilized.
- A positive test is sacroiliac joint pain.
- Because this test approximates a Patrick Fabere procedure, the examiner needs to be alert for coxa signs of disease.

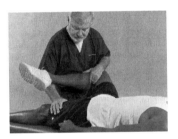

FIG. 9-10

9

CLINICAL PEARL

Osteitis condensans ilii causes a disturbance of the normal architecture of the ilium in which increased condensations of bone occur in the auricular portion of the ilium without a corresponding change in the sacroiliac joint or the sacrum. Osteitis condensans ilii must be differentiated from ankylosing spondylitis, which also causes condensations around the sacroiliac joint. Laguerre test reveals a mechanical problem of the sacroiliac joint. Involvement of the joint in osteitis condensans ilii can be confirmed only by diagnostic imaging.

LEWIN-GAENSLEN TEST

Assessment for a Sacroiliac Joint Abnormality

ORTHOPEDIC GAMUT 9-11
OBSERVATIONS OF GAIT

1. Equality of stride length
2. Excessive pelvic tilt or lean during ambulation
3. Antalgic lean of the lumbopelvic spine
4. Excessive swayback or hyperlordosis
5. Changes in pelvic inclination (tilt)

ORTHOPEDIC GAMUT 9-12
SACROILIAC JOINT DISORDERS

Classification of disorders of the sacroiliac joint include:
1. Inflammatory lesions
2. Infectious lesions
3. Mechanical lesions
4. Degenerative lesions
5. Osteitis condensans ilii

PROCEDURE

- Lewin-Gaenslen test is a modification of Gaenslen test.
- The patient lies on the unaffected side and pulls the knee of that side to the chest.
- The patient holds the affected thigh in extension for the examiner.
- The examiner, positioned behind the patient, then provides pressure by hyperextending the affected thigh (Fig. 9-11).
- Pain produced in the sacroiliac joint is a positive finding.
- The test is significant for sacroiliac lesions.

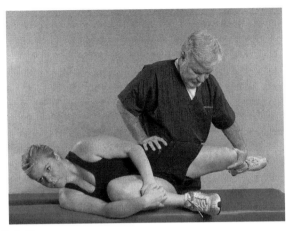

FIG. 9-11

CLINICAL PEARL

Because of the strength of the sacroiliac ligaments, sprain of these structures is uncommon. Bending movements—such as lifting and hyperextension, which produce a torsion sprain on the joint—are more likely to cause sprain of the thinner capsular ligaments in the small lumbosacral joints.

9

PIEDALLU SIGN

Assessment for Abnormal Torsion Movement of the Sacroiliac Joint

PROCEDURE

- The patient is seated to keep the hamstrings from affecting pelvic-flexion symmetry.
- The posterior superior iliac spines are located and compared for height.
- If one posterior-superior iliac spine (PSIS) is lower than the other, the patient flexes forward.
- If the lower PSIS becomes higher during forward flexion, the test is positive.
- The PSIS migration to a higher prominence is the positive sign (Fig. 9-12).
- An abnormality in the torsion motion of the sacroiliac joint is suggested by the positive finding.

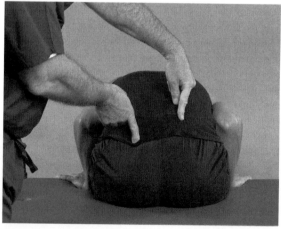

FIG. 9-12

CLINICAL PEARL

In the sacroiliac joint fixation complex, an irregular prominence of one articular surface becomes wedged on another prominence of the opposing articular surface. When reduction is successful, the pain is relieved immediately.

9

SACRAL APEX TEST

Assessment for Abnormal Rotational Shifting of the Sacroiliac Joint

PROCEDURE

- The patient is prone.
- The examiner places pressure at the apex of the patient's sacrum.
- Pressure is increased, causing a shear of the sacrum on the ilium (Fig. 9-13).
- If pain is produced over the joint, the test is positive.

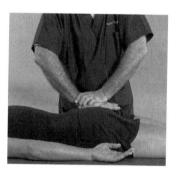

FIG. 9-13

CLINICAL PEARL

Sciatic neuritis is a term used to describe pain or other discomfort that is experienced anywhere along the distribution of the sciatic nerve and is caused primary by disease of the nerve or, more commonly, a mechanical disorder affecting the nerve. A sacroiliac subluxation-sprain may be the true cause of sciatic neuritis. The piriformis muscle is most often affected, and it may involve the L5–S1 and S2 distribution.

SACROILIAC RESISTED-ABDUCTION TEST

HIP-ABDUCTION STRESS TEST

Assessment for Generalized Abductor Muscular Weakness or Sprain or Subluxation of the Sacroiliac Joint

ORTHOPEDIC GAMUT 9-13

THREE ELEMENT COMPRISING PIRIFORMIS SYNDROME SYMPTOMS

1. Myofascial referred pain
2. Nerve compression
3. Sacroiliac joint dysfunction

ORTHOPEDIC GAMUT 9-14

FIVE CHARACTERISTICS OF PIRIFORMIS SYNDROME CAUSING SCIATIC PAIN

1. History of local trauma
2. Pain localized to the sacroiliac joint, greater sciatic notch, and piriformis muscle, which extend along the course of the sciatic nerve
3. Acute pain brought on by stooping or lifting and relieved somewhat by traction
4. Palpable spindle mass at the anatomical location of the piriformis muscle
5. Positive Lasègue sign

9

ORTHOPEDIC GAMUT 9-15

PIRIFORMIS MUSCLE

Trigger points in the piriformis muscle refer pain to the following:
1. Buttocks
2. Toward the hip
3. Posterior thigh
4. Calf
5. Sole of the foot

PROCEDURE

- The patient lies on the unaffected side with the affected leg extended and slightly abducted.
- The unaffected limb can be flexed at the hip and knee to provide stability.
- The examiner then exerts downward pressure on the abducted leg against the patient's resistance.
- The test is repeated on the opposite side.
- If the test elicits pelvic pain near the posterior superior iliac spine, it is positive (Fig. 9-14).
- The test is specific for a sacroiliac sprain or subluxation.

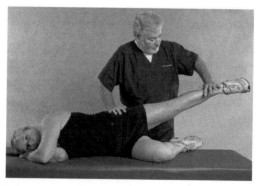

FIG. 9-14

CLINICAL PEARL

Slight, unilateral hip-abductor weakness is found in association with lateral pelvic tilt. The abductors are weak on the slightly elevated side of the pelvis. The beginning weakness in the abductors, as seen in nonparalytic individuals, is usually associated with handedness and is a strain weakness from postural or occupational causes.

9

SMITH-PETERSEN TEST

Assessment for Sacroiliac Joint Involvement versus Lumbosacral Spine Involvement

Comment

The Smith-Petersen test is often confused with and thought to be synonymous with the Goldthwait sign or Lasègue test.

ORTHOPEDIC GAMUT 9-16

INTERNATIONAL ASSOCIATION FOR THE STUDY OF PAIN DIAGNOSTIC CHARACTERISTICS FOR PATIENTS WITH SACROILIAC SYNDROME MUST POSSESS ALL OF THE FOLLOWING CHARACTERISTICS

1. Pain in the region of the sacroiliac joint, with possible radiation to the groin, medial buttocks, and posterior thigh
2. Reproduction of pain by physical examination techniques that stress the joint
3. Complete elimination of pain with intraarticular injection of local anesthetic
4. An ostensibly morphologically normal joint without demonstrable pathognomonic radiographic abnormalities

---

ORTHOPEDIC GAMUT 9-17

SACROILIAC JOINT INJURIES

Four forms of sacroiliac joint injuries include:

1. Dislocation, in which the articular surfaces are completely displaced from each other
2. Subluxation, in which the articular surfaces remain in contact although they are displaced
3. Sprain, in which a tear of the capsular ligament occurs without a disturbance in its relationship to the opposing surfaces
4. Fracture-dislocation, in which a fracture of part of one of the bones has taken place for the articular surfaces to be completely displaced from each other

PROCEDURE

- The Smith-Petersen test is performed with the patient in the supine posture.
- Straight leg raising is performed slowly while one hand is placed under the lower part of the patient's spine.
- As the hamstrings tighten, leverage is progressively applied to the sacroiliac joint and then to the lumbosacral articulation.
- If pain is brought on before the lumbar spine begins to move, Smith-Petersen considers that a sacroiliac condition is present (Fig. 9-15).
- If, however, pain does not come on until after the lumbar spine begins to move, either sacroiliac or lumbosacral involvement may be present.
- Straight leg raising of both sides should be accomplished.
- If, on the unaffected side, the leg can be raised much higher, sacroiliac involvement is likely.
- If discomfort is elicited when both legs are brought to the same level, lumbosacral involvement is likely.

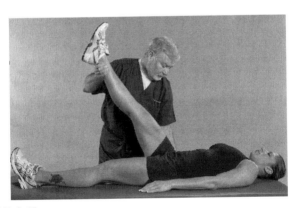

FIG. 9-15

CLINICAL PEARL

An acute sacroiliac flexion sprain is caused by lifting heavy objects. In many instances, however, the patient with chronic sacral pain has also sustained an ancient fall or flexion sprain. In cases of partial tearing of the sacroiliac ligaments, in which poor healing has taken place, a painful fibrous area persists, resulting in a chronic, weak area of the joint. This area becomes symptomatic when placed under tension and stress.

SQUISH TEST

Assessment for Posterior Sacroiliac Ligament Damage

ORTHOPEDIC GAMUT 9-18

FACTORS PREDISPOSING PATIENTS TO INSUFFICIENCY FRACTURE

- Female sex
- Osteoporosis
- Degenerative arthritis
- Inflammatory arthritis
- Radiation therapy
- Reconstructive surgery in the lower extremity
- Paget disease
- Regional disuse osteopenia

ORTHOPEDIC GAMUT 9-19

BONY PELVIS

Injuries to the bony pelvis are two types:
1. Isolated fractures of the pubic rami or ilium
2. Double fractures of the pelvic ring

ORTHOPEDIC GAMUT 9-20

PELVIC RING

The double fractures of the pelvic ring occur in three forms:
1. Type I: The anterior portion of the ring may be broken if all four pubic rami are broken, and the loose portion of the ring will get driven posteriorly.
2. Type II: One side of the pubis may be fractured anteriorly and posteriorly and may roll laterally.
3. Type III: One side of the pelvic ring may be fractured and it may roll laterally and be superiorly displaced as well.

ORTHOPEDIC GAMUT 9-21

YOUNG AND BURGESS PELVIC FRACTURE CLASSIFICATION

1. Anteroposterior compression injury
2. Injury that results from an anteroposteriorly directed force producing sacroiliac joint opening, which causes external rotation of the hemi pelvis
3. Lateral compression injuries
4. Injury that results from a force parallel to the trabeculae of the sacrum and applied to the lateral aspect of the pelvis (Different lateral compression injuries are found depending on the antero-posterior location of this lateral impacting force.)
5. Vertical shear injury
6. Injury that results from a vertically directed force causing fracture of the pubic rami and disruption of all the ligamentous structures

---

PROCEDURE

- The patient is supine.
- Pressure is placed on the patient's anterosuperior iliac spines. The examiner pushes down at a 45-degree angle (Fig. 9-16).
- Pain indicates a positive test and suggests injury of the posterior sacroiliac ligaments.

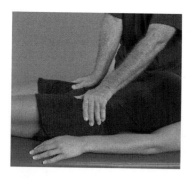

FIG. 9-16

CLINICAL PEARL

In elderly adults, fractures of the pubic rami and ischial rami are often caused by a trivial fall. The fractures usually occur in pairs. Fracture of one ramus alone is unusual. A positive squish test in an elderly patient indicates a possible fracture of a ramus and a posterior sacroiliac sprain. The fracture can be confirmed with diagnostic imaging.

9

YEOMAN TEST

Assessment for Anterior Sacroiliac Ligament Injury

PROCEDURE

- The patient is lying prone.
- With one hand, the examiner applies firm pressure over the suspect sacroiliac joint, fixing the pelvis to the table.
- With the other hand, the examiner flexes the patient's leg on the affected side and hyperextends the thigh by lifting the knee off the examining table (Fig. 9-17).
- If pain is increased in the sacroiliac area, this increase in pain indicates a sacroiliac lesion.
- This pain is caused by the strain placed on the anterior sacroiliac ligaments.
- In a patient without a sacroiliac lesion, pain will not be felt during this maneuver.

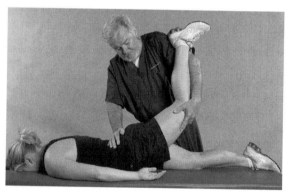

FIG. 9-17

CLINICAL PEARL

Ruptured sacroiliac ligaments do not heal soundly, even if they are accurately repaired, because the scar tissue, which forms at the site of the repair, stretches and is never as tough as the original. Surgical repair is often attempted after severe rupture of these ligaments, but conservative management may be equally effective.

9

HIP

INTRODUCTION

Hip pain is a common symptom with diverse etiologies. Typically, hip disease is characterized by pain in the groin. The pain may radiate to the anterior, lateral, or medial thigh and occasionally to the knee. Causes of pain in the groin and anterior thigh area include iliopsoas bursitis, adduction tendinitis, hernias, and pain from retroperitoneal structures, as well as femoroacetabular impingement.

Pain in the trochanteric area aggravated by lateral decubitus position is highly suggestive of trochanteric bursitis. Pain in the ischiogluteal area aggravated by the sitting position should suggest an ischiogluteal bursitis. Groin pain aggravated by walking and relieved by rest is suggestive of a degenerative hip arthropathy. Pain in the same location, when associated with morning stiffness lasting more than 30 minutes and relieved by activity, is typical of an inflammatory arthropathy. Vascular insufficiency tends to produce buttock pain aggravated by walking and relieved within minutes by rest (Table 10-3).

TABLE 10-1

HIP JOINT CROSS-REFERENCE TABLE BY ASSESSMENT PROCEDURE

Hip Joint

Disease Assessed	Actual leg-length test	Allis sign	Anvil test	Apparent leg-length test
Subluxation				
Coxa Vara				
Poliomyelitis				
Legg-Calvé-Perthes Disease				
Hip Flexion Contracture				
Gracilis Contracture				
Iliotibial Band				
Osteoarthritis				
Meningeal Irritation				
Pelvic Obliquity	•			•
Calcaneal Fracture			•	
Tibial/Fibular Fracture			•	
Coxa Abnormality			•	
Fracture			•	
Tibial Dysplasia		•		
Hip Dislocation		•		
Leg Length	•			•

Test/Sign

Continued

10

TABLE 10-1

HIP JOINT CROSS-REFERENCE TABLE BY ASSESSMENT PROCEDURE—cont'd

Disease Assessed

Hip Joint	Chiene test	Gauvain sign	Guilland sign	Hip telescoping test	Jansen test
Subluxation					
Coxa Vara					
Poliomyelitis					
Legg-Calvé-Perthes Disease					
Hip Flexion Contracture					
Gracilis Contracture					
Iliotibial Band					
Osteoarthritis					•
Meningeal Irritation			•		
Pelvic Obliquity					
Calcaneal Fracture					
Tibial/Fibular Fracture					
Coxa Abnormality		•			•
Fracture	•				
Tibial Dysplasia					
Hip Dislocation				•	
Leg Length					

Test/Sign

Ludloff sign

Ober test

Patrick test

Phelps test

Thomas test

Trendelenburg test

TABLE 10-2

HIP JOINT CROSS-REFERENCE TABLE FOR SYNDROME OR TISSUE

Calcaneal fractures	Anvil test
Coxa abnormality	Anvil test
	Gauvain sign
	Jansen test
	Patrick test
	Phelps test
	Thomas test
Coxa vara	Trendelenburg test
Fracture	Anvil test
	Chiene test
	Ludloff sign
	Trendelenburg test
Gracilis contracture	Phelps test
Hip dislocation	Allis sign
	Hip telescoping test
	Trendelenburg test
Hip flexion contracture	Thomas test
Iliotibial band	Ober test
Leg length	Actual leg-length test
	Apparent leg-length test
Legg-Calvé-Perthes disease	Trendelenburg test
Meningeal irritation	Guilland sign
Osteoarthritis	Jansen sign
	Trendelenburg test
Pelvic obliquity	Actual leg-length test
	Apparent leg-length test
Poliomyelitis	Trendelenburg test
Subluxation	Trendelenburg test
Tibial dysplasia	Allis sign
Tibial/fibular fracture	Anvil test

TABLE 10-3

HIP DIAGNOSTIC CONSIDERATIONS

Articular
Inflammatory joint diseases
    Rheumatoid arthritis
    Spondyloarthropathies
    Polymyalgia rheumatica
Degenerative joint diseases
    Primary osteoarthritis
    Secondary osteoarthritis
Metabolic joint diseases
    Gout
    Pseudogout
    Ochronosis
    Hemochromatosis
    Wilson disease
    Acromegaly
Infections
Tumors
    Benign
        Pigmented villonodular synovitis
        Osteochondromatosis
    Malignant
        Synovial sarcoma
        Synovial metastasis
Hemarthrosis
Juvenile
    Transient *toxic* synovitis
    Juvenile chronic arthritis

Periarticular
Bursitis
    Trochanteric
    Iliopsoas
    Ischiogluteal
Tendinitis
    Trochanteric
    Adductor
Acute calcific periarthritis
Heterotropic calcifications

10

Continued

TABLE 10-3

HIP DIAGNOSTIC CONSIDERATIONS—cont'd

Osseous
Bone lesions
  Fractures, neoplasms, infection, osteonecrosis of the femoral head,
  metabolic bone disease (Paget disease of bone, stress fractures,
  osteomalacia, hyperparathyroidism, renal osteodystrophy), reflex
  sympathetic dystrophy (transient migratory osteoporosis)
Juvenile
  Congenital dislocation of the hip
  Acetabular dysplasia
  Coxa vara
  Slipped capital femoral epiphysis
  Legg-Calvé-Perthes disease
  Rickets
Neurologic
Entrapment neuropathies
  Lateral femoral cutaneous nerve (meralgia paresthetica)
Lumbar nerve root compression L2, L3, and L4
Vascular
Atherosclerosis of aorta iliac vessels

Modified from Klippel JH, Dieppe PA: *Rheumatology*, vol 1-2, ed 2, London, 1998, Mosby.

Hip disease may result in adduction or abduction deformities. An adduction deformity is an upward tilt of the pelvis on the side of the adducted thigh. An abduction deformity is an elevation of the uninvolved side.

ORTHOPEDIC GAMUT 10-1

HIP

Loading forces acting on the hip:
1. Standing transfers one third of the body weight to the hip joint mechanism.
2. Standing on one limb transfers 2.4 to 2.6 times the body weight to the hip joint mechanism.
3. Walking transfers 1.3 to 5.8 times the body weight on the hip joint mechanism.

Pain in the posterior aspect of the hip is most often referred from the lumbar spine. Sacroiliac disorders can also cause buttock pain. Mechanical disorders of the thoracolumbar junction (T12 and L1) may refer pain to the greater trochanter area and thus may mimic trochanteric bursitis. Thrombosis or aneurysm formation of branches of the aorta or iliac vessels may give rise to buttock, thigh, or leg pain that may be confused with hip pain. The presence of pain at the extremes of abduction and internal rotation suggests early hip disease caused by arthritis or osteonecrosis. Limitation of hip movements in all directions in a diabetic patient suggests an adhesive capsulitis of the hip joint. The presence of systemic symptoms such as fatigue, fever, weight loss, or worsening of pain at night requires baseline laboratory tests and a radionuclide bone scan in search of a tumor or an indolent infectious process.

10

ESSENTIAL ANATOMY

The femur is the longest and strongest bone in the body. The femoral neck forms an *angle of inclination* with the femoral shaft on the frontal plane. In children, this angle may be up to 150 degrees; in adults, however, it is approximately 125 degrees. Variations in this angle commonly occur. An increase in the angle of inclination is known as *coxa valga*, and a reduction in this angle is coxa vara. The femoral neck is typically aligned anterior to the femoral shaft on the transverse plane. This *angle of anteversion* is approximately 15 degrees in adults. An increase in this angle is known as *excessive femoral anteversion;* a decrease is often called *femoral retroversion.*

ORTHOPEDIC GAMUT 10-2
PROXIMAL FEMUR

The four major components of the proximal femur are:
1. Greater trochanter
2. Lesser trochanter
3. Femoral neck
4. Femoral head

ORTHOPEDIC GAMUT 10-3

GENDER PREVALENCE FACTORS IN OSTEOPOROSIS

The prevalence of osteoporosis is lower in men than in women for several physiologic reasons:
- A greater accumulation of skeletal mass during growth
- Greater bone size
- Absence of midlife menopause
- A slower rate of bone loss
- A shorter male life expectancy

ORTHOPEDIC GAMUT 10-4

HIP BURSAE

The three most clinically important hip bursae are as follows:
1. Trochanteric bursa
2. Iliopsoas bursa
3. Ischiogluteal bursa

ESSENTIAL MOTION ASSESSMENT

When measuring the range of hip movement, the examiner must ensure that the patient's pelvis remains stationary. To accomplish this task, the examiner keeps a hand on the patient's anterosuperior iliac spine to detect any movement.

ORTHOPEDIC GAMUT 10-5

HIP RANGE OF MOTION

In testing range of motion of the hips, the patient performs the following:

WHILE SUPINE
1. Raises the leg above the body with the knee extended
2. Brings the knee to the chest while keeping the other leg straight
3. Swings the leg laterally and medially while keeping the knee straight
4. Places the side of the foot on the opposite knee and moves the flexed knee down toward the examination table (external rotation)
5. Flexes the knee and rotates the leg so that the flexed knee moves inward toward the opposite leg (internal rotation)

WHILE EITHER PRONE OR STANDING
Swings the straightened leg behind the body

Among all of the movements of the hip, abduction and internal rotation are usually the first ones to be painful or limited in the presence of a hip abnormality (Figs. 10-1 to 10-6).

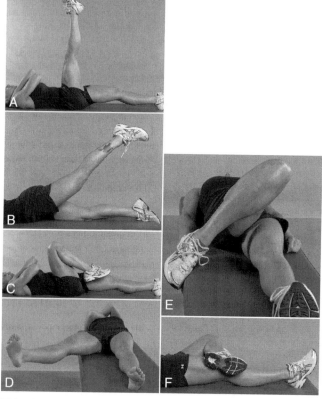

FIG. 10-1 Range of motion of the hip. **A,** Hip flexion with the leg extended. **B,** Hip hyperextension, knee extended. **C,** Hip flexion, knee flexed. **D,** Abduction **E,** Internal rotation. **F,** External rotation.

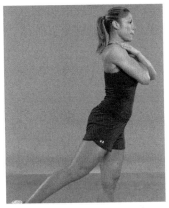

FIG. 10-2 Extension of the hip is defined as the upward (or backward) motion of the hip from the zero starting position. Motion beyond the neutral position (0 degrees) is sometimes alternatively called hyperextension.

With the available methods of eliminating exaggerated lumbar lordosis and accomplishing fixation of the pelvis, 15 degrees of extension or hyperextension of the hip may be obtained.

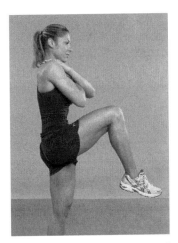

10

FIG. 10-3 The thigh can be flexed to 120 degrees from the neutral or extended position (0 degrees) if the knee has first been flexed to 90 degrees.

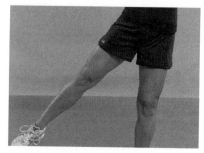

FIG. 10-4 Abduction and adduction are measured while both thighs and legs are in the extended position and are parallel to each other. Normally, when the leg and thigh are extended, the hip abducts to approximately 40 to 45 degrees from the neutral position.

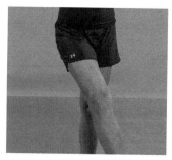

FIG. 10-5 Adduction with the leg straight out is limited by the legs and thighs, which come into contact with each other. Adduction is usually possible to approximate 20 to 30 degrees from the neutral (starting) position.

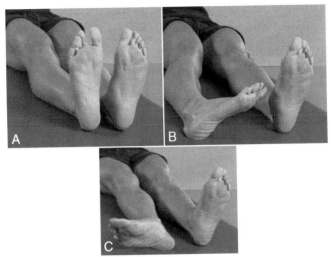

FIG. 10-6 **A,** External and internal rotation of the hip can be tested with the patient's hip and knee fully extended while the patient is supine. **B,** Rolling the thigh, leg, and foot inward. **C,** Rolling the thigh, leg, and foot outward. The hip normally rotates inward approximately 40 degrees and outward approximately 45 degrees.

ESSENTIAL MUSCLE FUNCTION ASSESSMENT

The innervation of the hip joint follows Hilton's law, which states that a joint is innervated by the same nerves that innervate the muscles acting on it. Thus, branches from the femoral, sciatic, obturator, and superior and inferior gluteal nerves innervate the hip joint. The sclerotome reference for the hip joint is generally considered to be L3. The cutaneous innervation of the hip, buttock, and thigh can be referenced to peripheral nerves or dermatomes (Figs. 10-7 to 10-12).

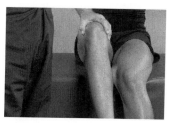

FIG. 10-7 The iliopsoas is the primary flexor of the hip, and it is innervated by the femoral nerve, which contains the L1, L2, and L3 nerve roots. The examiner asks the patient to flex the hip against manual resistance.

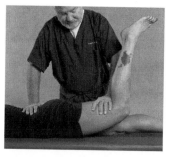

FIG. 10-8 Prime movers in extension of the hip are the gluteus maximus (inferior gluteal nerve, L5, S1, and S2), semitendinosus (tibial branch of sciatic nerve, L4, L5, S1, and S2), and semimembranosus (tibial branch of sciatic nerve, L5, S1, and S2) muscles, as well as the long head of the biceps femoris (tibial branch of the sciatic nerve, S1, S2, and S3) muscle. To measure the strength of the gluteus maximus, the patient is directed to extend the hip against the examiner's hand.

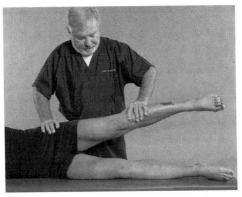

FIG. 10-9 The gluteus medius muscle (superior gluteal nerve, L4, L5, and S1) is the prime mover in abduction of the hip. An additional test can be performed by placing the patient in a side-lying position on the examination table and having the patient abduct the hip against resistance provided by the examiner.

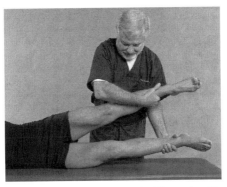

10

FIG. 10-10 Prime movers in adduction of the hip are the adductor magnus (obturator and sciatic nerves, L3, L4, L5, and S1), adductor brevis (obturator nerve, L3, and L4), adductor longus (obturator nerve, L3, and L4), pectineus (femoral nerve, L2, L3, L4, and occasionally obturator nerve, L3, and L4), and gracilis (obturator nerve, L3, and L4) muscles. The patient then adducts the lower leg off the table, toward the elevated leg. The examiner's free hand provides graded resistance proximal to the knee joint.

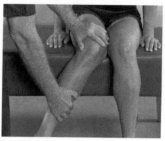

FIG. 10-11 Prime movers in external rotation of the hip are the obturator externus (obturator nerve, L3, and L4), obturator internus (sacral plexus, L4, L5, and S1), piriformis (sacral plexus, S1, and S2), gemellus superior (sacral plexus, L5, S1, and S2), gemellus inferior (sacral plexus, L4, L5, and S1), and the gluteus maximus (inferior gluteal nerve, L5, S1, and S2) muscles. The patient then rotates the hip and thigh laterally, and the lower leg rotates medially while the examiner's other hand applies graded resistance above the ankle against the motion being tested.

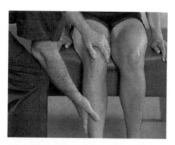

FIG. 10-12 Prime movers in internal rotation of the hip are the gluteus minimus (superior gluteal nerve, L4, L5, and S1) and the tensor fasciae latae (superior gluteal nerve, L4, L5, and S1) muscles. The patient then rotates the thigh medially and rotates the lower leg laterally while the examiner's other hand provides graded resistance above the ankle joint.

ESSENTIAL IMAGING

The major part of the pelvis is typically visualized with a single anteroposterior (AP) view. Both lower extremities are internally rotated approximately 20 degrees to elongate the femoral necks and take the trochanteric processes out of superimposition with the femoral necks.

ORTHOPEDIC GAMUT 10-6

BASIC HIP IMAGING STUDY

The basic hip plain-film imaging study:
1. AP pelvic view
2. AP spot hip view
3. Lateral (frog leg) spot view of the side of complaint

ORTHOPEDIC GAMUT 10-7

OSSEOUS DEFORMITIES OF THE PROXIMAL FEMUR

Four common osseous deformities of the proximal femur are:
1. Coxa vara
2. Coxa valga
3. Femoral anteversion
4. Femoral retroversion

ORTHOPEDIC GAMUT 10-8

COXA VARA

The developmental and acquired conditions that can resulting in coxa vara are:
1. Intertrochanteric fracture
2. Slipped capital femoral epiphysis
3. Legg-Calvé-Perthes disease
4. Congenital hip dislocation
5. Rickets
6. Paget disease

10

ACTUAL LEG-LENGTH TEST

Assessment for True Leg-Length Discrepancy

Comment

Methods of measuring the lower limbs are often confusing. Accuracy in measurement is of more than academic significance. Accurate measurement is of practical importance when corrective operations or adjustments to the shoes are contemplated. Limb length can be measured clinically within an error of 1 cm. If greater accurancy is needed, radiographic measurement (scanography) is recommended. The first required step is to measure the real, or true, length of each limb. Second, the examiner must determine the existence of any apparent, or false, discrepancy in the length of the limbs as a result of fixed pelvic tilt. Measuring the true leg length is always necessary. Also necessary is to measure apparent discrepancy only when a correctable pelvic tilt is observed.

ORTHOPEDIC GAMUT 10-9

LEG-LENGTH DEFICIENCY

Tests to determine leg-length deficiency occurring above the trochanteric level include:

1. Measurement of Bryant triangle
2. Construction of Nélaton line
3. Construction of Shoemaker line

PROCEDURE

- The patient is lying supine with the feet together, the knees and hips straight, and the anterosuperior iliac spines and the iliac crests exposed.
- The examiner, by way of palpation, marks the apex of the anterior iliac spines and the crests of the ilia.
- The examiner then measures the distance between these features and the medial malleolus (Fig. 10-13).
- The distance is recorded and compared with the opposite side.
- These distances represent the actual leg length.
- Actual leg-length discrepancies are caused by an abnormality above or below the trochanter level.

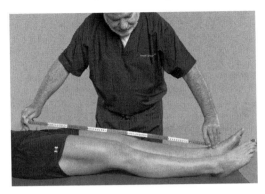

FIG. 10-13

CLINICAL PEARL

Causes of true shortening above the trochanter include (1) coxa vara, resulting from neck fractures, slipped epiphysis, Perthes disease, and congenital coxa vara; (2) loss of articular cartilage from infection or arthritis; and (3) dislocation of the hip. Rarely does lengthening of the other limb give relative, true shortening. This relative, true shortening may be caused by (1) stimulation of bone growth from increased vascularity, which may occur after long bone fracture in children or bone tumor, and (2) coxa valga, which follows polio.

10

ALLIS SIGN

ALSO KNOWN AS GALEAZZI SIGN

Assessment for Femoral Portion Structural Deficiency or Tibial Portion Structural Deficiency

---

ORTHOPEDIC GAMUT 10-10
FORMS OF CONGENITAL HIP DISLOCATION

1. Congenital hip dysplasia
2. Acetabular dysplasia
3. Congenital subluxation

ORTHOPEDIC GAMUT 10-11
DIAGNOSING CONGENITAL HIP DYSPLASIA

1. Neonatal (birth to 1 month): Barlow test, Ortolani test
2. Infancy (1 month to 2 years): limited hip abduction with the hips flexed to 45 degrees, shortening on the affected side with hips and knees flexed (Galeazzi sign), Trendelenburg sign
3. Age 2 to 6 years: obvious limp, Trendelenburg sign, limb shortening if unilateral
4. Older than 6 years: limp, limited hip abduction

ORTHOPEDIC GAMUT 10-12

CATEGORIES OF PEDIATRIC LIMPING

I. An antalgic limp is one that is painful, and a child with an antalgic limp spends a greater portion of the gait cycle on the asymptomatic leg than the symptomatic leg.

II. A Trendelenburg limp is not painful but is caused by muscle weakness or instability of the hip joint such as in unilateral developmental dysplasia of the hip. A child with a Trendelenburg gait tilts the pelvis away from the involved side. In a single-limb stance on the affected side, the patient shifts the trunk over the involved side to stabilize the hip.

III. A child with bilateral developmental dysplasia of the hip has a waddling gait.

PROCEDURE

- The patient is lying supine with the knees flexed and the soles of the feet flat on the table, the great toes and malleoli being approximated bilaterally.
- The examiner observes the heights of the knees from a viewpoint at the foot of table.
- If one knee is lower than the other, ipsilateral hip dislocation or severe coxa disorder is indicated (Fig. 10-14).
- Tibial length discrepancies are also discerned in this position.
- From viewing the position from the side, the examiner can assess femoral length discrepancies (Fig. 10-15).

10

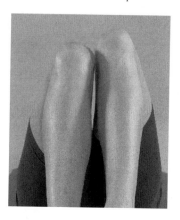

FIG. 10-14

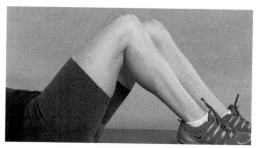

FIG. 10-15

CLINICAL PEARL

Congenital dislocation of the hip is a condition in which one or both hips are dislocated at birth or are dislocated in the first few weeks of life. The disorder has a familial tendency and a well-established geographic distribution. It may also occur with other congenital defects.

ANVIL TEST

Assessment for Fracture of the Femoral Neck or Head

ORTHOPEDIC GAMUT 10-13

MSCORE (MALE, SIMPLE CALCULATED OSTEOPOROSIS RISK ESTIMATION)

- MSCORE is based on bone mineral density at the femoral neck
- MSCORE is derived from five variables independently associated with osteoporosis
- MSCORE = [2 × (patient age in decades) − (weight in lb ÷ 10) + 4 with gastrectomy, + 4 with emphysema, + 3 with two or more prior fractures + 14]
- Increased osteoporosis risk is reflected in higher MSCORE values
  - low (<9)
  - moderate (9–13)
  - high (>13)

PROCEDURE

- While the patient is lying supine, the inferior calcaneus is struck with the examiner's fist (Fig. 10-16).
- Localized pain in the thigh indicates a femoral fracture or a severe pathologic condition of the joint.
- Localized pain in the leg indicates a tibial or fibular fracture.
- Pain localized to the calcaneus indicates calcaneal fracture.

10

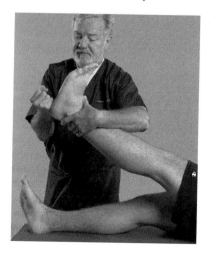

FIG. 10-16

CLINICAL PEARL

Two questions must be answered in the assessment of a hip fracture. Does a fracture exist? Is the fracture displaced? The break usually becomes obvious when viewed with diagnostic imaging, but an impacted fracture can be missed. The assessment is important because impacted or undisplaced fractures have a good prognosis. Displaced fractures have a high rate of non-union and avascular necrosis.

APPARENT LEG-LENGTH TEST

Assessment for Apparent Leg-Length Discrepancy

ORTHOPEDIC GAMUT 10-14

ANATOMIC LEG-LENGTH DIFFERENCE

Causes of an anatomic leg-length difference include:
1. Poliomyelitis of the lower limb
2. Fracture of the femur or tibia
3. Bone growth problems of the lower extremity (epiphyseal plate damage)

ORTHOPEDIC GAMUT 10-15

LEG-LENGTH MEASUREMENTS

Leg-length measurement landmarks include:
1. Iliac crest to greater trochanter to determine whether coxa vara is present
2. Greater trochanter to knee for femur length
3. Knee joint line to medial malleolus for tibial length

ORTHOPEDIC GAMUT 10-16

FUNCTIONAL LEG-LENGTH DIFFERENCE

Causes of a functional leg-length difference include:
1. One pronated foot or one supinated foot
2. Muscle spasms in one hip
3. Hip capsule tightness
4. Adductor muscle spasm on one side
5. More genu valgus on one side
6. Femoral anteversion on one side

10

PROCEDURE

- Measurement is made bilaterally from the umbilicus or xiphisternum to the apex of the medial malleolus (Fig. 10-17).
- This measurement is an index of the functional length of the lower extremities.

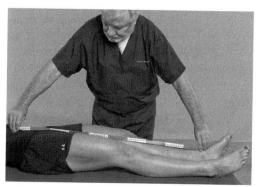

FIG. 10-17

CLINICAL PEARL

Pelvic tilting accompanied by a heel discrepancy indicates apparent shortening of the limb. This apparent shortening may be accompanied by some true shortening. The discrepancy at the heels provides a measure of its degree.

CHIENE TEST

Assessment for Fracture of the Neck of the Femur; Hip Dislocation

---

ORTHOPEDIC GAMUT 10-17

HIP FRACTURES

Typical locations of fractures of the hip include:
1. Extracapsular or trochanteric
2. Femoral neck or subcapital areas (These areas are intracapsular.)
3. Proximal femoral shaft or subtrochanteric areas

ORTHOPEDIC GAMUT 10-18

Subtrochanteric Fracture Complications
1. Malunion
2. Delayed union
3. Non-union

ORTHOPEDIC GAMUT 10-19

HIP FRACTURE MALUNION AND NON-UNION

Two factors associated with hip fracture malunion and non-union:
1. The subtrochanteric area of the proximal femur is cortical bone, with decreased blood supply.
2. The subtrochanteric area is prone to large biomechanical stresses that can lead to loosening of various fixation devices.

10

ORTHOPEDIC GAMUT 10-20

FEMORAL NECK FRACTURE NON-UNION

Non-union of femoral neck fractures occurs in approximately 15% of the cases. Reasons for non-union are:
1. Meager blood supply
2. Inaccurate approximation and rigid fixation of the fragments

ORTHOPEDIC GAMUT 10-21

FACTORS INFLUENCING THE OCCURRENCE OF AVASCULAR NECROSIS IN PEDIATRIC PROXIMAL FEMUR FRACTURE

- Ligamentum teres contributes very little blood supply to the head until the age of 8; as an adult, it serves only 20%.
- Medial and lateral circumflex metaphyseal vessels that traverse the femoral neck predominately supply the head at birth. These later become virtually nonexistent by the age of 4, owing to the development of the cartilaginous physis that forms a barrier to these penetrating vessels.
- As the metaphyseal vessels diminish, their supply to the femoral head, the lateral epiphyseal vessels, become the main blood supply as they bypass the physeal barrier. These vessels can be identified as the posteroinferior and posterosuperior branches of the medial circumflex artery that supply the femoral head throughout the rest of its life.

ORTHOPEDIC GAMUT 10-22

CLINICAL FEATURES OF NON-UNION OF FEMORAL NECK FRACTURES

1. Pain in the hip when bearing weight
2. Shortening and external rotation of the limb
3. Grating or crepitus in the hip during motion

PROCEDURE

- The examiner determines whether a fracture of the neck of the femur has occurred by using a tape measure.
- The patient is supine with the legs extended on the examination table.
- Using a tape measure, the examiner measures the circumference of the thigh, passing the tape over the level of the greater trochanter (Fig. 10-18).
- The distance is recorded and compared with that of the opposite leg.
- An increased diameter indicates that the trochanter has rolled laterally.
- This increased measurement correlates with fracture of the neck of the femur.

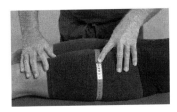

FIG. 10-18

CLINICAL PEARL

10

A fracture of the neck of the femur occurs mainly among elderly women whose bones are osteoporotic. The patient may fall, but the patient more often catches a foot on something and ends up twisting the hip. The femoral neck is broken by rotational force. In most cases, the fracture is markedly displaced and completely unstable. In some cases, the fragments are impacted, and the patient may even walk about, albeit with some pain.

GAUVAIN SIGN

Assessment for Tuberculous Arthritis of the Hip Joint or Adult-Onset Osteonecrosis of the Femoral Head

---

ORTHOPEDIC GAMUT 10-23

OSTEONECROSIS

Common causes of osteonecrosis include:
1. Steroid use
2. Alcohol use
3. Trauma
4. Gout
5. Metabolic problems
6. Genetic problems

ORTHOPEDIC GAMUT 10-24

HIP PAIN

Other causes of hip pain producing symptoms similar to osteonecrosis include:
1. Gout
2. Femoral or inguinal hernia
3. Pigmented villonodular synovitis
4. Stress fracture of femoral neck
5. Rheumatoid arthritis

> ### ORTHOPEDIC GAMUT 10-25
>
> ## RADIOGRAPHIC STAGES OF OSTEONECROSIS AIDING PROGNOSIS
>
> **Osteonecrosis is classified into several radiographic stages that aid with prognosis:**
>
> Stage 0: No change on plain-film radiographs but a positive magnetic resonance imaging scan
> Stage I: Mottled densities or osteopenia
> Stage II: Areas of increased density in the femoral head crescent sign with subchondral fracture
> Stage III: Depression of femoral head
> Stage IV: Flattening and collapse of femoral head
> Stage V: Degenerative arthrosis

PROCEDURE

- The patient is lying supine or in a side-lying position with the affected thigh extended.
- The examiner carefully rotates the thigh (Fig. 10-19).
- The sign is positive if contraction of the abdominal muscles is noted on the same side that is being maneuvered.
- The sign is significant for reflex muscle spasm, which is commonly elicited in tuberculosis of the coxa, or adult-onset osteonecrosis.

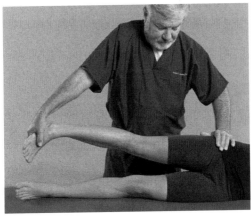

FIG. 10-19

CLINICAL PEARL

A resurgence in tuberculosis (TB) has occurred worldwide. Approximately 2 billion people have latent infection, 8 million develop active TB annually, and 2 to 3 million die as a result of TB. With this resurgence, cases with extrapulmonary TB have also shown an increase. Approximately 10% to 11% of extrapulmonary TB involves joints and bones, which is approximately 1% to 3% of all TB cases. The global prevalence of latent joint and bone TB is approximately 19 to 38 million. TB arthritis is most commonly associated with monoarthritis of weight-bearing joints in the hip or the knee. A child infected with this disease walks with a limp and often complains of pain in the groin or knee. Night pain is another feature. In early cases, complete resolution may be hoped for with antituberculous therapy, bed rest, and traction. In the advanced case, joint debridement is carried out with efforts to obtain a bony fusion of the joint.

GUILLAND SIGN

Assessment for Meningeal Irritation

Comment

The signs and symptoms of meningitis may develop explosively de novo or may appear in the waning stages of an infection that is localized elsewhere. Headache, backache, nausea, and vomiting are common symptoms, and nuchal rigidity occurs in more than 80% of patients. Kernig/Brudzinski sign is often present. Only in the neonate and very young infant is meningitis often unattended by evidence of increased pressure and meningeal irriation. At this stage, even fever may be absent. Photophobia may be a prominent, early symptom and is related in some way to the meningeal inflammation.

PROCEDURE

- While the patient is in a supine position, a brisk flexion of the hip and the knee occurs when the quadriceps muscle on the opposite limb is irritated, such as by a firm pinch (Fig. 10-20).
- The sign is present in cases of meningeal irritation.

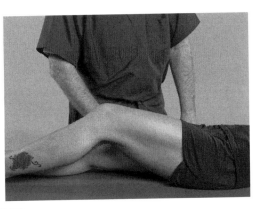

FIG. 10-20

10

CLINICAL PEARL

Acute meningitis (associated with cortical encephalitis and often with ventriculitis) is an emergency and should be suspected in any patient with the acute onset of nonlocalizing central nervous system signs. Fever, nuchal rigidity, headache, altered mental status, vomiting, and photophobia are typically present. The absence of fever is not uncommon. Meningeal signs are not usually present in infants younger than 6 months. Acute signs may also be less apparent in elderly, alcoholic, immunocompromised, or comatose patients.

HIP TELESCOPING TEST

Assessment for Congenital Dislocation of the Hip Articulation

---

ORTHOPEDIC GAMUT 10-26

SLIPPED FEMORAL CAPITAL EPIPHYSIS

Radiographic signs of slipped femoral capital epiphysis include the following:

1. Blurring of the epiphyseal line
2. Increased width of the epiphyseal plate
3. Prolongation of the superior neck fails to cut epiphysis
4. Loss of height of the epiphysis in comparison with a normal contralateral hip

---

PROCEDURE

- The patient is in a supine position.
- The hip and knee are both flexed to 90 degrees.
- The femur is pushed down toward the examination table (Fig. 10-21).
- The leg is lifted from the examination table.
- Movement in hip dislocation will be considerable.
- This is hip telescoping.

10

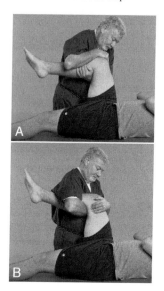

FIG. 10-21

CLINICAL PEARL

When treatment in childhood for congenital dislocation of the hip has been unsuccessful, or even where the condition has not been diagnosed, a patient may seek help during the third and fourth decades of life. Symptoms may arise from the hips or the spine. In the hips, secondary arthritic changes occur in the false joint that may form between the dislocated femoral head and the ilium. In the spine, osteoarthritic changes are the result of longstanding scoliosis. The telescoping test may remain positive for as long as the cause of the dislocation goes untreated.

JANSEN TEST

Assessment for Osteoarthritis of the Hip Joint

ORTHOPEDIC GAMUT 10-27

PIRIFORMIS SYNDROME AXIOMS

1. Symptoms of piriformis syndrome are not usually substantiated by clinical or electrophysiologic findings.
2. Denervation in the sciatic nerve distribution is usually caused by aberrant fascial bands, rather than piriformis muscle.

PROCEDURE

- In osteoarthritis deformans of the hip, the patient is asked to cross the legs, with a point just above the ankle resting on the opposite knee (Fig. 10-22).
- If significant disease exists, this test and motion are impossible.

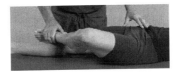

FIG. 10-22

10

CLINICAL PEARL

Primary osteoarthritis of the hip occurs in middle-age and elderly patients and is often associated with obesity and overuse. However, in many instances, no obvious cause can be found. The symptoms of secondary osteoarthritis of the hip are identical to those of primary osteoarthritis. The condition most commonly occurs as a sequel to congenital hip dislocation.

LUDLOFF SIGN

Assessment for Traumatic Separation of the Lesser Trochanter

ORTHOPEDIC GAMUT 10-28

MALIGNANT LESIONS

The 13 common malignant tissue lesions are:
1. Neuroblastoma
2. Ewing sarcoma
3. Lymphoma
4. Primary osteogenic sarcoma or chondroma
5. Secondary osteogenic sarcoma or chondroma
6. Metastatic carcinoma of the thyroid
7. Metastatic carcinoma of the breast in women
8. Metastatic carcinoma of the prostate in men
9. Metastatic carcinoma of the bronchus
10. Metastatic carcinoma of the kidneys
11. Hypernephroma
12. Myeloma
13. Neurogenic carcinoma

PROCEDURE

- In traumatic separation of the epiphysis of the lesser trochanter, swelling and ecchymosis are present at the base of Scarpa triangle, and the patient cannot raise the thigh when in the seated position (Fig. 10-23).

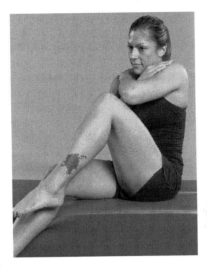

FIG. 10-23

10

OBER TEST

Assessment for Iliotibial Band Contracture

PROCEDURE

- The patient is in a side-lying position on the unaffected hip and thigh.
- The examiner places one hand on the patient's pelvis to steady it and grasps the patient's ankle lightly with the other hand, holding the knee flexed at a right angle.
- The thigh is abducted and extended in the coronal plane of the body.
- In the presence of iliotibial band contracture, the leg will remain abducted; the degree of abduction depends on the amount of contracture present (Fig. 10-24).
- The sign is present both in the conscious and in the anesthetized patient.
- Ober calls attention to the frequency of a negative roentgenogram in the presence of clinical signs and symptoms of irritation of the sacroiliac or lumbosacral joints.
- He refers to the importance of the iliotibial band as a factor to consider in the occurrence of lumbosacral spinal disorders with or without associated sciatica.

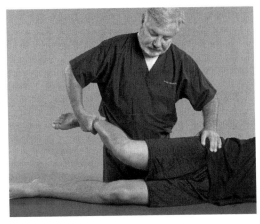

FIG. 10-24

CLINICAL PEARL

Transient synovitis of the hip is the most common cause of an irritable hip and can produce a limp and a positive Ober test. The patient sometimes has a history of preceding minor trauma, which in some cases is at least coincidental. Radiographs of the hip sometimes give confirmatory evidence of synovitis, but no other pathologic condition is demonstrable.

10

PATRICK TEST

Also Known As FABERE Sign (Flexion, Abduction, External Rotation, Extension)

Assessment for Intracapsular Coxa Pathologic Conditions

ORTHOPEDIC GAMUT 10-29

HIP OSTEOARTHRITIS

Classic radiographic findings of hip osteoarthritis include:
1. Loss of joint space
2. Sclerosis of subchondral bone of the femoral head
3. Osteophytes around the joint margins
4. Bone cysts in the subchondral bone

PROCEDURE

- Patrick test is of particular value in geriatric cases because it indicates hip joint disease.
- The patient lies supine, and the examiner grasps the patient's ankle and flexes the knee.
- The thigh is flexed, abducted, externally rotated, and extended (Fig. 10-25).
- The first letters of these words form the acronym FABERE.
- Pain in the hip during the maneuver, particularly on abduction and external rotation, is a positive sign of a coxa pathologic condition.

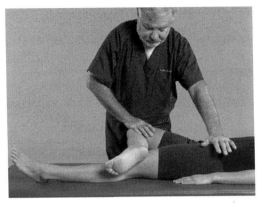

FIG. 10-25

CLINICAL PEARL

An intracapsular fracture, which can cause a positive Patrick test, can cut off the blood supply to the femoral head completely, which can lead to aseptic necrosis, non-union, or both. Because the fracture line is inside the capsule, blood is contained within it. This trapped blood raises the intracapsular pressure, damaging the femoral head still further, and prevents visible bruising because the blood cannot reach the subcutaneous tissues.

10

PHELPS TEST

Assessment for Contracture of the Gracilis Muscle, Associated with a Pathologic Condition of the Hip Joint

PROCEDURE

- The patient is lying prone, the knees are extended, and the thighs are maximally abducted.
- Pain and resistance should be used as criteria for maximal abduction.
- The patient's knees are flexed bilaterally to a right angle (Fig. 10-26).
- The examiner notes if the maneuver allows more hip abduction.
- The test is positive if knee flexion increases or knee extension decreases hip abduction.
- The test indicates contracture of the gracilis muscle.

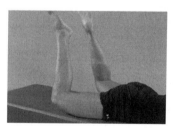

FIG. 10-26

CLINICAL PEARL

Two nonspecific gait abnormalities commonly result from hip disease. The antalgic gait usually indicates a painful hip. The patient shortens the stance phase on the affected hip, leaning over the affected side, to prevent painful contraction of the hip abductors. Trendelenburg gait, or abductor limp, indicates weakness of the abductors on the affected side. During the stance phase, on the affected side, the contralateral pelvis dips down, and the body leans to the unaffected side. If the condition is bilateral, a waddling gait is produced.

THOMAS TEST

Assessment for Flexion Contracture Involving the Iliopsoas

PROCEDURE

- The patient lies supine, and the thigh is flexed with the knee bent toward the abdomen.
- The patient's lumbar spine should normally flatten, or flex.
- If the spine maintains a lordosis, the test is positive and indicates hip flexion contracture, as from a shortened iliopsoas muscle (Fig. 10-27).

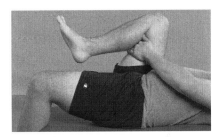

FIG. 10-27

10

CLINICAL PEARL

Restricted hip flexion may be compensated by an increase in lumbar lordosis. This increase masks the fixed flexion deformity. Fixed flexion, external rotation, and abduction accumulate sequentially as the hip disease progresses.

TRENDELENBURG TEST

**Assessment for Insufficiency of the
Hip Abductor System**

ORTHOPEDIC GAMUT 10-30

POSITIVE TRENDELENBURG TEST

Fundamental causes for a positive Trendelenburg test include:
1. Paralysis of the abductor muscles, which can occur with poliomyelitis
2. Marked approximation of the insertion of the muscles to their origin by upward displacement of the greater trochanter causing the muscles to be slack (This slackening may occur in severe coxa vara or congenital dislocation of the hip.)
3. Absence of a stable fulcrum causes a positive test (This result occurs in the ununited fracture of the femoral neck.)
4. Sometimes, a combination of two of the aforementioned factors

---

PROCEDURE

- The patient with a suspected hip involvement stands on one foot, on the side of the involvement, and raises the other foot and leg for thigh flexion and knee flexion.
- If the hip and its muscles are normal, the iliac crest will be low on the standing side and high on the side of the elevated leg.
- If hip joint involvement and muscle weakness are involved, the iliac crest will be high on the standing side and low on the side of the elevated leg (Fig. 10-28).
- The test is commonly positive in a developing Legg-Calvé-Perthes disease, poliomyelitis, muscular dystrophy, coxa vara, Otto pelvis, epiphyseal separation, coxa ankylosis, dislocation, fracture, or subluxation.

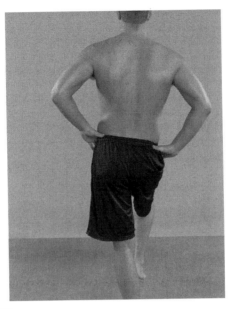

FIG. 10-28

10

CLINICAL PEARL

Trendelenburg test is positive as a result of (1) gluteal paralysis or weakness (from polio), (2) gluteal inhibition (from pain arising in the hip joint), (3) gluteal insufficiency from coxa vara, or (4) congenital dislocation of the hip. Nevertheless, false-positive results have been recorded in approximately 10% of the patients with hip pain.

CHAPTER ELEVEN

KNEE

AXIOMS IN ASSESSING THE KNEE

- The knee consists of two joints: the patellofemoral and the tibiofemoral.
- Knee pain can arise from the joint itself, from periarticular tissues, or from the hip or femur.

INTRODUCTION

Pain is the most common presenting symptom of knee abnormalities. The causes of knee pain tend to be age related. A convenient way to classify knee pain complaints is by age group and by whether the pain is intraarticular, periarticular, or referred (Table 11-3).

TABLE 11-1
KNEE JOINT CROSS-REFERENCE TABLE BY ASSESSMENT PROCEDURE

Disease Assessed

Knee Test/Sign	Osteochondritis	Quadriceps	Valgus Deformity	Effusion	Anterolateral Rotary Syndrome	Patellar Syndromes (Soft Tissue)	Patellar Fracture	Posterior Oblique Ligament	Arcuate-Popliteus Complex	Posterior Cruciate Ligament	Iliotibial Band	Posterior Capsule	Anterior Cruciate Ligament	Chondromalacia Patellae	Patellar Dislocation	Lateral Meniscus	Medial Meniscus	Lateral Collateral Ligament	Medial Collateral Ligament
Abduction stress test																			●
Adduction stress test																		●	
Apley compression/distraction test																●	●		

Continued

TABLE 11-1

KNEE JOINT CROSS-REFERENCE TABLE BY ASSESSMENT PROCEDURE —cont'd

Disease Assessed

Disease Assessed \ Test/Sign	Apprehension test for the patella	Bounce home test	Childress duck waddle test	Clarke test
Osteochondritis				
Quadriceps				
Valgus Deformity				
Effusion				
Anterolateral Rotary Syndrome				
Patellar Syndromes (Soft Tissue)				•
Patellar Fracture				
Posterior Oblique Ligament				
Arcuate-Popliteus Complex				
Posterior Cruciate Ligament				
Iliotibial Band				
Posterior Capsule				
Anterior Cruciate Ligament				
Chondromalacia Patellae				•
Patellar Dislocation	•			
Lateral Meniscus			•	•
Medial Meniscus			•	•
Lateral Collateral Ligament				
Medial Collateral Ligament				

Knee

Drawer test	Dreyer sign	Fouchet sign	Lachman test	Lateral pivot shift maneuver	Losee test	McMurray sign	Noble compression test	Patella ballottement test	Payr sign	Q-angle test	Slocum test	Steinmann sign	Thigh circumference test	Wilson sign
														●
													●	
										●				
							●							
										●				
		●								●				
	●													
●			●								●			
●			●	●							●			
●											●			
●			●				●				●			
●			●								●			
●			●	●							●			
		●							●					
									●					
						●						●		
						●		●				●		
			●											
●											●			

TABLE 11-2

KNEE CROSS-REFERENCE TABLE BY SUSPECTED SYNDROME OR TISSUE

Anterior cruciate ligament	Drawer test
	Lachman test
	Lateral pivot shift maneuver
	Slocum test
Arcuate-popliteus complex	Drawer test
	Lachman test
	Lateral pivot shift maneuver
	Slocum test
Anterolateral rotary syndromes	Losee test
	Q-angle test
Chondromalacia patella	Clarke test
	Fouchet sign
	Q-angle test
Effusion	Patella ballottement test
Iliotibial band	Drawer test
	Lateral pivot shift maneuver
	Noble compression test
	Slocum test
Lateral collateral ligament	Adduction stress test
	Lateral pivot shift maneuver
	Slocum test
Lateral meniscus	Apley compression/distraction test
	Bounce home test
	Clarke test
	McMurray sign
	Steinmann sign
Medial collateral ligament	Abduction stress test
	Drawer test
	Slocum test
Medial meniscus	Apley compression/distraction test
	Bounce home test
	Clarke test
	McMurray sign
	Payr sign
	Steinmann sign
Osteochondritis	Wilson sign
Patellar dislocation	Apprehension test for the patella
	Q-angle test
Patellar fracture	Dreyer sign
Patellar syndromes	Clarke test
	Fouchet sign
	Q-angle test

TABLE 11-2

KNEE CROSS-REFERENCE TABLE BY SUSPECTED SYNDROME OR TISSUE—cont'd

Posterior capsule	Drawer test
	Lateral pivot shift maneuver
	Slocum test
Posterior cruciate ligament	Drawer test
	Slocum test
Posterior oblique ligament	Drawer test
	Fouchet sign
	Slocum test
Quadriceps	Thigh circumference test
Valgus deformity	Q-angle test

TABLE 11-3

INTRAARTICULAR KNEE PAIN DIFFERENTIATED BY AGE

Age	Intraarticular
Juvenile (2-10 yrs)	Juvenile chronic arthritis
	Osteochondritis dissecans
	Septic arthritis
	Torn discoid lateral meniscus
Adolescent (10-18 years)	Osteochondritis dissecans
	Torn meniscus
	Anterior knee pain syndrome
	Patellar malalignment
Early adult (18-30 yrs)	Torn meniscus
	Instability
	Anterior knee pain syndrome
	Inflammatory conditions
Adult (30-50 yrs)	Degenerate meniscal tears
	Early degeneration after injury or meniscectomy
	Inflammatory arthropathies
Mature (>50 yrs)	Osteoarthritis
	Inflammatory arthropathies

11

Adapted from Klippel JH, Dieppe PA: *Rheumatology,* vol 1-2, ed 2, London, 1998, Mosby.

ORTHOPEDIC GAMUT 11-1

KNEE STABILITY

Knee stability depends on four ligaments:
1. Tibial collateral
2. Fibular collateral
3. Anterior cruciate
4. Posterior cruciate

The rounded contour of the femoral condyles furnishes little stability and the flat tibial plateaus, deepened by the semilunar cartilages. The quadriceps muscle and its tendinous expansions are great contributors to the stability and function of the knee. The earliest clinical indication of internal knee derangement is atrophy of the quadriceps.

The knee is not a true hinge joint. The tibia navigates a helical course on the condyles of the femur. Most traumatic arthritis of the knee in middle-age and elderly people results from minor derangements of the soft tissues, especially the menisci.

The knee lacks the stability of the hip, which has its ball and socket, or the ankle, which has its mortise and tendon. Both the hip and the ankle have structures that give some degree of bony stability. In the knee joint, the socket of the top of the tibia is so minimal that the lateral tibial plateau may be flat or even convex. The little bit of buffering provided by the menisci gives minimal increase in stability because the menisci are unstable themselves. For stability, the knee must depend largely on the soft tissues, ligaments, capsule, and muscles.

Making an accurate diagnosis about the exact nature of the patient's knee injury is extremely important. Examination must determine what part of the knee is injured and how bad the injury is.

ORTHOPEDIC GAMUT 11-2
KNEE

Parts of a knee vulnerable to injury:
1. Ligaments
2. Muscle tendon
3. Capsule
4. Meniscus
5. Cartilage
6. Bone
7. Bursae
8. Any combination of these

ESSENTIAL ANATOMY

The knee joint is the articulation of the femur, patella, and tibia. The fibula is not involved in this articulation. The knee allows for flexion and extension and for rotation when the knee is in complete flexion but not if the knee is fully extended.

ORTHOPEDIC GAMUT 11-3
FABELLA

A fabella can be a source of:
- Fabellar pain syndrome
- Chondromalacia
- Fractures
- Symptomatic dislocation
- Osteoarthritis
- Hypertrophy causing peroneal nerve paralysis

11

ESSENTIAL MOTION ASSESSMENT

The flexion-extension movement of the knee is not a simple hinge motion (Figs. 11-1 and 11-2). As the knee passes through its degrees of flexion and extensions, the imaginary mediolateral axis through which the movement occurs shifts up and down on the femur.

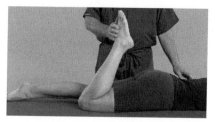

FIG. 11-1 The normal angle of knee flexion ranges from 130 to 150 degrees.

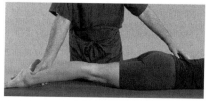

FIG. 11-2 The knee should normally extend to a straight line (0 degrees) and can occasionally be hyperextended up to 15 degrees.

ESSENTIAL MUSCLE FUNCTION ASSESSMENT

The examiner tests the muscles responsible for knee flexion and extension, the hamstrings and quadriceps, respectively (Figs. 11-3 and 11-4).

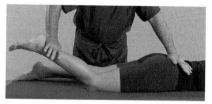

FIG. 11-3 The prime movers involved in flexion of the knee are the biceps femoris (sciatic nerve, tibial branch, S1, S2, and S3 to the long head; peroneal branch, L4, L5, S1, and S2 to the short head), semitendinosus (sciatic nerve, tibial branch, L4, L5, S1, S2, and S3), and the semimembranosus (sciatic nerve, tibial branch, L4, L5, S1, S2, and S3) muscles. The patient flexes the knee through its range of motion.

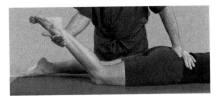

FIG. 11-4 The prime mover involved in extension of the knee is the quadriceps femoris (rectus femoris, vastus intermedius, vastus medialis, and vastus lateralis) muscle (innervated by the femoral nerve, L2, L3, and L4). Extension of the knee is tested while the patient extends the knee through its range of motion.

ORTHOPEDIC GAMUT 11-4

THIGH MUSCLES

The three thigh muscles that attach to the medial side of the tibia (supplied by three different nerves) are the following:

1. Gracilis (obturator nerve)
2. Sartorius (femoral nerve)
3. Semitendinosus (tibial nerve)

ORTHOPEDIC GAMUT 11-5

SCIATIC NERVE

The sciatic nerve innervates the following:

1. Hip joint
2. Biceps femoris
3. Semitendinosus
4. Semimembranosus
5. Ischial head of the adductor magnus

11

ESSENTIAL IMAGING

The typical knee study consists of an anteroposterior (or posteroanterior) and a lateral view. Many examiners will include tangential, tunnel, or oblique views for further evaluation. The tangential view provides an axial depiction of the patella and its relationship with the femur. The tunnel allows excellent visualization of the intercondylar region of the femoral-tibial articulation.

ABDUCTION STRESS TEST

ALSO KNOWN AS VALGUS STRESS TEST

Assessment for Medial Collateral Ligament Injury

ORTHOPEDIC GAMUT 11-6

MEDIAL COLLATERAL LIGAMENT INJURY CLASSIFICATIONS

Grade I:	0 to 5 mm of joint opening with no instability
Grade II:	5 to 10 mm of joint opening with some degree of instability
Grade III:	10 to 15 mm of joint opening with moderate instability
Grade IV:	Greater than 15 mm of joint opening with gross ligament instability

---

PROCEDURE

- While the patient is lying supine and the knee is in complete extension, the examiner, who is on the ipsilateral side, places one palm against the lateral aspect of the patient's knee, at the joint line.
- While the other hand is gripping the ankle, the examiner laterally draws the leg to open the medial side of the joint (Fig. 11-5).
- If the patient is indifferent to this action, the examiner repeats it while the knee is in approximately 30 degrees of flexion, a position of lesser stability.
- This maneuver makes the medial joint vulnerable to torsion stress.
- The production or increase of pain, especially below, above, or at the joint line, is evidence of medial collateral ligament injury.

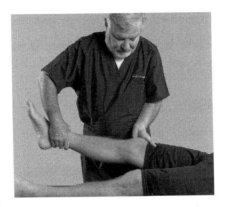

FIG. 11-5

CLINICAL PEARL

The knee is an unusual joint because it contains ligaments deep within the joint. Medial and lateral collateral menisci in the joint can also be damaged. Finally, the normal motions of the knee are very complex, including two planes of rotation. Multiple and complex injuries are common.

11

ADDUCTION STRESS TEST

Also Known as Varus Stress Test

Assessment for Lateral Collateral Ligament Injury

ORTHOPEDIC GAMUT 11-7

PROXIMAL TIBIOFIBULAR JOINT DYSFUNCTION SYMPTOMS

- Dull ache at the lateral aspect of the knee
- Pain radiating distally or proximally or both
- Hamstring tightness
- Knee and ankle movements that exacerbate the pain
- Pain that is relieved by rest
- Painful fibular head
- Full knee extension restricted or absent owing to hamstring tightness or pain

---

PROCEDURE

- While the patient is lying supine and the knee is in complete extension, the examiner, who is on the ipsilateral side, places one palm against the medial aspect of the patient's knee, at the joint line.
- While the examiner's other hand grasps the ankle, the examiner draws the leg medially to open the lateral side of the joint (Fig. 11-6).
- If the patient is indifferent to this procedure, the examiner repeats it with the knee in approximately 30 degrees of flexion.
- An initiation or increase of pain above, below, or at the joint line is evidence of lateral collateral ligament injury.

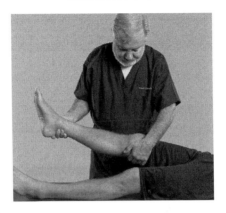

FIG. 11-6

CLINICAL PEARL

Little congruency exists between the articular surfaces of the tibia and the femur. As a result, the knee has a well-developed system of ligaments for stability and an arrangement of intraarticular menisci that reduce the contact loading between the femur and the tibia.

11

APLEY COMPRESSION TEST

ALSO KNOWN AS APLEY DISTRACTION TEST AND APLEY GRINDING TEST

Assessment for Collateral Ligament Injury and Meniscus Tears

ORTHOPEDIC GAMUT 11-8

INDICATIONS OF PATHOLOGIC CONDITIONS OF THE MENISCUS

1. Pain or tenderness on the lateral surfaces of the knee joint
2. Popping, snapping, or grating sounds with movement
3. Inability to fully extend the knee *(locking)*

PROCEDURE

- The test involves four steps, and if any or all of these steps elicit knee pain or clicking, the test is positive.
- The patient is lying prone with the lower limbs straight and the ankles hanging over the end of the examination table.
- The examiner grasps the foot of the involved lower extremity, strongly rotates the leg internally and flexes the knee past 90 degrees.
- This maneuver is repeated with the leg strongly rotated in external rotation (Fig. 11-7).
- The examiner anchors the patient's thigh to the examination table by placing a knee in the patient's popliteal space.
- A small pillow or towel should be used for cushioning.
- The examiner strongly distracts the patient's knee joint by lifting the foot.
- This move is followed by rapidly rotating the leg, both internally and externally (Fig. 11-8).
- This procedure is repeated with strong downward pressure on the patient's foot.
- An intermediate maneuver may be performed.

- The examiner flexes the patient's knee to 90 degrees and rapidly rotates the foot and leg both internally and externally without anchorage to rule out a rotational strain or collateral ligament tear.
- The test is significant for meniscus tear.

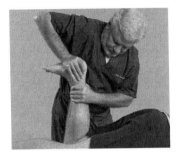

FIG. 11-7

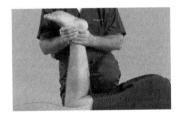

FIG. 11-8

CLINICAL PEARL

The phrase *internal derangement of the knee* is a common provisional diagnosis for any patient with mechanical symptoms of the knee. The initials of this phrase, *IDK*, also stands for "I don't know," and the temptation to use these initials, instead of making a complete diagnosis, must be avoided.

APPREHENSION TEST FOR THE PATELLA

Assessment for Vulnerability to Recurrent Dislocation of the Patella

ORTHOPEDIC GAMUT 11-9

PREDISPOSING FACTORS FOR PATELLAR DISLOCATION

- High Q-angle
- Patella dysplasia
- Shallow trochlea
- Patella alta
- Lateral structure tightness
- Vastus medialis insufficiency
- Generalized joint laxity
- Femoral or tibial torsion
- Valgus knee

PROCEDURE

- The apprehension test for the patella is a test for vulnerability to recurrent dislocation of the patella.
- For the test, the patient is either supine or seated, with the quadriceps muscles relaxed.
- The knee is flexed to 30 degrees.
- The examiner carefully and slowly pushes the patella laterally (Fig. 11-9).
- If the patella feels as if it is about to dislocate, the patient will contract the quadriceps muscles and bring the patella back into line.
- This action indicates a positive test.
- The patient will also exhibit a look of apprehension.

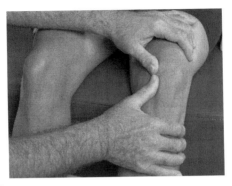

FIG. 11-9

CLINICAL PEARL

The examiner should observe for genu recurvatum and the position of the patella in relation to the femoral condyles. A high patella *(patella alta)* is a predisposing factor to recurrent lateral dislocation of the patella. The recurrent dislocation of the patella is also most common in women with the genu valgum deformity.

11

BOUNCE HOME TEST

Assessment for Meniscal Tears

ORTHOPEDIC GAMUT 11-10

CLASSIFICATIONS OF DISCOID MENISCUS

1. Complete, disk-shaped meniscus thin center; covers the tibial plateau
2. Incomplete, semilunar-shaped meniscus; partial tibial plateau coverage
3. Wrisberg-type, hypermobile meniscus caused by deficient posterior tibial attachment

---

PROCEDURE

- The patient is supine.
- The patient's knee is flexed completely.
- The knee is allowed to drop into extension (Fig. 11-10).
- If the extension is not complete, the test is positive.
- The positive finding suggests a torn meniscus.

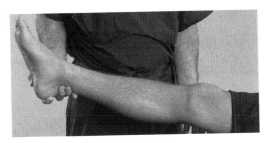

FIG. 11-10

CLINICAL PEARL

Meniscus lesions are the most common internal derangement. Although the menisci are damaged by trauma, the incident is often so trivial that the patient cannot remember any injury at all. Because of this circumstance, patients with meniscal injuries are rarely seen in emergency rooms.

11

CHILDRESS DUCK WADDLE TEST

Assessment for Medial or Lateral Meniscus Tears

ORTHOPEDIC GAMUT 11-11

COMMON MENISCAL TEARS TYPE

1. Type I: splitting of the meniscus, along its longitudinal axis, producing the so-called bucket-handle tear
2. Type II: a tear along transverse axis of the meniscus

PROCEDURE

- The patient stands with the feet somewhat apart and the legs in maximal internal rotation.
- A full squat is attempted (Fig. 11-11).
- During this maneuver, the patient's heels may come up from the floor, with weight bearing passing to the balls of the feet.
- The maneuver is repeated, with the lower limbs in maximal external rotation (Fig. 11-12).
- A positive test consists of pain, inability to fully flex the knee, or a clicking sound on either posterior side of the joint.
- The test is significant during internal rotation for a medial meniscus tear or during external rotation for a lateral meniscus tear.

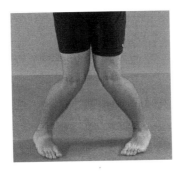

FIG. 11-11

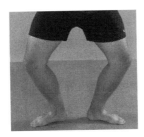

FIG. 11-12

CLINICAL PEARL

The menisci are important parts of the load-bearing mechanism of the knee because they absorb the downward thrust of the convex femoral condyles. The menisci are so effective that, if they are removed, the force that is taken by the articular cartilage during peak loading increases approximately five times. Therefore, a meniscectomy exposes the articular cartilage to much greater forces than normal. Evidence of degenerative osteoarthritis is seen in 75% of patients 10 years after a total meniscectomy.

11

CLARKE SIGN

Assessment for Chondromalacia Patellae

ORTHOPEDIC GAMUT 11-12

THREE GROUPS OF PATELLAR MALACIA

1. Group I is trauma related.
   a. A chondral fracture or infraction may exist caused either by acute trauma or by repeated, lesser traumata to the patella.
   b. Infraction of the patellar cartilage causes irritation of the patellar groove on the femur, and gradual changes supervene with fissuring, absorption, and fragmentation of the cartilage.
2. Group II is associated with a disturbance of the rhythm of the patellar function.
   a. These disturbances are commonly called *tracking disorders*.
   b. This is the type of malacia that accompanies intrinsic injury to the knee.
   c. Any condition that causes a disturbance in the rhythm of the knee action often results in involvement of the undersurface of the patella.
   d. The knee is checked abruptly, motion is reversed, and the patella is driven against the femur.
   e. A relationship exists between the locking of the knee and the degree of malacia present.
   f. These two factors are much more important for indicating the amount of malacia present than is the age of the patient.
   g. The exact mechanism of the breakdown of the patella has never been wholly explained.
   h. This condition also probably occurs as the result of various other causes, including direct trauma and synovitis of the joint and general chondrolytic changes.
   i. The particular pathologic changes described usually accompany other intrinsic conditions of the knee.

ORTHOPEDIC GAMUT 11-12

THREE GROUPS OF PATELLAR MALACIA—cont'd

3. Group III is primary malacia of the patella, usually a bilateral condition, without any demonstrable etiologic factor.
   a. These cases are puzzling.
   b. The examiner cannot rule out the effect of repeated trauma because young patients are usually very physically active.
   c. These patients should be expected to traumatize the patella repeatedly.
   d. However, the simultaneous involvement of both knees, with relative lack of involvement of other chondral surfaces equally susceptible to trauma, prompts the examiner to seek a cause other than a simple contusion.

ORTHOPEDIC GAMUT 11-13

ETIOLOGY OF CHONDROMALACIA PATELLA

1. Any injury or anatomic abnormality that predisposes the area to an irregular pattern of movement of the patella
2. Meniscus injuries that alter normal tibiofemoral motion
3. Recurrent subluxation of the patella
4. Quadriceps imbalance
5. Patella alta
6. Angular deformities of the knee
7. Direct trauma to the patella

11

PROCEDURE

- The patient's knee is extended fully.
- The examiner compresses the quadriceps muscles at the superior pole of the patella.
- The patient gently contracts the quadriceps muscles as the examiner resists the movement of the patella (Fig. 11-13).
- Retropatellar pain and failure to hold the contraction is considered positive.
- A positive test suggests chondromalacia patella.
- To test different parts of the patella, the knee should be tested in 30, 60, and 90 degrees of flexion and in full extension.

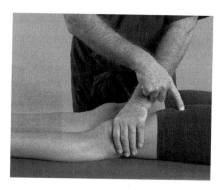

FIG. 11-13

CLINICAL PEARL

In examining the patella, the examiner should note any tenderness over the anterior surface and whether a bipartite ridge is present. Upper and lower pole tenderness occurs in Sinding-Larsen-Johansson disease and jumper's knee (an extensor apparatus traction injury).

DRAWER TEST

**Assessment for Injury to Some Degree of
(1) the Anterior Cruciate Ligament, Especially the
Anteromedial Bundle, (2) the Posterolateral Capsule,
(3) the Posteromedial Capsule, (4) the Medial
Collateral Ligament, Especially the Deep Fibers,
(5) the Iliotibial Band, (6) the Posterior Oblique
Ligament, (7) the Arcuate-Popliteus Complex, and
(8) the Posterior Cruciate Ligament
(in Testing Posterior Drawer Movements)**

ORTHOPEDIC GAMUT 11-14
GRADES OF KNEE LIGAMENT SPRAINS

1. Mild—grade I, first-degree ligament sprain: an incomplete stretching of collagen ligament fibers, resulting in minimal pain, minimal or no swelling, no loss of joint function, and no clinical or functional instability.
2. Moderate—grade II, second-degree ligament sprain: a partial loss of ligament fiber continuity. A few collagen ligament fibers may be completely torn; however, most of the ligament remains intact. This degree of sprain is characterized by moderate (more intense than a first-degree sprain) pain, moderate swelling, some loss of joint function, and some loss of joint stability.
3. Severe—grade III, third-degree sprain (rupture): the entire collagen ligament fiber bundles are completely torn. No continuity exists within the body of the ligament. This injury is usually characterized by profound pain, intense swelling, loss of joint function, and instability.

11

ORTHOPEDIC GAMUT 11-15

HUGHSTON KNEE INSTABILITIES INDEX

1. Mild instability: graded 1+ (5 mm or less of joint surface separation)
2. Moderate instability: graded 2+ (joint surface separation of 4 to 10 mm)
3. Severe instability: graded 3+ (joint surface separation of 10 mm or more)

ORTHOPEDIC GAMUT 11-16

POSITIVE ANTERIOR DRAWER TEST

In a positive anterior drawer test, the following structures may have been injured to some degree:
1. Anterior cruciate ligament, especially the anteromedial bundle
2. Posterolateral capsule
3. Posteromedial capsule
4. Medial collateral ligament, especially the deep fibers
5. Iliotibial band
6. Posterior oblique ligament
7. Arcuate-popliteus complex

ORTHOPEDIC GAMUT 11-17

COMMON TYPES OF POSTERIOR CRUCIATE LIGAMENT TEARS

1. The medial tibial condyle subluxates anteriorly (anteromedial instability).
2. The lateral tibial condyle subluxates anteriorly (anterolateral rotary instability).
3. The lateral tibial condyle subluxates posteriorly (posterolateral rotary instability).
4. Combinations of these lesions may be found.

ORTHOPEDIC GAMUT 11-18

POSITIVE POSTERIOR DRAWER TEST

In a positive posterior drawer test, the following structures may have been injured to some degree:
1. Posterior cruciate ligament
2. Arcuate-popliteus complex
3. Posterior oblique ligament
4. Anterior cruciate ligament

PROCEDURE

- The patient's knee is flexed to 90 degrees.
- The patient's foot is held on the table by the examiner.
- The tibia is pulled forward on the femur by placing hands around the tibia (Fig. 11-14).
- Normal movement is approximately 6 mm.
- When the tibia moves forward more than 6 mm on the femur, the test is positive.
- To test the posterior cruciate ligament (PCL), the tibia is pushed back on the femur (Fig. 11-15).
- The test is positive when excessive movement is noted.

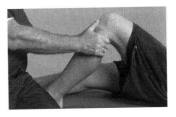

FIG. 11-14

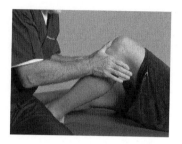

FIG. 11-15

CLINICAL PEARL

A tibia that is already displaced backward, as a result of a posterior cruciate tear, may give a false-positive result when the examiner is testing the anterior cruciate. This false-positive test may also occur with the Lachman test.

DREYER SIGN

Assessment for Fracture of the Patella

ORTHOPEDIC GAMUT 11-19

ORTIGUERA AND BERRY CLASSIFICATION OF PERIPROSTHETIC FRACTURES OF THE PATELLA

1. Type I: intact extensor mechanism; stable implant
2. Type II: disruption of extensor mechanism; with or without implant in place
3. Type III: intact extensor mechanism
a. Loosening of patellar component
b. Reasonable remaining bone stock
c. Poor bone stock

PROCEDURE

- While lying supine with the knee extended, the patient is unable to raise the leg.
- When the examiner applies compression to the thigh, by using the hands to give anchorage to the quadriceps, the patient is able to lift the leg (Fig. 11-16).
- When this force is removed, the patient is again unable to raise the leg.
- The test is significant for a fracture of the patella.

11

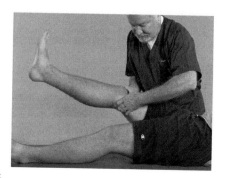

FIG. 11-16

CLINICAL PEARL

The quadriceps muscle gains insertion into the tibia through the medium of the patella, which is enclosed within the quadriceps expansion and the patellar tendon. Complete rupture may occur as a disruption through the patella. This area is the usual site of rupture for a common variety of fractured patella. The injury occurs mainly in adults of middle age.

FOUCHET SIGN

Assessment for Patellar Tracking Disorder, Peripatellar Syndrome, or Patellofemoral Dysfunction

---

ORTHOPEDIC GAMUT 11-20

PATHOMECHANICS OF PATELLOFEMORAL DISORDERS

1. Q-angle
2. Lateral retinacular tightness
3. Vastus medialis obliquus deficiency
4. Lateral deviation of the patella at terminal extension (J-sign)
5. Patella alta or infera
6. Trochlear depth
7. Congruence of the patellofemoral joint

ORTHOPEDIC GAMUT 11-21

DEJOUR'S CLASSIFICATION OF EXTENSOR MECHANISM MALALIGNMENT

- Major patellar instability; more than one documented dislocation
- Objective patellar instability; one dislocation with associated anatomic abnormalities
- Potential patellar instability; patellar pain with associated radiologic abnormalities

11

PROCEDURE

- While the patient is lying supine and the knee is in full extension, the examiner uses the flat of a hand to compress the patella against the femur (Fig. 11-17).
- If this action produces point tenderness and pain at the patellar margin, the sign is present.
- If pain is not produced by this maneuver, the examiner then rubs the patella transversely against the femur.
- Audible or palpable grating and pain confirm the presence of the sign.
- When the patella has peripheral tenderness on medial or lateral displacement, this is known as Perkins sign.
- Perkins sign is significant for patellar tracking disorder, peripatellar syndrome, or patellofemoral dysfunction.

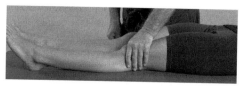

FIG. 11-17

CLINICAL PEARL

Placing a palm of the hand over the patient's patella and the thumb and index finger along the joint line as the joint is flexed and extended will distinguish the source of the crepitus from damaged articular surfaces.

LACHMAN TEST

**Assessment for Injury to Some Degree of
(1) the Anterior Cruciate Ligament, Especially the
Posterolateral Bundle, (2) the Posterior Oblique
Ligament, and (3) the Arcuate-Popliteus Complex**

PROCEDURE

- The patient is supine.
- The patient's knee is held between full extension and 30 degrees of flexion.
- The patient's femur is stabilized with one hand as the tibia is moved forward (Fig. 11-18).
- A mushy, or soft, end-feel when the tibia is moved forward on the femur and the infrapatellar tendon slope disappears is a positive sign.
- A positive sign suggests damage to (1) the anterior cruciate ligament (ACL), especially the posterolateral bundle, (2) the posterior oblique ligament, and (3) the arcuate-popliteus complex.

11

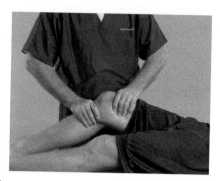

FIG. 11-18

CLINICAL PEARL

When medial and lateral or anterior and posterior, as well as the medial and lateral, compartments are torn, combined complex instability exists. Transitory dislocation, or at least subluxation of the knee, is a preliminary symptom. In many instances, the peroneal nerve has been injured.

LATERAL PIVOT SHIFT MANEUVER

ALSO KNOWN AS TEST OF MCINTOSH

Assessment for Injury to Some Degree of
(1) the Anterior Cruciate Ligament,
(2) the Posterolateral Capsule, (3) the Arcuate-Popliteus
Complex, (4) the Lateral Collateral Ligament, and
(5) the Iliotibial Band

PROCEDURE

- The patient is supine.
- The examiner flexes the knee slightly (5 degrees).
- A valgus stress is applied to the knee while maintaining a medial rotation torque on the tibia and at the ankle.
- The leg is flexed 30 to 40 degrees. The tibia reduces or jogs backward.
- The patient experiences the sensation of the knee *giving way* (Fig. 11-19).
- This sensation is the positive finding.
- To some degree, (1) the ACL, (2) the posterolateral capsule, (3) the arcuate-popliteus complex, (4) the lateral collateral ligament, or (5) the iliotibial band has been injured.

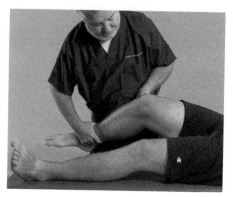

FIG. 11-19

CLINICAL PEARL

Normally, the knee's center of rotation changes constantly through its range of motion as a result of the shape of the femoral condyles, the ligamentous restraint, and the muscle pull. A positive pivot shift test usually suggests damage to the anterior cruciate, the posterior capsule, or the lateral collateral ligament.

LOSEE TEST

Assessment for Anterolateral Rotary Instability of the Knee

PROCEDURE

- The patient is in a supine position.
- The patient's leg is externally rotated.
- The patient's knee is flexed to 30 degrees.
- The examiner hooks a thumb behind the patient's fibular head.
- A valgus force is applied to the knee.
- The knee is extended, and forward pressure is applied behind the fibular head with the examiner's thumb (Fig. 11-20).
- The leg moves into medial rotation.
- If a *clunk* is felt forward just before full extension of the knee, the test is positive.
- This clunk means that the tibia has subluxed anteriorly and indicates injury to the same structures listed with the lateral pivot shift maneuver.
- The Losee test assesses anterolateral rotary instability.

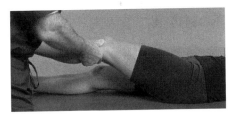

FIG. 11-20

11

CLINICAL PEARL

If rotary instability is present, then as full extension is reached, a dramatic clunk will occur as the lateral tibial condyle subluxates forward. The patient should relate this information to the sensations experienced during activity.

MCMURRAY SIGN

Assessment for Medial or Lateral Meniscus Injury

PROCEDURE

- The patient is lying supine, and the thigh and leg are flexed until the heel approaches the buttock.
- One of the examiner's hands is on the knee, and the other is on the heel.
- The examiner internally rotates and slowly extends the leg (Fig. 11-21).
- The examiner then externally rotates and slowly extends the leg.
- McMurray sign is present if, at some point in the arc, a painful click or snap is heard.
- This sign is significant in meniscal injury.
- The point in the arc at which the snap is heard locates the site of injury of the meniscus.
- If noted with internal rotation, the lateral meniscus will be involved.
- The higher the leg is raised when the snap is heard, the more posterior the lesion is in the meniscus.
- If noted with external rotation, the medial meniscus will be involved.

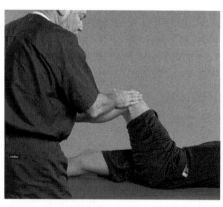

FIG. 11-21

CLINICAL PEARL

The examiner should observe for tenderness in the joint line and test for a springy block to full extension of the knee. These two signs, in association with evidence of quadriceps atrophy, are the most consistent and reliable signs of a torn meniscus.

NOBLE COMPRESSION TEST

Assessment for Iliotibial Band Friction Syndrome

ORTHOPEDIC GAMUT 11-22

EXTRINSIC AND INTRINSIC CAUSATIVE FACTORS OF ILIOTIBIAL BAND FRICTION SYNDROME

EXTRINSIC FACTORS

1. Running or cycling on an oblique surface causing a pelvic tilt
2. Sudden increase in running or cycling distance
3. Improper seating with cleats too far internally rotated or a saddle that is not well positioned

INTRINSIC FACTORS

1. Varus knee deformity that predisposes the area for this friction syndrome between the lateral femoral epicondyle and the overriding iliotibial band
2. Leg-length discrepancy
3. Forefoot pronation

PROCEDURE

- The patient is in a supine position.
- The patient's hip and knee are flexed 90 degrees.
- The examiner applies thumb pressure to the lateral femoral condyle.
- The patient's knee is extended as the thumb pressure is maintained.
- In the positive test, the patient will complain of severe pain over the lateral femoral condyle, near 30 degrees of flexion (Fig. 11-22).
- This pain indicates iliotibial band syndrome.

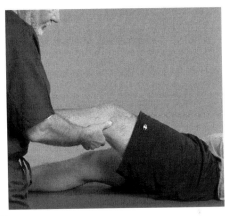

FIG. 11-22

CLINICAL PEARL

This syndrome produces a line of tenderness that extends from the anterolateral tibia, across the joint line, and up the side of the thigh. Tenderness is usually maximal over the lateral femoral condyle, and a painful arc occurs at approximately 30 degrees of flexion.

11

PATELLA BALLOTTEMENT TEST

Assessment for Joint Effusion

PROCEDURE

- The patient's knee is extended.
- A slight tap or pressure is applied over the patella (Fig. 11-23).
- This test is positive if a large amount of swelling in the knee is detected.

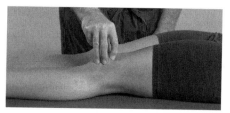

FIG. 11-23

CLINICAL PEARL

If popliteal swelling is found, confirming communication with the joint is possible by massaging its contents back into the main synovial cavity while the knee is in flexion. The examiner maintains pressure on the patient's popliteal fossa, extends the knee, and then removes the pressure. The swelling will not reappear until the patient flexes the knee several times, confirming a valve-like communication between the main cavity and the *cyst*.

PAYR SIGN

Assessment for Injury of the Posterior Horn of the Medial Meniscus

PROCEDURE

- The patient is in the cross-legged, yoga-seated position, with the feet and ankles crossed.
- The examiner applies downward pressure on the knee joint (Fig. 11-24).
- Pain is elicited on the medial side of the joint when the sign is present.
- The test is significant when a lesion of the posterior horn of the medial meniscus is present.

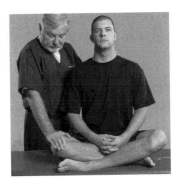

FIG. 11-24

11

CLINICAL PEARL

Meniscal cysts lie in the joint line, feel firm during palpation, and are tender to deep pressure. Cysts of the menisci may be associated with tears. Lateral meniscus cysts are by far the most common. Cystic swellings on the medial side are sometimes caused by ganglions that arise from the pes anserinus (insertion of the sartorius, gracilis, and semitendinosus).

Q-ANGLE TEST

Assessment for Patellofemoral Dysfunction, Patella Alta, Subluxating Patella, Increased Femoral Anteversion, Genu Valgum, or Increased Lateral Tibial Torsion

PROCEDURE

- To determine the Q-angle, a line is drawn from the anterosuperior iliac spine to the midpoint of the patella and from the tibial tubercle to the midpoint of the patella.
- The angle formed by the intersection of these two lines is the Q-angle (Fig. 11-25).
- Normally, the Q-angle is 13 to 18 degrees. The normal angle for men is 13 degrees, and for women it is 18 degrees.
- Less than 13 degrees suggests patellofemoral dysfunction or patella alta.
- Greater than 18 degrees suggests patellofemoral dysfunction, subluxating patella, increased femoral anteversion, genu valgum, or increased lateral tibial torsion.

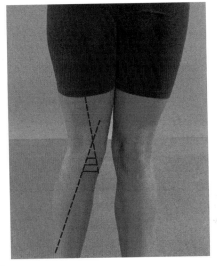

FIG. 11-25

CLINICAL PEARL

In children, an increased Q-angle is associated with genu valgum. The examiner must note whether the genu valgum is unilateral or, as is usual, bilateral. The severity of the deformity is recorded by measuring the intermalleolar gap. The examiner grasps the child's ankles and rotates the legs until the patellae are vertical. The legs are brought together to touch lightly at the knees. A measurement is made between the malleoli. Serial measurements, often every 6 months, are used to check progress. Note that, with growth, a static measurement is an angular improvement.

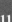
11

SLOCUM TEST

Assessment for Anterolateral Rotary Instability, with Injury to Some Degree of (1) the Anterior Cruciate Ligament, (2) the Posterolateral Capsule, (3) the Arcuate-Popliteus Complex, (4) the Lateral Collateral Ligament, (5) the Posterior Cruciate Ligament, and (6) the Iliotibial Band (Tensor Fascia Lata)

PROCEDURE

- The patient is setting in supine position.
- The knee is flexed to 80 or 90 degrees; the hip is flexed to 45 degrees.
- The foot is internally rotated.
- The foot is held as the tibia is pulled anteriorly.
- Movement will occur on the lateral side of the knee if the test is positive.
- This movement indicates anterolateral rotatory instability.
- Excessive movement suggests injury to (1) the ACL, (2) the posterolateral capsule, (3) the arcuate-popliteus complex, (4) the lateral collateral ligament, (5) the PCL, or (6) the iliotibial band.
- The test also may be performed while the patient is seated with the knees flexed over the edge of the examination table.
- The examiner pulls or pushes the tibia to the knee while medially or laterally rotating the foot (Fig. 11-26).
- Pulling on the tibia tests for anterior rotary instability. Pushing the tibia tests for posterior rotary instability.

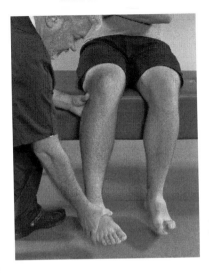

FIG. 11-26

CLINICAL PEARL

This maneuver tightens the lateral capsule, giving enough stability to eliminate the anterior drawer sign. If the anterior drawer sign is still positive while the patient is in this position (most anterior movement occurring on the lateral side), the lateral capsule (or lateral collateral ligament) is likely also damaged.

11

STEINMANN SIGN

ALSO KNOWN AS STEINMANN TENDERNESS DISPLACEMENT TEST

Assessment for Lateral or Medial Meniscus Tear

ORTHOPEDIC GAMUT 11-23
FACTORS CONTRIBUTING TO MENISCUS TEAR
1. The knee must be bearing weight.
2. The knee must be flexed.
3. A rotation strain is required.

PROCEDURE

- Knee pain moves anteriorly when the knee is extended and moves posteriorly when the knee is flexed (Fig. 11-27).
- The movement of pain is the positive sign.
- This sign indicates a meniscus tear.
- Medial pain is elicited by lateral rotation.
- Lateral pain is elicited by medial rotation.

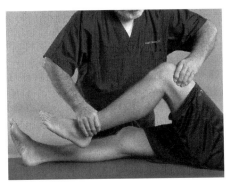

FIG. 11-27

CLINICAL PEARL

Patients use the term *locking* to describe episodes of severe pain in the knee or even collapsing of the knee. Curiously, the word is not applied in this way to any other joints. *Locking* denotes mechanical jamming of the knee joint and nothing more.

THIGH CIRCUMFERENCE TEST

**Assessment for Muscle Hypertonicity or
Hypotonicity of the Thigh**

ORTHOPEDIC GAMUT 11-24

RISK FACTORS FOR PATELLAR OR QUADRICEPS RUPTURE

- Diabetes mellitus
- Gout
- Repetitive microtrauma
- Endocrine disorders

PROCEDURE

- An area of the thigh 10 cm above the patella is identified.
- The circumference of the leg at that point is measured and compared with the opposite leg (Fig. 11-28).

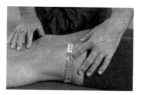

FIG. 11-28

CLINICAL PEARL

Although all the quadriceps muscle atrophies uniformly, atrophy of the bulky vastus medialis (particularly in a fit young man) may be the most conspicuous. Quadriceps atrophy is a difficult sign to detect, particularly in the middle-age, elderly, and female patients. Some asymmetry of muscle bulk is common.

WILSON SIGN

Assessment for Osteochondritis Dissecans of the Knee

ORTHOPEDIC GAMUT 11-25

COMMON ORIGINS OF A LOOSE BODY IN THE KNEE

- Osteochondritis dissecans at the lateral border of the medial femoral condyle (men)
- Marginal fracture that is from the lateral margin of the lateral femoral condyle and is secondary to direct trauma or patellar dislocation (men)
- Medial tangential osteochondral fracture of the patella from dislocation (men)
- This order is reversed in the female patient.

ORTHOPEDIC GAMUT 11-26

COMMON SITES FOR OSTEOCHONDRITIS DISSECANS

1. The lateral border of the medial femoral condyle
2. The inferior, central area of the lateral femoral condyle
3. The inferior, central region of the medial femoral condyle

---

ORTHOPEDIC GAMUT 11-27

POSSIBLE CONTRIBUTORY FACTORS FOR OSTEOCHONDRITIS DISSECANS

- Trauma
- Ischemia
- Ossification defects
- Epiphyseal dysplasia
- Family history

11

PROCEDURE

- The patient is in a supine position.
- The patient's knee is flexed to 90 degrees by the examiner.
- The knee is extended with the tibia medially rotated.
- Near 30 degrees of flexion, pain in the knee increases (the patient often stops the rotating movement).
- If the tibia is rotated laterally, the pain disappears, which is a positive test (Fig. 11-29).
- The positive test indicates osteochondritis dissecans of the femur.

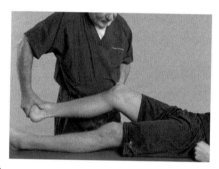

FIG. 11-29

CLINICAL PEARL

Patients often give a classic account of a loose fragment in the knee and are usually able to describe its size and shape. Loose bodies are sometimes called *joint mice,* which is an appropriate description because these loose bodies can be recognized instantly, but they disappear and may be impossible to find again. Loose bodies should not be called *foreign bodies.* Foreign bodies, including bullets and bits of gravel, come from outside the body and are rare in joints.

CHAPTER TWELVE

LOWER LEG, ANKLE, AND FOOT

AXIOMS IN ASSESSING THE LOWER LEG, ANKLE, AND FOOT

- Pain in the ankle and foot can arise from the bones and joints, periarticular soft tissues, nerve roots and peripheral nerves, or vascular structures.
- Pain in the foot can also be referred from the lumbar spine or knee joint.
- The greatest majority of painful foot conditions result from inappropriate footwear, weak intrinsic muscles, foot deformities, or static disorders.

INTRODUCTION

The leg, ankle, and foot are subject to static deformities more than any other skeletal unit. The weight-transmitting and propulsive functions of these structures are restricted daily by nonyielding foot coverings. Anatomic variations in the shape and stability of joint surfaces may predispose, resist, or modify the deforming force of common footwear.

Modern civilization disregards the physiologic features of the ankle and foot. Fashion and eye appeal rather than function determine shoe design, especially in the fore part of the shoe, where most disabilities and deformities of the foot occur.

ORTHOPEDIC GAMUT 12-1

IMPORTANT SHOE DESIGN FEATURES

1. The arch support can reduce muscle fatigue in the calf and disperse arch pressure.
2. Outsoles with 1.5-cm thickness in the metatarsal zone tend to produce lower metatarsal pressure and vertical impact force and to reduce low back discomfort.
3. A shoe upper with soft leather and mid-sole made with ethylene vinyl acetate or polyurethane materials are helpful to increase whole-body and foot comfort.
4. An outsole with heel height between 1.8 and 3.6 cm tends to generate lower heel pressure and vertical impact force in the forefoot and to reduce ankle discomfort.

The restrictive force of poorly fitting shoes produces little deformity on the tarsus because the tarsus is made up of short, heavy bones. Normal movement in the tarsal joints is limited because the articular surfaces of the tarsal joints are flat. However, the phalanges and metatarsals are long thin bones with a normally wide range of joint motion. Restrictive force on these bones produces most of the static deformities of the forefoot. These static deformities include first metatarsophalangeal joint deformities, hammertoe, tailor's bunion, overlapping toes, and many other conditions that are deviations from the normal (Table 12-3).

TABLE 12-1

LOWER LEG, ANKLE, AND FOOT CROSS-REFERENCE TABLE BY ASSESSMENT PROCEDURE

Lower Leg, Ankle, and Foot

Disease Assessed

Test/Sign	Tarsal Tunnel Syndrome	Achilles' Tendon	Metatarsalgia	Neuroma	Fibular Fracture	Thrombophlebitis	Calcaneus Fracture	Foot Pronation	Peroneal Nerve Paralysis	Atrophy	Vascular	Talofibular Ligament
Anterior drawer sign of the ankle												●
Buerger test											●	
Calf circumference test										●		
Claudication test											●	
Duchenne sign									●			

Continued

12

TABLE 12-1

LOWER LEG, ANKLE, AND FOOT CROSS-REFERENCE TABLE BY ASSESSMENT PROCEDURE—cont'd

Disease Assessed

Lower Leg, Ankle, and Foot

Test/Sign	Tarsal Tunnel Syndrome	Achilles' Tendon	Metatarsalgia	Neuroma	Fibular Fracture	Thrombophlebitis	Calcaneus Fracture	Foot Pronation	Peroneal Nerve Paralysis	Atrophy	Vascular	Talofibular Ligament
Foot tourniquet test											●	
Helbings sign								●				
Hoffa test							●					
Homans sign						●					●	
Keen sign					●							

	Morton test.	Moszkowicz test	Moses test	Perthes test	Strunsky sign	Thompson test	Tinel foot sign
							●
						●	
	●			●			
	●						
						●	
		●	●	●			

TABLE 12-2

LOWER LEG, ANKLE, AND FOOT CROSS-REFERENCE TABLE BY SYNDROME OR TISSUE

Achilles tendon	Thompson test
Atrophy	Calf circumference test
Calcaneus fracture	Hoffa test
	Thompson test
Fibular fracture	Keen sign
Foot pronation	Helbings sign
Metatarsalgia	Morton test
	Strunsky sign
Neuroma	Morton test
Peroneal nerve paralysis	Duchenne sign
Talofibular ligament	Anterior drawer sign of the ankle
Tarsal tunnel syndrome	Tinel foot sign
Thrombophlebitis	Homans sign
	Moses test
Vascular	Buergers test
	Claudication test
	Foot tourniquet test
	Homans sign
	Moszkowicz test
	Moses test
	Perthes test

TABLE 12-3

ANKLE AND FOOT DIFFERENTIATION BY ONSET

Articular	Trauma, sprain
	Arthritis
	Metatarsalgia
	Congenital disorders (e.g., clubfoot)
Neurologic	Entrapment of lumbosacral nerve roots form herniated lumbar disc
	Entrapment of the lateral popliteal nerve behind the neck of the fibula
	Tarsal tunnel syndrome (posterior tibial nerve)
	Interdigital (Morton) neuroma
	Peripheral neuropathy and insensitive foot
Periarticular	Cutaneous and subcutaneous
	Plantar fascia
	Tendons and tendon sheaths
	Bursitis
	Acute calcific periarthritis
Osseous	Fracture
	Epiphysitis (osteochondritis)
	Bone neoplasms, infection
	Painful accessory ossicles
Vascular	Ischemic foot pain
	Vasospastic disorders with Raynaud phenomenon
	Cholesterol embolization with *purple toes*

The human foot is uniquely specialized. The metatarsals and toes enable the body to stand erect. The versatility of the forefoot permits the human to retain an upright stance and allows for grace during walking, dancing, and athletics.

A well-developed and strong foot withstands surprising abuse. Morbid changes take place only when maltreatment becomes excessive. An underdeveloped and frail foot, ankle, and lower-leg mechanism may fail under ordinary stress and strain.

The ankle and foot are inspected in both the resting and standing positions for evidence of swelling, deformity, and skin abnormalities such as edema, erythema, tophi, subcutaneous nodules, or ulcers. Abnormalities of gait are observed while the patient is walking. The gait or walking cycle can be divided into two phases: the stance or weight-bearing phase and the swing or non–weight-bearing phase.

12

ORTHOPEDIC GAMUT 12-2

ETIOLOGY OF ACHILLES TENDON SWELLING

1. Tendon rupture
2. Calcaneal bursitis
3. Rheumatoid nodules
4. Urate tophi

In the standing position, the calcaneus normally maintains the line of the Achilles tendon. Deformities of the subtalar joint, resulting in eversion (calcaneovalgus) or inversion (calcaneovarus) of the heel, are best observed from behind. *Equinus* and *calcaneus* refer to angulation of the ankle in plantar and dorsiflexion, respectively. Inspection while the patient is standing may reveal lowering of the longitudinal arch (pes planus) or increased height of the arch (pes cavus).

ESSENTIAL ANATOMY

The leg is divided by fascial septa into posterior, lateral, and anterior compartments. Because they have a common nerve supply, the anterior and lateral compartments are often considered to be one. The posterior compartment is further divided into a superficial and deep area. Although each compartment of the leg has a specialized vascular and nerve supply, the nerves and vessels are sometimes not physically within the compartment they supply (e.g., the lateral compartment is supplied by the peroneal artery, which lies in the posterior compartment).

The anterior leg muscles attach to the area between the tibia and fibula.

ORTHOPEDIC GAMUT 12-3

MUSCLE OF THE ANTERIOR COMPARTMENT OF THE LEG

1. Tibialis anterior
2. Extensor hallucis longus
3. Extensor digitorum longus

ORTHOPEDIC GAMUT 12-4

ANKLE JOINT

Structures crossing the ankle joint:
ANTERIORLY
- Tendons of the tibialis anterior
- Extensor hallucis longus
- Anterior tibial vessels
- Deep peroneal nerve
- Extensor digitorum longus
- Peroneus tertius

POSTEROMEDIALLY
- Tibial vessels
- Tibial nerve
- Flexor hallucis longus

POSTEROLATERALLY
- Tendons of the peroneus longus and brevis

ESSENTIAL MOTION ASSESSMENT

For the sake of simplicity, motions are tested along three different axes. Dorsiflexion and plantar flexion are movements at the ankle joint that occur around a transverse axis that passes through the body of the talus. Inversion and eversion are movements of rotation of the foot along its long axis. Abduction and adduction of the forefoot, occurring along a vertical axis, are movements of the midtarsal joints. Pronation and supination refer to a weight-bearing foot. The complex movements of eversion and inversion indicate changes in the form of the whole foot when it is not bearing weight.

ORTHOPEDIC GAMUT 12-5

ANKLE AND FOOT

Activities for testing range of motion of the ankle and foot:
1. Point the foot up toward the ceiling.
2. Point the foot down toward the floor.
3. With the foot bent at the ankle, point the medial side of the foot toward the floor (eversion) and repeat with the lateral side (inversion).
4. Rotate the ankle, turning the foot away from and then toward the other foot.

Movements of the lesser toes can be measured in a similar manner. Clinically, the examiner should note whether fixed contractures exist or if the joints are supple. Restriction of joint motion can be the result of soft-tissue contractures, bony abutment, or intraarticular adhesions. Motion may be restricted because of pain that results from inflammation or injuries (Figs. 12-1 and 12-2).

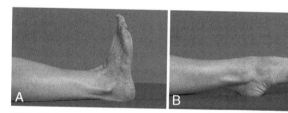

FIG. 12-1 A normal ankle allows 20 degrees of dorsiflexion (**A**) and 40 degrees of plantar flexion from this position (**B**).

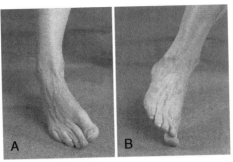

FIG. 12-2 A normal joint allows 20 degrees of eversion (**A**) and approximately 30 degrees of inversion (**B**).

ESSENTIAL MUSCLE FUNCTION ASSESSMENT

The main muscles of the calf are the soleus and gastrocnemius. The soleus acts purely as a flexor of the ankle, and the gastrocnemius flexes both the ankle and the knee. The flexor digitorum longus and flexor hallucis longus flex the toes and big toe, respectively. The anterior compartment muscles include the tibialis anterior, extensor digitorum longus, and extensor hallucis longus. The tibialis anterior inverts the foot and dorsiflexes the ankle.

The motions in the ankle joint are plantar flexion and dorsiflexion. The muscles in the posterior compartment, which are innervated by the tibial nerve, are responsible primarily for plantar flexion motion. The major muscles for plantar flexion are the gastrocnemius and soleus, and they are supplemented by the tibialis posterior, peroneus longus, flexor digitorum longus, and hallucis longus. The power of the gastrocnemius-soleus group is weakened when the knee is in flexion because the gastrocnemius is a two-joint muscle. However, while the knee is in flexion, the passive range of ankle dorsiflexion increases slightly. The muscles of the anterior compartment, innervated by the deep peroneal nerve, are responsible primarily for dorsiflexion motion. Dorsiflexion is performed by the tibialis anterior and the extensor digitorum longus. When these two muscles act together, their individual actions of inversion and eversion are neutralized. The extensor hallucis longus and peroneus tertius also aid in dorsiflexion (Figs. 12-3 to 12-6).

12

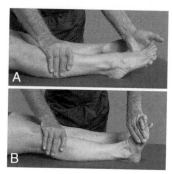

FIG. 12-3 The soleus is evaluated by applying a dorsiflexion force to the foot while the patient plantar flexes the foot (**A**). The tibialis anterior is tested by exerting a counterforce to the dorsiflexion and inversion movement of the foot and ankle (**B**).

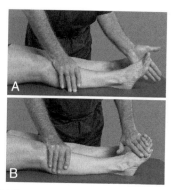

FIG. 12-4 The tibialis posterior is evaluated by exerting a counterforce to the foot while the patient inverts and plantar flexes the foot (**A**). The peroneus longus is tested by exerting a counterforce to a foot that is held in plantar flexion while the patient actively everts it (**B**).

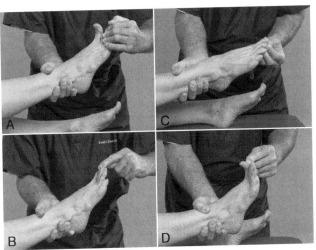

FIG. 12-5 Flexion of the metatarsophalangeal joint is achieved primarily by the lumbricales, interossei, and flexor hallucis brevis, which are augmented by the flexor hallucis longus and the flexor digitorum longus and brevis (**A**). Extension of these joints is achieved primarily by the extensor digitorum longus and the extensor hallucis longus, which are supplemented by the extensor digitorum brevis and the extensor hallucis brevis (**B**).

FIG. 12-6 The muscle power of the long toe extensors is tested by exerting a counterforce to the toes while the patient extends the metatarsophalangeal joints (**A** and **B**). The long toe flexors are tested by exerting a counterforce to the tip of the toes while the patient flexes the interphalangeal joints (**C** and **D**).

12

ESSENTIAL IMAGING

The standard views of the ankle are the anteroposterior (AP), medial oblique (Mortise view), and lateral views. The AP ankle view includes the collimate field from the distal tibia and fibula through the talocalcaneal junction. The primary purpose of the AP ankle view is to illustrate the coronal relationship of the talocrural articulation and its surrounding bony elements of the tibia, fibula, and talus. The AP and oblique projections of the ankle are sensitive for ruling out sites of injury along the lower tibia and fibula. The lateral ankle view includes the lower tibia and fibula. In cases of suspected ligamentous instability, eversion and inversion stress views can be performed. Inversion will test the lateral collateral ligament, whereas eversion will check the medial collateral (deltoid) ligament.

ORTHOPEDIC GAMUT 12-6

VIEWS OF THE FOOT

Three basic plain-film views of the foot are:
1. AP or dorsoplantar view
2. Oblique view
3. Lateral view

ANTERIOR DRAWER SIGN OF THE ANKLE

Assessment for Anterior Talofibular Ligament Sprain

ORTHOPEDIC GAMUT 12-7

ANKLE SPRAINS CLASSIFICATIONS

Grade I: Localized tenderness, minimal swelling or ecchymoses, and normal range of motion without instability

Grade II: Moderate to severe pain, swelling or ecchymoses and restricted range of motion, potential mild instability, and painful weight bearing

Grade III: Severe pain, edema, hemorrhage, loss of motion, and inability to ambulate; ankle instability common, with complete functional loss

---

ORTHOPEDIC GAMUT 12-8

OTTAWA ANKLE RULES FOR FOOT AND ANKLE IMAGING IN ACUTE ANKLE INJURY

1. An ankle diagnostic image is required if the patient complains of any pain along the lateral malleolus or medial malleolus and any of these findings:
   - Bone tenderness at posterior edge or tip of lateral malleolus OR
   - Bone tenderness at posterior edge or tip of medial malleolus OR
   - Inability to bear weight both immediately and later
2. A foot diagnostic image is required if the patient has any pain in the mid foot tarsal area and any of these findings:
   - Bone tenderness at the base of the fifth metatarsal OR
   - Bone tenderness at the navicular OR
   - Inability to bear weight immediately or later

PROCEDURE

- The patient may be seated or supine.
- The examiner places one hand around the anterior aspect of the patient's lower tibia, just above the ankle, while gripping the calcaneus in the palm of the other hand.
- While the tibia is pushed posteriorly, the calcaneus and talus are drawn anteriorly (Fig. 12-7).
- Normally, this action produces no movement.
- The sign is present when the talus slides anteriorly under the ankle mortise.
- The test indicates anterior talofibular ligament instability, which is usually secondary to rupture.

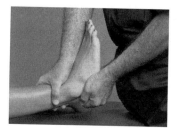

FIG. 12-7

CLINICAL PEARL

The drawer sign is a sensitive indicator of the amount of ligamentous damage in the ankle. Ankles with drawer sign will often require casting or rigid immobilization, at the least, in acute-stage management. Instability may sometimes follow tears of the anterior talofibular portion of the lateral ligament. This instability may be confirmed by radiographs after local anesthesia. The examiner supports the patient's heel on a sandbag and presses firmly downward on the tibia for 30 seconds before exposure. A gap that is between the talus and the tibia and is greater than 6 mm is a pathologic condition.

BUERGER TEST

Assessment for Vascular Compromise of the Lower Extremity

ORTHOPEDIC GAMUT 12-9

CATEGORIES OF PERIPHERAL VASCULAR DISEASE IN THE LOWER EXTREMITY

- Disease of the peripheral arterial system
- Disease of the peripheral venous system

PROCEDURE

- While the patient is lying supine, the examiner elevates the leg and extends the knee to a point of comfortable tolerance, approximately 45 degrees for no less than 3 minutes.
- The examiner lowers the limb, and the patient sits up with both legs dangling side by side over the examining table (Fig. 12-8).
- The test measures arterial blood supply to the lower limbs.
- The blood supply is deficient if the dorsum of the foot blanches and the prominent veins collapse when the leg is initially raised.
- The test is also positive if, when the leg is lowered, 1 to 2 minutes is required for a ruddy (reddish) cyanosis to spread over the affected part and for the veins to fill and become prominent.

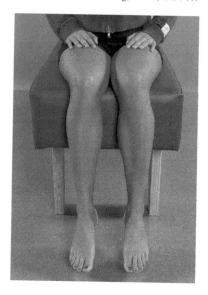

FIG. 12-8

CLINICAL PEARL

Sciatic-like pain is not uncommon in lower extremity vascular disorders. This test allows a quick determination of neurogenic versus vascular pain. The test demonstrates loss of vascular integrity, but as circulation diminishes, the primary complaint is produced.

CALF CIRCUMFERENCE TEST

Assessment for Muscular Atrophy or Hypertrophy of the Lower Extremity

ORTHOPEDIC GAMUT 12-10
FIVE LEG COMPARTMENTS

1. Anterior
2. Lateral
3. Posterior tibial
4. Deep posterior
5. Superficial posterior

ORTHOPEDIC GAMUT 12-11
CHARACTERISTIC OF VOLKMANN ISCHEMIA

1. Swelling
2. Edema
3. Extravasation of red blood cells
4. Destruction of blood cells
5. Replacement of muscle tissue by a fibrous scar

PROCEDURE

- While the patient is lying supine, the circumference of the bellies of the gastrocnemius and soleus muscles are measured (Fig. 12-9).
- The measurement is compared with the calf circumference of the opposite leg.
- Because the dominance of a leg is not established except in highly specialized sports or occupations, the measurements should be equal.
- A diminished calf circumference may represent simple loss of muscle tone, but it may also represent atrophy of muscle fibers.
- An increased calf circumference, corroborated with other pathologic findings, may indicate a fulminating compartment syndrome.

12

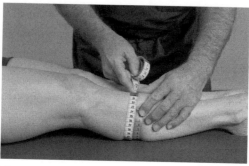

FIG. 12-9

CLINICAL PEARL

In knee injuries, the first sign of internal joint derangement is loss of tone in the quadriceps. Internal derangement of the ankle joint produces the same phenomenon in its controlling musculature. The gastrocnemius-soleus mechanism weakens and loses tone to a degree sufficient to be quantified with a tape measure. This measuring can help differentiate the degree of ankle involvement.

CLAUDICATION TEST

Assessment for Chronic Arterial Occlusive Disease

ORTHOPEDIC GAMUT 12-12

CONDITIONS AFFECTING THE POPLITEAL ARTERY

1. Popliteal artery entrapment syndrome
2. Adventitial cystic disease of the popliteal artery

PROCEDURE

- The patient walks at a rate of 120 steps per minute for 60 seconds.
- This goal can be accomplished by having the patient walk on a treadmill.
- The time that elapses between the start of the test and the occurrence of leg cramping is the claudication time (Fig. 12-10).
- The site of the cramping and often the color change (pallor) in the tissues identifies the level of the lesion.
- The test indicates peripheral vascular disease of chronic arterial occlusion.

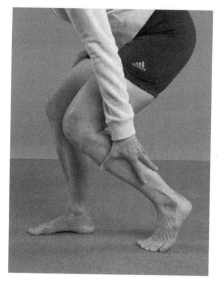

FIG. 12-10

CLINICAL PEARL

The claudication test may be an assumed finding in patients who complain of leg cramps during distance walking. The pain of neurogenic origin is differentiated from pain of arterial origin when the patient relates sitting with almost immediate cramp relief.

DUCHENNE SIGN

Assessment for Lesions of the Superficial Peroneal Nerve

ORTHOPEDIC GAMUT 12-13

ADDITIONAL ANTEROLATERAL COMPARTMENT SYNDROME TEST PROCEDURES

1. Resisted dorsiflexion and eversion with pressure applied over the tunnel
2. Passive plantar flexion and inversion
3. Stretching of the nerve, as in the second test, with percussion over the tunnel

PROCEDURE

- The examiner pushes up the head of the patient's first metatarsal with the thumb, and the patient plantar flexes the foot (Fig. 12-11).
- The sign is present when the medial border of the foot dorsiflexes, with the lateral border plantar flexing (Fig. 12-12).
- The head of the first metatarsal offers no resistance to the pushing thumb.
- The plantar crease runs laterally from the medial side of the big toe to the heel, and the arch disappears.
- This result is caused by paralysis of the peroneus longus, which results from a lesion of the superficial peroneal nerve or a lesion at or above the L4, L5, and S1 roots.

12

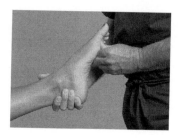

FIG. 12-11

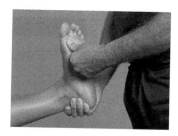

FIG. 12-12

CLINICAL PEARL

Before diagnosing pes planus that is caused by structural problems, the examiner should attempt to elicit Duchenne sign. The presence of this sign indicates a pes planus phenomenon that is caused by neural lesions at a much higher level than the arch itself.

FOOT TOURNIQUET TEST

Assessment for Arterial Insufficiency of the Lower Extremity

ORTHOPEDIC GAMUT 12-14

DIAGNOSTIC MANOMETER CRITERIA OF COMPARTMENT SYNDROME

1. Preexercise compartment pressures of 15 mm Hg or greater
2. One-minute postexercise compartment pressures of 30 mm Hg or greater
3. Compartment pressure measured 5 to 10 minutes after cessation of exercise of 15 mm Hg or greater

---

PROCEDURE

- Application of a pneumatic tourniquet, with pressure elevated to 20 mm Hg above the patient's resting diastolic blood pressure, to a normal extremity will obliterate arterial inflow and venous outflow, slow motor nerve conduction, decrease sensory conduction, and cause pain in the foot and at the site of tourniquet compression (Fig. 12-13).
- Anoxia and nerve compression occur simultaneously, and muscle weakness is evident within 3 to 5 minutes.
- Digital paresthesia occurs, and sensation diminishes gradually to anesthesia in approximately 30 minutes.
- These painful sensations are a combination of muscle and nerve ischemia and nerve compression.

12

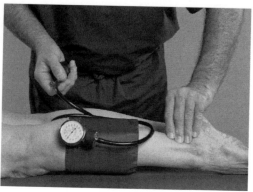

FIG. 12-13

CLINICAL PEARL

Tenderness at the front of the leg is characteristic in (1) Osgood-Schlatter disease, (2) Brodie abscess (or osteitis), (3) anterior tibial compartment syndrome, (4) stress fracture, and (5) shin splints. Tenderness at the back of the leg is characteristically situated (1) in the plantaris tendon in partial and complete ruptures, (2) over varicosities in superficial thrombophlebitis, and (3) over the tendocalcaneus in partial tears and complete ruptures.

HELBINGS SIGN

Assessment for Pes Planus

PROCEDURE

- Medial curving of the Achilles tendon, when viewed posteriorly, indicates foot pronation (Fig. 12-14).

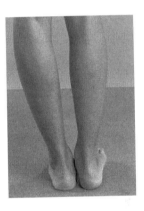

FIG. 12-14

CLINICAL PEARL

The arches of the foot do not become fully formed until a child has been walking for some years. The young child's foot is normally flat. If the arches fail to establish, an awkward gait and rapid, uneven wear and distortion of the shoes may occur; but it is rare for pain or other symptoms to develop. Persistent flatfoot may be associated with knock-knees, torsional deformities of the tibia, and valgus deformities of the heel.

12

HOFFA TEST

ALSO KNOWN AS HOFFA SIGN

Assessment for Fracture of the Calcaneus

PROCEDURE

- While the patient is lying prone, the ankles hang well over the edge of the examining table in a symmetric position.
- Hoffa test is positive if the examiner, using movement and palpation, finds the patient's Achilles tendon on the injured side less taut than that on the contralateral side.
- Dorsiflexion of the foot may also be increased in the relaxed position on the affected side (Fig. 12-15).
- A loose fragment may be observed and felt behind either malleolus.
- The test is significant for fracture of the calcaneus.

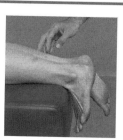

FIG. 12-15

CLINICAL PEARL

In geriatric patients, the Achilles tendon insufficiency that is caused by attrition also produces a positive Hoffa test. In this instance, the calcaneus remains intact.

HOMANS SIGN

Assessment for Thrombophlebitis of the Lower Extremity

PROCEDURE

- While the patient is lying in the supine position, the examiner dorsiflexes the patient's foot and squeezes the calf (Fig. 12-16).
- Deep-seated pain in the posterior leg or calf indicates thrombophlebitis.

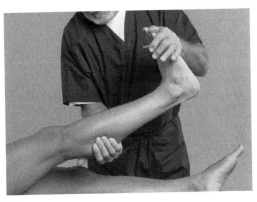

FIG. 12-16

CLINICAL PEARL

The use of Homans sign does not aid differentiation between a muscular lesion and thrombophlebitis. The differentiation occurs when the test is concluded. When the pain remits quickly, thrombophlebitis is suspected. When the pain persists or lags as an ache, calf strain is suspected.

12

KEEN SIGN

Assessment for Distal Fibular Fracture

ORTHOPEDIC GAMUT 12-15

DISTAL TIBIAL AND FIBULAR FRACTURES

Types of distal tibial or fibular fractures include the following:

1. *Bimalleolar fracture:* fractures of the medial and lateral malleoli
2. *Boot-top (skier) fracture:* spiral fracture of the distal diametaphyseal portions of the tibia and fibula
3. *Maisonneuve fracture:* fracture of the proximal fibula, as a result of severe inversion and external rotation of the ankle (often unobserved because of the severity of the ankle injury)
4. *Pott fracture:* fracture of the metadiaphyseal region of the distal fibula, with associated rupture of the distal tibiofibular ligament (Pott fracture that involves both the lateral and medial malleolus is highly likely to result in dislocation of the talus from the ankle mortise; isolated lateral [the more common] or medial malleolar fracture is less likely to destabilize the joint.)
5. *Toddler fracture:* spiral fracture of the distal diametaphyseal region of the tibia in a toddler
6. *Trimalleolar (Cotton) fracture:* fracture of the medial and lateral malleoli, in addition to the posterior tibial lip, often with tibiotalar dislocation

---

PROCEDURE

- If a fracture of the distal fibula exists (as in Pott fracture), the diameter around the malleoli area of the affected ankle is increased (Fig. 12-17).

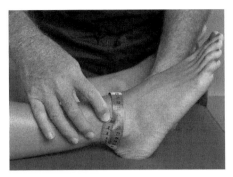

FIG. 12-17

CLINICAL PEARL

Keen sign is an early indicator of ankle fracture. When it is present, the sign mandates diagnostic imaging of the joint.

12

MORTON TEST

Assessment for Metatarsalgia or Morton Neuroma

Comment

Metatarsalgia, pain in the metatarsals, is very common in adults. This pain is caused by various foot deformities or arthritis of the metatarsophalangeal joints. This latter type of pain is most commonly caused by rheumatoid arthritis. The term *metatarsalgia* is used to refer to a pain syndrome and is not disease nomenclature per se (Table 12-4).

TABLE 12-4
CLASSIFICATION OF METATARSALGIA

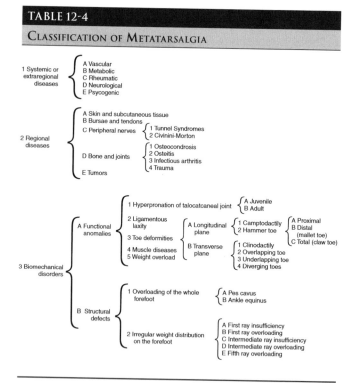

1 Systemic or extraregional diseases
- A Vascular
- B Metabolic
- C Rheumatic
- D Neurological
- E Psycogenic

2 Regional diseases
- A Skin and subcutaneous tissue
- B Bursae and tendons
- C Peripheral nerves
  - 1 Tunnel Syndromes
  - 2 Civinini-Morton
- D Bone and joints
  - 1 Osteocondrosis
  - 2 Osteitis
  - 3 Infectious arthritis
  - 4 Trauma
- E Tumors

3 Biomechanical disorders
- A Functional anomalies
  - 1 Hyperpronation of talocatcaneal joint
    - A Juvenile
    - B Adult
  - 2 Ligamentous laxity
  - 3 Toe deformities
    - A Longitudinal plane
      - 1 Camptodactily
      - 2 Hammer toe
        - A Proximal
        - B Distal (mallet toe)
        - C Total (claw toe)
    - B Transverse plane
      - 1 Clinodactily
      - 2 Overlapping toe
      - 3 Underlapping toe
      - 4 Diverging toes
  - 4 Muscle diseases
  - 5 Weight overload
- B Structural defects
  - 1 Overloading of the whole forefoot
    - A Pes cavus
    - B Ankle equinus
  - 2 Irregular weight distribution on the forefoot
    - A First ray insufficiency
    - B First ray overloading
    - C Intermediate ray insufficiency
    - D Intermediate ray overloading
    - E Fifth ray overloading

From Bardelli M, Turelli L, Scoccianti G: Definition and classification of metatarsalgia, *Foot Ankle Surg* 9(2):79-85, 2003.

PROCEDURE

- Transverse pressure across the heads of the metatarsals causes sharp pain in the forefoot (Fig. 12-18).
- This pressure indicates metatarsalgia or neuroma.

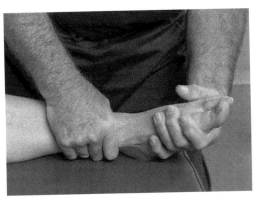

FIG. 12-18

CLINICAL PEARL

Anterior metatarsalgia is particularly common in middle-aged women and is also often associated with some splaying of the forefoot. Symptoms may be triggered by periods of excessive standing or by an increase in weight, and the patient often has concurrent flattening of the medial longitudinal arch. Weakness of the intrinsic muscles is usually present; thus, a tendency exists for clawing of the toes.

12

MOSZKOWICZ TEST

ALSO KNOWN AS MOSCHCOWITZ TEST

Assessment for Inadequacy of the Collateral Circulation as in an Arteriovenous Fistula in the Lower Extremity

---

ORTHOPEDIC GAMUT 12-16

THROMBOPHLEBITIS

Thrombophlebitis, or intravascular coagulation, is usually related to three critical factors of the Virchow's triad:
1. Venous stasis
2. Injury to the vein wall
3. Hypercoagulable state

ORTHOPEDIC GAMUT 12-17

COMMON CAUSES OF DEBILITATING PAIN IN PATIENTS WITH KLIPPEL TRENAUNAY SYNDROME

1. Chronic venous insufficiency
2. Cellulitis
3. Superficial thrombophlebitis
4. Deep-vein thrombosis
5. Calcification of vascular malformations
6. Intraosseous vascular malformation
7. Arthritis
8. Neuropathy
9. Unabated tissue growth

PROCEDURE

- The patient's lower extremity is elevated, and an elastic bandage is wrapped firmly around the limb.
- The elevated position is maintained for 5 minutes. Then the extremity is placed in a horizontal position, and the examiner quickly removes the applied bandage (Fig. 12-19).
- If the circulation is normal, a hyperemic blush occurs and rapidly flows into the area as the bandage is removed.
- The test is positive when the blush is absent or lags slowly behind the unbandaged area.
- The test demonstrates inadequacy of the collateral circulation as in an arteriovenous fistula.

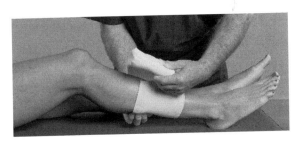

FIG. 12-19

CLINICAL PEARL

Thrombosis in the superficial veins of the calf and with local inflammatory changes is a common cause of recurrent calf pain, and the presence of tenderness and other inflammatory signs along the course of the calf vein makes diagnosis easy. Thrombosis in the deep veins is often silent, and its importance in the postoperative situation is well known.

MOSES TEST

Assessment for Arteriosclerosis Obliterans of the Lower Extremity

PROCEDURE

- Moses test is performed by grasping the patient's calf, which creates pain if phlebitis or vascular occlusion is present (Fig. 12-20).

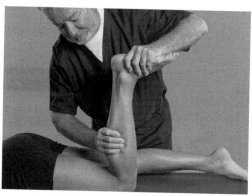

FIG. 12-20

CLINICAL PEARL

Pain in the calf is common for patients suffering from prolapsed intervertebral discs. Claudication pain is a feature of vascular insufficiency and spinal stenosis. Lesions of the foot and ankle that lead to protective muscle spasm during standing and walking often cause marked calf and leg pain.

PERTHES TEST

Assessment for Superficial Varicosities (Incompetency of the Valves of the Saphenous Vein) of the Lower Extremity

PROCEDURE

- While the patient is supine or standing, an elastic tourniquet is applied around the upper thigh to compress only the long saphenous vein.
- The patient then exercises the limb briskly, by walking, kicking, or twisting, for up to 60 seconds.
- The examiner then notes the prominence of the varicosities.
- Normally, the muscular action of the exercise should empty the blood from the superficial system (long saphenous) through the communicating veins into the deep system.
- If superficial varicosities disappear, the valves of the communicating and deep veins are competent.
- If superficial varicosities remain the same, both the superficial and communicating valves are incompetent.
- If the varicosities become distended and more prominent and pain develops, the deep veins are obstructed, and the valves of the communicating veins are incompetent (Fig. 12-21).

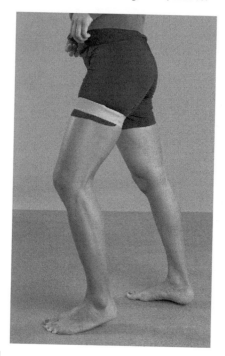

FIG. 12-21

CLINICAL PEARL

Vascular damage may lead to gangrene of the foot and ankle. The circulation must always be observed if the vessels have likely been traumatized seriously by stretching or contusion, and the findings must be recorded. Neurologic damage often accompanies vascular injury.

STRUNSKY SIGN

Assessment for Metatarsalgia

ORTHOPEDIC GAMUT 12-18
FOREFOOT DISORDERS

1. Lesser toe abnormalities
   a. Claw toes
   b. Mallet toes
   c. Hammertoes
   d. Hard and soft corns
2. More proximal problems
   a. Intractable plantar keratosis
   b. Bunionette
   c. Neuromas
   d. Metatarsophalangeal joint capsulitis and instability

PROCEDURE

- Sudden passive flexing of the toes is painless in a normal foot; however, if inflammation exists, pain is experienced in the anterior arch of the foot (Fig. 12-22).

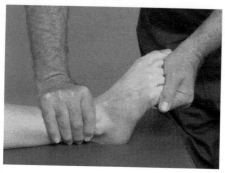

FIG. 12-22

CLINICAL PEARL

Pain in the forefoot (called *metatarsalgia*) has many origins. A prominent metatarsal head is a common cause of pain and can follow any operation on the forefoot, including Keller operation, or dislocation of the second toe.

THOMPSON TEST

Assessment for Achilles Tendon Rupture

ORTHOPEDIC GAMUT 12-19

PHYSICAL EXAMINATION PROCEDURES FOR A RUPTURED ACHILLES TENDON

1. The Thompson-Doherty squeeze test
2. Palpation of the medial head of the gastrocnemius
3. Palpation of a gap in the tendon
4. O'Brien needle test
5. Assessment of heel resistance strength

ORTHOPEDIC GAMUT 12-20

FACTORS PREDISPOSING ACHILLES TENDON RUPTURE

1. *Mechanical:* The patient rapidly pushes off with the knee extended.
2. *Vascular:* The tendon that ruptures usually will do so in the zone of relatively diminished blood supply.
3. *Quality of the tissue substance:* Many studies have revealed that the ruptured Achilles tendon will have preexisting degenerative pathologic changes.

12

PROCEDURE

- The patient is in a prone position with the feet hanging over the edge of the examination table.
- The examiner flexes the knee of the patient's affected leg to 90 degrees and squeezes the calf muscles just below the widest level of the posterior portion of the leg.
- Normally, this maneuver causes a reflex plantar flexion motion of the foot (Fig. 12-23).
- The test is positive when the foot does not respond.
- The test indicates a complete rupture of the Achilles tendon.

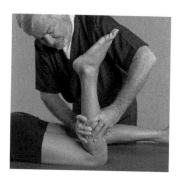

FIG. 12-23

CLINICAL PEARL

The Achilles tendon can be torn by the same movements, such as a forward lunge on the sports field or a squash court, that tear the medial head of the gastrocnemius. The patient will feel as though someone has kicked the Achilles tendon. Legendary stories have been told in which the victim of such a tear turns around and punches the person behind, in retribution.

TINEL FOOT SIGN

Assessment for Tarsal Tunnel Syndrome

ORTHOPEDIC GAMUT 12-21

TARSAL TUNNEL STRUCTURES

1. Posterior tibial nerve and its branches
2. Tendons of the posterior tibialis
3. Flexor digitorum longus
4. Flexor hallucis
5. Posterior tibial artery and vein

PROCEDURE

- Tapping the area over the posterior tibial nerve (medial plantar nerve) with a reflex hammer produces tingling distal to the percussion (Fig. 12-24).
- The paresthesia that radiates into the foot indicates tarsal tunnel syndrome.

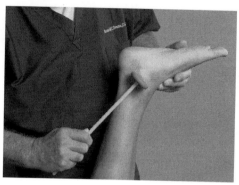

FIG. 12-24

CLINICAL PEARL

The medial plantar nerve enters the foot after passing beneath the medial ligament of the ankle, which it shares with the posterior tibial and flexor tendons. The structure of this feature is comparable to the carpal tunnel of the wrist. The medial plantar nerve is vulnerable to compression by swelling of the tendons or by space-occupying lesions, such as ganglia. Tarsal tunnel syndrome is not common, but it should be considered for patients who have neurologic symptoms in the hindfoot.

CHAPTER THIRTEEN

MALINGERING

INTRODUCTION

In a framework for disability, the examining physician needs to understand the interaction between the disability and the factors affecting a return to work. In this model of interaction, a *pathologic condition* is the disturbance of normal bodily processes at the cellular level. *Impairment* is a specific loss of function. *Functional limitation* is the lack of ability to perform an action or activity. *Disability* is the inability to perform socially defined activities. *Quality of life* refers to the patient's concept of total well-being. *Risk* or *cofactors* include biologic, environmental, lifestyle, and behavioral characteristics that are associated with musculoskeletal conditions. Whether people with specific physical limitations are disabled depends on their expectations, resources, and the demands of their physical environment.

Feigned illness, or malingering, is a sensitive medicolegal issue. Illness or injury that cannot be supported by medical fact confounds the physician's diagnostic procedures and health care delivery; it also serves as an element of fraud in the third-party payer system. Patients participating in this behavior are a bane.

ORTHOPEDIC GAMUT 13-1

COMMONLY USED PROCEDURES IN DETERMINING EXISTENCE OF COGNITIVE MALINGERING

- *Victoria Symptom Validity Test (VSVT):* The VSVT is a computer-administered and computer-scored test. It includes a total of 48 items, presented in three blocks of 16 items each. During the study trial, a single five-digit study number is presented for 5 seconds in the center of the computer screen. This presentation is followed by the retention interval and then by the recognition trial, in which the target and a five-digit distractor are displayed. The respondents are asked to choose the number they saw in the study trial. The retention interval is 5 seconds in the first block, 10 seconds in the second, and 15 seconds in the third.

- *Test of memory malingering (TOMM):* The TOMM is an instrument designed to provide an assessment whether an individual is falsifying symptoms of memory impairment. It consists of 50 pictures of common objects that the subject must remember. After the presentation of the 50 pictures, the individual has to recognize which one is the correct picture between two alternatives. The TOMM consists of two learning trials and an optional retention trial and has good face validity as a test of learning and memory.

- *The b test:* The b test is a measure to identify malingering requiring recognition of overlearned information. This test is a letter recognition and discrimination task that consists of a 15-page *stimulus booklet*. The examinee is asked to circle all instances of the letter *b* that appear on each page, working as quickly as possible.

Not all patients who feign an illness are completely aware of their actions. Some patients embellish symptoms and physical signs as learned responses or traits, whereas others describe physical problems with hysterical emotional overlays. The latter group is influenced mostly by fear of the unknown. Depression bears a significant relationship to pain (Box 13-1).

BOX 13-1

SYMPTOMS OF DEPRESSION

1. Depressed mood or irritable mood
2. Markedly diminished interest or pleasure in activities
3. Significant weight loss or weight gain when not dieting
4. Insomnia or hypersomnia nearly every day
5. Psychomotor agitation or retardation—observable by others
6. Fatigue or loss of energy
7. Feelings of worthlessness or excessive or inappropriate guilt, which may be delusional
8. Diminished ability to think or concentrate; indecisiveness
9. Recurrent thoughts of death, recurrent suicidal ideation without a plan, a suicide attempt, or a specific plan for committing suicide
10. Lack of reactivity to usually pleasurable stimuli
11. Depression worse in the morning
12. Early morning awakening

Data from *American Psychiatric Association Diagnostic and Statistical Manual of Mental Disorders,* ed 3, revised, Washington DC, 1987, American Psychiatric Association. In White AH, Schofferman JA: *Spine care,* vol. 1-2, St. Louis, 1995, Mosby.

ORTHOPEDIC GAMUT 13-2

DSM-IV* SYMPTOM SPECIFIC CATEGORIES IN EXCESSIVE COGNITIVE SYMPTOMS

A. *Somatization disorder* requires:
   a. At least four pain symptoms
   b. Two gastrointestinal symptoms
   c. One sexual symptom
   d. One pseudoneurologic symptom

B. *Undifferentiated somatoform disorder* requires one or more physical complaints, with no reference made to cognitive difficulties.

C. *Conversion disorder* requires one or more symptoms or deficits affecting voluntary motor or sensory function without mention of cognitive or memory difficulties.

D. *Pain disorder* requires only excessive pain symptoms.

E. *Somatoform disorder NOS* includes individuals with predominantly excessive cognitive symptoms.

F. *Dissociative amnesia* requires one specific type of cognitive problem, such as the inability to recall important personal information, usually of a traumatic or stressful nature.

G. *Dissociative fugue* requires one specific cognitive difficulty, such as the inability to recall some or all of one's past. This difficulty must surface in the context of a sudden, unexpected travel away from home or one's customary place of daily activities.

H. *Dissociative identity disorder* occurs in individuals with multiple personalities in which they exhibit an inability to recall important information about one or more personality states when they are in a different personality state.

I. *Dissociative disorder NOS* encompasses individuals with excessive cognitive complaints.

---

*DSM-IV, Diagnostic and Statistical Manual of Mental Disorders, fourth edition.
NOS, Not otherwise specified.

ORTHOPEDIC GAMUT 13-3

PREDICTORS OF WORK INCAPACITY AND WORK LOSS BECAUSE OF DEPRESSION

1. Incoherent presentation of pain localization and stable symptoms
2. Inability to influence pain and function by movement or change of position
3. Relapse of a preexisting condition and lack of response in previous episodes
4. Work dissatisfaction
5. Problems of communicating realistic treatment goals
6. Poor self-perceived prognoses with unrealistically high perception of impairment

---

Two major categories of hysterical disorders are identified: patients with a fictitious illness, such as in malingering, and patients with Munchausen syndrome. Both types of patients are those with signs and symptoms that have no organic basis but who are not deliberately attempting to mislead the examiner.

Trivial physical trauma or disease is often at the root of a portrayed illness or injury. In many instances, by the time symptom embellishment is clinically recognized, the complaints are of such a magnitude that they are completely incongruous with the original illness or injury. A patient who originally experienced a minor, clinically documented upper respiratory infection now describes symptoms and subjective complaints that resemble those for histoplasmosis or black lung disease. Yet another patient may complain of total leg disability after a minor thigh contusion. Both patients have in common the total lack of clinical findings to support the complaints, and some type of secondary gain serves as a driving force behind the medical charade.

Individuals may feign physical symptoms to continue in a less-strenuous job at work, or they may do so to receive a parking space closer to their place of employment. These individuals may also fake symptoms to gain control over family members or fellow workers. The injured party may also allow others to do work the patient would ordinarily do.

13

The diagnosis of hysteria should be established based only on positive evidence. Even if the patient has an obvious hysterical disorder, a serious organic illness may still be present.

Conversion symptoms have a physiologic or pathologic substrate. A conversion disorder denotes a process in which a patient's emotions become transformed into physical (motor or sensory) manifestations. These patients are asking for help but in an inappropriate way. Conversion symptoms often occur in mentally defective individuals or in adolescents as a way of coping (albeit inadequately) with the environment. Common presentations include blindness, deafness, paresis, sensory disturbances, ataxia, seizures, and unconsciousness.

Malingering is the conscious misrepresentation of thoughts, feelings, and facts, and it is a condition in which symptoms and signs associated with pain or dysfunction are either partially or entirely feigned for secondary gain. Most commonly, malingering occurs in the setting of the workplace, where workers' compensation is an issue.

Labeling patients as hysterics, frauds, or malingerers is difficult. This task is rarely accomplished without reaping the wrath of the patient or substantial legal repercussions.

The actual percentage of patients who are malingerers is undetermined. However, estimates suggest that 2% of all patients seeking health care are malingering. Obviously, the ascertainment of the inaccuracy of a patient's report of pain and disability is a difficult process, but the possibility of malingering should be raised in the mind of the treating physician when major discrepancies or inconsistencies appear in the patient's medical situation. In this effort, outcome measures for the assessment of work capacity, work tolerance, dependable ability, and task demand are useful tools (Table 13-3).

TABLE 13-1
MALINGERING CROSS-REFERENCE TABLE BY ASSESSMENT PROCEDURE

Malingering, Hysteria, and Embellishment

Test/Sign	Paresis	Stoicism	Consciousness	Anesthesia	Deafness	Facial Anesthesia	Blindness	Cerebellar Lesions	Trigeminal Nerve	Olfactory Nerve	Facial Pain	General Pain	Sciatica	Lower Back
Pain														
Axial trunk-loading test														●
Burns bench test														●
Flexed-hip test														●
Flip sign													●	
Libman sign												●		
Magnuson test														●

Continued

TABLE 13-1

Malingering Cross-Reference Table by Assessment Procedure—cont'd

Mannkopf sign

Marked part pain-suggestibility test

Plantar flexion test

Related joint motion test

Seeligmuller sign

Trunk rotational test

Sensory

Anosmia testing

Coordination-disturbance testing

Cuignet test

Facial anesthesia testing

Gault test

Janet test

Limb-dropping test (upper extremities)

Lombard test

Marcus Gunn sign

Midline tuning-fork test									●
Optokinetic nystagmus test									●
Position-sense testing									●
Regional anesthesia testing									●
Romberg sign									●
Snellen test	●	●							●
Stoicism indexing									●
Motor									
Bilateral limb-dropping test (lower extremities)									●
Hemiplegic posturing					●		●		●
Hoover sign									●
Simulated foot-drop testing									
Simulated forearm-and-wrist-weakness testing									
Simulated grip-strength-loss test									
Tripod test (bilateral leg-fluttering test)								●	

TABLE 13-2

MALINGERING, HYSTERIA, AND EMBELLISHMENT CROSS-REFERENCE TABLE BY SUSPECTED SYNDROME OR TISSUE

Anesthesia	Janet test
	Midline tuning-fork test
	Regional anesthesia testing
Blindness	Cuignet test
	Marcus Gunn sign
	Midline tuning-fork test
	Snellen test
Cerebellar lesions	Coordination-disturbance testing
	Position-sense testing
	Romberg sign
	Hemiplegic posturing
	Simulated foot-drop testing
Consciousness	Limb-dropping test (upper extremities)
	Stoicism indexing
Deafness	Gault test
	Limb-dropping test (lower extremities)
Facial anesthesia	Facial anesthesia testing
	Lombard test
Facial pain	Seeligmuller sign
General pain	Libman sign
	Mannkopf sign
	Marked part pain-suggestibility test
	Related joint motion test
Lower back	Axial trunk-loading test
	Burns bench test
	Flexed-hip test
	Magnuson test
	Plantar flexion test
	Trunk rotational test
	Tripod test (bilateral leg-fluttering test)
Olfactory nerve	Anosmia testing
Paresis	Bilateral limb-dropping test (lower extremities)
	Hemiplegic posturing
	Hoover sign
	Simulated foot-drop testing
	Simulated forearm-and-wrist-weakness testing
	Simulated grip-strength-loss testing
Sciatica	Flip sign
	Plantar flexion test
Stoicism	Stoicism indexing
Trigeminal nerve	Anosmia testing

TABLE 13-3

DISTINCTIONS AMONG WORK CAPACITY, WORK TOLERANCE, DEPENDABLE ABILITY, AND TASK DEMAND

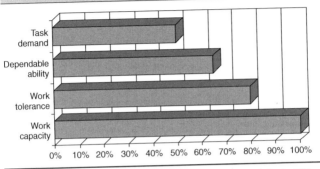

From Demeter SL, Andersson GBJ, Smith GM: *Disability evaluation,* St Louis, 1996, Mosby.

ORTHOPEDIC GAMUT 13-4

THE *FIVE Ds* OF GLOBAL HEALTH STATUS

1. Death
2. Disability—upper or lower limb functional problems
3. Discomfort—physical or psychologic
4. Drug reactions—or other medical or surgical iatrogenic problems
5. Dollars—both direct and indirect costs

> ### ORTHOPEDIC GAMUT 13-5
> ## IMPORTANCE OF MALINGERING ASSESSMENT
>
> **Examiners should be concerned about whether treatment-seeking patients are malingering for several important reasons:**
> - Diagnosis and treatment planning
> - Malingering needs to be ruled out before establishing a diagnosis.
> - If the diagnosis is incorrect, the resulting treatment may be misguided.
> - Threat to the therapeutic alliance with clinicians: Clinicians routinely working with traumatized populations that have high rates of suspected but undetected malingering often become suspicious of the motives of all patients.
> - Economic impact
> - In 1995, the total cost of insurance fraud in the United States was estimated to be $85.3 billion.
> - Most of this cost was the result of health insurance fraud, including (but not limited to) the malingering of posttraumatic stress disorder.
> - Threat to research databases: Researchers commonly recruit people studies from treatment-seeking populations.

OUTCOMES ASSESSMENTS

The health assessment questionnaire (HAQ) is a self-administered instrument that assesses discomfort and disability. It is used to measure outcome in many different neuromusculoskeletal diseases. Disease-specific instruments have been produced to help follow outcomes in several other neuromusculoskeletal diseases. This area includes a *fibromyalgia impact questionnaire*. The activity of inflammatory neuromusculoskeletal diseases can be assessed through *serologic* measures. Separate measures of both tender and swollen joints can be charted on a *homunculus*. A generic measure of anxiety and depression, such as the *hospital anxiety and depression* (HAD) scale, allows psychologic variables to be assessed independently from orthopedic disease-related outcomes. The EuroQuol® thermometer is one of the instruments that uses a simple visual technique to allow people to assess their own health status; the *disease repercussion profile* is another such resource (Box 13-2).

BOX 13-2

DISEASE IMPACT INDEX

Patients report severity of problems on a 0-to-10 scale in six dimensions:
- Functional activities
- Social activities
- Relationships
- Emotions
- Socioeconomic factors
- Body image

From Carr AJ, Thompson PW: Towards a measure of patient-perceived handicap in rheumatoid arthritis, *Br J Rheumatol* 33:378, 1994.

Armed with Borg pain scales, Oswestry disability indices, symptom magnification indexing, Dallas Pain Questionnaire, Waddell indexing (Table 13-4), and neuroorthopedic malingering tests, the physician is able to substantiate or refute the existence of malingering in any given case. These tests and indices are usually used in combination with the more traditional neuroorthopedic physical examinations. A singular positive finding or test does not indicate that the patient is magnifying or faking symptoms. Rather, the malingering diagnosis is based on the preponderance of positive malingering test findings and the absence of findings from traditional neuroorthopedic tests. Any positive findings must be further correlated with the medical history of the patient. The constellation of positive malingering tests, normal findings in traditional tests, and medical history discrepancies form the malingering diagnosis. Malingering and psychogenic rheumatism patients complain primarily of pain, sensory losses, or paralysis in any combination.

TABLE 13-4

NONORGANIC PHYSICAL SIGNS INDICATING
ILLNESS BEHAVIOR

	Physical Disease/ Normal Illness Behavior	Abnormal Illness Behavior
Symptoms		
Pain	Anatomic distribution	Whole leg pain
		Tailbone pain
Numbness	Dermatomal	Whole leg numbness
Weakness	Myotomal	Whole leg giving way
Time pattern	Varies with time and activity	Never free of pain
Response to treatment	Variable benefit	Intolerance of treatments
		Emergency admissions to hospital
Signs		
Tenderness	Anatomic distribution	Superficial
		Widespread nonanatomic
Axial loading	No lumbar pain	Lumbar pain
Simulated rotation	No lumbar pain	Lumbar pain
Straight-leg-raising	Limited on distraction	Improves with distraction
Sensory	Dermatomal	Regional
Motor	Myotomal	Regional, jerky, giving way

From Waddell G, et al: Symptoms and signs: physical disease or illness behavior?
Br Med J 289:739, 1984, British Medical Association.

CLINICAL PEARL

Standardized instruments are often used in survey research. Many of these instruments are devised in clinic settings where trained health care professionals complete health assessments. However, prohibitive cost and relative ease make participant-assessed outcome measures a more feasible approach to obtain constructs describing functional and mental health outcomes. With these more-convenient measures of health increasingly used as primary outcomes in epidemiologic studies, selecting an appropriate assessment tool involves careful review of the many standard survey instruments available. The Millennium Cohort, the largest cohort study ever undertaken by the U.S. Department of Defense, was launched in 2001 to gather health outcome information along with occupational and environmental exposures employing a longitudinal approach. In the first panel of enrollment, more than 77,000 participants joined the 22-year-long study, filling out either a mailed survey or an identical Web-based survey.

GENERAL PROCEDURES

General Patient Observation

Consensus has been reached among physicians that malingering is readily detected with appropriate medical and psychologic tests. Most patients who have remained conscious during an injury can give an adequate description of what happened. A malingerer is vague and on guard while describing the incidents of an injury or accident. However, some patients who also remain conscious at the time of injury are not as observant as others are, and these patients will be somewhat vague.

A malingerer often appears quarrelsome, nervous, and ill at ease. General observation of the patient before and after the physical examination may reveal that the patient is fully capable of movements or activities that were claimed to be impossible in the physical examination. The examiner should note how the patient enters and behaves in the reception room. It is helpful if a nonprofessional staff person takes the patient's history and engages the claimant in conversation.

13

Detailed History

Occasionally, the physician is asked to distinguish fraud or exaggeration from organic injury. As should be apparent by now, this task is not an easy one. An examination, when deception or exaggeration is suspected, should be completed with a strictly impartial attitude on the part of the examiner. The patient must be accorded all the tact and courtesy that is ordinarily extended to any other patient. If the physician-patient rapport is compromised, confidence is destroyed, and questions and tests, which are constructed to evoke sincerity on the part of the patient, become unreliable.

In many instances, the patient grudgingly gives the history. The malingering patient may remark, "I've told this to the last doctor, and I don't see any reason to repeat it."

The patient may also deny permission to review previous X-ray findings or case histories, stating that only the attorney can grant such permission. The genuine patient will not usually hesitate to furnish all patient information or permissions in this regard.

Malingerers will give an involved and long history, most of which is often discovered to be false. When the patient's history, actions, and examination findings suggest that symptoms are exaggerated, one of the duties of the physician to make the examination so complete that no question will remain as to the actual extent of any organic disease or injury.

Psychogenic Rheumatism Profile

Patients with psychiatric disorders may develop pain as part of the symptoms associated with mental illness. Patients with pain may also develop psychiatric disorders as part of the symptoms associated with the physical illness. Pain associated with neurosis is more common than pain associated with schizophrenia or endogenous depression.

ORTHOPEDIC GAMUT 13-6

REASONS FOR PSYCHOLOGIC ILLNESS THAT CAUSE THE APPEARANCE OR EXACERBATION OF PAIN

1. Anxiety
2. Psychiatric hallucination
3. Increased tension in the muscles, with associated inadequate circulation and the accumulation of metabolic byproducts (lactic acid)
4. Hysteria with conversion reactions

ORTHOPEDIC GAMUT 13-7

PSYCHOGENIC RHEUMATISM*

Symptoms and signs of psychogenic rheumatism are:

1. Dramatic urgency for an appointment that is not justified by the severity of the disease
2. A list (in writing) of complaints so long and detailed that no fact is left out
3. Multiple test results, including electrocardiogram, electromyelogram, electroencephalogram, barium enema, upper gastrointestinal series, computed tomography scans, myelograms, and magnetic resonance imaging, with no positive findings
4. Patient demands to review the laboratory data first to determine the cause of the symptoms; patient highlights any minor abnormalities
5. Preoccupation with future disability from minor physical changes
6. Persons who accompany the patient may be entirely separated from the patient's condition or intensely supportive; the companion may be highlighting every abnormality, often using the pronoun *we* during the description of tests or treatments
7. Inability of the patient to relax during the examination (Boxes 13-3 and 13-4)
8. Marked theatrical responses to questions concerning pain
9. The patient often holds onto the physician during the examination, as a gesture of seeking support

*From Rotes-Querol J: The syndrome of psychogenic rheumatism, *Clin Rheum Dis* 5:797, 1979.

BOX 13-3

CLINICAL SYMPTOMS OF ANXIETY

Motor tension
- Trembling, twitching, or feeling shaky
- Muscle tension, aches, or soreness
- Restlessness
- Easy fatigability

Autonomic hyperactivity
- Shortness of breath or smothering sensation
- Palpitations or accelerated heart rate
- Sweating or cold clammy hands
- Dry mouth
- Dizziness or light-headedness
- Nausea, diarrhea, or other abdominal distress
- Flushes (hot flashes) or chills
- Frequent urination
- Trouble swallowing or *lump in throat*

Vigilance and scanning
- Feeling keyed up or on edge
- Exaggerated startle response
- Difficulty concentrating or *mind going blank* because of anxiety
- Trouble falling or staying asleep
- Irritability

From White AH, Schofferman JA: *Spine care,* vol 1-2, St Louis, 1995, Mosby.

BOX 13-4

DSM-III-R* CRITERION FOR ANXIETY

300.02 Generalized anxiety disorder—unrealistic or excessive anxiety and worry more days than not

Other anxiety disorders

Panic disorder

300.21 with agoraphobia or

300.01 without agoraphobia

300.22 Agoraphobia without history of panic disorder

300.23 Social phobia

300.29 Obsessive compulsive disorder

300.89 Posttraumatic stress disorder

300.00 Anxiety disorder not otherwise specified

*DSM-III-R, *Diagnostic and Statistical Manual of Mental Disorders*, third edition, revised.
Data from *American Psychiatric Association Diagnostic and Statistical Manual of Mental Disorders*, ed 3, revised, Washington DC, 1987, American Psychiatric Association. In White AH, Schofferman JA: *Spine care*, vol. 1-2, St. Louis, 1995, Mosby.

ORTHOPEDIC GAMUT 13-8

COMBINED EMORY AND ELLARD INCONSISTENCY PROFILES*

1. Discrepancies become apparent between a patient's complaints of terrible pain and an attitude of calmness and well-being.
2. A complete work-up for organic disease by two or more physicians is negative.
3. The patient makes dramatized complaints that are vague or have global implications. "It just hurts," or "I hurt bad." This statement may be further attested by malingering hand signals.
4. The patient exaggerates a trivial pathologic condition (e.g., a mild strain, muscular cramp, contusion) and embellishes it with medical terms learned from previous contact with physicians. "My back spasms paralyze my legs."

Continued **13**

ORTHOPEDIC GAMUT 13-8

COMBINED EMORY AND ELLARD INCONSISTENCY PROFILES*—cont'd

5. The patient overemphasizes gait or posture abnormalities that develop suddenly, persist, and cannot be substantiated objectively. For example, the patient complains of a limp that is not confirmed by a specific pattern of wear on old shoes; or the patient reports daily use of a cane or back brace, but these items show little wear.

6. The patient resists evaluation or rehabilitation when the stated goal of therapy is a return to gainful employment.

7. The patient exhibits a lack of motivation to learn new coping skills, despite verbal reports of compliance with treatment. For instance, the patient will show no increase in back motion despite claims of completing range-of-motion exercise daily.

8. The patient misses appointments for objective studies that measure function, motion, or vocational capabilities.

9. The patient has an unconventional response to treatment, such as reports of increased symptoms after therapy that follows no anatomic or physiologic pattern. For example, the patient may respond to tranquilizers as if they are stimulants and vice versa.

10. The patient shows resistance to treatment procedures, especially in the presence of intense complaints of pain.

11. Psychologic or emotional disturbances are absent (Box 13-5).

12. Psychologic tests are inconsistent and without clinical presentations. For example, the Minnesota Multiphasic Personality Index profile indicates a psychotic disorder, but no clinical signs of psychosis are present (Box 13-6).

13. Discrepancies arise between reports by the patient and spouse or other close relatives.

14. Personal and occupational history appears unstable.

15. The patient's personal history reflects a character disorder that might include drug or alcohol abuse, criminal or compulsive behavior, erratic personal relationships, and violence.

---

*From Evans RC: Malingering/symptoms exaggeration. In Sweere JJ, editor: *Chiropractic family practice*, Gaithersburg, Md, 1992, Aspen.
Data from Ellard J: Psychological reaction to compensable injury, *Med J Australia* 2:349-55, 1970; and Brena SF, Chapman SL: *Pain and litigation: textbook of pain*, London, 1984, Churchill Livingstone.

CLINICAL PEARL

In distinguishing psychogenic rheumatism from primary fibromyalgia, the patients with primary fibromyalgia are usually women, 25 to 40 years of age, who complain of diffuse musculoskeletal aches, pains or stiffness associated with tiredness, anxiety, poor sleep, headaches, irritable bowel syndrome, subjective swelling in the articular and periarticular areas, and numbness. Physical examination reveals the presence of multiple tender points at specific sites and the absence of joint swelling. Symptoms are influenced by weather and activities, as well as by time of day (worse in the morning and the evening). In contrast, symptoms of psychogenic rheumatism have little fluctuation, if any, and are modulated by emotional rather than physical factors. Psychogenic rheumatism produces diffuse tenderness rather than tender points at specific sites.

Special Hand Signals by the Patient

How a patient uses the hands to describe the area of pain is useful in determining the validity of the complaints. At first, malingering patients take care not to touch the area they claim experiences pain. Because the complaint is a sham, touching of the part abets the lie. The examiner often inadvertently aids this process by physically touching the area of complaint before the patient has. The patient now only has to agree with the frustrated examiner concerning the exact location of the pain (Fig. 13-1).

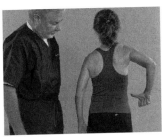

FIG. 13-1 At first, the malingering patient takes care to avoid touching the area of claimed pain.

The psychogenic rheumatic patient uses the whole hand to paint the area of involvement with pain. Because this type of patient perceives the lesion abnormally, the distribution is painted to cover a whole body part. This pain crosses more than one dermatome boundary, and this patient's discomfort is real. The discomfort may have origin in an organic lesion, but because of learned responses or fear, the patient rubs the whole part with the hand to indicate its extent. Careful questioning and guidance will help this patient better define the most focal trigger areas (Fig. 13-2).

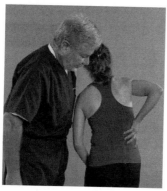

FIG. 13-2 The hysteric patient, or the patient with psychogenic rheumatism, paints the area of complaint with the whole hand. The discomfort is real, but the borders of the complaint exceed the known anatomic distributions.

Patients with organic, pain-producing lesions are concerned that the source of the pain might be missed. When directed to point to the pain, this type of patient will touch the part with one or two fingers, which is representative of a more focal appreciation of the discomfort. In severe expression of the symptoms, this patient also may place the examiner's hand on the exact location of the pain. These patients do not want to risk having the source missed and not treated (Fig. 13-3).

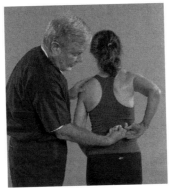

FIG. 13-3 Patients experiencing organic pain for the first time are concerned that the lesion will be missed. This patient will touch the part, precisely locating it with one or two fingers. The patient may also hold the examiner's finger on the spot of worst complaint.

PAIN QUALIFICATION AND QUANTIFICATION

Overview

Pain disrupts the life of the individual in terms of relationships with others, self-esteem, ability to complete tasks of daily living and to work, and ability to function as a member of the community. Disability is strongly correlated with attitude to illness; these considerations underlie the importance of assessing patients' beliefs regarding the nature and prognosis of their pain (Table 13-5).

ORTHOPEDIC GAMUT 13-9

RELAY STATIONS

Three main relay stations for sensory stimuli from the periphery to the sensory cortex include:
1. The peripheral sensory nervous system, with its cell station in the spinal ganglia
2. The pathways and centers in the spinal cord and medulla
3. The sensory centers of the diencephalon, especially the thalamus

---

13

TABLE 13-5

ACTIVITIES OF DAILY LIVING AND VISUAL ANALOG QUESTIONNAIRE

A. How often is it painful for you to:

	Never	Sometimes	Most of the Time	Always
Dress yourself?				
Get in and out of bed?				
Lift a cup or glass to your lips?				
Walk outdoors on flat ground?				
Wash and dry your entire body?				
Bend down to pick up clothing from the floor?				
Turn faucets on or off?				
Get in and out of a car?				

B. How much pain have you had in the past week (mark the scale):

Pain as bad as it could be

No pain _____ 100

0

From Callahan LF, et al: Quantitative pain assessment for routine care of rheumatoid arthritis patients, using a pain scale on activities of daily living and a visual analog pain scale, *Arthritis Rheum* 30:630, 1987.

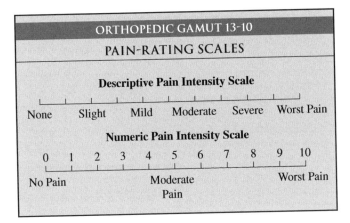

ORTHOPEDIC GAMUT 13-11

CLINICAL FEATURES OF BURNING MOUTH SYNDROME

Pain
Descriptors: burning
Intensity: variable, weak to intense
Pattern: continuous, not paroxysmal
Localization:
- Independent of a nervous pathway
- Often bilateral and symmetrical

Paroxysmal: not
Pain during sleep: infrequent

Associated signs and symptoms:
Dysgeusia
Xerostomia
Thirst

Sensory:
Chemosensory anomalies
Psychological changes

Adapted from Patton LL et al: Management of burning mouth syndrome: systematic review and management recommendations, *Oral Surg Oral Med Oral Pathol Oral Radiol Endodontol* 103(suppl 1):S39.e1-S39.e13, 2007.

ORTHOPEDIC GAMUT 13-12

CATEGORIES OF PAIN

1. Pure nerve pain
2. Pain associated with nerve and vascular insufficiency
3. Pain related to numerous local alterations, such as inadequate skin coverage, fibrosis, bone pressure, tendon irritation, and collagen fibrosis

ORTHOPEDIC GAMUT 13-13

OSWESTRY-TYPE PAIN-DISABILITY QUESTIONNAIRE*

This questionnaire has been designed to give the examiner information about pain and how it affects your ability to manage in everyday life. Please circle, in each section, only one statement that most closely applies to you.

SECTION 1: PAIN INTENSITY

1. I can tolerate the pain I have without having to use painkillers.
2. The pain is bad, but I manage without taking painkillers.
3. Painkillers give complete relief from pain.
4. Painkillers give moderate relief from pain.
5. Painkillers give very little relief from pain.
6. Painkillers have no affect on the pain, and I do not use them.

SECTION 2: PERSONAL CARE (E.G., WASHING, DRESSING)

1. I can look after myself normally without causing extra pain.
2. I can look after myself normally, but it causes extra pain.
3. Looking after myself is painful, and I am slow and careful.
4. I need some help, but I manage most of my personal care.
5. I need help every day in most aspects of self-care.
6. I do not get dressed. I wash with difficulty and stay in bed.

SECTION 3: LIFTING

1. I can lift heavy weights without increased pain.
2. I can lift heavy weights, but it gives added pain.
3. Pain prevents me from lifting heavy weights off the floor, but I can manage if they are conveniently positioned, such as on a table.
4. Pain prevents me from lifting heavy weights, but I can manage light to medium weights if they are conveniently positioned.
5. I can lift only very light weights.
6. I cannot lift or carry anything at all.

SECTION 4: WALKING

1. Pain does not prevent me from walking any distance.
2. Pain prevents me from walking more than 1 mile.
3. Pain prevents me from walking more than ½ mile.
4. Pain prevents me from walking more than ¼ mile.
5. I can walk only using a cane or crutches.
6. I am in bed most of the time and have to crawl to the toilet.

13

Continued

ORTHOPEDIC GAMUT 13-13

OSWESTRY-TYPE PAIN-DISABILITY QUESTIONNAIRE*—cont'd

SECTION 5: SITTING

1. I can sit in any chair as long as I like.
2. I can sit only in my favorite chair as long as I like.
3. Pain prevents me from sitting more than 1 hour.
4. Pain prevents me from sitting for more than 30 minutes.
5. Pain prevents me from sitting more than 10 minutes.
6. Pain prevents me from sitting at all.

SECTION 6: STANDING

1. I can stand as long as I want without added pain.
2. I can stand as long as I want, but it gives me added pain.
3. Pain prevents me from standing for more than 1 hour.
4. Pain prevents me from standing for more than 30 minutes.
5. Pain prevents me from standing for more than 10 minutes.
6. Pain prevents me from standing at all.

SECTION 7: SLEEPING

1. Pain does not prevent me from sleeping well.
2. I can sleep well only by using sleeping tablets.
3. Even when I take sleeping tablets, I have less than 6 hours of sleep.
4. Even when I take sleeping tablets, I have less than 4 hours of sleep.
5. Even when I take sleeping tablets, I have less than 2 hours of sleep.
6. Pain prevents me from sleeping at all.

SECTION 8: SEXUAL ACTIVITY

1. My sexual activity is normal and causes no extra pain.
2. My sexual activity is normal but causes some extra pain.
3. My sexual activity is nearly normal but is very painful.
4. My sexual activity is severely restricted by pain.
5. My sexual activity is nearly absent because of pain.
6. Pain prevents any sexual activity at all.

ORTHOPEDIC GAMUT 13-13

OSWESTRY-TYPE PAIN-DISABILITY QUESTIONNAIRE*—cont'd

SECTION 9: SOCIAL LIFE
1. My social life is normal and gives me no extra pain.
2. My social life is normal but increases the degree of pain.
3. Pain has no significant effect on my social life other than limiting my more energetic interests, such as dancing.
4. Pain restricts my social life, and I do not go out often.
5. Pain has restricted my social life to my home.
6. I have no social life because of pain.

SECTION 10: TRAVELING
1. I can travel anywhere without added pain.
2. I can travel anywhere, but it gives me added pain.
3. Pain is bad, but I manage journeys of more than 2 hours.
4. Pain restricts me to a journey of less than 1 hour.
5. Pain restricts me to short, necessary journeys that take no longer than 30 minutes.
6. Pain prevents me from traveling, except to the physician or hospital.

SCORING
Each item is given a point value ranging from 0 to 5, from top to bottom, for a potential total score of 0 to 50. The score is doubled for a total percentage score. If an item is not answered or the patient makes up an answer, it is dropped from the total potential score, and the total percentage is calculated using the remaining answers. The percentages are interpreted as follows: 0% to 20% indicates minimal disability in the activities of daily living (ADL), 20% to 40% represents moderate ADL disability, 40% to 60% is severe ADL disability, 60% to 80% is crippled ADL disability, and 80% to 100% represents symptom magnification or bed bound.

*From Fairbank JTC: The Oswestry low back disability questionnaire, *Physiotherapy* 66:271, 1980, Chartered Society of Physiotherapy.

ORTHOPEDIC GAMUT 13-14

CHARACTERISTICS OF PURE MALINGERING

- The simulation of a nonexistent illness or injury
- The voluntary provocation, aggravation, and protraction of disease by artificial means
- False allegations about the existence of some malady, such as epilepsy

---

CLINICAL PEARL (ASSESSMENT OF PAIN)

Feigning or pretense of nonexistent symptoms by word, gesture, action, or behavior is simulation *(positive malingering)* or dissimulation *(negative malingering)*. The deliberate and designed feigning of disease or disability or the intentional concealment of disease, if it exists, is pure malingering. The magnification or intensification of symptoms that already exist is partial malingering or exaggeration. Ascribing morbid phenomena or symptoms to a definite cause, although the cause may be recognized or ascertained to have no relationship to the symptoms, is false imputation. The six areas of psychological forensic practice are (1) mental state at the offense, (2) risk for violence, (3) risk for sexual violence, (4) competency to stand trial, (5) competency to waive *Miranda* rights, and (6) *malingering*.

AXIAL TRUNK-LOADING TEST

Assessment for Lumbar Spine Malingering

Comment

In the valid patient, any antalgic position can be taken as a sign that pain can be alleviated or abolished. The Quebec Task Force Classification System for categorizing spinal disorders lends in the differentiation of spinal pain validity (Table 13-6).

TABLE 13-6

THE QUEBEC CLASSIFICATION SYSTEM

Classification	Symptoms	Duration of Symptoms from Onset	Working Status at Time of Evaluation
		a (<7 days)	W (working)
		b (7 days–7 weeks)	I (idle)
		c (>7 weeks)	
1	Pain without radiation		
2	Pain radiation to extremity, proximally		
3	Pain radiation to extremity, distally		
4	Pain radiation to upper or lower limb neurologic signs		
5	Presumptive compression of a spinal nerve root on a simple roentgenogram (i.e., spinal instability or fracture)		
6	Compression of a spinal nerve root confirmed by (1) specific imaging techniques (i.e., computed axial tomography, myelography, or magnetic resonance imaging) or (2) other diagnostic techniques (e.g., electromyography, venography)		
7	Spinal stenosis		
8	Postsurgical status, 1–6 mos after intervention		
9	Postsurgical status, >6 mos after intervention		
	9.1 Asymptomatic		
	9.2 Symptomatic		
10	Chronic pain syndrome		W (working)
11	Other diagnoses		I (idle)

From Spitzer WO et al: Scientific approach to the assessment and management of activity related spinal disorders: a monograph for clinicians. Report of the Quebec Task Force on Spinal Disorders, *Spine* 12(suppl 7):S1, 1987.

PROCEDURE

- The examiner presses the patient's cranium in a downward direction (Fig. 13-4).
- The existing antalgic positioning must not be disturbed during the axial loading.
- The axial loading may elicit pain in the neck, but it should not elicit pain in the lower back.
- Malingering should be suspected if the patient indicates that pain is felt in the lower back.

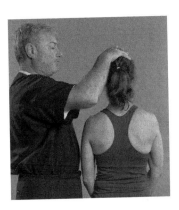

FIG. 13-4

CLINICAL PEARL

People with back pain express a fear that the reality of their pain is being questioned. Many of these individuals strive and frequently fail to achieve clinical and social characteristics that make up appropriate sickness behavior. A lack of proof that they are sick, including a lack of medical diagnosis, appropriate health care treatment, and visible disabilities, often leads to accusations, both felt and enacted, of malingering, hypochondria, mental illness, or any combination.

13

BURNS BENCH TEST

Assessment for Lumbar Spine Malingering

ORTHOPEDIC GAMUT 13-15
COMMON LUMBAR SPINE DISORDERS

- Herniated lumbar discs
  - Younger patients
  - Causes radicular type symptoms in the lower extremities
- Spinal stenosis
  - Elderly patients
  - Most common diagnoses in Medicare patients undergoing lumbar spine surgery
  - Back pain
  - Radicular type symptoms
  - Problems walking secondary to neurogenic claudication
- Degenerative spondylolisthesis
  - Segmental instability
  - Occurs in conjunction with spinal stenosis
  - Affects patients in their fifth and sixth decades of life
  - May cause symptoms of neurogenic claudication and radiculopathy
- Lumbar disc degeneration or collapse
  - Observed at one or more levels in the vast majority of all patients by the age of 50
  - May begin as early as age 20

PROCEDURE

- The patient is instructed to kneel on a stool and bend the trunk forward far enough to allow touching of the floor with fingertips or hands (Fig. 13-5).
- Patients who may be expected to perform this test successfully include those afflicted with sciatica, sacralization, spondylolisthesis, compression fractures of vertebra, and so on.
- A malingerer will fail to perform the maneuver and usually states, "I can't do it," or words to that effect, even before attempting the move.

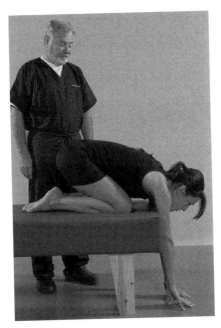

FIG. 13-5

CLINICAL PEARL

Patients with lumbar disc degeneration can cause back pain without associated radiculopathy or neurologic dysfunction in the lower extremities and represent a much greater challenge in terms of presentation, clinical imaging, and management than the other three diagnoses.

FLEXED-HIP TEST

Assessment for Lumbar Spine Malingering

PROCEDURE

- The examiner places one hand under the patient's lumbar spine and the other hand under the patient's knee.
- The examiner lifts the knee while flexing the hip (Fig. 13-6).
- If the patient indicates that lower back, or if leg pain is felt in the lower back before the lumbar spine moves, malingering should be suspected.

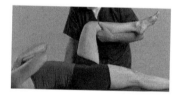

FIG. 13-6

CLINICAL PEARL

The causes of lower back pain in most people are unclear. Serious structural lesions such as tumors, infection, fractures, and severe deformities are frequently painful and are diagnosed with modern imaging studies. Such patients with serious structural problems are uncommon in outpatient clinical settings. Much more often, people have back pain episodes of varying degrees and either do not seek care or are treated symptomatically without a diagnosis.

FLIP SIGN

Assessment for Feigned Low Back Pain

PROCEDURE

- While the patient is lying in a supine position on the examining table, the examiner raises the patient's affected leg, keeping the patient's knee straight.
- If this movement is limited by pain or muscle resistance, the examiner then directs the patient to sit up, making sure the legs are kept flat on the table.
- If the patient can sit in this manner without pain, the test is positive.
- Sitting with the legs straight out reproduces the same maneuver as a straight-leg-raising test (Fig. 13-7).

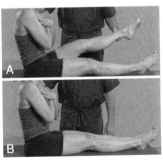

FIG. 13-7 In a modification of this test, the patient is directed to sit up, with the legs extended and flat on the examination table. If the patient can sit up in this manner, the test is positive (**A**); in a final move, the examiner performs a leg lift of the affected part. If this can be accomplished without pain, the test is positive (**B**).

13

LIBMAN SIGN

Assessment for Hypersensitivity of Mastoid Process

PROCEDURE

- The examiner applies finger pressure to the mastoid process (Fig. 13-8).
- The pressure is gradually increased until the patient states that it is becoming noticeably uncomfortable.
- This point is an indication of that patient's pain threshold, which varies from patient to patient.
- The threshold gives the examiner an idea if this patient has a low, high, or moderate pain threshold.
- The threshold is not to be used specifically as a criterion for malingering.
- Identifying a patient's pain threshold will quantify discomfort in this patient and applies to this patient only.
- This testing procedure will be useful during interpretation of palpation findings or subjective statements concerning pain or discomfort.

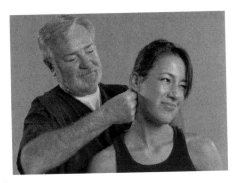

FIG. 13-8

CLINICAL PEARL

Chronic pain patients are typically more impaired on more complex attention-demanding tasks; however, tasks that require fewer attentional resources are unaffected even when pain levels were high. However, the relationship between pain and cognitive impairment is complex.

MAGNUSON TEST

Assessment for Feigned Low Back Pain

PROCEDURE

- The patient with lower back pain is directed to point to the site of the pain.
- The examiner marks the site.
- The examiner then distracts the patient by performing an examination away from the marked site of pain and later resumes the examination of the lower back.
- The test is positive with any change in the location of the pain of greater than 1 to 2 cm (Fig. 13-9).
- The test is significant as evidence of simulated pain, hysteria, or malingering.

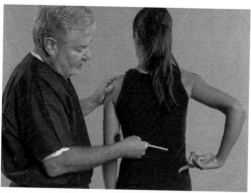

FIG. 13-9

MANNKOPF SIGN

Assessment for Simulated Pain

PROCEDURE

- The examiner establishes the patient's resting pulse rate, and the patient is made as comfortable as possible.
- Then, without changing the patient's position, the examiner applies mechanical pressure or electrical stimulation over the painful area while monitoring the pulse rate (Fig. 13-10).
- An increase in pulse rate of 10 or more beats per minute constitutes a positive sign.
- The sign is absent in simulated pain.

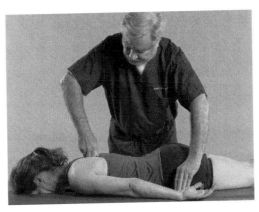

FIG. 13-10

MARKED PART PAIN-SUGGESTIBILITY TEST

Assessment for Pain Exaggeration

PROCEDURE

- The examiner applies pressure to the described painful point and marks it.
- The patient is distracted by examination of some other part of the body and pressing on new, tender areas.
- The examiner returns to the area of original complaint and asks the patient to close the eyes and then locate the tender points.
- If the patient cannot place the points of pain or tenderness closer than 2 in from the marked area, exaggeration is suspected (Fig. 13-11).

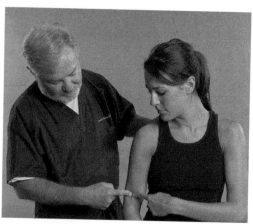

FIG. 13-11

CLINICAL PEARL

Human babesiosis was first recognized in Europe in 1957. In 1999, the southern-most range of human babesiosis on America's Atlantic coast was reported to be northwestern New Jersey. Other agents such as *Borrelia burgdorferi*, the Lyme disease spirochete, the rickettsiae of ehrlichiosis, and bacterial rods of *Bartonella* spp. within tick saliva often accompany *Babesia* spp.; increasingly, patients are coinfected with Lyme disease and babesiosis. If the disease is misdiagnosed as influenza, for example, and therefore goes untreated, infected humans tend to decompensate, often mislabeled as depressed or *hypochondriacal*, among others, rarely receiving optimal treatment for smoldering but active babesiosis—a sometimes fatal disease, especially if the patient is older or becomes immunocompromised.

PLANTAR FLEXION TEST

Assessment for Feigned Low Back Pain

ORTHOPEDIC GAMUT 13-16

ACTIVE PLANTAR FLEXION

Active plantar flexion stresses the calf muscles similarly to the treadmill test but with less effect on the cardiovascular system. The procedure is as follows:

- Both feet are placed in an adjustable brace, stabilizing and isolating the lower limbs.
- The patient pushes with both feet against pedals simultaneously until the pedals stop and holds the position for two seconds.
- The patient releases the pedals gently over 2 seconds.
- The patient presses the pedals in time to an audible signal set at 30 beats per minute; one signal to push is followed by a signal to release the pedals.
- The time in which the patient feels pain in the calf muscles is recorded (pain-free exercise time).
- The time at which the patient claims to reach their limit of exercise is recorded (maximal exercise time).
- The patient is allowed to stop for other symptoms; as in the treadmill test, symptoms, as well as blood pressure and heart rate before and after exercise, are recorded.

PROCEDURE

- The patient is instructed to raise the legs, one at a time, until pain is felt in the lower back or the leg.
- The angle at which the pain occurs is noted, and the patient lowers the leg.
- The examiner places one hand under the patient's knee and one hand under the patient's foot and raises the lower extremity, keeping the patient's knee slightly flexed.
- The leg is raised to one half of the height at which the pain was originally elicited.
- The foot is passively plantar flexed at this point (Fig. 13-12).
- If the patient indicates that this move causes lower back pain, malingering should be suspected.

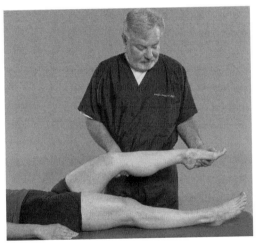

FIG. 13-12

RELATED JOINT MOTION TEST

Assessment for Feigned Pain

PROCEDURE

- The painful part is either actively or passively moved.
- This move is performed with isometric resistance of a muscle group that is nearby but is in no way associated with the pain.
- If the patient complains of pain, the examiner moves the muscle group or related joint later, judging the inaccuracy of the statements and the correlated reactions (Fig. 13-13).
- This assessment is accomplished by using a flexor group where an extensor group may produce pain in the joint.
- In cases in which the same muscle serves more than one movement, all movements should be tested.

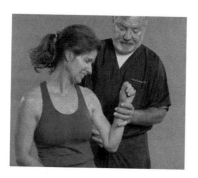

FIG. 13-13

SEELIGMULLER SIGN

Assessment for Hysterical Face Pain

PROCEDURE

- Mydriasis (dilated pupil) is present on the side of the face that is afflicted with neuralgia.
- The sign is present as long as pain is present.
- The sign is absent in cases of hysteria and malingering (Fig. 13-14).

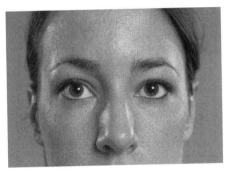

FIG. 13-14

TRUNK ROTATIONAL TEST

Assessment for Nonorganic Low Back Pain

ORTHOPEDIC GAMUT 13-17

SEQUENCE OF MUSCULAR RECRUITMENT DURING LATERAL FLEXION

1. Quadratus
2. Ligamentum flavum
3. Interspinous ligament

PROCEDURE

- The patient rotates the trunk.
- The examiner ensures that the patient's pelvis rotates as well (Fig. 13-15).
- If the patient indicates that this causes lower back pain, malingering should be suspected.
- The lumbar spine is not moving.
- Instead, the whole spine is rotated from the hips and thighs.

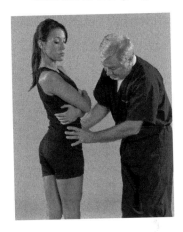

FIG. 13-15

CLINICAL PEARL

Although episodes of acute low back pain are a nearly universal human experience, the subsequent development of chronic disability and diminished work capacity occurs in only a limited percentage of individuals. In 1987, the Quebec Task Force on Spinal Disorders reported that 7% of individuals with work-related low back pain accounted for 76% of compensation costs and work absence as a result of low back pain.

SENSORY DEFICIT QUALIFICATION AND QUANTIFICATION

Overview

The nervous system does not perceive external events directly. Instead, the brain receives an abstract picture that is a composite of nerve impulses that originate at the periphery. The transformation of external stimuli into conductible impulses is called *transduction. Sensibility* is the reception or encoding of external stimuli and the transmission of impulses along nerve fibers.

13

ORTHOPEDIC GAMUT 13-18

SPECIFIC ASPECTS OF POSTINJURY NEUROPATHIC PAIN SYNDROMES

1. Mechanoallodynia and thermal allodynia
   a. Allodynia refers to pain provoked by an innocuous mechanical or thermal stimulus.
   b. Dynamic mechanoallodynia and hyperalgesia refers to a gentle moving stimulus over the skin surface that elicits pain, whereas static mechanoallodynia and hyperalgesia is pain produced by a stationary pressure stimulus.
2. Mechanohyperalgesia and thermal hyperalgesia—hyperalgesia signifies a lowered threshold to a normally painful stimulus and enhanced pain perception.
3. Hyperpathia—hyperpathia is a reflection of disordered central pain processing in which the pain threshold is increased but once exceeded pain reaches maximal intensity too rapidly, is more severe than expected, and is not stimulus bound.

ORTHOPEDIC GAMUT 13-19

NEURAL SENSIBILITY

Neural sensibility encompasses:
1. Sight
2. Smell
3. Sound
4. Taste
5. Temperature change
6. Pain
7. Touch-pressure
8. Movement or change in position

ORTHOPEDIC GAMUT 13-20

SENSATION

Sensation is divided into three groups:
1. Superficial
2. Deep
3. Combined

ORTHOPEDIC GAMUT 13-21

TWO GROUPS OF CUTANEOUS SENSIBILITY

1. Epicritic
2. Protopathic

CLINICAL PEARL
(SENSORY DEFICIT ASSESSMENT)

In the evaluation of what appears to be psychogenic changes in sensation, the examiner must remember that some variation in the nerve supply exists in normal individuals. Furthermore, hysterical or malingered changes may be superimposed on organic anesthesia in peripheral nerve lesions and other neurologic disorders. An ipsilateral decrease or loss of the senses of vision, hearing, smell, and taste may occasionally accompany hysterical (or malingered) hemianesthesia, which almost invariably occurs on the left side.

ANOSMIA TESTING

Assessment for Feigned Anosmia

ORTHOPEDIC GAMUT 13-22

CAUSE OF DISORDERS OF THE SENSE OF SMELL

1. Inflammatory and other lesions of the nasal cavity
2. Fracture of the anterior fossa of the skull
3. Tumors of the frontal lobe and pituitary region
4. Meningitis
5. Hydrocephalus
6. Posttraumatic cerebral syndrome
7. Arteriosclerosis
8. Cerebrovascular accidents
9. Certain drug intoxications
10. Psychoses
11. Neuroses
12. Congenital defects

ORTHOPEDIC GAMUT 13-23

SPECIAL SYNDROMES INVOLVING THE OLFACTORY NERVE

1. Foster-Kennedy syndrome (unilateral optic atrophy, with or without anosmia and contralateral papilledema)
2. Aura of epilepsy

PROCEDURE

- With complaints involving the loss of the sense of smell, the patient is directed to index various odors by smelling aromatics such as peppermint, clove, vanilla, coffee grounds (uncooked), and then, finally, spirit of ammonia (Fig. 13-16).
- An individual with psychogenic loss of smell often claims the inability to smell any of these substances.
- Ammonia is extremely pungent and actually irritates the trigeminal nerve endings in the nose, rather than being smelled by the olfactory nerve proper.
- Hence, a damaged olfactory nerve does not impair a patient's ability to notice (smell) the pungent ammonia fumes.

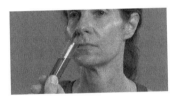

FIG. 13-16

CLINICAL PEARL

One challenge to the implementation of the olfactory event-related potential in a clinical setting is the need for measurement of habituation-free brain potentials. The neuronal recovery time for the olfactory system is significantly longer than that of both the auditory and the visual systems. Specifically, the presentation of two olfactory stimuli 45 seconds apart results in habituation to the second presentation, which does not completely recover even after 90 seconds. This phenomenon is the result, in part, of adaptation of olfactory receptor cells and, in part, of habituation to the original presentation of the stimulus.

13

COORDINATION-DISTURBANCE TESTING

Assessment for Nonorganic Loss of Coordination

ORTHOPEDIC GAMUT 13-24

PRINCIPLES OF ESSENTIAL TREMOR

- Essential tremor (ET) is the most common tremor disorder and ranks among the most common neurologic movement disorders.
- Because the tremor persists, the prevalence of ET in older adults is much higher, estimated at 4% to 37% in people older than 40 to 55 years, many of whom are never formally diagnosed.
- The principal criterion for diagnosing ET is the clinical observation of postural or kinetic tremor involving the hands and forearms that is visible and persistent; additional or isolated tremor of the head may also be present.
- Tremor in the voice, jaw, or lower extremities may also be present.
- In addition, other common causes of tremor (e.g., enhanced physiologic tremor, altered thyroid function, Parkinson disease, dystonia, other neurologic disorders) must be ruled out.

PROCEDURE

- The patient with coordination disturbances is instructed to touch the tip of the nose while the eyes are open.
- The patient is then instructed to close the eyes and again touch the tip of the nose.
- With organic cerebellar lesions, an intention crescendo tremor is demonstrated as the finger approaches the nose.
- The malingerer will move the finger in a guided but devious course toward the nose without exhibiting the intention tremor (Fig. 13-17).

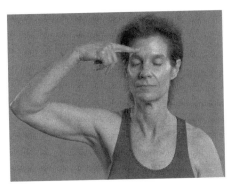

FIG. 13-17

CUIGNET TEST

Assessment for Simulated Blindness

ORTHOPEDIC GAMUT 13-25	
SUMMARY OF CLINICAL TESTS FOR FUNCTIONAL VISUAL LOSS	
Clinical tests	**Principle**
Total Binocular Blindness	
Observation	Clue to true or simulated difficulties in visual tasks
Finger tip test	Proprioceptive tasks and does not require vision
Signature test	
Mirror test	Convergence, miosis and accommodation reflex
Optokinetic test	Optokinetic reflex of smooth pursuit
Pupil response	Detection of afferent and efferent pathway
Menace reflex	Shock value
Tearing reflex	Tearing with bright light
Monocular Blindness	
Pupil response	Direct afferent visual pathway light testing
Fogging test	Elicit better vision than claimed
Stereopsis testing	Require binocular vision
Prism shift test	Demonstrates binocular vision
Reduced Visual Acuity	
Fogging test and stereoacuity	As above
Reduced Visual Field	
Visual field to confrontation, kinetic and static perimetry	Physiological visual field characteristics

Adapted from Chen CS et al: Practical clinical approaches to functional visual loss, *J Clin Neurosci* 14(1):1-7, 2007.

PROCEDURE

- The examination starts from the moment the patient walks into the consulting room; much information can be gained by careful observation. A truly blind patient will move cautiously and bump into objects naturally. A functionally blind patient will deliberately bump into objects or exaggerate movements. The examiner observes hand shaking. Furthermore, the examiner observes the accompanying person and their behavior toward the patient. It provides a very strong clue to the *overall picture*.
- Without a positive Marcus Gunn phenomenon but with continued complaint of unilateral blindness, the examiner places a refractive lens over the *good* eye, ostensibly to test it.
- The lens actually deprives the eye of any effective vision.
- The malingering patient is directed to read a Snellen chart (Fig. 13-18).
- This task is accomplished perfectly with the blind eye.

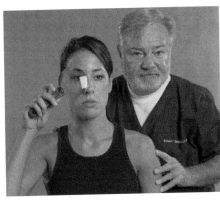

FIG. 13-18

FACIAL ANESTHESIA TESTING

Assessment for Hysterical or Simulated Face Anesthesia

ORTHOPEDIC GAMUT 13-26
LESIONS INVOLVING THE TRIGEMINAL COMPLEX
• Trigeminal nerve branches
• Isolated idiopathic trigeminal neuropathy
• Vasculitis
• Traumatism
• Lymphoma, bone tumors, metastasis
• Trigeminal tumors
• Trigeminal ganglion
• Herpes zoster
• Immunological aggressions to Gasserian ganglia neurons
• Trigeminal neuralgia surgery
• Trigeminal nerve roots
• Meningioma, acoustic neurinoma, trigeminal neurinoma
• Aneurysms, vascular malformations
• Polyradiculoneuritis
• Vascular compression
• Trigeminal nuclei
• Infarcts, other vascular lesions in the brainstem
• Encephalitis and intraaxial tumors
• Demyelinating diseases of the central nervous system
• Syringobulbia
• Changes in excitability in trigeminal nerve mediated reflexes
• Parkinson disease and other parkinsonisms
• Cranial and cervical dystonia
• Huntington disease
• Various movement disorders (tics, head tremor; hemifacial spasm)

Adapted from Valls-Sole J: Neurophysiological assessment of trigeminal nerve reflexes in disorders of central and peripheral nervous system, *Clin Neurophysiol* 116(10):2255-2265, 2005.

ORTHOPEDIC GAMUT 13-27

CLINICALLY APPLICABLE BRAINSTEM REFLEXES MEDIATED BY THE TRIGEMINAL NERVE

- Blink reflex
- Corneal reflex
- Masseteric inhibitory reflex
- Mandibular reflex

PROCEDURE

- In a patient with symptoms of facial anesthesia, the examiner applies a vibrating tuning fork to the numb side of the patient's forehead near the midline (Fig. 13-19).
- The malingerer or hysteric will state that no sensation is felt.
- When the examiner moves the application of the tuning fork just across the midline, the patient now reports sensing the vibrations immediately.
- The lack of vibration sense on the *numb* side is impossible because the bone tissue conducts the vibration that is applied to the area of claimed anesthesia to the normal side.
- This test is valid even for a pathologic bone condition or an organic bone disease.

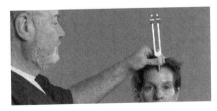

FIG. 13-19

GAULT TEST

Assessment for Simulated Deafness

ORTHOPEDIC GAMUT 13-28
CAUSES OF IMPAIRED HEARING

1. Involvement of the auditory structures in infectious diseases such as meningitis, syphilis, typhoid, mumps, measles, and hemolytic streptococcal infection
2. Tumors of the cerebellopontine angle, temporal lobe, eighth nerve, or cochlea
3. Trauma, such as from skull fracture
4. Injury by such toxic substances as quinine, arsenic, alcohol, salicylates, mercury, or aminoglycoside antibiotics (kanamycin)
5. Psychogenic disturbances
6. Physiologic dysfunction that may occur in senility and from excessive noise

---

ORTHOPEDIC GAMUT 13-29
COMPONENTS OF REFLEX BLINKING

- The inhibition of the basal tonic levator palpebrae superioris muscles, which keeps the eyes open
- The concurrent activation of the orbicularis oculi muscles

ORTHOPEDIC GAMUT 13-30

CONSIDERATIONS IN BLINKING

- Levator palpebrae superioris inhibition precedes and outlasts the orbicularis oculi activation
- This normal configuration is impaired in parkinsonism and blepharospasm
- Spontaneous blinking demonstrates a highly interindividual rate variation (among 10 to 20 per minute in adults)
- Abnormal blink rates occur in neurologic diseases related to dopaminergic transmission impairments

---

PROCEDURE

- The examiner can gain a crude estimate of the patient's hearing ability by using the auditory-palpebral reflex.
- When a patient hears a loud sound, an involuntary blink is the response.
- With the patient's normal ear covered, an assistant standing behind the patient (out of the patient's line of sight) can clap the hands or pop a bag.
- The examiner observes the patient for blinking or a startled response (Fig. 13-20).
- If the patient has a response, the examiner can be certain that the patient heard something.
- If the patient does not respond, the significance of the test is doubtful.

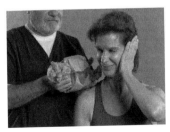

FIG. 13-20

JANET TEST

Assessment for Simulated Anesthesia

PROCEDURE

- If anesthesia is the complaint, the patient is instructed to close the eyes.
- The patient is then directed to answer *yes* if a pinprick is felt on the skin or *no* if not (Fig. 13-21).
- Obviously, the only appropriate answer is silence when the supposedly anesthetic area is touched.

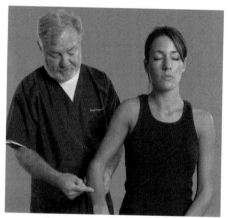

FIG. 13-21

LIMB-DROPPING TEST
(UPPER EXTREMITIES)

Assessment for Feigned Unconsciousness

ORTHOPEDIC GAMUT 13-31

THREE COMPONENTS OF THE GLASGOW COMA SCALE

- *Motor response:* The ease with which motor responses can be elicited in the limbs, together with the wide range of different patterns that can occur, makes motor activity a suitable guide to the functioning state of the central nervous system.
- *Verbal response:* Probably the commonest definition of the end of a coma, or the recovery of consciousness, is the patient's first understandable utterance.
- *Eye opening:* Spontaneous eye opening indicates that the arousal mechanisms in the brainstem are active.

ORTHOPEDIC GAMUT 13-32

GLASGOW COMA SCALE

Eye Opening

Spontaneous	4
To speech	3
To pain	2
None	1

Best Verbal Response

Oriented	5
Confused conversation	4
Inappropriate words	3
Incomprehensible sounds	2
None	1

Best Motor Response

Obeys commands	6
Localizes pain	5
Withdrawal (normal flexion)	4
Abnormal flexion (decorticate)	3
Extension (decerebrate)	2
None	1

ORTHOPEDIC GAMUT 13-33

LEVEL OF CONSCIOUSNESS

Diseases producing disturbances of the level of consciousness fall into the following four main categories:

1. Supratentorial mass lesions that secondarily compress deep midline structures
2. Infratentorial lesions that directly damage the central brainstem core
3. Metabolic disorders that widely depress or interrupt cortical function
4. Psychiatric disorders resembling coma

ORTHOPEDIC GAMUT 13-34

GLASGOW-LIEGE SCALE

The five brainstem reflexes selected disappear in descending order during rostral-caudal deterioration. The disappearance of the last, the oculocardiac, coincides with brain death.

Brainstem Reflex	Points
Frontoorbicular	5
Vertical oculovestibular	4
Pupillary light	3
Horizontal oculovestibular	2
Oculocardiac	1
No response	0

PROCEDURE

- In many instances, when the examiner holds up the hand of a patient who is feigning reduced consciousness and lets the hand drop over the patient's face, the arms will consciously swerve to keep the hand from striking the face.
- A patient with an organically reduced level of consciousness will not make this movement of avoidance and will usually have pupillary abnormalities and other positive neurologic signs (Fig. 13-22).

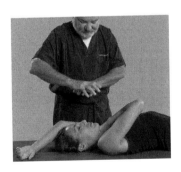

FIG. 13-22

13

LOMBARD TEST

Assessment for Simulated Deafness

PROCEDURE

- Lombard auditory test is a test of hearing that relies on the effect of induced noise on a subject's hearing responses (auditory brain response).
- The test is used in the investigation of nonorganic hearing loss.
- The patient with hearing loss is seated for this examination.
- The examiner engages the patient in conversation or has the patient read aloud from a page.
- As the reading progresses or the conversation continues, background noise is induced and amplified (Fig. 13-23).
- If the patient's voice grows louder with the background noise, the testing is positive and indicates nonorganic hearing loss.

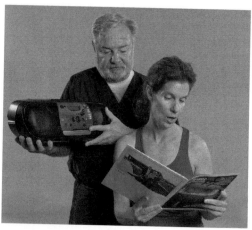

FIG. 13-23

MARCUS GUNN SIGN

Assessment for Normal Optic Neural Function

PROCEDURE

- If an organic basis for unilateral blindness is found, the lesion must be situated anteriorly to the optic chiasm, and the pupillary reaction is usually abnormal.
- Marcus Gunn sign is especially useful for evaluating the existence of unilateral blindness.
- To elicit the Marcus Gunn sign, the patient's eyes are fixed at a distant point and a strong light shone on the intact eye.
- A crisp, bilateral contraction of the pupils is noted.
- When the light is moved to the affected eye, both pupils dilate for a brief period.
- When the light is returned to the intact eye, both pupils contract promptly and remain contracted (Fig. 13-24).
- This response indicates damage to the optic nerve on the affected side.

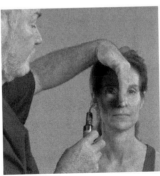

FIG. 13-24 On return of the light to the intact eye, both pupils contract promptly and remain contracted. This response indicates damage to the optic nerve on the affected side. The absence of Marcus Gunn sign in unilateral blindness indicates a nonorganic basis for the complaint.

MIDLINE TUNING-FORK TEST

Assessment for Simulated Anesthesia

PROCEDURE

- Patients with organic sensory disturbances are able to perceive a vibrating tuning fork placed on either side of the head or on either side of the sternum because the conduction vibrates through the bone (Fig. 13-25).
- In a conversion reaction, the sternum or head is split.
- For example, vibration is perceived on one side of the midline of the forehead or sternum but not on the other.

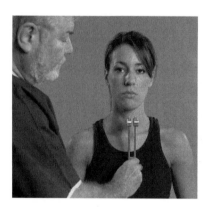

FIG. 13-25

OPTOKINETIC NYSTAGMUS TEST

Assessment for Feigned Blindness

PROCEDURE

- With faked blindness, the patient will often avoid personal injury when walking and will blink to unexpected physical threats.
- Pupillary reactions are normal, and optokinetic nystagmus is normal.
- To demonstrate optokinetic nystagmus, the examiner instructs the patient to keep the eyes open.
- The examiner holds a ruler or a tape measure 10 inches in front of the patient's face, ostensibly to measure pupillary distances.
- As the pupils constrict, which demonstrates attempted focusing, the ruler is moved from left to right across the patient's field of vision (Fig. 13-26).
- A patient who can see the ruler will fix the vision on the vertical markings and develop an involuntary eye movement called optokinetic nystagmus.
- This phenomenon is a similar to the one a person exhibits while riding in a vehicle and looking out the window watching telephone poles go by.
- This test is used when routine eye examination reveals a normal fundus and intact pupillary reactions to light.
- With organic blindness, pupillary reflexes are abnormal, and optokinetic nystagmus is absent.
- Hysterical field defects, when plotted out on a tangent screen, will not change with the varying distance between the patient and the screen.

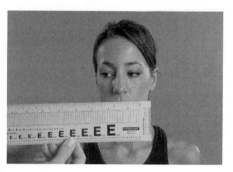

FIG. 13-26

POSITION-SENSE TESTING

Assessment for Feigned Loss of Position Sense

PROCEDURE

- If a patient claims that the position of a body part cannot be differentiated, the patient is directed to close the eyes, and the examiner bends the patient's fingers or toes up or down.
- The patient is instructed to state what direction the examiner is bending the digit.
- A patient may report contrary findings by saying *up* when the examiner is bringing the digit down, and vice versa (Fig. 13-27).
- With organic sensory loss, the patient has a 50% chance of correctly guessing the digit position.
- The malingerer's reporting average is always contrary to the actual digit position and therefore incorrect a majority of the time.

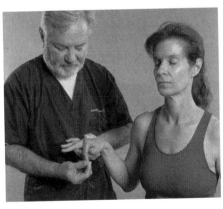

FIG. 13-27

REGIONAL ANESTHESIA TESTING

Assessment for Feigned Anesthesia

ORTHOPEDIC GAMUT 13-35

THALAMIC PAIN

Patients with thalamic pain exhibit the following characteristics:

- Ipsilateral, constant, severe pain, described as "crushing, aching, or burning"
- Paroxysmal episodes of hypersensitivity to stimulation, making sensory examinations difficult if not impossible
- Increased sensory threshold; and referred pain over a wide area
- A distinct lag between the time of application and the subsequent recognition of a stimulus is also noted
- Coupled with this delayed appreciation, stimulus-induced pain is described as having a more prolonged duration than that of the stimulus duration itself

---

PROCEDURE

- To define a regional complaint of numbness, the examiner uses a straight pin or a Wartenberg pinwheel and delineates the areas where the claimed numbness ceases.
- The usual organic cause of anesthesia or paresthesia is peripheral neuritis.
- With peripheral neuritis, the upper border of the anesthesia is blurry and usually different for each different sensation tested, such as pain, touch, heat, and vibration.
- In the hysterical or malingering patient, the border of anesthesia is extremely abrupt, stopping at a wrist crease or some other external anatomic area that is unrelated to the dermatome pattern (Fig. 13-28).
- This numbness landmark may even vary from examination to examination.
- Most malingerers claim a simultaneous loss of all forms of sensation, including touch, pain, temperature, and vibratory sensation.
- All losses are identical as to extent and accurate neural distribution or dermatome patterns are not present.

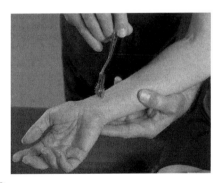

FIG. 13-28

13

ROMBERG SIGN

ALSO KNOWN AS STATION TEST

Assessment for Nonorganic Ataxia

PROCEDURE

- With this disorder of balance loss, the patient is instructed to stand with the feet together, first with the eyes open, then with the eyes closed.
- With organic sensory ataxia, the patient will sway the body from the ankles.
- Swaying from the hips toward a wall to catch one's self in the nick of time suggests malingering (Fig. 13-29).

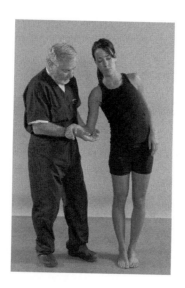

FIG. 13-29

SNELLEN TEST

Assessment for Feigned Color Blindness

ORTHOPEDIC GAMUT 13-36

COLOR BLINDNESS

Color blindness may be hereditary or acquired. Hereditary types are transmitted as recessive characteristics, sometimes X-linked. These characteristics include the following:

1. Achromatopsia (total color blindness)
2. Monochromatism (partial color blindness, with ability to recognize one of the three basic colors remaining)
3. Dichromatism (ability to recognize two of the three basic colors)

In normal (trichromatic) vision, the eye can perceive three light primaries (red, blue, and green) and can mix these in suitable portions. Thus white or any color of the spectrum can be matched. Color blindness can result from a lessened capacity to match three primary colors. It can be dichromatic vision, in which only one pair of the primary colors is perceived, the two colors being complementary to each other. Most dichromats are red-green blind and confuse red, yellow, and green (Table 13-7).

TABLE 13-7

COMPARISON OF ACQUIRED AND CONGENITAL COLOR VISION DEFICIENCIES

Acquired Color Vision Defect	Congenital Color Vision Defect
Onset after birth	Onset at birth
Monocular differences in the type and severity of the defect occur frequently	Both eyes are equally affected
Color alterations are frequently associated with other visual problems such as low acuity and reductions in the useful visual (except in rod monochromatism) or visual field	The visual problems are specific to color perception; there are no problems with acuity field
The type and severity of the deficiency fluctuate throughout life	The type and severity of the defect are the same
The type of defect might not be easy to classify; combined or nonspecific defects occur frequently	The type of defect can be classified precisely
Predominantly either protan or deutan	Predominantly tritan
Higher incidence in men	Same incidence in both sexes

Adapted from Lillo JA, Moreira H, Charles S: Color blindness. In *Encyclopedia of applied psychology*, New York, 2004, Elsevier.

PROCEDURE

- For pretended color blindness in one eye, the patient is requested to look at alternate red and green letters.
- The admittedly good eye is covered with a red glass (Fig. 13-30).
- If the green letters are read, evidence of fraud is present.

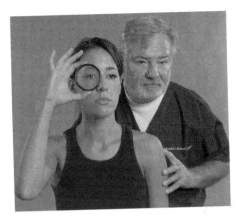

FIG. 13-30

STOICISM INDEXING

Assessment for Congenital Insensitivity to Pain

PROCEDURE

- The interval between eye blinks in the average patient is 25 to 30 seconds.
- A 60-second lapse between blinks while staring straight ahead indicates a patient who is stoic (Fig. 13-31).
- A stoic patient can be described as impassive and calm in the face of pain and discomfort.
- Stoic patients may also be cool and indifferent to the sensations elicited in testing.

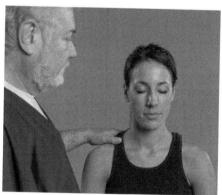

FIG. 13-31

PARALYSIS QUALIFICATION AND QUANTIFICATION

Overview

Motion is a fundamental property of most animal life. The lowest multicellular animals possess rudimentary neuromuscular mechanisms. In higher forms, motion is based on the transmission of impulses from a receptor through an afferent neuron and ganglion cell to muscle. This same principle is found in the reflex arc of higher animals, including humans, in whom the anterior spinal cord has developed into a central regulating mechanism. This central regulating mechanism is involved in initiating and integrating movements.

Motor disturbances include weakness and paralysis, which may result from lesions of the voluntary motor pathways or of the muscles themselves. Impaired motor functioning may result from involvement of muscle, myoneural junction, peripheral nerve, or the central nervous system.

The types of paralysis or paresis are based on the location. Hemiplegia is a spastic or flaccid paralysis of one side of the body and extremities, limited by the median line sagittally. Monoplegia is a paralysis of one extremity only. Diplegia is a paralysis of any two corresponding extremities, both of which are usually lower extremities, but may be upper extremities. Paraplegia is a symmetric paralysis of both lower extremities. Quadriplegia, or tetraplegia, is a paralysis of all four extremities. Hemiplegia alternans (crossed paralysis) is a paralysis of one or more ipsilateral cranial nerves and contralateral paralysis of the arm and leg.

ORTHOPEDIC GAMUT 13-37

MOVEMENT DISORDERS OF ORGANIC ORIGIN

- Tremor
- Dystonia
- Chorea
- Bradykinesia
- Myoclonus
- Tics
- Athetosis
- Ballism
- Incoordination

13

ORTHOPEDIC GAMUT 13-38
PSYCHOGENIC MOVEMENT DISORDERS

Psychogenic movement disorders in order of clinical frequency:
- Action tremor
- Resting tremor
- Dystonia
- Bradykinesia
- Myoclonus
- Incoordination resembling cerebellar dysfunction
- Tics
- Chorea
- Athetosis
- Ballism

Distractibility and variability are especially common in psychogenic tremor (80% of cases) and commonly coexist with entrainment and coactivation signs (Table 13-8).

TABLE 13-8
CLINICAL CHARACTERISTICS OF PSYCHOGENIC MOVEMENT DISORDERS

Mode of onset	• Abrupt
	• Precipitating event
	• Fast progression to maximal symptom severity and disability
Clinical signs	• Signs incongruent with organic disease
	• Distractibility and variability
	• Multiple abnormal movements
	• Increased movement with attention to the affected body part
	• Deliberate slowness of movement
	• Entrainment, coactivation
	• Association with false weakness, sensory loss, and pain
	• Unresponsiveness to drugs for organic movement disorders, response to placebo drugs and suggestion

Adapted from Hinson VK, Haren WB: Psychogenic movement disorders, *Lancet Neurol* 5(8):695-700, 2006.

CLINICAL PEARL (PARALYSIS ASSESSMENT)

Abnormalities of the motor system, which may be manifestations of both hysteria and malingering, include disturbances of muscle strength and power, disorders of tone, dyskinesia, and abnormalities of coordination, station, and gait. Rarely do changes in volume or contour occur (except for wasting from disuse), and no abnormalities are found on electromyographic examination. These motor changes of psychic origin may resemble almost any type of motor disturbance that is brought about by organic disease of the nervous system.

In both hysterical and malingered paralyses, the patient makes little effort to contract the muscles necessary for executing the desired movement. The patient may remain calm and indifferent while demonstrating the lack of strength. The patient may also show little sign of alarm at the presence of complete paralysis and may smile cheerfully during the examination. Reliable evidence that the patient is not exerting all available power in an attempt to carry out a voluntary movement can be elicited by watching and palpating the contraction of the antagonists, as well as the agonists.

13

BILATERAL
LIMB-DROPPING TEST
(LOWER EXTREMITIES)

Assessment for Feigned Paresis of Lower Extremity

ORTHOPEDIC GAMUT 13-39

FUNCTIONAL AMBULATION CLASSIFICATION

Level 0: Nonambulation
Level 1: Nonfunctional or dependent ambulation
Level 2: Household ambulation
Level 3: Surroundings of the house ambulation (neighborhood)
Level 4: Community ambulation
Level 5: Normal ambulation

ORTHOPEDIC GAMUT 13-40

THE BARTHEL INDEX

Full credit is not given for an activity if the patient needs even minimal help/supervision. A score of 0 is given when the patient cannot meet the criteria as defined.

Patient Name: _____
Rater Name: _____
Date: _____

Activity	Score

Feeding
0 = unable
5 = needs help cutting, spreading butter, etc., or requires modified diet
10 = independent   _____

Bathing
0 = dependent
5 = independent (or in shower)   _____

Grooming
0 = needs to help with personal care
5 = independent face/hair/teeth/shaving (implements provided)   _____

Dressing
0 = dependent
5 = needs help but can do about half unaided
10 = independent (including buttons, zips, laces, etc.) _____

Bowels
0 = incontinent (or needs to be given enemas)
5 = occasional accident
10 = continent   _____

Bladder
0 = incontinent, or catheterized and unable to manage alone
5 = occasional accident
10 = continent   _____

Toilet Use
0 = dependent
5 = needs some help, but can do something alone
10 = independent (on and off, dressing, wiping)   _____

Continued

13

ORTHOPEDIC GAMUT 13-40

THE BARTHEL INDEX—cont'd

Transfers (bed to chair and back)
  0 = unable help (one or two people, physical), can sit
 10 = minor help (verbal or physical)
 15 = independent _____

Mobility (on level surfaces)
 0 = immobile or < 50 yards
 5 = wheelchair independent, including corners, > 50 yards
 10 = walks with help of one person (verbal or physical)
   > 50 yards
 15 = independent (but may use any aid; for example, stick)
   > 50 yards

Stairs
 0 = unable
 5 = needs help (verbal, physical, carrying aid)
 10 = independent _____

Total (0–100)   SCORE _____

1. The index should be used as a record of what a patient does, not as a record of what a patient could do.
2. The main aim is to establish degree of independence from any help, physical or verbal, however minor and for whatever reason.
3. The need for supervision renders the patient not independent.
4. A patient's performance should be established using the best available evidence. Asking the patient, friends or relatives, and nurses are the usual sources, but direct observation and common sense are also important. However direct testing is not needed.
5. Usually, the patient's performance over the preceding 24 to 48 hours is important, but occasionally longer periods will be relevant.
6. Middle categories imply that the patient supplies over 50% of the effort.
7. Use of aids to be independent is allowed.

The advantage of the BI is its simplicity. It is useful in evaluating a patient's state of independence before treatment, patient progress undergoing treatment, and patient status when reaching maximum benefit. The total score is not as significant or meaningful as the breakdown into individual items, because these indicate where the deficiencies are.

PROCEDURE

- Lower extremities are usually portrayed to be either weak or completely paralyzed.
- To determine whether the patient has a weak hip or leg, the patient is placed on the examination table in a supine position.
- The examiner flexes the patient's legs at the hip, keeping the knees straight.
- The examiner holds the legs in an elevated position by cradling the patient's feet in a hand and instructs the patient to push the legs downward and hard against the examiner's hand.
- The examiner suddenly pulls the hand away (Fig. 13-32).
- If leg weakness is of an organic origin, the affected leg will fall to the examination table.
- If the weakness is faked, the leg may move up or hang in midair for a moment before falling because of hip muscle flexor actuation.

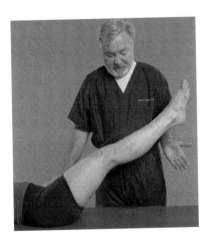

FIG. 13-32

HEMIPLEGIC POSTURING

Assessment for Nonorganic Hemiplegia

ORTHOPEDIC GAMUT 13-41

HEMIPLEGIC MOVEMENT PATTERNS IN CHILDREN WITH CEREBRAL PALSY

Movement Patterns for the Task of Rising from a Supine Position to a Standing Position	Segmental Score
I. Upper Limb Categories	
a. Push and reach to bilateral push	1
b. Push and reach to asymmetric push	2
c. Symmetric push	3
d. Symmetric reach	4
e. Push and reach followed by pushing on one leg	5
f. Push and reach to bilateral push followed by pushing on leg	6
II. Axial Categories	
a. Full rotation with abdomen down	1
b. Full rotation with abdomen up	2
c. Partial rotation	3
d. Forward with rotation	4
e. Symmetric	5
III. Lower Limb Categories	
a. Pike	1
b. Pike jump to squat	2
c. Kneel	3
d. Jump to squat	4
e. Half-kneel	5
f. Asymmetric wide based squat	6
g. Narrow based symmetric squat	7

PROCEDURE

- Paralysis is yet another symptom presentation from the repertoire of the hysteric, psychogenic, rheumatic, or malingering patient.
- A patient with a feigned paralyzed leg and arm may incorrectly assume the existence of difficulty in turning the head toward the paralyzed side (Fig. 13-33).
- Pronation drift (the inability to hold the pronated arms still) is absent on station and gait.

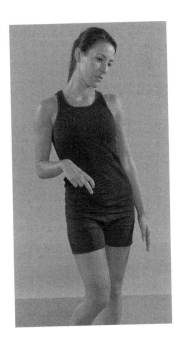

FIG. 13-33

HOOVER SIGN

Assessment for Feigned Leg Paresis

Neurologic loss is usually described as a sensory or motor deficit. The sensory loss may produce hypoesthesia, paresthesia, or hyperesthesia and may produce pain or numbness over a specific area. The motor deficits may be described as a weakness, as stiffness, or, more commonly, as difficulty in walking far, running, or jumping. If outright paralysis is present, the onset may have been sudden or insidious (Table 13-9). The paralysis may be flaccid or spastic. Flaccidity is associated with lower motor neuron disorders and spasticity with upper motor neuron disorders. The examiner must determine whether the symptoms have increased or decreased and to what degree the patient is disabled. The examiner must also determine whether a loss of sphincter control of the bladder and rectum has occurred.

TABLE 13-9

COMMON CAUSES OF HYPOKALEMIC PARALYSIS

Potassium Deficit

Group 1

Hypochloremic metabolic alkalosis	Excessive vomiting
	Diuretics
	Licorice ingestion
	Mineralocorticoid syndromes
	Bartter or Gitelman syndrome
	Liddle syndrome

Group 2

Hyperchloremic metabolic acidosis and low NH_4^+ excretion	Distal renal tubular acidosis (medullary-sponge kidney, Sjögren syndrome)
	Proximal renal tubular acidosis, Fanconi syndrome

Group 3

Hyperchloremic metabolic acidosis and high NH_4^+ excretion	Toluene abuse
	Diarrheal state
	Urethral diversion

Intracellular potassium shift

Group 4

Normal acid–base balance	Thyrotoxic periodic paralysis
	Familial periodic paralysis
	Sporadic periodic paralysis
	Hypernatremic hypokalemic paralysis
	Barium poisoning

NH_4^+, Ammonium.
From Pompeo A et al: Thyrotoxic hypokalemic periodic paralysis: an overlooked pathology in Western countries, *Eur J Intern Med* 18(5):380–390, 2007.

PROCEDURE

- Hoover sign is helpful in differentiating between organic and hysterical paralysis.
- When a supine patient is directed to lift the paralyzed or affected one leg, normally the patient unconsciously presses the heel of the unaffected leg against the examination table.
- In organic hemiplegia, this downward pressure is accentuated on the healthy side as the patient attempts to raise the paretic leg.
- If the examiner places a hand under the patient's heel, this pressure can be felt (Fig. 13-34).
- In malingering, the patient will feel no, or very little, pressure on the opposite side of the affection as the patient attempts to raise the involved extremity.

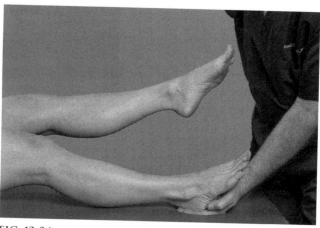

FIG. 13-34

SIMULATED FOOT-DROP TESTING

Assessment for Feigned Steppage Gait or Foot Drop

PROCEDURE

- With feigned total leg weakness or paralysis, a patient may pretend to be unable to raise the forefoot while walking.
- This complaint must be separated from organic foot drop.
- The patient is standing, and the examiner is positioned behind the patient (Fig. 13-35).
- The patient is instructed to maintain a rigid and narrow-based posture, with the feet close together.
- In a surprise move, the examiner grasps the shoulders of the patient and pulls the patient's body backward (Fig. 13-36).
- The examiner notes the movement of the patient's toes and forefoot.
- If the forefoot rises, the test is positive.
- A positive test indicates feigned foot drop.

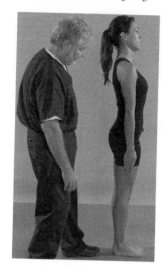

FIG. 13-35

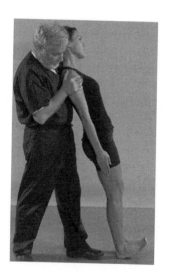

FIG. 13-36

SIMULATED FOREARM-AND-WRIST-WEAKNESS TESTING

Assessment for Simulated Weakness of Forearm and Wrist

ORTHOPEDIC GAMUT 13-42

LAMB BILATERAL HAND ACTIVITY INDEX OF ACTIVITIES PERFORMED WITH BOTH HANDS ACTING SIMULTANEOUSLY AND TOGETHER*

- Unscrew the top from a bottle.
- Fill a cup or glass and drink.
- Open a can with a manual can opener.
- Remove a match from a box or book and light it.
- Use a knife and fork for eating.
- Apply toothpaste to a toothbrush and clean teeth.
- Put on a jacket.
- Close buttons on clothing.
- Fasten a belt around the waist.
- Tie shoelaces.
- Sharpen a pencil in a manual sharpener.
- Write messages.
- Use a dial telephone.
- Staple papers together.
- Wrap string around a package.
- Use playing cards.

When progress is being measured, each of these items listed may be scored on a scale of 0 to 5, or 0 to 10, and added. A total score of 80 or 160, respectively, represents a return to normal bilateral hand functions.

---

*Modified from McRae R: *Clinical orthopaedic examination*, ed 3, Edinburgh, 1990, Churchill Livingstone.

PROCEDURE

- If the complaint is persisting forearm or wrist weakness that is not associated with grip strength loss, the patient is directed to dorsiflex the wrist, usually by making a fist.
- If this task cannot be performed, the patient is then asked to squeeze a dynamometer while the examiner palpates the patient's forearm (Fig. 13-37).
- In functional or feigned weakness, the examiner will feel the patient's forearm extensors contract synergistically and will see the wrist extend when the patient squeezes.

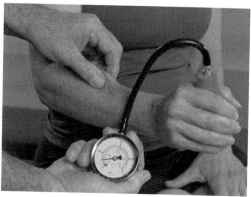

FIG. 13-37

SIMULATED GRIP-STRENGTH-LOSS TESTING

Assessment for Simulated Grip Strength Loss

ORTHOPEDIC GAMUT 13-43

NEUROPATHY

The differential diagnosis of neuropathy includes many diseases that present with similar symptoms (symmetric distal sensory losses). However, patients with neuropathy occasionally may complain of the following symptoms:

1. Thickened nerves (hypertrophic neuropathy)
2. Mononeuritis
3. Radiculopathy
4. Cranial nerve involvement
5. Autonomic disturbances
6. Ascending neuritis
7. Weakness without sensory findings

PROCEDURE

- When grip strength loss is the complaint, the patient is directed to squeeze the examiner's fingers with the paralyzed hand as hard as possible.
- While the patient performs this task, the examiner suddenly tears the fingers away.
- If grip weakness is caused by organic disease, a sudden tug will break the grasp easily.
- If the weakness is being faked, strong resistance is likely to be encountered before the malingerer realizes the error or contradiction and releases the grip (Fig. 13-38).

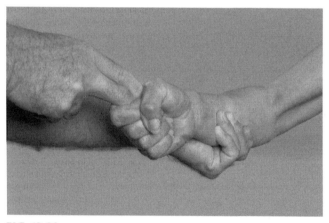

FIG. 13-38

TRIPOD TEST
(BILATERAL LEG-FLUTTERING TEST)

Assessment for Simulated Lumbar Pain

PROCEDURE

- A patient may attempt to fake a leg paralysis as the result of a further faked lumbar intervertebral disc syndrome.
- In this instance, the patient is instructed to sit on the examination table with the knees flexed at 90 degrees and the legs hanging dependent.
- The patient is directed to extend and relax, or flex, the legs rapidly and repeatedly.
- If lumbar disc involvement exists, the patient will need to lean back to perform this maneuver, if able to do it at all (Fig. 13-39).
- The patient feigning disc involvement can accomplish the maneuver without assuming such a tripod posture (Fig. 13-40).

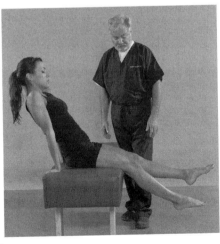

FIG. 13-39

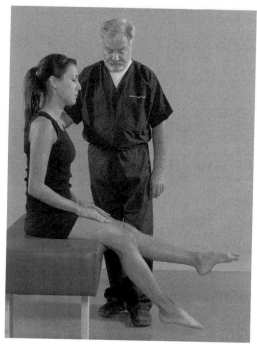

FIG. 13-40

TABLE 13-10

CAUSES OF UNILATERAL FOOT DROP AND BILATERAL FOOT DROP

I. Unilateral foot drop	a. Deep peroneal mononeuropathy
	b. Common peroneal mononeuropathy
	c. Anterior compartmental syndrome of the leg
	d. Sciatic mononeuropathy
	e. Lumbosacral plexopathy (lumbosacral trunk)
	f. L5 radiculopathy
	g. L4 radiculopathy
	h. Multifocal motor neuropathy
	i. Hereditary neuropathy with liability to pressure palsy
	j. Amyotrophic lateral sclerosis
	k. Poliomyelitis and postpoliomyelitis syndrome
	l. Cortical or subcortical parasagittal cerebral lesion
II. Bilateral foot drop	a. Myopathies
	b. Distal myopathies
	c. Scapuloperoneal muscular dystrophy
	d. Facioscapulohumeral muscular dystrophy
	e. Myotonic dystrophy
	f. Neuropathies
	g. Multifocal motor neuropathy with conduction block
	h. Chronic inflammatory demyelinating polyneuropathy
	i. Bilateral peroneal neuropathies
	j. Bilateral sciatic neuropathies
	k. Bilateral lumbosacral plexopathies
	l. Radiculopathies
	m. Bilateral L5 radiculopathies
	n. Conus medullaris lesion
	o. Anterior horn cell disorders
	p. Amyotrophic lateral sclerosis
	q. Poliomyelitis and the postpoliomyelitis syndrome
	r. Cerebral lesions
	s. Bilateral cortical or subcortical parasagittal lesions

(Adapted from Katirji B, Michael JA, Robert BD: Causes of unilateral foot drop and bilateral foot drop. In: *Encyclopedia of the neurological sciences*. New York, 2003, Academic Press.)

13

BOX 13-5

Mood Disorders—DSM-III-R* Classifications

Bipolar Disorders
296.6x Mixed—both manic and depressed features
296.4x Manic
296.5x Depressed
301.13 Cyclothymia
296.70 Bipolar disorder not otherwise specified

Depressive Disorders—Major Depression
296.6x Single episode
296.3x Recurrent
300.40 Dysthymia

*DSM-III-R, Diagnostic and Statistical Manual of Mental Disorders, third edition, revised.
Fifth digit (x) allows coding of current state of disorder: 1 = mild; 2 = moderate;
3 = severe, without psychotic features; 4 = with psychotic features; 5 = in partial
remission; 6 = in full remission; 0 = unspecified
Data from American Psychiatric Association Diagnostic and Statistical Manual of Mental
Disorders, ed 3, revised, Washington DC, 1987, American Psychiatric Association. In
White AH, Schofferman JA: Spine care, vol. 1-2, St. Louis, 1995, Mosby.

BOX 13-6

Description of MMPI-2*

L, F, and K are validity scales.

L is called the *lie scale* and measures willingness to admit minor
social faults. It gives information about social conformity, self-
image and self-insight, and denial.

F refers to infrequency and consists of items that are socially unac-
ceptable or have disturbing content. Persons scoring on the low
end of this scale are usually conventional and unassuming.
Those with elevations are admitting to severe emotional distress or psychopathologic condition or both. Very high scores
suggest an invalid profile.

K refers to correction, and the items measure personal resources
required to cope with life. Low scores suggest exaggeration of
problems or severe emotional distress. Higher scores can result
when patients are very confident and in charge or when they
are being defensive in their efforts to present themselves as
adequate and in control when in fact their lives are in disarray.

BOX 13-6

DESCRIPTION OF MMPI-2*—cont'd

Scales 1 through 10 are the basic clinical scales of the MMPI-2. The information is presented using T scores. A T score of 50 is average; T scores over 65 are in the abnormal range.

Scale 1 is also known as the *Hypochondriasis (HS) scale*. This scale consists of items that concern bodily functioning. Many of the items are vague in their content. Persons scoring low on this scale do not have or are denying that they have any physical complaints. Those whose scores are elevated have many physical complaints and concerns. If scores are above 65, physical complaints are often the major focus of the person's life.

Scale 2 is known as the *Depression (D) scale*. It consists of items that measure subjective depression, psychomotor slowing and immobilization, physical complaints, mental dullness, and brooding. High scores indicate the presence of depression, and low scores indicate persons whose affective functioning is within normal limits.

Scale 3 is known as *Hysteria (Hy)*. It consists of items that indicate whether the individual tends to avoid emotional and social unpleasantness. Those that do may then experience their emotions and stress as somatic complaints. High scorers will often deny psychologic problems and look for concrete solutions to their problems.

Scale 4 is known as *psychopathic deviate (Pd)*. Eight items refer to authority conflicts, and the rest of the items deal with family conflicts, denial of social and dependency needs, social alienation, and self-integration. High scorers are often angry, impulsive, in conflict with authority figures in their lives, and are feeling isolated and despondent. High scorers who are not psychopathic are often undergoing stressful transitions in their lives.

Scale 5 is known as *Masculinity-Femininity (Mf)*. Scores on this reflect traditional versus nontraditional masculine or feminine interests and beliefs, conflicts about sexuality, and interests in aesthetics. Low scores for women suggest feelings of helplessness and dependency, whereas low scores for men suggest an action-oriented *macho* approach to life. High-scoring men often hold interests in activities usually considered as feminine and may be experiencing insecurity, helplessness, and conflicts of sexuality. High-scoring women report interest in traditional male patterns and are often seen as unfriendly, dominating, and aggressive.

13

Continued

BOX 13-6

DESCRIPTION OF MMPI-2*—cont'd

Scale 6 is known as *Paranoia (Pa)*. In addition to paranoia and externalization of blame, this scale contains items related to hypersensitivity, subjectivity, naiveté, righteousness, and denial of hostility and distrust. Very high scorers are outright paranoid and may have a thought disorder, whereas low scorers may be insensitive to others and unaware of others' motives. They may also be denying the presence of paranoid thoughts.

Scale 7 is known as *Psychasthenia (Pt)*. Items center on the presence of worries, brooding, and rumination. High scorers are seen as anxious and insecure, and may be indecisive. If scores are very high, the individual may be compulsive and agitated with feelings of guilt and fear disrupting everyday functioning.

Scale 8 is known as *Schizophrenia (Sc)*. High scorers are having difficulty with their thinking and feelings. They often feel out of control and unable to take positive action in their own behalf. Extremely high scores are suggestive of severe situational stress. More moderate elevations are seen in those with thought disorders with difficulties in logic concentration and judgment common.

Scale 9 is known as *Hypomania (Ma)*. This scale provides information about motivation, physical and emotional activity levels, confidence in social situations, and feelings of self-importance. High scorers are restless, agitated, emotionally labile and may have racing thoughts. They may also have difficulty delaying gratification and can be impulsive. Manic features appear as scores elevate.

Scale 10 is known as *Social Introversion (Si)*. This scale provides information about social interests, interpersonal skills, self-consciousness, and feelings of alienation from self or others. High scorers are often depressed. They withdraw from social interactions and feel shy and insecure. Low scorers are usually socially extroverted and outgoing.

MMPI-2, Minnesota Multiphasic Personality Inventory, second edition.
From White AH, Schofferman JA: *Spine care,* vol 1-2, St Louis, 1995, Mosby.

APPENDIX

These tables are taken from Chapter 1 of the companion to this book, *Illustrated Orthopedic Physical Assessment, Third Edition.*

TABLE A-1

SUMMARY OF GLUCOSE TOLERANCE TESTS AND INTERPRETATIONS

Fasting Blood Glucose

From 70 to 99 mg/dL (3.9 to 5.5 mmol/L)	Normal glucose tolerance
From 100 to 125 mg/dL (5.6 to 6.9 mmol/L)	Impaired fasting glucose (prediabetes)
126 mg/dL (7.0 mmol/L) and above on more than one testing occasion	Diabetes

Oral Glucose Tolerance Test (OGTT) [except pregnancy] (2 hours after a 75-gram glucose drink)

Less than 140 mg/dL (7.8 mmol/L)	Normal glucose tolerance
From 140 to 200 mg/dL (7.8 to 11.1 mmol/L)	Impaired glucose tolerance (prediabetes)
Over 200 mg/dL (11.1 mmol/L) on more than one testing occasion	Diabetes

Gestational Diabetes Screening: Glucose Challenge Test (1 hour after a 50-gram glucose drink)

Less than 140* mg/dL (7.8 mmol/L)	Normal glucose tolerance
140* mg/dL (7.8 mmol/L) and over	Abnormal, needs OGTT (see below)

Gestational Diabetes Diagnostic: OGTT (100-gram glucose drink)

Fasting[†]	95 mg/dL (5.3 mmol/L)
1 hour after glucose load[†]	180 mg/dL (10.0 mmol/L)
2 hours after glucose load[†]	155 mg/dL (8.6 mmol/L)
3 hours after glucose load[†‡]	140 mg/dL (7.8 mmol/L)

*Some use a cutoff of >130 mg/dL (7.2 mmol/L) because that identifies 90% of women with gestational diabetes, compared to 80% identified using the threshold of >140 mg/dL (7.8 mmol/L).

[†]If two or more values are above the criteria, gestational diabetes is diagnosed.

[‡]A 75-gram glucose load may be used, although this method is not as well validated as the 100-gram OGTT; the 3-hour sample is not drawn if 75 grams is used

TABLE A-2

SUMMARY OF CBC COMPONENTS AND INTERPRETATIONS

Test	Name	Increased/Decreased
WBC	White blood cell	May be increased with infections, inflammation, cancer, leukemia; decreased with some medications (such as methotrexate), some autoimmune conditions, some severe infections, bone marrow failure, and congenital marrow aplasia (marrow doesn't develop normally)
% Neutrophil	Neutrophil/Band/Seg	This is a dynamic population that varies somewhat from day to day depending on what is going on in the body. Significant increases in particular types are associated with different temporary/acute and/or chronic conditions. An example of this is the increased number of lymphocytes seen with lymphocytic leukemia. For more information, see Blood Smear and WBC.
% Lymphs	Lymphocyte	
% Mono	Monocyte	
% Eos	Eosinophil	
% Baso	Basophil	
Neutrophil	Neutrophil/Band/Seg	
Lymphs	Lymphocyte	
Mono	Monocyte	
Eos	Eosinophil	
Baso	Basophil	
RBC	Red blood cell	Decreased with anemia; increased when too many made and with fluid loss due to diarrhea, dehydration, burns
Hgb	Hemoglobin	Mirrors RBC results
Hct	Hematocrit	Mirrors RBC results
MCV	Mean corpuscular volume	Increased with B_{12} and Folate deficiency; decreased with iron deficiency and thalassemia
MCH	Mean corpuscular hemoglobin	Mirrors MCV results
MCHC	Mean corpuscular hemoglobin concentration	May be decreased when MCV is decreased; increases limited to amount of Hgb that will fit inside a RBC
RDW	Red blood cell distribution width	Increased RDW indicates mixed population of RBCs; immature RBCs tend to be larger

TABLE A-2

SUMMARY OF CBC COMPONENTS AND INTERPRETATIONS—cont'd

Platelet	Platelet	Decreased or increased with conditions that affect platelet production; decreased when greater numbers used, as with bleeding; decreased with some inherited disorders (such as Wiskott-Aldrich, Bernard-Soulier), with Systemic lupus erythematosus, pernicious anemia, hypersplenism (spleen takes too many out of circulation), leukemia, and chemotherapy
MPV	Mean platelet volume	Vary with platelet production; younger platelets are larger than older ones

TABLE A-3

CATEGORIES OF SYNOVIAL FLUID BASED UPON CLINICAL AND LABORATORY FINDINGS

Measure	Normal	Noninflammatory	Inflammatory	Septic	Hemorrhagic
Volume, mL (knee)	<3.5	Often >3.5	Often >3.5	Often >3.5	Usually >3.5
Clarity	Transparent	Transparent	Translucent-opaque	Opaque	Bloody
Color	Clear	Yellow	Yellow to opalescent	Yellow to green	Red
Viscosity	High	High	Low	Variable	Variable
WBC, per mm3	<200	200-2,000	2000-10,000	>100,000*	200-2,000
PMNs, percent	<25	<25	≥50	≥75	50-75
Culture	Negative	Negative	Negative	Often positive	Negative
Total protein, g/dL	1-2	1-3	3-5	3-5	4-6
LDH (compared to levels in blood)	Very low	Very low	High	Variable	Similar
Glucose, mg/dL	Nearly equal to blood	Nearly equal to blood	>25, lower than blood	<25, much lower than blood	Nearly equal to blood

LDH, Lactic dehydrogenase; PMN, polymorphonuclear cell; WBC, white blood cell.
*Lower with infections caused by partially treated or low virulence organisms

TABLE A-4

SUMMARY OF THYROID-STIMULATING HORMONE TEST RESULTS AND INTERPRETATIONS

TSH	T4	T3	Interpretation
High	Normal	Normal	Mild (subclinical) hypothyroidism
High	Low	Low or normal	Hypothyroidism
Low	Normal	Normal	Mild (subclinical) hyperthyroidism
Low	High or normal	High or normal	Hyperthyroidism
Low	Low or normal	Low or normal	Rare pituitary (secondary) hypothyroidism

T3, Triiodothyronine; *T4*, thyroxine; *TSH*, thyroid-stimulating hormone.

TABLE A-5

SUMMARY OF THYROXINE (T4) TEST RESULTS AND INTERPRETATIONS

T4	TSH	T3	Interpretation
Normal	High	Normal	Mild (subclinical) hypothyroidism
Low	High	Low or normal	Hypothyroidism
Normal	Low	Normal	Mild (subclinical) hyperthyroidism
High or normal	Low	High or normal	Hyperthyroidism
Low or normal	Low	Low or normal	Rare pituitary (secondary) hypothyroidism

T3, Triiodothyronine; *T4*, thyroxine; *TSH*, thyroid-stimulating hormone.

TABLE A-6

SUMMARY OF TRIIODOTHYRONINE (T3) TEST RESULTS AND INTERPRETATIONS

T3	T4	TSH	Interpretation
Normal	Normal	High	Mild (subclinical) hypothyroidism
Low or normal	Low	High	Hypothyroidism
Normal	Normal	Low	Mild (subclinical) hyperthyroidism
High or normal	High or normal	Low	Hyperthyroidism
Low or normal	Low or normal	Low	Rare pituitary (secondary) hypothyroidism

T3, Triiodothyronine; *T4,* thyroxine; *TSH,* thyroid-stimulating hormone.

GLOSSARY OF ABBREVIATIONS

A

a	artery, before
aa	equal part of each
AA	affected area
AAA	abdominal aortic aneurysm
A2	aortic second sound
AAL	acute lymphoblastic, leukemia, anterior axillary line
ab	antibody
abd	abdomen
ABG	arterial blood gasses
ABN	abnormal
ABP	arterial blood pressure
abs	absent
a/c.	before meals (ante sebum)
Ac	acute
AC	anterior chamber
acc	accident
accom	accommodation
acid phos	acid phosphate
ACL	anterior cruciate ligament
ACTH	adrenocorticotrophic hormone
AD	right ear
add.	abductor or abduction
ADH	antidiuretic hormone
ADL	activates of daily living
ad lib	as desired
adm.	admission
AE	above elbow
AEA	above elbow amputation
AF	atrial fibrillation, afebrile
AFB	acid fast bacilli
AFO	ankle-foot orthosis
A/G	albumin globulin ratio (blood)
AI	aortic insufficiency
AIDS	acquired immunodeficiency syndrome
AJ	ankle jerk
a.k.	above knee
aka	alcoholic ketoacidosis

AKA	above knee amputation
alb.	albumin
alc.	alcohol
alk. phos.	alkaline phosphate
ALL	acute lymphocytic leukemia
ALS	amyotrophic lateral sclerosis
ALT	alternating with, alanine aminotransferase (formerly serum glutamate pyruvate transaminase [SGPT])
AMA	against medical advice
amb.	ambulating, ambulatory
AMI	acute myocardial infarction
AML	acute myeloid leukemia
amp.	amputation, ampule
ANA	antinuclear antibody
anes.	anesthesia
ann. fib.	annulus fibrosis
ANS	autonomic nervous system
ant.	anterior
ante	before
Anxty	anxiety
A/O	alert and oriented
AOB	alcohol on breath
AODM	adult onset diabetes mellitus
A&P	auscultation and percussion
AP	anteroposterior
APC	atrial premature contractions
aph	aphasia
AP & lat	anteroposterior and lateral
aq.	water
AR	aortic regurgitation
ARD	acute respiratory distress
ARDS	adult respiratory distress syndrome
ARF	acute respiratory failure, acute rheumatic fever
art	arterial
AS	left ear, aortic stenosis
ASA	acetylsalicylic acid, aspirin
A.S.A. 1	normal healthy patient
A.S.A. 2	patient with mild systemic disease
A.S.A. 3	patient with severe systemic disease
A.S.A. 4	patient with incapacitating systemic disease that is constant threat to life

ASAP	as soon as possible
ASCVD	atherosclerotic cardiovascular disease
ASD	atrial septal defect
ASHD	arteriosclerotic heart disease
ATNR	asymmetrical tonic neck reflex
AU	both ears
aud.	auditory
Aur. Fib	auricular fibrillation
A-V	arteriovenous
AVF	arteriovenous fistula
AVR	aortic valve replacement
Ax.	axilla, axillary

B

B.	bath
BA	barium
Bab.	Babinski sign
Ba.E	barium enema
Bas.	basal, basilar
baso	basophile
BBB	bundle branch block
BBT	basal body temperature
BCA	basal cell atypia
BCD	basal cell dysplasia
BCE	basal cell epithelioma
BDC	burn dressing change
BE	below elbow, barium enema
BEA	below elbow amputation
BFP	biological false positive
Bic.	biceps
b.i.d.	twice daily
BIH	bilateral inguinal hernia
bilat.	bilateral, bilaterally
bili	bilirubin
b.i.n.	twice a night
BiW	twice weekly
BJ	biceps reflex
bk.	back
BK	below knee
BKA	below knee amputation
bl cult	blood culture

bld.	blood
Bl.T	bleeding time
BM	black male, bone marrow, bowel movement
BMR	basal metabolic rate
body wt.	body weight
BOMA	otitis media, both ears, acute
BP	blood pressure
BPD	bronchopulmonary dysplasia
BPH	benign prostatic hypertrophy
BPM	beats per minute
BR	bedrest, bathroom
brach.	brachial
broncho	bronchoscopy
BS	blood sugar, bowel sounds
B.S.	breath sounds
BSA	body surface area
BST	blood serologic test
BT	bleeding time
BUN	blood urea nitrogen
Bx.	biopsy

C

c.	with
C	cervical, Caucasian
C.	centigrade, Celsius complement
CI-XII	first to twelfth cranial nerve
C–1 to C–7	cervical vertebrae
Ca	calcium
CA	carcinoma, cancer
CABG	coronary artery bypass graft
CAD	coronary artery disease
CAHD	coronary atherosclerotic heart disease
Cal	calorie, calories
CAPD	continuous ambulatory peritoneal dialysis
Caps	capsules
car.	carotid
card.	cardiac
Card Cath	cardiac catheterization
CAT	computerized axial tomography
cath	catheterization, catheter
CBC	complete blood count
CBD	common bile duct

CBF	cerebral blood flow
CBG	capillary blood gas
CBR	complete bed rest
cc.	cubic centimeter
CC	chief complaint
CCU	coronary care unit
CD	cardiac disease, contagious disease
CEA	carcinoembryonic antigen
Cerv.	cervix, cervical
CF	cardiac failure, cystic fibrosis
CHD	congenital heart disease, coronary heart disease
Chem.	chemotherapy
CHF	congestive heart failure
CHO	carbohydrate
Chol	cholesterol
Chr	chronic
C.I	color index
CI	cardiac insufficiency, cardiac index
CIS	carcinoma in situ
CK	creatinine kinase
Cl	chlorine, chloride
Clav.	clavicle
cldy	cloudy
CLL	chronic lymphocytic leukemia
Cl.T	clotting time
cm.	centimeter
CML	chronic myeloid leukemia
CMV	cytomegalovirus
CN	cranial nerve
CNS	central nervous system
cnst.	constipation
c/o	complains of, complaints
CO_2	carbon dioxide
comb.	combine, combination
comm.	communicable
comp.	compound, compress
conc.	concentrated
cons.	consultation
cont.	contractions, continued
COPD	chronic obstructive pulmonary disease
Cor	heart
CPAP	continuous positive airway pressure

CPC	clinicopathological conference
CPK	creatinine phosphokinase
CPPB	continuous positive pressure breathing
CPR	cardiopulmonary resuscitation
CPT	chest physical therapy
CR	closed reduction
cran.	cranial
CRD	chronic respiratory disease
creat.	creatinine
CRF	chronic renal failure
C/S, CS	cesarean section
C&S	culture and sensitivity
CSF	cerebrospinal fluid
C-spine	cervical spine
CT	computed axial tomography
CV	cardiovascular
CVA	cerebrovascular accident, costovertebral angle
CVL	central venous line
CVP	central venous pressure
CVS	cardiovascular system
Cx	cervix, culture
CxR	chest x-ray
Cysto	cystoscopy

D

DAP	distal airway pressure
db.	decibel
DBE	deep breathing exercise
d/c	discontinue
DC	discharges, discontinue
DD	discharge diagnosis
DDx	differential diagnosis
decr.	decreased
dehyd.	dehydrated
Derm.	dermatology
DES	diethylstilbestrol
DI	diabetes insipidus, diagnostic imaging
DIAG.	diagnosis
diam.	diameter
DIC	disseminated intravascular coagulation, disseminated coagulopathy
diff.	differential

dil.	dilute
dim.	diminished
DIP	distal interphalangeal (joint)
dis.	disease
disch.	discharge
disp.	disposition
dist.	distilled, distal
div.	divorced
DJD	degenerative joint disease
DKA	diabetic ketoacidosis
DLE	disseminated lupus erythematosus
D/L DI	deciliter
DM	diabetes mellitus, diastolic murmur
DNA	deoxyribonucleic acid
DNKA	did not keep appointment
DOB	date of birth
DOE	dyspnea on exertion
Dors	dorsal
D.P.	dorsal pedia
DPT	diphtheria, pertussis, tetanus vaccine
drsg.	dressing
D/S	discharge summary
DTR	deep tendon reflexes
DTs	delirium tremens
DUI	driving under influence
Dx	diagnosis

E

e	without
EBV	Epstein-Barr virus
ECG	electrocardiogram
ECHO	enterocytopathogenic human orphan virus
E. coli	*Escherichia coli*
ED	emergency department
EEG	electroencephalogram
EENT	eyes, ears, nose, throat
EEX	electrodiagnosis
EKG	electrocardiogram
elev.	elevated
EMG	electromyogram
ENT	ears, nose, throat
Eoc.	eosinophiles

EOM	extraocular movement
ESR	erythrocyte sedimentation rate
ETIOL.	etiology
ETOH	ethanol
EVAL	evaluation
ex.	exercise, example
ext.	extremities, external

F

F	finger, female, Fahrenheit
FA	fluorescent antibody
F.A.	first aid
F.B.	foreign body
FBS	fasting blood sugar
FDP	flexor digitorum profundus
Fe def.	iron deficiency
FEF	forced expiratory flow
fem.	femoral
fem. pop.	femoral popliteal
FEV	forced expiratory volume
f.f.	force fluid
FH	family history, fetal heart
Fio_2	faction of inspired oxygen concentration
fl.	fluids
flac.	flaccid
flex.	flexor, flexion
fl. oz.	fluid ounce
FM	finger movement
fract.	fractional
FRC	functional residual capacity
FS	finger stick
FSH	follicle stimulating hormone
F/U, F-U, F.U.	follow-up
FUO	fever of unknown origin
FVC	forced vital capacity
Fx	fracture

G

G.A.	general anesthesia
GB	gallbladder
GBS	gallbladder series

G.C.	gonococcus
GCS	Glasgow Coma Scale
GE	gastroenterology
G/E	gastroenteritis
gen, genl.	general
GFR	glomerular filtration rate
GI	gastrointestinal
gluc	glucose
gm	gram
Gm+	gram positive
Gm–	gram negative
gm.%	grams per 100 cc
GMA	grand mal attack
Gt.tr.	gait training
GSW	gunshot wound
GTT	glucose tolerance test
GU	genitourinary
G/W	glucose and water

H

h	hour
H	hydrogen history, hour, hypodermic
H/A	headache
HASCVD	hypertensive arteriosclerotic cardiovascular disease
Hb., Hgb	hemoglobin
HB	heart block
HBP	high blood pressure
H&C	hot and cold
HCO_3	bicarbonate
Hct.	hematocrit
HCVD	hypertensive cardiovascular disease
h.d.	at bedtime
Hd	head, Hodgkin disease
HDL	high density lipids
HEENT	head, eyes, ears, nose, throat
hern.	hernia
Hem	hematology
Hem Pro	hematology profile
HH	hard of hearing
hist.	history, histology
HIV	human immunodeficiency virus

HKAFO	hip knee ankle foot orthosis
HLA	human leukocyte group A, histocompatibility leukocyte focus
HM	hand movement
HNP	herniated nucleus pulposus
h/o	history of
HOB	head of bed
horiz.	horizontal
H&P	history and physical
HPI	history of present illness
HR	heart rate
H.R.S.T.	heat, reddening, swelling, tenderness
HS	bedtime
H_2O	water
H_2O_2	hydrogen peroxide
Ht	height, heart
HVD	hypertensive vascular disease
Hx	history
Hz	hertz (cycles/second)

I

I	radioactive iodine
IA	intra-arterially
IABP	intra-aortic balloon pump
i.c.	intracutaneous(ly)
ICCU	intensive coronary care unit
ICF	intracellular fluid
ICS	intercostal space
ICU	intensive care unit
i.d.	during the day
ID	intradermal, identification, infectious disease
IDDM	insulin dependent diabetes mellitus
I/E	inspiratory, expiratory
Ig	immunoglobulin
IGA	immunoglobulin A
IGE	immunoglobulin E
IGG	immunoglobulin gamma
G	globulin
IGM	immunoglobulin M
IH	infectious hepatitis
IHD	ischemic heart disease

IM	intramuscular, intramedullary
imp.	impression
In.	inches
incr.	increased (ing)
inf	infusion, inferior
inj	injured, injection
inspir	inspiration, inspiratory
int.	internal
INTHC	intrathecally
IO	inferior oblique
IPJ	interphalangeal joint
irreg.	irregular
IS	intercostal space
IST	insulin shock therapy
ITP	idiopathic thrombocytopenic purpura
I, U., IU	International Unit
IV	intravenous(ly)
IVD	intervertebral disc

J

J	joint
JRA	juvenile rheumatoid arthritis
jt.	joint
JVP	jugular venous pulse

K

K	potassium, kidney
KC1	potassium chloride
Kcal.	kilocalorie, calorie
Kg.	kg. kilogram
KJ, K-J	knee jerk
KK	knee kick
17 KS	17 keto steroids
KUB	kidney, ureter, bladder (x-rays)

L

L	left, liver, liter, lower, light, lumbar
L2, L3	second, third lumbar vertebrae
LA	left antrum
lab.	laboratory
lac.	laceration

LAD	left anterior descending coronary artery
lam.	laminectomy
lat.	lateral
lb.	pound
LBP	lower back pain
LCA	left coronary artery
L.D.	lethal dose
LDH	lactic dehydrogenase
LDL	low density lipids
LE	lupus erythematosus
L.E.	lower extremities
leuc.	leukocytes
lg	large, leg
LICS	left intercostal space
lig.	ligament
LIH	left inguinal hernia
liq.	liquid
LKS	liver, kidneys, spleen
LLE	left lower extremity
LLG	left lateral gaze
LLL	left lower lobe
LLQ	left lower quadrant
LMA	left mentoanterior
l/min	liter per minute
LML	left mediolateral
LMP	left mentoposterior, last menstrual period
LMT	left mentotransverse
L.N.	lymph node
LNMP	last normal menstrual period
L.O.C.	loss of consciousness, level of consciousness, laxative of choice
LOM	left otitis media
LOP	left occipital posterior
LOS	length of stay
LP	lumbar puncture, light perception
LRQ	lower right quadrant
L.S.	lumbosacral
LSA	lateral sacrum anterior
LSK	liver, spleen, kidneys
LSP	left sacrum posterior
LST	left sacrum transverse
Lt.	left, light

LUE	left upper extremity
LUL	left upper lobe
LUQ	left upper quadrant
Lymphs	lymphocytes
lytes	electrolytes

M

m.	minimum
m, M	married, male, mother murmur, meter, mass, molar
MA	mental age
macro.	macrocytic, macroscopic
MAP	mean arterial pressure
max.	maximum, maxillary
mcg.	microgram
MCH	mean corpuscular hemoglobin
MCHC	mean corpuscular hemoglobin concentration
MCL	midclavicular line
MCP	metacarpophalangeal joint
MCV	mean corpuscular volume
MD	muscular dystrophy
Mdnt.	midnight
ME	middle ear, medical examiner
Med.	medicine
MEq/L	milliequivalents per liter
Mets.	metastasis
mg.	milligram
Mg.	magnesium
MG	myasthenia gravis
mg/dl	milligrams per deciliter
mg.%	milligrams per 100 cc
Ml	myocardial infarction, mitral insufficiency
micro	microcytic, microscopic
Min	minute
ml.	milliliter
mm	millimeter
mm.	muscles
MMPI	Minnesota Multiphasic Personality Inventory
mod	moderate
mono.	monocyte
MP	metacarpophalangeal
MRI	magnetic resonance imaging
mss	massage

MT	metacarpophalangeal (joint)
M.T.	muscles and tendons
MVA	motor vehicle accident

N

n.	nerve
N2	nitrogen
N_2O	nitrous oxide (anesthetic)
Na	sodium
NaCl	sodium chloride
NED	no evidence of disease
neg.	negative
NER	no evidence of recurrence
NERD	no evidence of recurrent disease
Neur.	neurology
NKA	no known allergies
NM	neuromuscular
NMR	nuclear magnetic resonance
noct.	nocturnal
NOS	not otherwise specified
Ns.	nerves
N.S.	nervous system
NSA	no significant abnormality
NSAID	nonsteroidal anti-inflammatory drug
N&V	nausea and vomiting
NS	neurosurgery
NTP	normal temperature and pressure
NVD	nausea, vomiting, diarrhea
NWB	non–weight-bearing
NYD	not yet diagnosed

O

o	none, without
O	oral
O2	oxygen
O_2 cap.	oxygen capacity
O_2 sat.	oxygen saturation
OA	osteoarthritis
Obs	observation
OCC.	occipital, occasional
O/E	on examination
OH	occupational history

OOB	out of bed
Op.	operation
OR	operating room, open reduction
OR-IF	open reduction with internal fixation
Ortho.	orthopedic surgery
os	opening, mouth, bone
OTC	over-the-counter (pharmaceuticals)
O.T.	occupational therapy, old tuberculin
oz.	ounce

P

P	after, phosphorus pulse
PA	posteroanterior
p & a	percussion and auscultation
palp.	palpate, palpated, palpable
Path.	pathology
PA view	posterior-anterior view on x-ray
Pb	lead
PBI	protein bound iodine
p/c., p.c.	after meals
PCL	posterior cruciate ligament
PCo_2	carbon dioxide concentration
PCV	packed cell volume (of blood)
PE	physical examination, pulmonary embolism
PERRLA	pupils equal, round, reactive to light and accommodation (normal)
PET	positron emission tomography
PH	past history
PID	pelvic inflammatory disease
PIP	proximal interphalangeal
plts.	platelets
P.M.	afternoon, post-mortem
PMH	past medical history
PMN	polymorphonuclear (leukocytes)
PM&R	physical medicine and rehabilitation
PNI	peripheral nerve injury
POMR	problem oriented medical record
poplit.	popliteal
pos.	positive
post.	posterior
PRE	progressive resistive exercise
p.r.m.	according to circumstances

p.r.n., PRN	as often as necessary
prod.	productive
Prog.	prognosis
PROM	passive range of motion, premature rupture of membranes
pron.	pronator, pronation
pros.	prostate, prostatic
prosth.	prosthesis
prot.	protein, Protestant
pro.time	prothrombin time
PSH	past surgical history
psi	pounds per square inch
PSMA	progressive spinal muscular atrophy
pt., Pt.	patient
PT	physical therapy
P.T.	physical therapy, posterior tibial artery pulse
PTB	patellar tendon bearing
PTCA	percutaneous transvenous coronary angioplasty (balloon angioplasty)
PVD	peripheral vascular disease
PVT	previous trouble
PWB%	partial weight bearing with percent
Px, PX	physical examination

Q

q	every
q.d.	every day
q.h.	every hour
q2h	every two hours
q4h	every four hours
q.i.d.	four times a day
q.i.w.	four times a week
q.l.	as much as desired
qn, q.n.	every night
q.n.s., QNS	quantity not sufficient
q.o.d.	every other day
q.o.n.	every other night
q.p.	as much as you please
q.q., Q.Q.	each, every
q.q.h.	every four hours
q.s.	quantity, sufficient
qt.	quart

qts.	drops
quad.	quadriplegic
quant.	quantitative or quantity
q.v.	as much as you wish
q.w.	every week

R

r., R	right, rectal, roentgen, x-ray
RA	rheumatoid arthritis, right atrium
rad.	radial
r.a.m.	rapid alternating movements
R.A.S.	right arm sitting
rbc, RBC	red blood count, red blood cell
RE	reconditioning exercise
reg.	regular
rehab.	rehabilitation
resp.	respiratory, respirations
RF	rheumatic fever
R to L&A	react to light and accommodation
RLE	right lower extremity
RMSF	Rocky Mountain spotted fever
RNA	ribonucleic acid
RO, R/O	rule out
ROM	range of motion, rupture of membranes,
ROS	review of systems
RRE, RR&E	round, regular, and equal
RSD	reflex sympathetic dystrophy
Rt.	right
RUE	right upper extremity
Rx	therapy, prescription

S

s	without
S	sensation, sensitive, serum
sec	second
sed.	rate erythrocyte sedimentation rate
Sens.	sensory, sensation
Serol.	serology, serological test
SGOT, SGO-T	serum glutamic oxalacetic transaminase
SH	social history, serum hepatitis
SI	sacroiliac joint, stroke index
SIDS	sudden infant death syndrome

skel.	skeletal
SLE	systemic lupus erythematosus
SLR	straight leg raising
sm	small
SMA-14	routine admission chemistry
SNS	sympathetic nervous system
S.O.A.P.	subjective, objective assessment plan
SOB	shortness of breath
sp.	spine, spinal
sp.cd.	spinal cord
stat., STAT	immediately
STD	sexually transmitted disease
sup.	superior
supin.	supination
SWD	short wave diathermy
Sx	symptoms
sys.	system

T

T3	triiodothyronine
T4	total serum thyroxine
TA	tendon Achilles
T&A	tonsils and adenoids, tonsillectomy and adenoidectomy
tab.	tablet
TB	tuberculosis
tbsp.	tablespoon
TCDB	turn, cough, deep breathe
temp	temperature
TENS	transient electric nerve stimulation
T.F.	tuning fork
THERAP.	therapy, therapeutic
thor.	thorax, thoracic
THR	total hip replacement
TIA	transient ischemic shock, transient ischemic attack
t.i.d.	three times a day
TIP	terminal interphalangeal (joint)
t.i.w.	three times per week
TJ	triceps reflex
TKR	total knee replacement
TMJ	temporomandibular joint
TPR	temperature, pulse, respiration

tr	trace
TSH	thyroid stimulating hormone
tsp.	teaspoon
TSS	toxic shock syndrome
Tx	treatment, traction

U

U.	unit
U/A	urinalysis
UCD	usual childhood diseases
UCHD	usual childhood diseases
uln	ulnar
ULQ	upper left quadrant
unilat.	unilateral
Ur.	urine
URD	upper respiratory disease
URI	upper respiratory infection
Urol.	urology
URQ	upper right quadrant
u/s, US	ultrasound
UTI	urinary tract infection
UVL	ultraviolet light

V

V	vein
VA	visual acuity
VC, (vit.cap)	vital capacity
VD	venereal disease
VDRL	venereal disease research laboratory test; blood test for syphilis
vert.	vertical
Via	by way of
vit.	vitamin
VLDL	very-low-density lipoproteins
vol	volume
VS, V.S.	vital signs

W

W	widowed, white
wbc, WBC	white blood count, white blood cell
WBT	weight bearing to tolerance
WF	white female

wk	week
WM	white male
w/n	within
WN	well nourished
WNL	within normal limits
WP	whirlpool
wt.	weight
w/u	workup

X

x	times

Y

y.o.	years old
yrs.	years

BIBLIOGRAPHY

Abenhaim L et al: The prognostic consequences in the making of the initial medical diagnosis of work-related back injuries, *Spine* 20:791, 1994.

Abrahams S, H Kern J: Anterior knee pain: plica syndrome, the forgotten pathology? *Physiotherapy* 87(10):523-528, 2001.

Abramowitz JS, Moore EL: An experimental analysis of hypochondriasis, *Behav Res Ther* 45(3):413-424, 2007.

Abrams WB, Berkow R: *The Merck manual of geriatrics,* Rahway, NJ, 1990, Merck Sharp & Dohme Research Laboratories.

Adachi N et al: The complete type of suprapatellar plica in a professional baseball pitcher: consideration of a cause of anterior knee pain, *Arthroscopy* 20(9):987-991, 2004.

Adams JA: Transient synovitis of the hip joint in children, *J Bone Joint Surg* 45B:471, 1963.

Adams JC, Hamblen DL: *Outline of orthopaedics,* ed 11, Edinburgh, 1990, Churchill Livingstone.

Adams JC: *Standard orthopaedic operations,* Edinburgh, 1985, Churchill Livingstone.

Adams RD, Victor M: *Principles of neurology,* ed 3, New York, 1985, McGraw-Hill.

Adams RD: *Diseases of muscle,* ed 3, London, 1975, Henry Kimpton.

Adolfsson L: Ganglion cyst communicating with the elbow joint presenting as a distal forearm tumour, *J Hand Surg* 22(4):552-554, 1997.

Aegerter E, Kirkpatrick JA: *Orthopaedic diseases,* ed 3, Philadelphia, 1968, WB Saunders.

Agee JM et al: Endoscopic release of the carpal tunnel: a randomized prospective multicenter study, *J Hand Surg* 17A:987, 1992.

Agency for Health Care Policy and Research, Public Health Service, U.S. Department of Health and Human Services: Diagnostic imaging for low back pain gets mixed review, *Res Activities* 12:3, 1990.

Agency for Health Care Policy and Research, Public Health Services, U.S. Department of Health and Human Services: *Acute low back pain in adults, Clinical Practice Guideline. Number 14,* Rockville, 1994, AHCPR Publication No. 95-0642, The Agency.

Agnew LRC, editor: *Dorland's illustrated medical dictionary,* ed 27, Philadelphia, 1988, WB Saunders.

Agur A, editor: *Grant's atlas of anatomy,* Baltimore, 1991, Williams & Wilkins.

Ahmad CS et al: Factors affecting dropped biceps deformity after tenotomy of the long head of the biceps tendon, *Arthroscopy* 23(5):537-541, 2007.

Ahwee Leftwich S et al: High incidence disabilities: placement determinants and implications for instruction and service delivery. In *Advances in learning and behavioral disabilities,* vol 18, Greenwich, Conn, 2005, JAI.

Akbas M, Yegin A, Karsli B: 778 reflex sympathetic dystrophy in a 10 year old pediatric, *Eur J Pain* 10(suppl 1):S202-S203, 2006.

Alaranta H et al: A prospective study of patients with sciatica: a comparison between conservatively treated patients and patients who have undergone operation, III, results after one year follow-up, *Spine* 15:1245, 1990.

Alario AJ: *Practical guide to the care of the pediatric patient,* St Louis, 1997, Mosby.

Albeck MJU et al: A controlled comparison of myelography, computed tomography, and magnetic resonance imaging in clinically suspected lumbar disc herniation, *Spine* 20:443, 1995.

Alberti A: Headache and sleep, *Sleep Med Rev* 10(6):431-437, 2006.

Alexander CJ: The etiology of femoral epiphyseal slipping, *J Bone Joint Surg* 48B:299, 1966.

Alexander E Jr, Davis CH: Reduction and fusion of fracture of the odontoid process, *J Neurosurg* 31:580, 1969.

Allaire SH et al: Management of work disability, resources for vocational rehabilitation, *Arthritis Rheum* 36:1663, 1993.

Allen AA, Warner JJP: Management of the stiff shoulder, *Oper Tech Orthop* 5(3): 238-247, 1995.

Allen BL et al: A mechanistic classification of closed indirect fractures and dislocations of the lower cervical spine, *Spine* 7:1, 1982.

Allison D, Strickland N: *Acronyms & synonyms in medical imaging,* Oxford, UK, 1996, ISIS Medical Media.

Allman LF: *Back school program: introduction to back injuries,* Atlanta, 1990, Atlanta Sports Medicine Clinic, PC.

Alricsson M, Werner S: Young elite cross-country skiers and low back pain—a 5-year study, *Phys Ther Sport* 7(4):181-184, 2006.

Altchek DW et al: Arthroscopic acromioplasty: technique and results, *J Bone Joint Surg* 72A:1198, 1990.

Altman RD: Musculoskeletal questions and answers, *J Musculoskeletal Med* 7:10, 1990.

Amadio PC: The Mayo Clinic and carpal tunnel syndrome, *Mayo Clin Proc* 67:42, 1992.

American Academy of Orthopaedic Surgeons: *Atlas of limb prosthetics,* St Louis, 1981, Mosby.

American Academy of Orthopaedic Surgeons: *Instructional course lectures,* vol 37, Chicago, 1988, AAOS.

American Academy of Orthopaedic Surgeons: *Joint motion: method of measuring and recording,* Edinburgh, 1965, British Orthopaedic Association.

American Board of Chiropractic Orthopedists: *Proceedings 1997,* New Orleans, 1997, American Board of Chiropractic Orthopedists.

American College of Sports Medicine: *Guidelines for exercise testing and prescription,* ed 4, Philadelphia, 1991, Lea & Febiger.

American Medical Association: *Guides to the evaluation of permanent impairment,* ed 4, Chicago, 1993, American Medical Association.

American Medical Association: *How to use guides to the evaluation of permanent impairment,* ed 4, Falmouth, Conn, 1993, SEAK.

American Orthopaedic Association: *Manual of orthopaedic surgery,* Chicago, 1972, American Orthopaedic Association.

American Psychiatric Association: *Diagnostic and statistical manual of mental disorders,* ed 3, Washington, 1980, American Orthopaedic Association.

American Society for Surgery of the Hand: *The hand examination and diagnosis,* Aurora, Colo, 1978.

Ames MD, Schut L: Results of treatment of 171 consecutive myelomeningoceles, *Pediatrics* 50:466, 1972.

Aminoff MJ: *Electrodiagnosis in clinical neurology,* ed 2, New York, 1986, Churchill Livingstone.

Ammann W, Matheson GO: Radionuclide bone imaging in the detection of stress fractures, *Clin J Sport Med* 1:115, 1991.

Amundsen T: Lumbar spinal stenosis: clinical and radiologic features, *Spine* 10:1178, 1995.

Amyes EW, Anderson FM: Fracture of the odontoid process of the axis, *J Bone Joint Surg* 56A:1663, 1974.

Anderson B, Kayes S: Treatment of flexor tenosynovitis of the hand trigger finger with corticosteroids: a prospective study of the response to local injection, *Arch Intern Med* 151:153, 1991.

Anderson GH et al: Preoperative skin traction for fractures of the proximal femur, a randomized prospective trial, *J Bone Joint Surg* 75B:794, 1993.

Anderson KN, Anderson LE: *Mosby's pocket dictionary of medicine, nursing, & allied health,* ed 2, St Louis, 1994, Mosby.

Anderson PA et al: Flexion distraction and chance injuries to the thoracolumbar spine, *J Orthop Trauma* 5:153, 1991.

Andersson G: The epidemiology of spinal disorders. In Frymoyer J, editor: *The adult spine,* New York, 1991, Raven.

Andersson GBJ: Occupational biomechanics. In Weinstein J, Wiesel SW, editors: *The lumbar spine,* Philadelphia, 1990, WB Saunders.

Andersson GBJ: The epidemiology of spinal disorders. In Frymoyer JW, editor: *The adult spine: principles and practice,* New York, 1990, Raven.

Andrews JR, Whiteside JA, Buettner CM: Clinical evaluation of the elbow in throwers, *Oper Tech Sports Med* 4(2):77-83, 1996.

Andrikoula SI et al: Intra-articular ganglia of the knee joint associated with the anterior cruciate ligament: a report of 4 cases in 3 patients, *Arthroscopy* (in press, corrected proof).

Andrish JT: The leg. In DeLee JD, Drez D editors: *Orthopaedic sports medicine, principles and practice,* vol 2, Philadelphia, 1994, WB Saunders.

Angelo RL, Soffer SR: Elbow anatomy relative to arthroscopy. In Andrews Jr, Soffer SR, editors: *Elbow arthroscopy,* St Louis, 1994, Mosby.

Aniel DM, Fritschy D: Anterior cruciate ligament injuries. In DeLee JC, Drez D, editors: *Orthopaedic sports medicine: principles and practice,* vol 2, Philadelphia, 1994, WB Saunders.

Ankarath S: Chronic wrist pain: diagnosis and management, *Curr Orthop* 20(2):141-151, 2006.

Ansel BM: Rheumatic disorders in childhood, *Clin Rheum Dis* 2:303, 1976.

Aoki M, Okamura K, Yamashita T: Snapping annular ligament of the elbow joint in the throwing arms of young brothers, *Arthroscopy* 19(8):e89-e92, 2003.

Aoki M et al: Magnetic resonance imaging findings of refractory tennis elbows and their relationship to surgical treatment, *J Shoulder Elbow Surg* 14(2):172-177, 2005.

Apfelberg DB, Larson SJ: Dynamic anatomy of the ulnar nerve at the elbow, *Plast Reconstr Surg* 51:76, 1973.

Apley AG, Solomon L: *Concise system of orthopaedics and fractures,* London, 1988, Butterworth-Heinemann.

Appelrouth D, Gottlieb NL: Pulmonary manifestations of ankylosing spondylitis, *J Rheumatol* 2:446, 1975.

Apps BK, Cohen BB, Steel CM: *Biochemistry, a concise test for medical students,* ed 5, Iowa City, Iowa, 1992, Bailliere Tindall.

Aprill C: Diagnostic disc injection. In Frymoyer JW, editor: *The adult spine: principles and practice,* New York, 1991, Raven.

Arabi A et al: Discriminative ability of dual-energy x-ray absorptiometry site selection in identifying patients with osteoporotic fractures, *Bone* 40(4):1060-1065, 2007.

Arbisi PA, Butcher JN: Failure of the FBS to predict malingering of somatic symptoms: response to critiques by Greve and Bianchini and Lees Haley and Fox, *Arch Clin Neuropsychol* 19(3):341-345, 2004.

Arnbjornson A et al: The natural history of recurrent dislocation of the patella, long-term results of conservative and operative treatment, *J Bone Joint Surg* 74B:140, 1992.

Arner M, Jonsson K, Aspenberg P: Complete palmar dislocation of the lunate in rheumatoid arthritis: avascularity without avascular changes, *J Hand Surg* 21(3): 384-387, 1996.

Arntz CT, Jackins S, Matsen FA III: Prosthetic replacement of the shoulder for the treatment of defects in rotator cuff and the surface of the glenohumeral joint, *J Bone Joint Surg* 75A:485, 1993.

Arokoski JPA et al: Postural control in male patients with hip osteoarthritis, *Gait Posture* 23(1):45-50, 2006.

Aronoff GM et al: Pain treatment programs: do they run workers to the workplace? *Spine* 2:123, 1987.

Aronoff GM: *Evaluation and treatment of chronic pain,* Baltimore, 1985, Urban and Schwartzenberg.

Arrigoni P, Brady PC, Burkhart SS: Calcific tendonitis of the subscapularis tendon causing subcoracoid stenosis and coracoid impingement, *Arthroscopy* 22(10):1139. e1-1139.e3, 2006.

Asbury AK, McKhann GM, McDonald WI: *Disease of the nervous system,* Philadelphia, 1986, WB Saunders.

Ashford RF, Nagelburg S, Adkins R: Sensitivity of the Jamar dynamometer in detecting submaximal grip effort, *J Hand Surg* 21(3):402-405, 1996.

Askenasy HM, Braham MJ, Kosary IZ: Delayed spinal myelopathy after atlanto-axial fracture dislocation, *J Neurosurg* 17:1100, 1960.

Assimakopoulos A et al: The innervation of the human meniscus, *Clin Orthop* 275:232, 1992.

Aston JN: *A short textbook of orthopaedics and traumatology,* Philadelphia, 1967, JB Lippincott.

Atkinson G, Davenne D: Relationships between sleep, physical activity and human health, *Physiol Behav* 90(2-3):229-235, 2007.

Atkinson G, Nevill A, Hopkins WG: Typical error versus limits of agreement, *Sports Med* 30(5):375-381, 2000.

Atkinson G, Nevill AM: Statistical methods for assessing measurement error (reliability) in variables relevant to sports medicine, *Sports Med* 26(4):217-238, 1998.

Aulicino P: Neurovascular injuries in the hands of athletes, *Hand Clin* 6:455, 1990.

Auvin S et al: Neuropathological and MRI findings in an acute presentation of hemiconvulsion-hemiplegia: a report with pathophysiological implications, *Seizure* 16(4):371-376, 2007.

Avioli LV: Osteoporosis, pathogenesis and therapy. In Avioli LV, Vrane SM, editors: *Metabolic bone disease,* New York, 1977, Academic Press.

Avioli LV: Senile and post-menopausal osteoporosis, *Adv Intern Med* 21:391, 1976.

Avioli LV: Significance of osteoporosis: a growing national health care problem, *Orthop Rev* 21:1126, 1992.

Avramov AI et al: The effects of controlled mechanical loading on group II, III, and IV afferent units from the lumbar facet joint and surrounding tissue: an in vitro study, *J Bone Joint Surg* 74A:1465, 1992.

Aydogan M et al: Severe erosion of lumbar vertebral body because of a chronic ruptured abdominal aortic aneurysm, *Spine J* (in press, corrected proof).

Ba AM, LoTempio MM, Wang MB: Pharyngeal diverticulum as a sequela of anterior cervical fusion, *Otolaryngol Head Neck Surg* 131(2):P256-P257, 2004.

Bailey RW, Badgley CE: Stabilization of the cervical spine by anterior fusion, *J Bone Joint Surg* 42A:565, 1960.

Baird KS, Crossan JF, Ralston SH: Abnormal growth factor and cytokine expression in Dupuytren's contracture, *J Clin Pathol* 46:425, 1993.

Baird KS et al: T-cell-mediated response in Dupuytren's disease, *Lancet* 341:1622, 1993.

Baker AB, Joynt RJ: *Clinical neurology,* New York, 1985, Harper & Row.

Baker CL, Norwood LA, Hughston JC: Acute combined posterior and posterolateral instability of the knee, *Am J Sports Med* 12:204, 1984.

Baker PA, Watson SB: Functional gracilis flap in thenar reconstruction, *J Plast Reconstr Aesthet Surg* (in press, corrected proof).

Bakkum B, Cramer G: Muscles that influence the spine. In Cramer G, Darby S: *Basic and clinical anatomy of the spine, spinal cord, and ANS,* St Louis, 1995, Mosby.

Ballinger PW, editor: *Merrill's atlas of roentgenographic positions and standard radiologic procedures,* ed 8, St Louis, 1995, Mosby.

Ballou SP, Kushner I: C-reactive protein and the acute phase response, *Adv Intern Med* 37:313, 1992.

Barabis J: Therapist's management of thoracic outlet syndrome. In Hunter JM et al, editors: *Rehabilitation of the hand: surgery and therapy,* ed 3, St Louis, 1990, Mosby.

Barboi AC, Barkhaus PE: Electrodiagnostic testing in neuromuscular disorders, *Neurol Clin* 22(3):619-641, 2004.

Barkauskas VH et al: *Health & physical assessment,* ed 2, St Louis, 1998, Mosby.

Barker S et al: Guidance for pre-manipulative testing of the cervical spine, *Physiotherapy* 87(6):318-321, 2001.

Barlow TG: Congenital dislocation of the hip, *Hosp Med* 2:571, 1968.

Barnes R: Fracture of the neck of the femur, *J Bone Joint Surg* 49B:607, 1967.

Barnett CH, Davies DV, MacConaill MA: *Synovial joints: their structure and mechanics,* New York, 1961, Longmans Green.

Barnsley L, Lord S, Bogduk N: Whiplash injury, *Pain* 59:283, 1994.

Barnsley L et al: The prevalence of chronic cervical zygapophyseal joint pain after whiplash, *Spine* 10:20, 1995.

Barrack RL, Skinner HB: The sensory function of knee ligaments. In Daniel D et al, editors: *Knee ligaments: structure, function, injury and repair,* New York, 1990, Raven.

Barre JA: Le syndrome sympathique cervical posterieur et sa cause frequente, l'artherite cervicale, *Rev Neurol (Paris)* 33:1246, 1926.

Barton NJ: Arthroplasty of the forefoot in rheumatoid arthritis, *J Bone Joint Surg* 55B:126, 1973.

Bassett FH III et al: Talar impingement by the anteroinferior tibiofibular ligament: a cause of chronic pain in the ankle after inversion sprain, *J Bone Joint Surg* 72A:55, 1990.

Bateman JE: The diagnosis and treatment of ruptures of the rotator cuff, *Surg Clin North Am* 43:1523, 1963.

Bateman JE: *The shoulder and neck,* ed 2, Philadelphia, 1978, WB Saunders.

Bateman JE: *The shoulder and neck,* Philadelphia, 1972, WB Saunders.

Bateman JE: *Trauma to nerves in limbs,* Philadelphia, 1962, WB Saunders.

Batson OV: The function of the vertebral veins and their role in the spread of metastasis, *Ann Surg* 112:138, 1940.

Batt AK, Braham RA, Goodman C: Selected physical capacity norms for Australian football players at the non-elite level, *J Sci Med Sport* 10(2):119-126, 2007.

Battie MC, Bigos SJ: Industrial back pain complaints, *Orthop Clin North Am* 22:273, 1991.

Battie MC et al: Managing low back pain: attitudes and treatment preferences of physical therapist, *Phys Ther* 74:219, 1994.

Bauer DC et al: Factors associated with appendicular bone mass in older women, *Ann Intern Med* 118:657, 1993.

Baxter DE, Pfeiffer GB: Treatment of chronic heel pain by surgical release of the first branch of the lateral plantar nerve, *Clin Orthop* 279:229, 1992.

Baxter DE: *The foot and ankle in sport,* St Louis, 1995, Mosby.

Beal MC: The sacroiliac problem, review of anatomy, mechanics and diagnosis, *J Am Osteopath Assoc* 82:667, 1982.

Beals RK: The normal carrying angle of the elbow, *Clin Orthop* 119:194, 1976.

Beaman D et al: *Substance P innervation of lumbar facet joints.* Proceedings of the seventh annual meeting of North American Spine Society, Boston, July 9-11, 1991.

Beaton DE, O'Driscoll SW, Richards RR: Grip strength testing using the BTE work simulator and the Jamar dynamometer: a comparative study, *J Hand Surg* 20(2): 293-298, 1995.

Beattie P et al: Validity of derived measurements of leg-length differences obtained by the use of a tape measure, *Phys Ther* 70:150, 1990.

Bechman H et al: Getting the most from a 20-minute visit, *Am J Gastroenterol* 89: 662, 1994.

Bechtel R: Physical characteristics of the axial interosseous ligament of the human sacroiliac joint, *Spine J* 1(4):255-259, 2001.

Beckenbaugh RD et al: Kienbock's disease: the natural history of Kienbock's disease and consideration of lunate fractures, *Clin Orthop* 149:98, 1980.

Bednar DA, Orr FW, Simon GT: Observations on the pathomorphology of the thoracolumbar fascia in chronic mechanical back pain: a microscopic study, *Spine* 20:1161, 1995.

Beekman RA et al: Extensor mechanism slide for the treatment of proximal interphalangeal joint extension lag: an anatomic study, *J Hand Surg* 29(6):1063-1068, 2004.

Beeson PB, McDermott W: *Textbook of medicine,* ed 13, Philadelphia, 1971, WB Saunders.

Beetham WP et al: *Physical examination of the joints,* Philadelphia, 1965, WB Saunders.

Bell GR, Modic MT: Radiology of the lumbar spine. In Rothman RA, Sinecone FA, editors: *The spine,* ed 3, Philadelphia, 1992, WB Saunders.

Bell JA: Sensibility evaluation. In Hunter JM et al, editors: *Rehabilitation of the hand,* St Louis, 1978, Mosby.

Bellah RD et al: Low-back pain in adolescent patients: detection of stress injury to the pars interarticularis with SPECT, *Radiology* 180:509, 1991.

Belsole RJ et al: Computed analyses of the pathomechanics of scaphoid waist nonunions, *J Hand Surg* 16A:899, 1991.

Ben-Galim P et al: Hip-spine syndrome: the effect of total hip replacement surgery upon low back pain in patients with severe osteoarthritis of the hip, *Spine J* 6(5, suppl 1):31S-32S, 2006.

Benito MB, Gorricho BP: Acute mastoiditis: Increase in the incidence and complications, *Int J Pediatr Otorhinolaryngol* 71(7):1007-1011, 2007.

Benjamin HJ, Hang BT: Common acute upper extremity injuries in sports, *Clin Pediatr Emerg Med* 8(1):15-30, 2007.

Bennell K et al: The nature of anterior knee pain following injection of hypertonic saline into the infrapatellar fat pad, *J Orthop Res* 22(1):116-121, 2004.

Bennett JB, Tullos HS: Acute injuries to the elbow. In Nicholas JA, Hershman EB, editors: *The upper extremity in sports medicine,* St Louis, 1990, Mosby.

Bennett JG: Rehabilitation of patellofemoral joint dysfunction. In Greenfield BH, editor: *Rehabilitation of the knee: a problem solving approach,* Philadelphia, 1994, FA Davis.

Bennett JT, MacEwen GD: Congenital dislocation of the hip: recent advances and current problems, *Clin Orthop* 247:15, 1989.

Bennett RM et al: A multidisciplinary approach to fibromyalgia treatment, *J Musculoskel Med* 8:21, 1991.

Bennett WF: Arthroscopic bicipital sheath repair: two-year follow-up with pulley lesions, *Arthroscopy* 20(9):964-973, 2004.

Benson DF, Blumer D: *Psychiatric aspect of neurologic disease,* New York, 1975, Grune & Stratton.

Benson MKD, Byrnes DP: The clinical syndromes and surgical treatment of thoracic intervertebral disc prolapse, *J Bone Joint Surg* 57B:471, 1975.

Benson MKD, Evans DCJ: The pelvis osteotomy of Chiari, *J Bone Joint Surg* 58B:164, 1976.

Benzon HT et al: Piriformis syndrome: anatomic considerations, a new injection technique, and a review of the literature, *Anesthesiology* 98(6):1442-1448, 2003.

Berens DL: Roentgen features of ankylosing spondylitis, *Clin Orthop* 74:20, 1971.

Berg EE: The sternal-rib complex: a possible fourth column in thoracic spine fractures, *Spine* 18:1916, 1993.

Berger RA: Endoscopic carpal tunnel release, a current perspective, *Hand Clin* 10:625, 1994.

Bergfeld JA: Acromioclavicular complex. In Nicholas JA, Hershman EB, editors: *The upper extremity in sports medicine*, St Louis, 1990, Mosby.

Berghs H et al: Diagnostic value of sacroiliac joint scintigraphy with 99m technetium pyrophosphate in sacroiliitis, *Ann Rheum Dis* 37:190, 1978.

Berkeley ME et al: Surgical therapy for congenital dislocation of the hip in patients who are twelve to thirty-six months old, *J Bone Joint Surg* 66A:412, 1984.

Berkowitz JF, Kier R, Rudicel S: Plantar fasciitis: MR imaging, *Radiology* 179:665, 1991.

Bernat JL: A dangerous backache, *Hosp Pract (Off Ed)* 12:36, 1977.

Bernstein EF: *Vascular diagnosis*, ed 4, St Louis, 1993, Mosby.

Berquist T: *MRI of the musculoskeletal system*, ed 3, Philadelphia, 1996, JB Lippincott.

Berry JD, Rowbotham MC, Petersen KL: Complex regional pain syndrome-like symptoms during herpes zoster, *Pain* 110(1-2):8-9, 2004:

Berthelot J-M et al: Contribution of centralization phenomenon to the diagnosis, prognosis, and treatment of diskogenic low back pain, *Joint Bone Spine* (in press, uncorrected proof).

Berthelot J-M et al: Provocative sacroiliac joint maneuvers and sacroiliac joint block are unreliable for diagnosing sacroiliac joint pain, *Joint Bone Spine* 73(1):17-23, 2006.

Berthelot J-M: Current management of reflex sympathetic dystrophy syndrome (complex regional pain syndrome type I), *Joint Bone Spine* 73(5):495-499, 2006.

Bettmane EH, Neudorfer RJ: Cervical disc pathology resulting in dysphagia in an adolescent boy, *N Y State J Med* 60:2465, 1960.

Beynnon BD et al: Anterior cruciate ligament strain behavior during rehabilitation exercises in vivo, *Am J Sports Med* 23:24, 1995.

Bhagavan NV: *Medical biochemistry*, Boston, 1992, Jones and Bartlett.

Bharam S: Labral tears, extra-articular injuries, and hip arthroscopy in the athlete, *Clin Sports Med* 25(2):279-292, 2006.

Bianchini K et al: Detection and diagnosis of malingering in electrical injury, *Arch Clin Neuropsychol* 20(3):365-373, 2005.

Bianchini KJ, Greve KW, Glynn G: On the diagnosis of malingered pain-related disability: lessons from cognitive malingering research, *Spine J* 5(4):404-417, 2005.

Bierbaum BE et al: Late complications of total hip replacement. In Steinberg ME, editor: *The hip and its disorders*, Philadelphia, 1991, WB Saunders.

Bijlsma JWJ, Knahr K: Strategies for the prevention and management of osteoarthritis of the hip and knee, *Best Pract Res Clin Rheumatol* 21(1):59-76, 2007.

Binak K et al: Arteriovenous fistula: hemodynamic effect of occlusion and exercise, *Am Heart J* 60:495, 1960.

Birch R: The place of microsurgery in orthopaedics. In *Recent advances in orthopaedics*, ed 5, Edinburgh, 1987, Churchill Livingstone.

Birchard D, Pichora D: Experimental corrective scaphoid osteotomy for scaphoid malunion with abnormal wrist mechanics, *J Hand Surg* 15A:863, 1990.

Birklein F, Kunzel W, Sieweke N: Despite clinical similarities there are significant differences between acute limb trauma and complex regional pain syndrome I (CRPS I), *Pain* 93(2):165-171, 2001.

Bischoff RJ et al: A comparison of computed tomography-myelography, magnetic resonance imaging and myelography in the diagnosis of herniated nucleus pulposus and spinal stenosis, *J Spinal Disord* 6:289, 1993.

Black HC: *Black's law dictionary,* St Paul, Minn, 1990, West Publishing.

Blackwell JR, Cole KJ: Wrist kinematics in expert and novice tennis players performing the backhand stoke: implications for tennis elbow, *J Biomech* 27:509, 1994.

Bland JH, Merrit JA, Boushey DR: The painful shoulder, *Semin Arthritis Rheum* 7:21, 1977.

Bland JH: *Disorders of the cervical spine diagnosis and medical management,* Philadelphia, 1987, WB Saunders.

Bland JH: Rheumatoid arthritis of the cervical spine, *J Rheumatol* 1:319, 1974.

Bland JM, Altman DG: Measurement error and correlation coefficients. *BMJ* 313(7048): 41-42, 1996.

Blockey NJ: Derotation osteotomy in the management of congenital dislocation of the hip, *J Bone Joint Surg* 66B:485, 1984.

Bloom RA: The active abduction view: a new maneuver in the diagnosis of rotator cuff tears, *Skeletal Radiol* 20:255, 1991.

Blount WP, Moe JH: *The Milwaukee brace,* Baltimore, 1973, Williams & Wilkins.

Bocchi L, Orso CA: Whiplash injuries of the cervical spine, *Ital J Orthop Traumatol* 9:171, 1983.

Boden S et al: Abnormal magnetic resonance scans of the spine in asymptomatic patients, *J Bone Joint Surg* 72A:403, 1990.

Boden SD et al: *The aging spine: essentials of pathophysiology, diagnosis and treatment,* Philadelphia, 1991, WB Saunders.

Bodley R: Imaging in chronic spinal cord injury—indications and benefits, *Eur J Radiol* 42(2):135-53, 2002.

Bogduk N, Amevo B, Pearcy M: A biological basis for instantaneous centers of rotation of the vertebral column, *Proc Inst Mech Eng* 209:177, 1995.

Bogduk N, Aprill C, Derby R: Discography. In White AH, Schofferman JA, editors: *Spine care,* vol 1, St Louis, 1995, Mosby.

Bogduk N, Macintosh JE, Pearcy MJ: A universal model of the lumbar back muscles in the upright position, *Spine* 17:897, 1992.

Bogduk N, Twomey LT: *Clinical anatomy of the lumbar spine,* ed 2, New York, 1991, Churchill Livingstone.

Bogduk N, Valencia F: Innervation and pain patterns of the thoracic spine. In Grant R, editor: *Physical therapy of the cervical and thoracic spine,* ed 2, New York, 1994, Churchill Livingstone.

Bogduk N: *Pathogenesis of degenerative disc disease,* Toronto, 1991, American Back Society.

Bogduk N: Pathology of lumbar disc pain, *Man Med* 5:72, 1990.

Bohlman HH et al: Spinal cord monitoring of experimental incomplete cervical spinal cord injury, *Spine* 6:428, 1981.

Bohlman HH, Ducker TB, Lucas JT: Spine and spinal cord injuries. In Rothman RH, Simeone FA, editors: *The spine,* ed 2, Philadelphia, 1982, WB Saunders.

Bohlman HH, Eismont FJ: Surgical techniques of anterior decompression and fusion for spinal cord injuries, *Clin Orthop* 138:154, 1981.

Bohlman HH, Riley L Jr, Robinson RA: Anterolateral approaches to the cervical spine. In Ruge D, Wiltse LL, editors: *Spinal disorders,* Philadelphia, 1977, Lea & Febiger.

Bohlman HH: Indications for late anterior decompression and fusion for cervical spinal cord injuries. In Tator CH, editor: *Early management of acute cervical spinal cord injury,* New York, 1982, Raven Press.

Bohlman HH: Late anterior decompression and fusion for the spinal cord injuries: review of 100 cases with long term results, *Orthop Trans* 4:42, 1980.

Bohlman HH: The neck. In D'Ambrosia R, editor: *Regional examination and differential diagnosis of musculoskeletal disorders,* Philadelphia, 1977, JB Lippincott.

Boileau P, Chuinard C: Arthroscopic biceps tenotomy: technique and results, *Oper Tech Sports Med* 15(1):35-44, 2007.

Boisen WR, Staples OS, Russell SW: Residual disability following acute ankle sprains, *J Bone Joint Surg* 37A:1237, 1955.

Boling MC et al: Outcomes of a weight-bearing rehabilitation program for patients diagnosed with patellofemoral pain syndrome, *Arch Phys Med Rehabil* 87(11): 1428-1435, 2006.

Bombelli R: *Osteoarthritis of the hip: pathogenesis and consequent therapy,* New York, 1976, Springer-Verlag.

Bonalaski JS, Schumacher HR: Arthritis and allied conditions. In Steinberg M, editor: *The hip and its disorders,* Philadelphia, 1991, WB Saunders.

Bond MR: *Pain: its nature, analysis and treatment,* Edinburgh, 1979, Churchill Livingstone.

Bondilla KK: Back pain: osteoarthritis, *J Am Geriatr Soc* 25:62, 1977.

Bone biopsy of the parasymphyseal region of athletes with osteitis pubis diagnosed by MRI demonstrates new woven bone formation, *J Sci Med Sport* 6(4, suppl 1): 95-84, 2003.

Bongers PM et al: Psychosocial factors at work and musculoskeletal disease, *Scand J Work Environ Health* 19:297, 1993.

Bordelon RL: Heel pain. In DeLee JD, Drez D, editors: *Orthopaedic sports medicine: principles and practice,* vol 2, Philadelphia, 1994, WB Saunders.

Bordurant FJ et al: Acute spinal cord injury: a study using physical examination and magnetic resonance imaging, *Spine* 15:161, 1990.

Borenstein D: Prevalence and treatment outcome of primary and secondary fibromyalgia in patients with spinal pain, *Spine* 20:1055, 1995.

Borenstein DG, Burton JR: Lumbar spine disease in the elderly, *J Am Geriatr Soc* 41:167, 1993.

Borenstein DG et al: *Low back pain: medical diagnosis and comprehensive management,* ed 2, Philadelphia, 1995, WB Saunders.

Borg G: Psychophysical bases of perceived exertion, *Med Sci Sport Exercise* 14:377, 1982.

Bottin A et al: Non-invasive assessment of the gracilis muscle by means of surface electromyography electrode arrays, *J Surg Res* 134(2):265-269, 2006.

Botwin KP, Gruber RD, Savarese R: Lumbar discography, *Tech Reg Anesth Pain Manag* 9(1):3-12, 2005.

Bough B et al: Degeneration of lumbar facet joints, *J Bone Joint Surg* 72B:275, 1990.

Boukhris S et al: Pain as the presenting symptom of chronic inflammatory demyelinating polyradiculoneuropathy (CIDP), *J Neurol Sci* 254(1-2):33-38, 2007.

Bourdillon JR: *Spinal manipulation,* ed 3, New York, 1982, Appleton-Century-Crofts.

Bourne G: *The structure and function of nervous tissue,* New York, 1968, Academic Press.

Bowen JR, Foster BK, Hartzell C: Legg-Calve-Perthes disease, *Clin Orthop* 185:97, 1984.

Bowen V, Cassidy JD: Macroscopic and microscopic anatomy of the sacroiliac joint from embryonic life until the eighth decade, *Spine* 6:620, 1981.

Bowlus B: *Mosby's regional atlas of human anatomy,* St Louis, 1997, Mosby.

Boyd HB, McLeod AC: Tennis elbow, *J Bone Joint Surg* 55A:1183, 1973.

Boytim MJ, Fischer DA, Neuman L: Syndesmotic ankle sprains, *Am J Sports Med* 19: 294, 1991.

Bozyk Z: Shoulder-hand syndrome in patients with antecedent myocardial infarctions, *Revmatologiia (Mosk)* 6:103, 1968.

Bozzae A et al: Lumbar disc herniation: MR imaging assessment of natural history in patients treated without surgery, *Radiology* 185:135, 1992.

Bradford DS et al: Scheuermann's kyphosis and roundback deformity: results of Milwaukee brace treatment, *J Bone Joint Surg* 56A:740, 1974.

Bradford DS et al: Scheuermann's kyphosis: results of surgical treatment by posterior spine arthrodesis in 22 patients, *J Bone Joint Surg* 57A:439, 1975.

Bradford DS: Juvenile kyphosis, *Clin Orthop* 128:45, 1977.

Bradford FK: Low back sprain and ruptured intervertebral disc, *Med Times* 88:797, 1960.

Bradley GW et al: Resurfacing arthroplasty: femoral head viability, *Clin Orthop* 220:137, 1987.

Bradley JP, Tibone JE, Watkins RC: History, physical examination, and diagnostic tests for neck and upper extremity problems. In Watkins RG, editor: *The spine in sports,* St Louis, 1996, Mosby.

Bradley JP, Tibone JE: Percutaneous and open surgical repairs of Achilles tendon ruptures, *Am J Sports Med* 18:188, 1990.

Bradley LA: Multivariate analysis of the MMPI profiles of low back pain patients, *J Behav Med* 1:253, 1978.

Bradley WG: *Disorders of peripheral nerves,* Oxford, UK, 1974, Blackwell Scientific.

Brahms MA: Common foot problems, *J Bone Joint Surg* 49A:1653, 1967.

Brain WR: Some unsolved problems in cervical spondylosis, *Br Med Bull* 1:711, 1963.

Braithwaite IJ, Jones WA: Scapho-lunate dissociation occurring with scaphoid fracture, *J Hand Surg* 17B:286, 1992.

Brand C et al: Cryptococcal sacroiliitis: case report, *Ann Rheum Dis* 44:126, 1985.

Brannan SR, Jerrard DA: Synovial fluid analysis, *J Emerg Med* 30(3):331-339, 2006.

Brashear HR Jr, Raney RB: *Shands' handbook of orthopaedic surgery,* St Louis, 1978, Mosby.

Braun J, Bollow M, Sieper J: Radiologic diagnosis and pathology of the spondyloar-thropathies, *Rheum Dis Clin North Am* 24(4):697-735, 1998.

Brav EA: The diagnosis of low back pain of orthopedic origin: an analysis of sixty-two cases, *Am J Surg* 55(1):57-66, 1942.

Breen A: The reliability of palpation and other diagnostic methods, *J Manipulative Physiol Ther* 15:54, 1992.

Breig A, Troup JDG: Biomechanical considerations in straight-leg-raising test: cadaveric and clinical studies of the effects of medial hip rotation, *Spine* 4:242, 1979.

Brems JJ: Degenerative joints disease of the shoulder. In Nicholas J, Hershman E, editors: *The upper extremity in sports medicine,* St Louis, 1990, Mosby.

Brena SF, Chapman SL: *Pain and litigation, textbook of pain,* Edinburgh, 1984, Churchill Livingstone.

Brieg A, Turnbull IM, Hassler O: Effects of mechanical stresses in the spinal cord in cervical spondylosis, *J Neurosurg* 25:45, 1966.

Brieg A: *Biomechanics of the central nervous system,* Chicago, 1960, Mosby.

Brier SR, Nyfield B: A comparison of hip and lumbopelvic inflexibility and low back pain in runners and cyclists, *J Manipulative Physiol Ther* 18:25, 1995.

Brier SR: *Primary care orthopedics,* St Louis, 1999, Mosby.

Bringnall CG, Stainsby GD: The snapping hip: treatment by Z-plasty, *J Bone Joint Surg* 73B:253, 1991.

Brody IA, Williams RH: The signs of Kernig and Brudzinski, *Arch Neurol* 21:215, 1969.

Brondum V, Larsen CF, Skov O: Fracture of carpal scaphoid: frequency and distribution in a well-defined population, *Eur J Radiol* 15:118, 1992.

Brook I: Superficial suppurative thrombophlebitis in children, caused by anaerobic bacteria, *J Pediatr Surg* 33(8):1279-1282, 1998.

Brooks M, Evans R, Fairclough J: *Sports injuries,* ed 2, London, 1992, Gower Medical.

Brotzman SB: *Clinical orthopaedic rehabilitation,* St Louis, 1996, Mosby.

Brown CW et al: The natural history of thoracic disc herniation, *Spine* 17:597, 1992.

Brown DE, Neumann RD: *Orthopedic secrets,* Philadelphia, 1995, Hanley & Belfus.

Brown DE: Ankle and leg injuries. In Mellion MB, Walsh M, Shelton GL, editors: *The team physician's handbook,* Philadelphia, 1990, Hanley & Belfus.

Brown M: The well elderly. In Guccione A, editor: *Geriatric physical therapy,* St Louis, 1993, Mosby.

Brown MD: Diagnosis of pain syndromes of the spine, *Orthop Clin North Am* 6:233, 1975.

Brown MG, Keyser B, Rothenberg ES: Endoscopic carpal tunnel release, *J Hand Surg* 17A:1009, 1992.

Brown RA et al: Carpal tunnel release: a prospective, randomized assessment of open and endoscopic methods, *J Bone Joint Surg* 75A:1265, 1993.

Brucini M et al: Pain thresholds and electromyographic features of periarticular muscles in patients with osteoarthritis of the knee, *Pain* 10(1):57-66, 1981.

Brudzinski J: A new sign of the lower extremities in meningitis of children (neck sign), *Arch Neurol* 21:216, 1969.

Brunner C, Kissling R, Jacob HAC: The efforts of morphology and histopathologic findings on the mobility of the sacroiliac joint, *Spine* 16:1111, 1991.

Bruno PA, Bagust J: An investigation into motor pattern differences used during prone hip extension between subjects with and without low back pain, *Clin Chiropractic* 10(2):68-80, 2007.

Buchler U: *Wrist instability,* St Louis, 1996, Mosby.

Bucholz RW: *Orthopaedic decision making,* ed 2, St Louis, 1996, Mosby.

Buckwalter J: Spine update: aging and degeneration of the human intervertebral disc, *Spine* 20:1307, 1995.

Budgell B, Noda K, Sata A: Innervation of posterior structures in the lumbar spine of the rat, *J Manipulative Physiol Ther* 20:359, 1997.

Buirski G: Magnetic resonance signal pattern of lumbar discs in patients with low back pain: a prospective study with discographic correlation, *Spine* 17:1205, 1992.

Bunker TD, Schranz PJ: *Clinical challenges in orthopaedics: the shoulder,* Oxford, UK, 1998, ISIS Medical Media.

Bunker TD: Frozen shoulder, *Curr Orthop* 12(3):193-201, 1998.

Bunnell S: Surgery of the rheumatic hand, *J Bone Joint Surg* 27:759, 1955.

Bunnell WP: Treatment of idiopathic scoliosis, *Orthop Clin North Am* 10:813, 1979.

Burgess A et al: Pelvic ring disruptions: effective classification system and treatment protocols, *J Trauma* 30:848, 1990.

Burkhart SS: Arthroscopic treatment of massive rotator cuff tears, *Clin Orthop* 26:45, 1991.

Burkus JK: Spine. In Loth T, editor: *Orthopaedic boards review,* St Louis, 1993, Mosby.

Burnett W: *Clinical science for surgeons,* London, 1981, Butterworth.

Burns J, Crosbie J: Weight bearing ankle dorsiflexion range of motion in idiopathic pes cavus compared to normal and pes planus feet, *Foot* 15(2):91-94, 2005.

Burton RI: Extensor tendons-late reconstruction. In Green DP, editor: *Operative hand surgery,* ed 3, New York, 1993, Churchill Livingstone.

Burwell RG, Harrison HM, editors: Perthes disease (symposium), *Clin Orthop* 209:2, 1986.

Busa R et al: Acute posterior interosseous nerve palsy caused by a synovial haemangioma of the elbow joint, *J Hand Surg* 20(5):652-654, 1995.

Buschbacher RM: *Musculoskeletal disorders, a practical guide for diagnosis and rehabilitation,* Boston, 1994, Andover Medical Publishers.

Bush LH: The torn shoulder capsule, *J Bone Joint Surg* 57A:256, 1975.

Bush SS et al: Symptom validity assessment: practice issues and medical necessity: NAN Policy & Planning Committee, *Arch Clin Neuropsychol* 20(4):419-426, 2005.

Bushong SC: *Radiologic science for technologist: physics, biology, and protection,* ed 5, St Louis, 1993, Mosby.

Butler D: *Mobilisation of the nervous system,* New York, 1991, Churchill Livingstone.

Butler DL, Noyes FR, Grood ES: Ligamentous restraints to anterior-posterior drawer in the human knee, *J Bone Joint Surg* 622A:259, 1980.

Butler WT et al: Diagnostic and prognostic value of clinical and laboratory findings in cryptococcal meningitis, *N Engl J Med* 270:59, 1964.

Butt S, Saifuddin A: The imaging of lumbar spondylolisthesis, *Clin Radiol* 60(5): 533-546, 2005.

Byung-June J et al: Solitary lumbar osteochondroma causing sciatic pain, *Joint Bone Spine* (in press, uncorrected proof).

Caffey J: The early roentgenographic changes in essential coxa plana, their significance in pathogenesis, *AMJ Am J Roentgenol* 103:620, 1968.

Cahalan T et al: Biomechanics of the golf swing in players with pathologic conditions of the forearm, wrist, and hand, *Am J Sports Med* 19:288, 1991.

Cahill DR: The anatomy and function of the contents of the human tarsal sinus and canal, *Anat Rec* 153:1, 1965.

Cailliet R: *Foot and ankle pain,* Philadelphia, 1979, FA Davis.

Cailliet R: *Hand pain and impairment,* ed 2, Philadelphia, 1975, FA Davis.

Cailliet R: *Head and face pain syndromes,* Philadelphia, 1992, FA Davis.

Cailliet R: *Knee pain and disability,* ed 2, Philadelphia, 1983, FA Davis.

Cailliet R: *Low back pain syndrome,* ed 3, Philadelphia, 1981, FA Davis.

Cailliet R: *Scoliosis: diagnosis and management,* Philadelphia, 1975, FA Davis.

Cailliet R: *Shoulder pain,* Philadelphia, 1966, FA Davis.

Cailliet R: *Soft tissue pain and disability,* Philadelphia, 1977, FA Davis.

Cain EL, Dugas JR: History and examination of the thrower's elbow, *Clin Sports Med* 23(4):553-566, 2004.

Callaghan JJ: The clinical results and basic science of total hip arthroplasty with porous coated prosthesis, *J Bone Joint Surg* 75A:299, 1993.

Calvino B, Grilo RM: Central pain control, *Joint Bone Spine* 73(1):10-16, 2006.

Cambridge CA: Range of motion measurements of the hand. In Hunter JM et al, editors: *Rehabilitation of the hand,* ed 3, St Louis, 1990, Mosby.

Cameron HU: *The technique of total hip arthroplasty,* St Louis, 1992, Mosby.

Cammisa M, De Serio A, Guglielmi G: Diffuse idiopathic skeletal hyperostosis, *Eur J Radiol* 27(suppl 1):S7-S11, 1998.

Camp WA: Sarcoidosis of the central nervous system: a case with postmortem studies, *Arch Neurol* 7:432, 1962.

Campbell JB, Campbell JM: *Mosby's survival guide to medical abbreviations & acronyms prefixes & suffixes symbols Greek alphabet,* St Louis, 1995, Mosby.

Campbell JN, Meyer RA: Mechanisms of neuropathic pain, *Neuron* 52(1):77-92, 2006.

Campbell WC: *Operative orthopaedics,* ed 7, London, 1981, Henry Kimpton.

Campion GV, Dixon A: *Rheumatology,* Oxford, UK, 1989, Blackwell.

Canale ST: *Campbell's operative orthopaedics,* vol 1-4, ed 9, St Louis, 1998, Mosby.

Canoso JJ: Bursitis, tenosynovitis, ganglions, and painful lesions of the wrist, elbow and hand, *Curr Opin Rheumatol* 2:276, 1990.

Carbayo JA et al: Using ankle-brachial index to detect peripheral arterial disease: prevalence and associated risk factors in a random population sample, *Nutr Metab Cardiovasc Dis* 17(1):41-49, 2007.

Carcone SM, Keir PJ: Effects of backrest design on biomechanics and comfort during seated work, *Appl Ergon* (in press, corrected proof).

Cardinal E, Lafortune M, Burns P: Power Doppler US in synovitis: reality or artifact? *Radiology* 200:868, 1996.

Cardon LJ, Toh S, Tsubo K: Traumatic boutonniere deformity of the thumb, *J Hand Surg* 25(5):505-508, 2000.

Carman DL et al: Measurement of scoliosis and kyphosis radiographs, intraobserver and interobserver variation, *J Bone Joint Surg* 72A:328, 1990.

Carney BT, Weinstein SL, Nuhe J: Long term follow up of slipped capital femoral epiphysis, *J Bone Joint Surg* 73A:667, 1991.

Carragee E et al: Surgical treatment for unstable low-grade isthmic spondylolisthesis in adults: a prospective controlled study of posterior instrumented fusion compared with combined anterior-posterior fusion, *Spine J* 6(5, suppl 1):47S, 2006.

Carrera GF et al: CT of sacroiliitis, *AJR Am J Roentgenol* 136:41, 1981.

Carson WG, Meyer JF: Diagnostic arthroscopy of the elbow: surgical techniques and arthroscopic portal anatomy. In McGinty JB, editor: *Operative arthroscopy,* New York, 1991, Raven.

Carter CO, Wilkinson JA: Genetic and environmental factors in the etiology of congenital dislocation of the hip, *Clin Orthop* 33:119, 1964.

Carver G, Willits J: Comparative study and risk factors of a CVA, *J Am Chiro Assoc* 32:65, 1996.

Cashley MAP: Basilar artery migraine or cerebral vascular accident? *J Manip Physiol Ther* 16:112, 1993.

Cassidy JD et al: Quebec task force on whiplash-associated disorders, redefining "whiplash" and its management (abridged), *Spine* 20(suppl):S1, 1995.

Cassidy JD: *The pathoanatomy and clinical significance of the sacroiliac joints,* Toronto, 1991, World Chiropractic Congress.

Castelli P et al: Endovascular repair of traumatic injuries of the subclavian and axillary arteries, *Injury* 36(6):778-782, 2005.

Castro FP: Adolescent idiopathic scoliosis, bracing, and the Hueter-Volkmann principle, *Spine J* 3(3):180-185, 2003.

Cats A, Linder SM: Spondyloarthropathies: an overview, *Spine* 4:497, 1990.

Catterall A: *Recent advances in orthopaedics,* ed 5, Edinburgh, 1987, Churchill Livingstone.

Catterall A: The natural history of Perthes disease (symposium), *J Bone Joint Surg* 53B:37, 1971.

Catterall M: Perthes disease. In Steinberg ME, editor: *The hip and its disorders,* Philadelphia, 1991, WB Saunders.

Cervical Spine Research Society: *The cervical spine,* Philadelphia, 1983, JB Lippincott.

Chahidi N et al: Gracilis free muscle flap for coverage of palmar defects, *J Hand Surg: Eur Vol* 32(suppl 1):59, 2007.

Chan CK et al: Ocular features of west Nile virus infection in North America: a study of 14 eyes, *Ophthalmology* 113(9):1539-1546, 2006.

Chance PF: Survey of inherited peripheral nerve diseases, *Electroencephalogr Clin Neurophysiol* 103(1):12, 1997.

Chandler TJ et al: Shoulder strength, power and endurance in college tennis players, *Am J Sports Med* 20:455, 1992.

Chandnani VP et al: Knee hyaline cartilage evaluated with MR imaging: a cadaveric study involving multiple imaging sequences and intraarticular injection of gadolinium and saline solution, *Radiology* 178:557, 1991.

Chansky HA, Iannotti JP: The vascularity of the rotator cuff, *Clin Sports Med* 10:807, 1991.

Chao EY et al: Biomechanics of malalignment, *Orthop Clin North Am* 25:379, 1994.

Chapman S, Nakielny R: *Aids to radiological differential diagnosis,* ed 3, London, 1995, Bailliere Tindall.

Chappuis JL, Johnson GD, Gines AM: *A source guide for spine care,* Atlanta, 1994, Grater Atlanta Spine Center.

Chard MD et al: Shoulder disorders in the elderly: a community survey, *Arthritis Rheum* 34:766, 1991.

Charnley J: Total hip replacement by low-friction arthroplasty, *Clin Orthop* 72:7, 1970.

Chavanet P et al: Performance of a predictive rule to distinguish bacterial and viral meningitis, *J Infect* 54(4):328-336, 2007.

Cheetham DR et al: Is the Stresst'er a reliable stress test to detect mild to moderate peripheral arterial disease? *Eur J Vasc Endovasc Surg* 27(5):545-548, 2004.

Chell J, Dhar S: Perthes disease, *Surgery (Oxford)* 22(1):18-20, 2004.

Chemmanam T et al: Anhidrosis: a clue to an underlying autonomic disorder, *J Clin Neurosci* 14(1):94-96, 2007.

Chen Y-G et al: Innervation of the metacarpophalangeal and interphalangeal joints: a microanatomic and histologic study of the nerve endings, *J Hand Surg* 25(1): 128-133, 2000.

Chen Y-L: Effectiveness of a new back belt in the maintenance of lumbar lordosis while sitting: a pilot study, *Int J Industr Ergon* 32(4):299-303, 2003.

Chhabra A et al: The arthroscopic appearance of a normal anterior cruciate ligament in a posterior cruciate ligament-deficient knee: the posterolateral bundle (PLB) sign, *Arthroscopy* 21(10):1267.e1-1267.e3, 2005.

Chibnall JT, Tait R: The pain disability index: factor structure and normative data, *Arch Phys Med Rehabil* 75:1082, 1994.

Childress HM: Popliteal cysts associated with undiagnosed posterior lesions of the medial meniscus, *J Bone Joint Surg* 52A:1487, 1970.

Chin CH, Chew KC: Lumbosacral nerve root avulsion, *Injury* 28(9-10):674-678, 1997.

Chin KR, Eiszner J, Persaud K: Impact of obesity on the incidence of surgery, outcomes, and complications in low back pain patients, *Spine J* 6(5, suppl 1):158S, 2006.

Chin KR et al: Changes in the iliac crest-lumbar relationship from standing to prone, *Spine J* 6(2):185-189, 2006.

Chiodo A, Chadd E: Ulnar neuropathy at or distal to the wrist: traumatic versus cumulative stress cases, *Arch Phys Med Rehabil* 88(4):504-412, 2007.

Chiodo A et al: Needle EMG has a lower false positive rate than MRI in asymptomatic older adults being evaluated for lumbar spinal stenosis, *Clin Neurophysiol* 118(4): 751-756, 2007.

Chiu M-C, Wang M-JJ: Professional footwear evaluation for clinical nurses, *Appl Ergon* 38(2):133-141, 2007.

Cho K-J et al: A case of an inflammatory myofibroblastic tumor of the mastoid presenting with chronic suppurative otitis media, *Auris Nasus Larynx* (in press, corrected proof).

Chobanian AV, Gavras H: *Hypertension,* Summit, Colo, 1990, CIBA Pharmaceutical.

Choi IS et al: Clinical characteristics of brachial plexopathy, *Clin Neurophysiol* 117 (suppl 1):188-189, 2006.

Chow JW et al: Reliability of a technique for determining sagittal knee geometry from lateral knee radiographs, *Knee* 13(4):318-323, 2006.

Christiansen TG et al: Diagnostic value of ultrasound in scaphoid fractures, *Injury* 22: 397, 1991.

Chusid JG, McDonald JJ: *Correlative neuroanatomy and functional neurology,* Los Altos, Calif, 1962, Lange Medical.

Cinquegranao D: Chronic cervical radiculitis and its relationship to "chronic bursitis," *Am J Phys Med Rehabil* 47:23, 1968.

Cipriano JJ: *Photographic manual of regional orthopaedic and neurological test,* ed 3, Baltimore, 1997, Williams & Wilkins.

Clain MR, Baxter DE: Achilles tendonitis, *Foot Ankle* 13:482, 1992.

Clancy WG: Repair and reconstruction of the posterior cruciate ligament. In Chapman MW, editor: *Operative orthopaedics,* vol 2, Philadelphia, 1993, JB Lippincott.

Clancy WG: Tendon trauma and overuse injuries. In Leadbetter WB, Buckwalter JA, Gordon SL, editors: *Sports-induced inflammation: clinical and basic science concepts,* Park Ridge, Ill, 1990, AAOS.

Clanton TO, Schon LC: Athlete injuries to the soft tissues of the foot and ankle. In Mann RA, Coughlin MJ, editors: *Surgery of the foot and ankle,* ed 6, St Louis, 1993, Mosby.

Clark J, Sidles JA, Matsen FF: The repair of the glenohumeral joint capsule to the rotator cuff, *Clin Orthop* 254:29, 1990.

Clarke NMP, Clegg J, Al-Chalabi AN: Ultrasound screening of hips at risk for congenital dislocation, *J Bone Joint Surg* 71B:9, 1989.

Cleeman E, Auerbach JD, Springfield DS: Tumors of the shoulder girdle: a review of 194 cases, *J Shoulder Elbow Surg* 14(5):460-465, 2005.

Cloward RB: Lesions of the intervertebral disc and their treatment by interbody fusion methods: the painful disc, *Clin Orthop* 27:51, 1963.

Cloward RB: The clinical significance of the sinu-vertebral nerve or the cervical spine in relation to the cervical disc syndrome, *J Neurol Neurosurg Psychiatry* 23:321, 1960.

Coates CJ, Paterson JM, Woods KR: Femoral osteotomy in Perthes disease: results at maturity, *J Bone Joint Surg* 72B:581, 1990.

Cobb TK et al: Anatomy of the flexor retinaculum, *J Hand Surg* 18A:91, 1993.

Codman EA: *The shoulder,* Boston, 1934, Author.

Coffman JD, Mannick JA: An objective test to demonstrate the circulatory abnormality in intermittent claudication, *Circulation* 33:177, 1966.

Cofield R: Degenerative and arthritic problems of the glenohumeral joint. In Rockwood C, Matsen F, editors: *The shoulder,* Philadelphia, 1990, WB Saunders.

Cohen HL, Brumlik J: *A manual of electroneuromyography,* New York, 1968, Harper and Row.

Cohen MS et al: Acute compartment syndrome: effect of dermotomy on fascial decompression in the leg, *J Bone Joint Surg* 73A:287, 1991.

Cohn RE: *Impairment rating examination and disability evaluation,* ed 3, Wilkesboro, NC, 1994, R Ernest Cohn.

Colachis SC: Movement of sacroiliac joint in adult male, *Arch Phys Med Rehabil* 44:490, 1963.

Coldham F, Lewis J, Lee H: The reliability of one vs. three grip trials in symptomatic and asymptomatic subjects, *J Hand Ther* 19(3):318-327, 2006.

Cole AJ, Herring SA: *The low back pain handbook: a practical guide for the primary care examiner,* Philadelphia, 1997, Hanley & Belfus.

Cole AJ, Herring SA: *The low back pain handbook: a practical guide for the primary care clinician,* Philadelphia, 1997, Hanley & Belfus.

Cole MH, Grimshaw PN: Electromyography of the trunk and abdominal muscles in golfers with and without low back pain, *J Sci Med Sport* (in press, corrected proof).

Colli BO et al: Neurogenic thoracic outlet syndromes: a comparison of true and nonspecific syndromes after surgical treatment, *Surg Neurol* 65(3):262-271, 2006.

Collins DN, Nelson CL: Infections of the hip. In Steinberg M, editor: *The hip and its disorders,* Philadelphia, 1991, WB Saunders.

Collo MC et al: Evaluating arthritic complaints, *Nurse Pract* 15:9, 1991.

Colloca CJ, Keller TS: Stiffness and neuromuscular reflex response of the human spine to posteroanterior manipulative thrusts in patients with low back pain, *J Manipulative Physiol Ther* 24(8):489-500, 2001.

Colman WW, Strauch RJ: Physical examination of the elbow, *Orthop Clin North Am* 30(1):15-20, 1999.

Colosimo AJ, Ireland ML: Thigh compartment syndrome in a football athlete: a case report and review of the literature, *Med Sci Sports Exerc* 24:958, 1992.

Colter JM: Lateral ligamentous injuries of the ankle. In Hamilton WC, editor: *Traumatic disorder of the ankle,* New York, 1984, Springer-Verlag.

Colvin LA, Power I: Neurobiology of chronic pain states, *Anesth Intensive Care Med* 6(1):10-13, 2005.

Compson JP, Waterman JK, Spencer JD: Dorsal avulsion fractures of the scaphoid: diagnostic implications and applied anatomy, *J Hand Surg* 18B:58, 1993.

Concannon MJ: *Common hand problems in primary care,* Philadelphia, 1999, Hanley & Belfus.

Conlon PW, Isdale IC, Rose BS: Rheumatoid arthritis of the cervical spine: an analysis of 333 cases, *Ann Rheum Dis* 25:120, 1966.

Connelly C: Easing low back pain, *Postgrad Med* 100, 1996.

Conway JE et al: Medial instability of the elbow in throwing athletes: treatment by repair or reconstruction of the ulnar collateral ligament, *J Bone Joint Surg* 74A:67, 1992.

Conwell TD: *Documenting patient progress "daily office charting seminar" thorough accurate quick procedures,* ed. 11, Lakewood, Colo, 1990, Clinical Advancement Plus Seminars.

Cook C et al: Interrater reliability and diagnostic accuracy of pelvic girdle pain classification, *J Manipulative and Physiol Ther* 30(4):252-258, 2007.

Cooke TDV, Lehmann PO: Intermittent claudication of neurogenic origin, *Can J Surg* 11:151, 1968.

Cooney WP III, Dobyns JH, Linscheid RL: Complications of Colles' fracture, *J Bone Joint Surg* 62A:613, 1980.

Cooney WP III, Linscheid RL, Dobyns JH: External pin fixation for unstable Colles' fracture, *J Bone Joint Surg* 61A:840, 1979.

Cooney WP III, Linscheid RL, Dobyns JH: *The wrist diagnosis and operative treatment,* vol 1-2, St Louis, 1998, Mosby.

Cooney WP, Dobyns JH, Linscheid RL: Arthroscopy of the wrist: anatomy and classification of carpal instability, *Arthroscopy* 6(2):133-140, 1990.

Cooper DE et al: Anatomy, histology and vascularity of the glenoid labrum, *J Bone Joint Surg* 74A:46, 1992.

Cooper DE, Warren RF, Barnes R: Traumatic subluxation of the hip resulting in aseptic necrosis and chondrolysis in a professional football player, *Am J Sports Med* 19:322, 1991.

Copeland SA et al: *Joint stiffness of the upper limb,* St Louis, 1997, Mosby.

Copperman DR, Stulberg SD: Ambulatory containment treatment in Perthes disease, *Clin Orthop* 203:289, 1986.

Coppes MH et al: Innervation of annulus fibrosis in low back pain, *Lancet* 336:189, 1988.

Cormack DH: *Essential histology,* Philadelphia, 1993, Lippincott.

Corso SJ, Thal R, Forman D: Locked patellar dislocation with vertical axis rotation, *Clin Orthop* 279:190, 1992.

Coughlin MJ: Conditions of the forefoot. In DeLee JD, Drez D, editors: *Orthopaedic sports medicine: principles and practice,* vol 2, Philadelphia, 1994, WB Saunders.

Cousins MJ, Phillips GD: *Acute pain management,* New York, 1986, Churchill Livingstone.

Coutaux A et al: Hyperalgesia and allodynia: peripheral mechanisms, *Joint Bone Spine* 72(5):359-371, 2005.

Covey DC, Sapega AA: Current concepts review, injuries of the posterior cruciate ligament, *J Bone Joint Surg* 75A:1376, 1993.

Cox JM: *Low back pain mechanism, diagnosis and treatment,* ed 5, Baltimore, 1990, Williams & Wilkins.

Coy JT et al: Pyogenic arthritis of the sacroiliac joint: long-term follow-up, *J Bone Joint Surg* 58A:845, 1976.

Craig Humphreys S et al: Assessing lumbar sagittal motion using videography in an in vivo pilot study, *Int J Industr Ergon* (in press, corrected proof).

Craik RL, Oatis CA: *Gait analysis theory and application,* St Louis, 1995, Mosby.

Cramer G et al: Comparison of computed tomography to magnetic resonance imaging in the evaluation of the lumbar intervertebral foramina, *Clin Anat* 7:173, 1994.

Cramer GD, Darby SA: *Basic and clinical anatomy of the spine, spinal cord, and ANS,* St Louis, 1995, Mosby.

Crawford EJ, Emery RJ, Archrogh PM: Stable osteochondritis dissecans. Does the lesion unite? *J Bone Joint Surg* 72B:320, 1990.

Crellin RQ, MacCabe JJ, Hamilton EB: Surgical management of the cervical spine in rheumatoid arthritis, *J Bone Joint Surg* 52B:244, 1970.

Crenshaw AH editor: *Campbell's operative orthopaedics,* vol 3, ed 8, St Louis, 1992, Mosby.

Crisco JJ, Fujita L, Spenciner DB: The dynamic flexion/extension properties of the lumbar spine in vitro using a novel pendulum system, *J Biomech* (in press, corrected proof).

Crisco JJ, Panjabi MM: The intersegmental and multisegmental muscles of the lumbar spine: a biomechanical model comparing lateral stabilizing potential, *Spine* 16:793, 1991.

Croft P, Schollum J, Silman A: Population study of tender point counts and pain as evidence of fibromyalgia, *BMJ* 309:696, 1994.

Crosby EB, Insall J: Recurrent dislocation of the patella, *J Bone Joint Surg* 58A:9, 1976.

Crosby EC, Humphrey T, Lauer EW: *Correlative anatomy of the nervous system,* New York, 1962, Macmillan.

Cruess RL, Rennie W: *Adult orthopaedics,* New York, 1987, Churchill Livingstone.

Cullinan AM: *Optimizing radiographic positioning,* Philadelphia, 1992, Lippincott.

Currey HLF: *Essentials of rheumatology,* ed 2, Edinburgh, 1988, Churchill Livingstone.

Curtis P: In search of the "back mouse," *J Fam Pract* 36:657, 1993.

Curwin S, Stanish WD: *Tendinitis: its etiology and treatment,* Lexington, 1984, The Collamore Press.

Cynn H-S et al: Effects of lumbar stabilization using a pressure biofeedback unit on muscle activity and lateral pelvic tilt during hip abduction in sidelying, *Arch Phys Med Rehabil* 87(11):1454-1458, 2006.

Cyrias JH: Lesions discals lombaires, *Acta Orthop Belg* 27:442, 1961.

Cyriax J: *Textbook for orthopaedic medicine,* vol 1: diagnosis of soft tissue lesions, London, 1975, Bailliere Tindall.

Cyriax J: *Textbook of orthopaedic medicine,* vol 1: diagnosis of soft tissue lesions, London, 1982, Bailliere Tindall.

Cyriax JH, Cyriax PJ: *Illustrated manual of orthopaedic medicine,* London, 1983, CM Publications.

Cyriax JH: *Textbook of orthopaedic medicine,* ed 8, London, 1983, Bailliere, Tindall.

Dacre JE, Worrall JG: Rheumatological Examination, *Medicine* 30(8):6-10, 2002.

Daffner RH et al: The radiology assessment of post-traumatic vertebral stability, *Skeletal Radiol* 19:103, 1990.

Daffner RH: *Clinical radiology, the essentials,* Baltimore, 1993, Williams & Wilkins.

Daffner RH: Thoracic and lumbar vertebral trauma, *Orthop Clin North Am* 21:463, 1990.

Dalinka MK, Neustadter LM: Radiology of the hip. In Steinberg ME, editor: *The hip and its disorders,* Philadelphia, 1991, WB Saunders.

Dalton S et al: Human shoulder tendon biopsy samples in organ culture produce procollagenase and tissue inhibitor of metalloproteinases, *Ann Rheum Dis* 54:571, 1995.

Dambro MR, Griffith JA: *Griffith's 5 minute clinical consult,* Baltimore, 1997, Williams & Wilkins.

D'Ambrogio KJ, Roth GB: *Positional release therapy assessment & treatment of musculoskeletal dysfunction,* St Louis, 1997, Mosby.

D'Ambrosia RD: *Musculoskeletal disorders regional examination and differential diagnosis,* Philadelphia, 1977, JB Lippincott.

Dandy DJ, Jackson RW: The impact of arthroscopy on the management of disorders of the knee, *J Bone Joint Surg* 57B:346, 1975.

Dandy DJ: *Essential orthopaedics and trauma,* Edinburgh, 1989, Churchill Livingstone.

Daniels DM, Stone ML: KT-1000 anterior-posterior displacement measurements. In Daniels DM, Akeson WH, O'Connor JJ, editors: *Knee ligament: structure, function, injury and repair,* New York, 1990, Raven.

Daniels L, Worthington C: *Muscle testing: techniques of manual examination,* Philadelphia, 1980, WB Saunders.

Darby S, Cramer G: Pain generators and pathways of the head and neck. In Curl D, editor: *Chiropractic approach to head pain,* Baltimore, 1994, Williams & Wilkins.

Daruwalla P, Darcy S: Personal and societal attitudes to disability, *Ann Tourism Res* 32(3):549-570, 2005.

Dasch B et al: Fracture-related hip pain in elderly patients with proximal femoral fracture after discharge from stationary treatment, *Eur J Pain* (in press, corrected proof).

Datz FL: *Handbook of nuclear medicine,* ed 2, St Louis, 1993, Mosby.

Davidson RI, Dunn EJ, Metzmaker W: The shoulder abduction test in the diagnosis of radicular pain in cervical extradural compressive monoradiculopathies, *Spine* 6:441, 1981.

Dawes HN et al: Borg's Rating of Perceived Exertion Scales: do the verbal anchors mean the same for different clinical groups? *Arch Phys Med Rehabil* 86(5):912-916, 2005.

Dawson DM, Hallett M, Millender LH: *Entrapment neuropathies,* Boston, 1983, Little, Brown.

Dawson DM, Hallett M, Millender LH: Pathology of nerve entrapment. In Dawson DM, Hallett M, Wilbourn A, editors: *Entrapment neuropathies,* ed 2, Boston, 1990, Little & Brown.

Day MO: Spondylolytic spondylolisthesis in an elite athlete, *Chiro Sports Med* 5:91, 1991.

de Groot IB et al: Validation of the Dutch version of the hip disability and osteoarthritis outcome score, *Osteoarthr Cartil* 15(1):104-109, 2007.

de Groot M et al: The active straight leg raising test (ASLR) in pregnant women: Differences in muscle activity and force between patients and healthy subjects, *Man Ther* (in press, corrected proof).

De Hertogh WJ et al: The clinical examination of neck pain patients: the validity of a group of tests, *Man Ther* 12(1):50-55, 2007.

de Kleyn A, Nieuwenhuyse P: Schwindelanfaelle und nystagmus bei einer bestimmten stellung des dopfes, *Acta Otolaryng* 11:155, 1927.

de Kleyn A, Versteegh C: Uber verschledene formen von nemieres syndrome, *Dtsch Z Nervenheilkd* 132:157, 1933.

De Smet L: Avascular necrosis of multiple carpal bones: A case report, *Ann Chir Main* 18(3):202-204, 1999.

De Smet L: The distal radioulnar joint in rheumatoid arthritis, *Int Congr Ser* 129:63-68, 2006.

Debeyre J, Patte D, Elmelik E: Repair of ruptures of the rotator cuff of the shoulder, *J Bone Joint Surg* 47B:36, 1965.

deBlecourt JJ et al: Hereditary factors in rheumatoid arthritis and ankylosing spondylitis, *Ann Rheum Dis* 20:215, 1961.

DeBosset P et al: Comparison of osteitis condensans ilii and ankylosing spondylitis in female patients: clinical, radiological and HLA typing characteristics, *J Chron Dis* 31:171, 1978.

Deen HG et al: Assessment of bladder function after lumbar decompressive surgery for spinal stenosis: a prospective study, *J Neurosurg* 80:971, 1994.

DeJong RN: *The neurologic examination,* ed 4, New York, 1978, Harper & Row.

Dejong RN: *The neurological examination incorporating the fundamentals of neuroanatomy and neurophysiology,* ed 3, New York, 1967, Harper & Row.

Del Notaro C, Hug T: Intra-articular hemangioma of the knee as a cause of knee pain, *Arthroscopy* 19(6):e12-e4, 2003.

Delagi E et al: *An anatomic guide for the electromyographer,* Springfield, Ill, 1975, Charles C Thomas.

Delahunt E: Neuromuscular contributions to functional instability of the ankle joint, *J Bodywork Mov Ther* (in press, corrected proof).

Delamarter RB et al: Experimental lumbar spinal stenosis, *J Bone Joint Surg* 72A:110, 1990.

Delauche-Cavallier MC et al: Lumbar disc herniation: computed tomography scan changes after conservative treatment of nerve root compression, *Spine* 17:927, 1992.

Delbarre F et al: Pyogenic infection of the sacroiliac joint, *J Bone Joint Surg* 57A:819, 1975.

DeLee JC, Drez D, editors: *Orthopedic sports medicine: principles and practice,* Philadelphia, 1994, WB Saunders.

Delitto A, Snyder-Mackler L: The diagnostic process: examples in orthopedic physical therapy, *Phys Ther* 75:203, 1995.

Dellon AL, Curtis RM, Edgerton MT: Evaluating recovery of sensation in the hand following nerve injury, *Johns Hopkins Med J* 130:235, 1972.

Dellon AL, Curtis RM, Edgerton MT: Reeducation of sensation in the hand after nerve injury and repair, *Plast Reconstr Surg* 53:297, 1974.

Dellon AL, Hament W, Gittelshon A: Nonoperative management of cubital tunnel syndrome: an 8 year prospective study, *Neurology* 43:1673, 1993.

Dellon AL et al: Diagnosis of compressive neuropathies in patients with fibromyalgia, *J Hand Surg* 28(6):894-897, 2003.

Deltoff MN, Kogon PL: *The portable skeletal x-ray library,* St Louis, 1998, Mosby.

DeMaio M et al: Plantar fasciitis, *Orthopedics* 16:1153, 1993.

Demeter SL, Anderson GBJ, Smith GM: *Disability evaluation,* St Louis, 1996, Mosby.

DeMeyer W: *Technique of the neurologic examination: a programmed text,* New York, 1969, McGraw-Hill.

Demoulin C et al: Spinal muscle evaluation using the Sorensen test: a critical appraisal of the literature, *Joint Bone Spine* 73(1):43-50, 2006.

DePalma AF, Rothman RH: *The intervertebral disc,* Philadelphia, 1970, WB Saunders.

DePalma AF: *Surgery of the shoulder,* ed 2, Philadelphia, 1973, JB Lippincott.

Derby R et al: The influence of pain tolerance and psychological factors on discography in chronic axial LBP patients, *Spine J* 5(4, suppl 1):S184-S185, 2005.

DeRosa C, Porterfield JA: A physical therapy model for the treatment of low back pain, *Phys Ther* 72:261, 1992.

DeRosa GP, Feller N: Treatment of congenital dislocation of the hip, management before walking age, *Clin Orthop* 225:77, 1987.

Deshpande JK, Tobias JD: *The pediatric pain handbook,* St Louis, 1996, Mosby.

Detenbeck LC: Function of the cruciate ligaments in knee stability, *Am J Sports Med* 2:217, 1974.

Dettenmeier PA: *Radiographic assessment for nurses,* St Louis, 1995, Mosby.

DeVellis B: The psychological impact of arthritis: prevalence of depression, *Arthritis Care Res* 8:284, 1995.

Deyerle WM, May VR: Sciatic tension test, *South Med J* 49:999, 1956.

Deyo R: Nonoperative treatment of low back disorders: differentiating useful therapy. In Frymoryer JW, editor: *The adult spine: principles and practice,* New York, 1991, Raven.

Deyo RA, Loeser JD, Bigos SJ: Herniated lumbar intervertebral disk, *Ann Intern Med* 112(8):598-603, 1990.

Deyo RA, Rainville J, Kent DL: What can the history and physical examination tell us about low back pain? *JAMA* 268:760, 1992.

Di Marzo L et al: Diagnosis of popliteal artery entrapment syndrome: the role of duplex scanning, *J Vasc Surg* 13:434, 1991.

Diamantopoulos A et al: The posterolateral corner of the knee: evaluation under microsurgical dissection, *Arthroscopy* 21(7):826-833, 2005.

Dias J, Buch K: Palmar wrist ganglion: does intervention improve outcome? A prospective study of the natural history and patient-reported treatment outcomes, *J Hand Surg* 28(2):172-176, 2003.

Dias JJ et al: Suspected scaphoid fractures, the value of radiographs, *J Bone Joint Surg* 72B:98, 1990.

Dickenson AH: Spinal cord pharmacology of pain, *Br J Anaesth* 75:193, 1995.

Dickinson WH, Duwelius PJ, Colville MR: Muscle strength following surgery for acetabular fractures, *J Orthop Trauma* 7:39, 1993.

Dickson RA: Conservative treatment for idiopathic scoliosis, *J Bone Joint Surg* 67B:176, 1985.

Dihlmann W: *Diagnostic radiology of the sacroiliac joints,* New York, 1980, George Thieme Verlag.

Dijkstra PU et al: Phantom pain and risk factors: a multivariate analysis, *J Pain Symptom Manage* 24(6):578-585, 2002.

Dilley DF, Tonkin MA: Acute calcific tendinitis in the hand and wrist, *J Hand Surg* 16B:215, 1991.

Dilsen N et al: A comparative roentgenologic study of rheumatoid arthritis and rheumatoid (ankylosing) spondylitis, *Arthritis Rheum* 5:341, 1962.

Dimitriou CG, Chalidis B, Pournaras J: Bilateral volar lunate dislocation, *J Hand Surg* (in press, corrected proof).

Dimitru D: *Electrodiagnostic medicine,* Philadelphia, 1995, Hanley & Belfus.

Dinham, JM: Popliteal cysts in children, *J Bone Joint Surg* 57B:69, 1975.

Dionysian E et al: Proximal interphalangeal joint stiffness: measurement and analysis, *J Hand Surg* 30(3):573-579, 2005.

Disler DG et al: Fat-suppressed three-dimensional spoiled gradient-echo MR imaging of hyaline cartilage defects in the knee: comparison with standard MR imaging and arthroscopy, *AJR Am J Roentgenol* 167:127, 1996.

Dixon AS et al: A double-blind controlled trial of Rumalon in the treatment of painful osteoarthrosis of the hip, *Ann Rheum Dis* 29:193, 1970.

Dobbs HS: Survivorship of total hip replacements, *J Bone Joint Surg* 62B:168, 1980.

Dodge PR, Swartz MN: Bacterial meningitis: special neurologic problems, postmeningitic complications and clinicopathologic correlations, *N Engl J Med* 272:954, 1965.

Doherty M et al: The "GALS" locomotor screen, *Ann Rheum Dis* 51:1165, 1992.

Doherty M, Doherty J: *Clinical examination in rheumatology,* London, 1992, Wolfe.

Doherty M, George E: *Self-assessment picture tests in rheumatology,* London, 1995, Mosby-Wolfe.

Doherty M: *Color atlas and text of osteoarthritis,* London, 1994, Wolfe.

Dommisse GF, Grobler L: Arteries and veins of the lumbar nerve roots and cauda equina, *Clin Orthop* 115:22, 1976.

Dommisse GF, Louw JA: Anatomy of the lumbar spine. In Floman Y, editor: *Disorders of the lumbar spine,* Rockville, Md, and Tel Aviv, Israel, s1990, Aspen and Freund Publishing House.

Donell S: Patellofemoral dysfunction—extensor mechanism malalignment, *Curr Orthop2* 20(2):103-111, 006.

Donelson R, McKenzie R: Mechanical assessment and treatment of spinal pain. In Frymoyer JW, editor: *The adult spine: principles and practice,* New York, 1991, Raven.

DonTigny RL: Anterior dysfunction of sacroiliac joint as a major factor in the etiology of idiopathic low back pain syndrome, *Phys Ther* 70:250, 1990.

Doody C, McAteer M: Clinical reasoning of expert and novice physiotherapists in an outpatient orthopaedic setting, *Physiotherapy* 88(5):258-268, 2002.

Doria AS et al: Contrast-enhanced power Doppler sonography: assessment of revascularization flow in Legg-Calve-Perthes' disease, *Ultrasound Med Biol* 28(2):171-182, 2002.

Dossett AB, Watkins RG: Stinger injuries in football. In Watkins RG, editor: *The spine in sports,* St Louis, 1996, Mosby.

Doucette SA, Goble EM: The effect of exercise on patellar tracking in lateral patellar compression syndrome, *Am J Sports Med* 20:434, 1992.

Doward DA, Troxell ML, Fredericson M: Synovial chondromatosis in an elite cyclist: a case report, *Arch Phys Med Rehabil* 87(6):860-865, 2006.

Doyle JR: Extensor tendons-acute injuries. In Green DP, editor: *Operative hand surgery,* ed 3, New York, 1993, Churchill Livingstone.

Dray A: Inflammatory mediators of pain, *Br J Anesth* 75:125, 1995.

Dray GJ, Eaton RG: Dislocation and ligament injuries in the digits. In Green DP, editor: *Operative hand surgery,* ed 3, New York, 1993, Churchill-Livingstone.

Dreyfus P, Michaelsen M, Fletcher D: Atlanto-occipital and atlantoaxial joint pain patterns, *Spine* 19:1125, 1994.

Duchenne GB: *Physiology of motion (translated by Emanuel B. Kaplan),* Philadelphia, 1975, WB Saunders.

Duhamel P: Criterion, construct and concurrent validity of a norm-referenced measure of malingering in pain patients, *Journal Pain* 6(3, suppl 1):S70, 2005.

Dulhunty JA: Sacroiliac subluxation, facts, fallacies and illusions, *J Aust Chiro Assoc* 15:91, 1985.

Dunaway DJ et al: The sartorial branch of the saphenous nerve: its anatomy at the joint line of the knee, *Arthroscopy* 21(5):547-551, 2005.

Dunk NM, Callaghan JP: Gender-based differences in postural responses to seated exposures, *Clin Biomech* 20(10):1101-1110, 2005.

Dunk NM et al: The reliability of quantifying upright standing postures as a baseline diagnostic clinical tool, *J Manipulative Physiol Ther* 27(2):91-96, 2004.

Dunn DJ et al: Pyogenic infections of the sacroiliac joint, *Clin Orthop* 118:113, 1976.

Dupoux E et al: Persistent stress `deafness': the case of French learners of Spanish, *Cognition* (in press, corrected proof).

Durrett LC: Management of patients with vertebrobasilar ischemia, *Chiropr Tech* 6:95, 1994.

Dussault R, Lander P: Imaging of the facet joints, *Radiol Clin North Am* 28:1033, 1990.

Duthie RB, Bentley G, editors: *Mercer's orthopaedic surgery,* ed 8, London, 1983, Edward Arnold.

Dutkowski JP: Nontraumatic bone and joint disorders. In Crenshaw AH, editor: *Campbell's operative orthopaedics,* ed 8, vol 3, St Louis, 1992, Mosby.

DuVries HL: Five myths about your feet, *Today's Health* 45:49, 1967.

DuVries HL: *Surgery of the foot,* ed 2, St Louis, 1965, Mosby.

Dvorak J, Dvorak V: *Manual medicine: diagnostics,* New York, 1990, Thieme.

Dworkin RH et al: Symptom profiles differ in patients with neuropathic versus non-neuropathic pain, *J Pain* 8(2):118-126, 2007.

Dyck P: The femoral nerve traction test with lumbar disc protrusion, *Surg Neurol* 6:163, 1976.

Dyck P: The stoop-test in lumbar entrapment radiculopathy, *Spine* 4:89, 1979.

Early PJ, Sodee DB: *Principles and practice of nuclear medicine,* St Louis, 1995, Mosby.

Eastcott HHG: *Arterial surgery,* ed 2, London, 1973, Pitman.

Eastwood DM, Gregg PJ, Atkins RM: Intra-articular fractures of the calcaneum, *J Bone Joint Surg* 75B:183, 1993.

Ebraheim N et al: Percutaneous computed tomography guided stabilization of posterior pelvis fractures, *Clin Orthop* 307:222, 1994.

Echternach J, editor: *Clinics in physical therapy of the hip,* New York, 1990, Churchill Livingstone.

Edeiken J: *Roentgen diagnosis of diseases of bone,* ed 4, Baltimore, 1990, Williams & Wilkins.

Edelson G et al: Bony changes at the lateral epicondyle of possible significance in tennis elbow syndrome, *J Shoulder Elbow Surg* 10(2):158-163, 2001.

Edgar MA, Ghadially JA: Innervation of the lumbar spine, *Clin Orthop* 115:35, 1976.

Edgar MS, Park WM: Induced pain patterns on passive straight-leg-raising in lower lumbar disc protrusion, *J Bone Joint Surg* 56B:658, 1974.

Edwards RR et al: Symptoms of distress as prospective predictors of pain-related sciatica treatment outcomes, *Pain* 130(1-2):47-55, 2007.

Eftekhar NS, editor: Low friction arthroplasty, *Clin Orthop* 211:2, 1986.

Egund N, Wingstrand H: Legg-Calve-Perthes disease: imaging with MR, *Radiology* 179:89, 1991.

Ehrlich M, Hulstyn M, D'Amoto C: Sports injuries in children and the clumsy child, *Pediatr Clin North Am* 39:433, 1992.

Eifert-Mangine M et al: Patellar tendinitis in the recreational athlete, *Orthopedics* 15:1359, 1992.

Eisele SA, Sammarco GL: Fatigue fractures of the foot and ankle in the athlete, *J Bone Joint Surg* 75:290, 1993.

Elattrache N, Fadale PD, Fu F: Thoracic spine fracture in a football player, *Am J Sports Med* 21:157, 1984.

Elattrache NS, Thompson B: Clinical impact of elbow magnetic resonance imaging, *Oper Tech Sports Med* 5(1):33-36, 1997.

Elias DA, White LM: Imaging of patellofemoral disorders, *Clin Radiol* 59(7):543-557, 2004.

Ellard J: Psychological reactions to compensable injury, *Med J Aust* 8:349, 1970.

Ellenberg ME et al: Prospective evaluation of the course of disc herniation in patients with radiculopathy, *Arch Phys Med Rehabil* 74:3, 1993.

Elliott FA, Schutta HS: The differential diagnosis of sciatica, *Orthop Clin North Am* 2:477, 1971.

Elliott J et al: MRI study of the cross-sectional area for the cervical extensor musculature in patients with persistent whiplash associated disorders (WAD), *Man Ther* (in press, corrected proof).

Elster AD: *Questions and answers in magnetic resonance imaging,* St Louis, 1994, Mosby.

Elstorm, Pankovich A: Muscle and tendon surgery of the leg. In Evarts CM, editor: *Surgery of the musculoskeletal system,* ed 2, New York, 1990, Churchill Livingstone.

Engelman EG, Engleman EP: Ankylosing spondylitis: recent advances in diagnosis and treatment, *Med Clin North Am* 61:347, 1977.

Engelman RM: Shoulder pain as a presenting complaint in upper lobe bronchogenic carcinoma: report of 21 cases, *Conn Med* 30:273, 1966.

Engesaeter LB et al: Ultrasound and congenital dislocation of the hip, *J Bone Joint Surg* 72B:202, 1990.

Engle RP, Meade TD, Canner BC: Rehabilitation of posterior cruciate ligament injuries. In Greenfield BH, editor: *Rehabilitation of the knee: a problem solving approach,* Philadelphia, 1993, FA Davis.

Epstein BS: *The spine, a radiological text and atlas,* ed 3, Philadelphia, 1969, Lea & Febiger.

Epstein MC: Cause of low back problem, *Dig Chiro Econ* 26:52, 1983.

Epstein O et al: *Clinical examination,* ed 2, London, 1997, Mosby.

Epstein O et al: *Clinical examination,* ed 2, London, 1997, Mosby.

Ericksen MF: Aging in the lumbar spine, *Am J Phys Anthropol* 48:241, 1974.

Ernst CW et al: Prevalence of annular tears and disc herniations on MR images of the cervical spine in symptom free volunteers, *Eur J Radiol* 55(3):409-414, 2005.

Eslam Pour A et al: Back pain and total hip arthroplasty: a prospective natural history study, *J Arthroplasty* 22(2):314, 2007.

Espinola-Klein C et al: Inflammation, atherosclerotic burden and cardiovascular prognosis, *Atherosclerosis* (in press, corrected proof).

Esposito MD et al: Thoracic outlet syndrome in a throwing athlete diagnosed with MRI and MRA, *J Magn Reson Imaging* 7:598, 1997.

Esterhai JL et al: Adult septic arthritis, *Orthop Clin North Am* 22:503, 1991.

Etherton JL et al: Pain, malingering and the WAIS-III Working Memory Index, *Spine J* 6(1):61-71, 2006.

Evangelisti S, Realve VF: Fibroma of tendon sheath as a cause of carpal tunnel syndrome, *J Hand Surg* 17A:1026, 1992.

Evans RC: Malingering/symptoms exaggeration. In Sweere JJ, editor: *Chiropractic family practice, a clinical manual,* Gaithersburg, Md, 1992, Aspen.

Evans RC: *Overview of orthopedic malingering. CAPIT homecoming and educational symposium,* Rotorura, New Zealand, 1986, Phillip Institute of Science and Technology.

Eyigor S, Durmaz B, Karapolat H: Monoparesis with complex regional pain syndrome-like symptoms due to brachial plexopathy caused by the varicella zoster virus: a case report, *Arch Phys Med Rehabil* 87(12):1653-1655, 2006.

Eyler VA, Diehl KW, Kirkhart M: Validation of the Lees-Haley Fake Bad scale for the MMPI-2 to detect somatic malingering among personal injury litigants, *Arch Clin Neuropsychol* 15(8):834-835, 2000.

Eyre-Brook A: Septic arthritis of the hip and osteomyelitis of upper end of the femur in infants, *J Bone Joint Surg* 42B:11, 1960.

Eyre-Brook AL, Jones DA, Harris FC: Pemberton's acetabuloplasty for congenital dislocation of subluxation of the hip, *J Bone Joint Surg* 60B:18, 1978.

Fahrni WH: Observations on straight-leg raising with special reference to nerve root adhesions, *Can J Surg* 9:44, 1966.

Faik A et al: Spinal cord compression due to vertebral osteochondroma: report of two cases, *Joint Bone Spine* 72(2):177-179, 2005.

Failinger MS, McGanety PL: Current concepts review, unstable fractures of the pelvic ring, *J Bone Joint Surg* 74A:781, 1992.

Fairbank JTC: The Oswestry low back pain disability questionnaire, *Physiotherapy* 8:66, 1980.

Fanelli GC, Orcutt DR, Edson CJ: The multiple-ligament injured knee: evaluation, treatment, and results, *Arthroscopy* 21(4):471-486, 2005.

Farasyn A: Referred muscle pain is primarily peripheral in origin: the "barrier-dam" theory, *Med Hypotheses* 68(1):144-150, 2007.

Farfan HF: *Mechanical disorders of the low back,* Philadelphia, 1973, Lea & Febiger.

Farin PU et al: Shoulder impingement syndrome; sonographic evaluation, *Radiology* 176:845, 1990.

Farnum CE et al: Volume increase in growth plate chondrocytes during hypertrophy: the contribution of organic osmolytes, *Bone* 30(4):574-581, 2002.

Farr D et al: Arthroscopic bursectomy with concomitant iliotibial band release for the treatment of recalcitrant trochanteric bursitis, *Arthroscopy* (in press, corrected proof).

Farrar WE: *Atlas of infections of the nervous system,* London, 1993, Wolfe.

Fayssoux RS et al: Spinal injuries after falls from hunting tree stands, *Spine J* (in press, uncorrected proof).

Feagin JA: *The crucial ligaments: diagnosis and treatment of ligamentous injuries about the knee,* New York, 1988, Churchill Livingstone; 1988.

Federico DJ, Lynch JK, Jokl P: Osteochondritis dissecans of the knee: a historical review of etiology and treatment, *Arthroscopy* 6:190, 1990.

Fedorczyk JM: Tennis elbow: blending basic science with clinical practice, *J Hand Ther* 19(2):146-153, 2006.

Fegan WG, Fitzgerald DE, Beesley WH: A modern approach to the injection treatment of varicose veins and its applications in pregnant patients, *Am Heart J* 68:757, 1964.

Feipel V, Berghe MV, Rooze MA: No effects of cervical spine motion on cranial dura mater strain, *Clin Biomech* 18(5):389-392, 2003.

Feldmann E: *Current diagnosis in neurology,* St Louis, 1994, Mosby.

Ferezy JS: *The chiropractic neurological examination,* Gaithersburg, Md, 1992, Aspen.

Ferguson AB Jr: The pathology of degenerative arthritis of the hip and the use of osteotomy in its treatment, *Clin Orthop* 77:118, 1971.

Ferkel RD et al: Arthroscopic treatment of anterolateral impingement of the ankle, *Am J Sports Med* 19:440, 1991.

Fernandez-de-las-Penas C et al: Referred pain from trapezius muscle trigger points shares similar characteristics with chronic tension type headache, *Eur J Pain* 11(4):475-482, 2007.

Fernandez-Palazzi F, Rivas S, Mujica P: Achilles tendinitis in ballet dancers, *Clin Orthop* 257:257, 1990.

Fernstrom U, Goldie I: Does granulation tissue in the intervertebral disc provoke back pain? *Acta Orthop Scand* 30:202, 1960.

Ferraz MB et al: EPM-ROM scale: an evaluative instrument to be used in rheumatoid arthritis trials, *Clin Exp Rheumatol* 8:491, 1990.

Ferris B, Edgar M, Leyshon A: Screening for scoliosis, *Acta Orthop Scand* 59:417, 1988.

Fetto JF, Marshall JL: Injury to the anterior cruciate ligament producing the pivot shift sign: an experimental study on cadaver specimens, *J Bone Joint Surg* 61A:710, 1979.

Ficat RP, Hungerford DS: *Disorders of the patello-femoral joint,* Baltimore, 1977, Williams & Wilkins.

Field T et al: Lower back pain and sleep disturbance are reduced following massage therapy, *J Bodywork Mov Ther* 11(2):141-145, 2007.

Finke J: Neurologic differential diagnosis: the lower cervical region, *Dutsch Med Wochenschr* 90:1912, 1965.

Finkelstein H: Stenosing tendovaginitis at the radial styloid process, *J Bone Joint Surg* 12:509, 1930.

Finneson BE: *Diagnosis and management of pain syndromes,* Philadelphia, 1969, WB Saunders.

Finneson BE: *Low back pain,* ed 2, Philadelphia, 1980, JB Lippincott.

Firer P: Etiology and results of treatment of iliotibial band friction syndrome, *J Bone Joint Surg* 72B:742, 1990.

Fisher M: Basilar artery embolism after surgery under general anesthesia: a case report, *Neurology* 43:1856, 1993.

Fisk JW, Balgent ML: Clinical and radiological assessment of leg length, *N Z Med J* 81:477, 1975.

Fitzpatrick TB et al: *Color atlas and synopsis of clinical dermatology common and serious diseases,* ed 2, New York, 1992, McGraw-Hill.

Flatt AE: *The care of minor hand injuries,* St Louis, 1972, Mosby.

Flores LP, Carneiro JZ: Peripheral nerve compression secondary to adjacent lipomas, *Surg Neurol* 67(3):258-262, 2007.

Fokkema DS et al: Different breathing patterns in healthy and asthmatic children: responses to an arithmetic task, *Respir Med* 100(1):148-156, 2006.

Folberg CR, Weiss AP, Akelman E: Cubital tunnel syndrome, part 1: presentation and diagnosis, *Orthop Rev* 23:136, 1994.

Foldes K et al: Nocturnal pain correlates with effusions in diseased hips, *J Rheumatol* 19:1756, 1992.

Fomby EW, Mellion MB: Identifying and treating myofascial pain syndrome, *Phys Sports Med* 25, 1997.

Forbes CD, Jackson WF: *A color atlas and text of clinical medicine,* Aylesbury, UK, 1993, Wolfe.

Ford JS: *Posttraumatic headache,* Chicago, 1985, Med Recertification Associates.

Foreman SM, Croft AC: *Whiplash injuries: the cervical acceleration/deceleration syndrome,* Baltimore, 1992, Williams & Wilkins.

Foreman SM, Stahl MJ, Sportelli L: *Medical-legal issues in chiropractic,* Palmerton, Pa, 1993, PracticeMakers Products.

Forestier R et al: French version of the Copenhagen neck functional disability scale, *Joint Bone Spine* 74(2):155-159, 2007.

Fornage B: *Musculoskeletal ultrasound,* New York, 1995, Churchill Livingstone.

Franz WB III: Overuse syndromes in runners. In Mellion MB, Walsh WM, Shelton GL, editors: *Sports injuries and athletic problems,* Philadelphia, 1990, Hanley & Belfus.

Freeman MD, Fox D, Richards T: The superior intracapsular ligament of the sacroiliac joint: confirmation of Ill's ligament, *J Manipulative Physiol Ther* 13:374, 1990.

Freemont AJ, Denton J: *Atlas of synovial fluid cytopathology,* vol 18, Dordrecht, 1991, Kluwer Academic.

Freemont FJ et al: The diagnostic value of synovial fluid cytoanalysis: a reassessment, *Ann Rheum Dis* 50:101, 1991.

French HP: Physiotherapy management of osteoarthritis of the hip: a survey of current practice in acute hospitals and private practice in the Republic of Ireland, *Physiotherapy* (in press, corrected proof).

Frey C, Shereff M, Greenridge N: Vascularity of the posterior tibial tendon, *J Bone Joint Surg*884,1990, 72A.

Frick SL: Evaluation of the child who has hip pain, *Orthop Clin North Am* 37(2):133-140, 2006.

Fricker PA, Taunton JE, Ammann W: Osteitis pubis in athletes; infection, inflammation, or injury, *Sports Med* 12:266, 1991.

Friedman SA, Holling HE, Roberts B: Etiologic factors in aortoiliac and femoro-popliteal vascular disease, *N Engl J Med* 271:1382, 1964.

Fries JF: *Arthritis, a take care of yourself health guide for understanding your arthritis,* ed 4, 1995, Addison-Wesley.

Fritz RC, Brody GA: MR imaging of the wrist and elbow, *Clin Sports Med* 14:315, 1995.

Froissart A, Pagnoux C, Cherin P: Lymph node paradoxical enlargement during treatment for tuberculous spondylodiscitis (Pott's disease), *Joint Bone Spine* 74(3):292-295, 2007.

Frost A, Bauer M: Skier's hip: a new clinical entity? proximal femur fractures sustained in cross-country skiing, *J Orthop Trauma* 5:47, 1991.

Frykman G: Fracture of the distal radius including sequelae-shoulder-hand-finger syndrome, disturbance in the distal radioulnar joint and impairment of nerve function: a clinical and experimental study, *Acta Orthop Scand Suppl* 108:1, 1967.

Frykman GK: *The orthopedic clinics of North America,* vol 12(2), Philadelphia, April 1981 and April 1984, WB Saunders.

Frymoyer J, editor: *Orthopedic knowledge update No. 4,* Rosemont, Ill, 1993, American Academy of Orthopedic Surgery.

Frymoyer J: *The adult spine,* New York, 1991, Raven.

Frymoyer JW, Cats-Baril WI: An overview of the incidences and costs of low back pain, *Orthop Clin North Am* 22:263, 1991.

Fu FH, Baratz M: Meniscal injuries. In DeLee JC, Drez D, editors: *Orthopaedic sports medicine: principals and practice,* vol 2, Philadelphia, 1994, WB Saunders.

Fulkerson JP, Hungerford DS: *Disorders of the patellofemoral joint,* Baltimore, 1990, Williams & Wilkins.

Fulkerson JP, Shea KP: Current concepts review disorders of patellofemoral alignment, *J Bone Joint Surg* 72A:1424, 1990.

Fulton M: *Lower-back pain: a new solution for an old problem,* Rolling Meadows, NJ, 1992, MedX.

Furman W, Marshall JL, Girgis FG: The anterior cruciate ligaments: a functional analysis based on postmortem studies, *J Bone Joint Surg* 58A:179, 1976.

Fuss FK, Bacher A: New aspects of the morphology and function of the human hip joint ligaments, *Am J Anat* 192:1, 1991.

Gabel G, Bishop AT, Wood MB: Flexor carpi radialis tendinitis. part II: results of operative treatment, *J Bone Joint Surg* 76A:1015, 1994.

Gabriel DA, Basford JR, An K-N: Vibratory facilitation of strength in fatigued muscle, *Arch Phys Med Rehabil* 83(9):1202-1205, 2002.

Gage JR, Winter RB: Avascular necrosis of the capital femoral epiphysis as a complication of closed reduction of congenital dislocation of the hip, *J Bone Joint Surg* 54A: 373, 1972.

Gaine WJ, Mohammed A: Osteophyte impingement of the popliteus tendon as a cause of lateral knee joint pain, *Knee* 9(3):249-252, 2002.

Galasko CSB, editor: *Neuromuscular problems in orthopaedics,* Oxford, UK, 1987, Blackwell.

Galasko CSB, Nobel J, editors: *Current trends in orthopaedic surgery,* Manchester, UK, 1988, Manchester University Press.

Galland O et al: An anatomical and radiological study of the femoropatellar articulation, *Surg Radiol Anat* 12:119, 1990.

Galpin RD et al: One-stage treatment of congenital dislocation of the hip in older children, *J Bone Joint Surg* 71A:734, 1989.

Galvez R et al: Cross-sectional evaluation of patient functioning and health-related quality of life in patients with neuropathic pain under standard care conditions, *Eur J Pain* 11(3):244-255, 2007.

Galway HR, MacIntosh DL: The lateral pivot shift: symptoms and sign of anterior cruciate ligament insufficiency, *Clin Orthop* 147:45, 1980.

Gamstorp I: Normal conduction velocity of ulnar, median, and peroneal nerves in infancy, childhood and adolescence, *Acta Paediatra Suppl* 146:68, 1963.

Ganguly DN, Roy KKS: A study on the craniovertebral joint in man, *Anat Anz* 114:433, 1964.

Ganz PA: The quality of life after breast cancer. Solving the problem of lymphedema, *N Engl J Med* 340(5):383-385, 1999.

Garbuz DS, Xu M, Sayre EC: Patients' outcome after total hip arthroplasty: a comparison between the Western Ontario and McMaster Universities Index and the Oxford 12-item Hip Score, *J Arthroplasty* 21(7):998-1004, 2006.

Garcia F, Florez MT, Conejero JA: A butterfly vertebra or a wedge fracture? *Int Orthop* 17:7, 1993.

Garcia JH: *Neuropathology the diagnostic approach,* St Louis, 1997, Mosby.

Garcia-Borreguero D et al: Diagnostic standards for dopaminergic augmentation of restless legs syndrome: report from the World Association of Sleep Medicine— International Restless Legs Syndrome Study Group Consensus Conference at the Max Planck Institute, *Sleep Med* (in press, corrected proof).

Garden RS: Tennis elbow, *J Bone Joint Surg* 43B:100, 1961.

Gardner E, Gray DJ, O'Rahilly R: *Anatomy: a regional study of human structure,* ed 4, Philadelphia, 1975, WB Saunders.

Gardner E, Gray DJ: The innervation of the joints of the foot, *Anat Rec* 161:141, 1968.

Gardner E: *Fundamentals of neurology,* ed 4, Philadelphia, 1963, WB Saunders.

Gargan MF, Fairbank JCT: Anatomy of the spine. In Watkins RG, editor: *The spine in sports,* St Louis, 1996, Mosby.

Garn AN, Thorsen H, Lonnberg F: The effect of low-level laser therapy on musculoskeletal pain: a meta-analysis, *Pain* 52:63, 1993.

Garret JC: Osteochondritis dissecans, *Clin Orthop Sports Med* 10:569, 1991.

Garrick J, Webb DR: Pelvis, hip, thigh injuries. In Garrick J, Webb DR, editors: *Sports injuries: diagnosis and management,* Philadelphia, 1990, WB Saunders.

Garth W: Evaluating and treating brachial plexus injuries, *J Musculoskeletal Med* 55, 1994.

Garth WB: Current concepts regarding the anterior cruciate ligament, *Orthop Rev* 21:565, 1992.

Gartland JJ: *Fundamentals of orthopaedics,* ed 2, Philadelphia, 1974, WB Saunders.

Gartland JJ: *Fundamentals of orthopaedics,* London, 1968, E & S Livingstone.

Gartland JJ: Orthopaedic clinical research, *J Bone Joint Surg* 70A:1357, 1988.

Gartsman GM: Arthroscopic acromioplasty for lesions of the rotator cuff, *J Bone Joint Surg* 72A:169, 1990.

Gascon J: A current problem: diagnosis of the shoulder pain syndrome, *Union Med Can* 94:463, 1965.

Gatehouse PD et al: Magnetic resonance imaging of the knee with ultrashort TE pulse sequences, *Magn Reson Imaging* 22(8):1061-1067, 2004.

Gatterman MI: Disorders of the pelvic ring. In Gatterman MI, editor: *Chiropractic management of spine-related disorders,* Baltimore, 1990, Williams & Wilkins.

Gatts SK, Woollacott MH: How Tai Chi improves balance: biomechanics of recovery to a walking slip in impaired seniors, *Gait Posture* 25(2):205-214, 2007.

Gavin TM, Shurr DG, Patwardhan AG: Orthotic treatment for spinal disorders. In Weinstein SL, editor: *The pediatric spine,* New York, 1993, Raven.

Ge H-Y et al: Hypoalgesia to pressure pain in referred pain areas triggered by spatial summation of experimental muscle pain from unilateral or bilateral trapezius muscles, *Eur J Pain* 7(6):531-537, 2003.

Gelberman RH et al: The vascularity of the lunate bone and Kienbock's disease, *J Hand Surg* 5A:272, 1980.

Gemmell H, Miller P: Should chiropractors recommend provocative discography for diagnostic purposes in patients with chronic low back pain? *Clin Chiropr* 8(1):20-26, 2005.

George M, Wall EJ: Locked knee caused by meniscal subluxation: magnetic resonance imaging and arthroscopic verification, *Arthroscopy* 19(8):885-888, 2003.

George VA et al: Morton's neuroma: the role of MR scanning in diagnostic assistance, *Foot* 15(1):14-16, 2005.

Gerard JA, Kleinfield SL: *Orthopaedic testing,* New York, 1993, Churchill Livingstone.

Gerber C, Krushell FJ: Isolated rupture of the tendon of the subscapularis muscle: clinical features in 16 cases, *J Bone Joint Surg* 73B:389, 1991.

Gertzbein SD: Spine update: classification of thoracic and lumbar fractures, *Spine* 19:626, 1994.

Geven LI, Smit AJ, Ebels T, Vascular thoracic outlet syndrome. Longer posterior rib stump causes poor outcome, *Eur J Cardiothorac Surg* 30(2):232-236, 2006.

Ghanem N et al: MRI and discography in traumatic intervertebral disc lesions, *Clin Imaging* 31(2):147, 2007.

Gianakopoulos G et al: Inversion devices: their role in producing lumbar distraction, *Arch Phys Med Rehabil* 66:100, 1985.

Gibbon WW, Cassar-Pullicino VN: Heel pain, *Ann Rheum Dis* 53:344, 1994.

Gibbons K, Soloniuk D, Razack N: Neurological injury and patterns of sacral fractures, *J Neurosurg* 72:889, 1990.

Gifford DB et al: Septic arthritis due to pseudomonas in heroin addicts, *J Bone Joint Surg* 57A:631, 1975.

Gilani SA, Fazal N: Role of TVS in diagnosis of female genital tuberculosis, *Ultrasound Med Biol* 32(5, suppl 1):P92-P93, 2006.

Giles LGF, Kaveri MJP: Some osseous and soft tissue causes of lumbar stenosis, *J Rheumatol* 17:1374, 1990.

Gilkey DP: Injury prevention in the workplace: a closer look at OSHA's proposed ergonomic standard, *J Am Chiropractic Assoc* 33:25, 1996.

Gilliatt RW: Normal conduction in human and experimental neuropathies, *Proc R Soc Lond B Biol* Sci 59:989, 1966.

Gillis L: *Diagnosis in orthopaedics,* London, 1969, Butterworths.

Gilula LA editor: *The traumatized wrist and hand: radiographic and anatomic correlation,* Philadelphia, 1992, Saunders.

Gilula LA, Yin Y: *Imaging of the wrist and hand,* Philadelphia, 1996, WB Saunders.

Gips H, Yannai U, Hiss J: Self-inflicted gunshot wound mimicking assault: a rare variant of factitious disorder, *J Forensic Leg Med* 14(5):293-296, 2007.

Girgis FG, Marshall JL, Al Monajem ARS: The cruciate ligaments of the knee joint: anatomical, functional and experimental analysis, *Clin Orthop* 106:216, 1975.

Giuliani G et al: CT scan and surgical treatment of traumatic iliacus hematoma with femoral neuropathy: case report, *J Trauma* 30:229, 1990.

Glenton C: Chronic back pain sufferers—striving for the sick role, *Soc Sci Med* 57(11):2243-2252, 2003.

Glick JM: Hip arthroscopy. In Mcginty JB et al, editors: *Operative arthroscopy,* New York, 1991, Raven.

Goddard BS, Reid JD: Movements induced by straight-leg-raising in the lumbo-sacral roots, nerves, and plexus and in the intra pelvic section of the sciatic nerve, *J Neurol Neurosurg Psychiatry* 28:12, 1965.

Godfrey J et al: Reliability, validity, and responsiveness of the simple shoulder test: psychometric properties by age and injury type, *J Shoulder Elbow Surg* 16(3): 260-267, 2007.

Gohlke F, Essigkrug B, Schmiz F: The pattern of the collagen fiber bundles of the capsule of the glenohumeral joint, *J Shoulder Elbow Surg* 3:111, 1994.

Goker B et al: The effects of minor hip flexion, abduction or adduction and x-ray beam angle on the radiographic joint space width of the hip, *Osteoarthr Cartil* 13(5): 379-386, 2005.

Goldberg, J, Kovarsky J: Tuberculous sacroiliitis, *South Med J* 76:1175, 1983.

Goldenberg DL: Fatigue in rheumatic disease, *Bull Rheum Dis* 44:4, 1995.

Goldie BS: *Orthopaedic diagnosis and management a guide to the care of orthopaedic patients,* ed 2, Oxford, UK, 1998, ISIS Medical Media.

Goldie I: Calcified deposits in the shoulder joint produced by calciphylaxis and their inhibition by triamcinolone: an experimental model, *Bull Soc Int Chir* 23:91, 1965.

Goldman GA et al: Idiopathic transient osteoporosis of the hip in pregnancy, *Int J Gynaecol Obstet* 46:317, 1994.

Goldner JL, Bright DS: The effect of extremity blood flow on pain and cold tolerance. In Omer G, Spinner M, editors: *Peripheral nerve injuries,* Philadelphia, 1979, WB Saunders.

Goldner JL et al: Metacarpophalangeal joint arthroplasty with silicone-Dacron prosthesis, Niebauer type, six and a half years experience, *J Bone Joint Surg* 2:200, 1977.

Goldner JL: Musculoskeletal aspects of emotional problems, editorial, *South Med J* 69:1, 1976.

Goldner JL: Volkmann's ischemic contracture. In Flynn JE, editor: *Hand surgery,* ed 2, Baltimore, 1975, Williams & Wilkins.

Goldstein JD et al: Spine injuries in gymnasts and swimmers, *Am J Sports Med* 19:463, 1991.

Goldstein LA, Waugh TR: Classification and terminology of scoliosis, *Clin Orthop* 93:10, 1973.

Goldstein MJ et al: Osteomyelitis complicating regional enteritis, *Gut* 10:264, 1969.

Goldstein RS: Geriatric orthopaedics, rehabilitative management of common problems. In Lewis CB, editor: *Aspen series in physical therapy,* Gaithersburg, Md, 1991, Aspen.

Goldstein TS: Treatment of common problems of the hip joint. In Goldstein TS, Lewis CB, series editors: *Geriatric orthopaedics rehabilitative management for common problems,* Gaithersburg, Md, 1991, Aspen.

Golightly YM et al: Relationship of limb length inequality with radiographic knee and hip osteoarthritis, *Osteoarthr Cartil* (in press, corrected proof).

Gombatto SP et al: Gender differences in pattern of hip and lumbopelvic rotation in people with low back pain, *Clin Biomech* 21(3):263-271, 2006.

Gomez D, Jha K, Jepson K: Ultrasound scan for the diagnosis of interdigital neuroma, *Foot Ankle Surg* 11(3):175-177, 2005.

Gondipalli P, Tobias JD: Anesthetic implications of Mobius syndrome, *J Clin Anesth* 18(1):55-59, 2006.

Goodfellow J, Hungerford DS, Woods C: Patello-femoral joint mechanics and pathology: chondromalacia patella, *J Bone Joint Surg* 58B:291, 1976.

Goodfellow J, Hungerford DS, Zindel M: Patello-femoral joint mechanics and pathology: functional anatomy of the patello-femoral joint, *J Bone Joint Surg* 58B:287, 1976.

Goodman CG, Snyder TE: *Systemic origins of musculoskeletal pain: associated signs and symptoms. In Differential diagnosis in physical therapy,* Philadelphia, 1990, WB Saunders.

Gordon G, Kabins SA: Pyogenic sacroiliitis, *Am J Med* 69:50, 1980.

Gordon M: *Nursing diagnosis: process and application,* ed 3, St Louis, 1994, Mosby.

Gorse GJ et al: Tuberculous spondylitis: a report of six cases and a review of the literature, *Medicine (Baltimore)* 62:178, 1978.

Goshi K et al: Thoracic scoliosis fusion in adolescent and adult idiopathic scoliosis using posterior translational corrective techniques (Isola): is maximum correction of the thoracic curve detrimental to the unfused lumbar curve? *Spine J* 4(2):192-201, 2004.

Goulet J et al: Comminuted fractures of the posterior wall of the acetabulum: a biomechanical evaluation of fixation methods, *J Bone Joint Surg* 76A:1457, 1994.

Gowers WR: *Diseases of the nervous system,* ed 2, London, 1969, Churchill.

Gracely RH, Undem BJ, Banzett RB: Cough, pain and dyspnea: similarities and differences, *Pulm Pharmacol Ther* 20(4):433-437, 2007.

Gracovetsky S: Biomechanics of the spine. In White AH, Schofferman JA, editors: *Spine care: diagnosis and conservative treatment,* St Louis, 1995, Mosby.

Gracovetsky S: The spine as a motor in sports: application to running and lifting, *Spine* 4:267, 1990.

Graham S et al: The Chiari osteotomy, *Clin Orthop* 208:249, 1986.

Gramaglia L et al: Worsening of chronic pain: the treatment, *Arch Gerontol Geriatr* 44(suppl 1):207-211, 2007.

Granata KP, Rogers E: Torso flexion modulates stiffness and reflex response, *J Electromyogr Kinesiol* 17(4):384-392, 2007.

Grant JCB, Basmajian JV: *Grant's method of anatomy,* ed 7, Baltimore, 1965, Williams & Wilkins.

Grassi L et al: Psychosomatic characterization of adjustment disorders in the medical setting: some suggestions for DSM-V, *J Affect Disord* 101(1-3):251-254, 2007.

Grauer JD et al: Resection arthroplasty of the hip, *J Bone Joint Surg* 71A:669, 1989.

Gray H: *Anatomy of the human body,* ed 28, Philadelphia, 1966, Lea & Febiger.

Green DP: Carpal dislocations and instabilities. In Green DP, editor: *Operative hand surgery,* ed 3, New York, 1993, Churchill-Livingstone.

Greenman PE: Innominate shear dysfunction in sacroiliac syndrome, *J Manual Med* 2:114, 1986.

Greenspan A, Montesano P: *Imaging of the spine in clinical practice,* London, 1993, Wolfe.

Greenspan A: *Orthopedic radiology,* ed 2, Philadelphia, 1992, JB Lippincott.

Greenstein GM: *Clinical assessment of neuromusculoskeletal disorders,* St Louis, 1997, Mosby.

Greenwald AS: Biomechanics of the hip. In Steinberg ME, editor: *The hip and its disorders,* Philadelphia, 1991, WB Saunders.

Gregersen GG, Lucas DB: An in vivo study of the axial rotation of the human thoracolumbar spine, *J Bone Joint Surg* 49A:247, 1967.

Gregory DE, Brown SHM, Callaghan JP: Trunk muscle responses to suddenly applied loads: do individuals who develop discomfort during prolonged standing respond differently? *J Electromyogr Kinesiol* (in press, corrected proof).

Grelsamer RP, Meadows S: The modified Insall-Salvati ratio for assessment of patellar height, *Clin Orthop* 282;170, 1992.

Grelsamer RP, Proctor CS, Bazos AN: Evaluation of patellar shape in the sagittal plane: a clinical analysis, *Am J Sports Med* 22:61, 1994.

Grelsamer RP, Tedder JL: The lateral trochlear sign: femoral trochlear dysplasia as seen on a lateral view roentgenograph, *Clin Orthop* 281:159, 1992.

Greve KW, Bianchini KJ, Ameduri CJ: Use of a forced-choice test of tactile discrimination in the evaluation of functional sensory loss: a report of 3 cases, *Arch Phys Med Rehabil* 84(8):1233-1236, 2003.

Grieve GP: *Common vertebral joint problems,* New York, 1981, Churchill Livingstone.

Grilo RM et al: Clinically relevant VAS pain score change in patients with acute rheumatic conditions, *Joint Bone Spine* (in press, uncorrected proof).

Grobler LS, Wiltse LC: Classification, non-operative, and operative treatment of spondylolisthesis. In Frymoyer JW, editor: *The adult spine: principles and practice,* New York, 1991, Raven.

Groen GJ, Baljet B, Drukker J: Nerves and nerve plexuses of the human vertebral collum, *Am J Anat* 188:282, 1990.

Grootboom MJ, Govender S: Acute injuries of the upper dorsal spine, *Injury* 24:389, 1993.

Gross ML, Nasser S, Finnerman GAM: Hip and pelvis. In DeLee JC, Drez D, editors: *Orthopaedic sports medicine: principles and practice,* vol 2, Philadelphia, 1994, WB Saunders.

Grossman ZD et al: *Cost-effective diagnostic imaging the clinician's guide,* ed 3, St Louis, 1995, Mosby.

Gruebel-Lee DM: *Disorders of the hip,* Philadelphia, 1983, JB Lippincott.

Grundberg AB, Reagan DS: Pathologic anatomy of the forearm: Intersection syndrome, *J Hand Surg* 10(2):299-302, 1985.

Guanche CA, Jones DC: Clinical testing for tears of the glenoid labrum, *Arthroscopy* 19(5):517-523, 2003.

Guckel C, Nidecker A: Diagnosis of tears in rotator-cuff-injuries, *Eur J Radiol* 25(3):168-176, 1997.

Guermazi M et al: Traduction en arabe et validation de l'indice d'Oswestry dans une population de lombalgiques Nord-Africains, *Ann Readapt Med Phys* 48(1):1-10, 2005.

Guiheneuc P, Ginet J: Etude du reflexe de Hoffmann obtenu au niveau du muscle quadriceps de sujets humains normaux, *Electroencephalogr Clin Neurophysiol* 3:225-231, 1974.

Guimberteau JC, Panconi B: Recalcitrant non-union of the scaphoid treated with a vascularized bone graft based on the ulnar artery, *J Bone Joint Surg* 72A:88, 1990.

Gunn CC, Milbrandt WE: Early and subtle signs in low-back sprain, *Spine* 3:267, 1978.

Gunther M, Blickhan R: Joint stiffness of the ankle and the knee in running, *J Biomech* 35(11):1459-1474, 2002.

Gurwood AS, Drake J: Guillain-Barre syndrome, *J Am Optometr Assoc* 77(11):540-546, 2006.

Gustilo RB, Kyle RF, Templeman DC: *Fractures and dislocations,* St Louis, 1993, Mosby.

820　BIBLIOGRAPHY

Guyton AC: *Structure and function of the nervous system,* Philadelphia, 1972, WB Saunders.

Guzzanti V et al: Patellofemoral malalignment in adolescents: computerized tomographic assessment with or without quadriceps contraction, *Am J Sports Med* 22:55, 1994.

Haack E, Tkach J: Fast MR imaging: techniques and clinical applications, *AJR Am J Roentgenol* 155:951, 1990.

Hadlow V: Neonatal screening for congenital dislocation of hip, *J Bone Joint Surg* 70B:740, 1988.

Haher TR, Felmly WT, O'Brien M: Thoracic and lumbar fractures: diagnosis and management. In Bridwell KH, DeWald RL, editors: *The textbook of spinal surgery,* Philadelphia, 1991, JB Lippincott.

Halbach JW, Tank RT: The shoulder. In Gould JA, editor: *Orthopaedic and sports physical therapy,* ed 2, St Louis, 1990, Mosby.

Hale BS, Raglin JS, Koceja DM: Effect of mental imagery of a motor task on the Hoffmann reflex, *Behav Brain Res* 142(1-2):81-87, 2003.

Hale MS: *A practical approach to arm pain,* Springfield, Ill, 1971, Charles C Thomas.

Hall AJ: Perthes disease: progression in etiological research. In Catterall P, editor: *Recent advances in orthopaedics,* ed 5, Edinburgh, 1987, Churchill Livingstone.

Hall CW, Danoff D: Sleep attacks-apparent relationship to atlantoaxial dislocation, *Arch Neurol* 32:57, 1975.

Hall LD, Tyler JA: Can quantitative magnetic resonance imaging detect and monitor the progression of early osteoarthritis? In Kuetner KE, Goldberg VM, editors: *Osteoarthritic disorders,* Rosemont, Ill, 1995, American Academy of Orthopaedic Surgeons.

Halland AM et al: Avascular necrosis of the hip in systemic lupus erythematosus: the role of magnetic resonance imaging, *Br J Rheumatol* 32:972, 1993.

Halperin JL: Evaluation of patients with peripheral vascular disease, *Thromb Res* 106(6): V303-V311, 2002.

Hamilton J, Manrique L, Scarborough N: Development of an intervertebral disc model for testing a new discography system, *J Pain* 7(4, suppl 1):S26-S73, 2006.

Hamilton MG, Thomas HG: Intradural herniation of a thoracic disc presenting as flaccid paraplegic: case report, *Neurosurgery* 27:482, 1990.

Hamilton WC: Anatomy. In Hamilton WC, editor: *Traumatic disorder of the ankle,* New York, 1984, Springer-Verlag.

Hammer WI: *Functional soft tissue examination and treatment by manual methods the extremities,* Gaithersburg, Md, 1991, Aspen.

Hammerberg KW: Kyphosis. In Bridwell DH, DeWald RL, editors: *The textbook of spinal surgery,* Philadelphia, 1991, JB Lippincott.

Hananouchi T et al: Interventional therapy for hip ganglion using open MRI, *Eur J Radiol Extra* 60(1):43-47, 2006.

Handelberg FM, Shahabpour M, Casteleyn PP: Chondral lesions of the patella evaluated with computed tomography, magnetic resonance imaging, and arthroscopy, *Arthroscopy* 6:24, 1990.

Hanley EN, Phillips ED: Profiles of patients who get spine infections and the type of infections that have a predilection for the spine. In Wiesel SW, editor: *Seminars in spine surgery,* vol 2, Philadelphia, 1990, WB Saunders.

Hanley MA et al: Self-reported treatments used for lower-limb phantom pain: descriptive findings, *Arch Phys Med Rehabil* 87(2):270-277, 2006.

Hanley MA et al: Preamputation pain and acute pain predict chronic pain after lower extremity amputation, *J Pain* 8(2):102-109, 2007.

Hann CL: Retropharyngeal-tendinitis, *AJR Am J Roentgenol* 130:1137, 1978.

Hansson G et al: Radiographic assessment of coxarthrosis following slipped capital femoral epiphysis, *Acta Radiol* 34:117, 1993.

Hansson G: Congenital dislocation of the hip joint: problems in diagnosis and treatment, *Curr Orthop* 2:104, 1988.

Hansson T et al: The lumbar lordosis in acute and chronic low-back pain, *Spine* 10:154, 1985.

Hardinge K: The etiology of transient synovitis of the hip in childhood, *J Bone Joint Surg* 52B:100, 1970.

Hardy RW, editor: *Lumbar disc disease,* ed 2, New York, 1992, Raven.

Harner CD et al: Loss of motion after anterior cruciate ligament reconstruction, *Am J Sports Med* 20:499, 1992.

Harris CM, Baum J: Involvement of the hip in juvenile rheumatoid arthritis, *J Bone Joint Surg* 70A:821, 1988.

Harris J, Fallat L: Effects of isolated Weber B fibular fractures on the tibiotalar contact area, *J Foot Ankle Surg* 43(1):3-9, 2004.

Harris R, Piller N: Three case studies indicating the effectiveness of manual lymph drainage on patients with primary and secondary lymphedema using objective measuring tools, *J Bodywork Mov Ther* 7(4):213-221, 2003.

Harris WH: Etiology of osteoarthritis of the hip, *Clin Orthop* 213:20, 1986.

Harrison DE et al: Cervical coupling during lateral head translations creates an S-configuration, *Clin Biomech* 15(6):436-440, 2000.

Harryman DJ et al: The role of the rotator internal capsule in passive motion and stability of the shoulder, *J Bone Joint Surg* 74A:53, 1992.

Harryman DT II et al: Repairs of the rotator cuff, *J Bone Joint Surg* 73A:982, 1991.

Harryman DT, Matsen FA, Sidles JA: Arthroscopic management of refractory shoulder stiffness, *Arthroscopy* 13(2):133-147, 1997.

Hart FD: *French's index of differential diagnosis,* ed 10, Baltimore, 1973, Williams & Wilkins.

Hartley A: *Practical joint assessment lower quadrant,* ed 2, St Louis, 1995, Mosby.

Harty M: Hip anatomy. In Steinberg ME, editor: *The hip and its disorders.* Philadelphia, 1991, WB Saunders.

Harvey FJ, Harvey PM, Horsely MW: De Quervain's disease: surgical or nonsurgical treatment, *J Hand Surg* 15A:83, 1990.

Harvey J, Tanner S: Low back pain in young athletes: a practical approach, *Sports Med* 12:394, 1991.

Harvey MA, James B: *Differential diagnosis,* Philadelphia, 1972, WB Saunders.

Hashiba Y et al: A comparison of lower lip hypoesthesia measured by trigeminal somato-sensory-evoked potential between different types of mandibular osteotomies and fixation, *Oral Surg Oral Med Oral Pathol Oral Radiol Endod* (in press, corrected proof).

Hass CJ et al: Gait initiation and dynamic balance control in Parkinson's disease, *Arch Phys Med Rehabil* 86(11):2172-2176, 2005.

Hassell AB et al: The relationship between serial measures of disease activity and outcome in rheumatoid arthritis, *Q J Med* 86:601, 1995.

Hassoun A et al: Female genital tuberculosis: uncommon presentation of tuberculosis in the United States, *Am J Med* 118(11):1295-1296, 2005.

Hassouna HZ, Singh D: The variation in the management of Morton's metatarsalgia, *Foot* 15(3):149-153, 2005.

Hastings D, McNab I, Lawson V: Neoplasms of the atlas and axis, *Can J Surg* 11:290, 1968.

Haustgen T, Bourgeois ML: L'evolution du concept de mythomanie dans l'histoire de la psychiatrie, *Ann Medicopsychol Rev Psychiatr* 165(5):334-344, 2007.

Hawkins RJ, Bokor D: Clinical evaluation of shoulder problems. In Rockwood C, Matshe F, editors: *The shoulder,* Philadelphia, 1990, WB Saunders.

Hawkins RJ, Kennedy JC: Impingement syndrome in athletics, *Am J Sports Med* 8:141, 1980.

Hawkins RJ, Mohtadi N: Rotator cuff problems in athletes. In DeLee JC, Drez D, editors: *Orthopaedic sports medicine: principals and practice,* vol 1, Philadelphia, 1994, WB Saunders.

Hawkins RJ: *An organized approach to musculoskeletal examination and history taking,* St Louis, 1995, Mosby.

Hayes KW, Petersen C, Falconer J: An examination of Cyriax's passive motion tests with patients having osteoarthritis of the knee, *Phys Ther* 74:697, 1994.

Hede A, Hempel-Poulson S, Jensen JS: Symptoms and level of sports activity in patients awaiting arthroscopy for meniscal lesions of the knee, *J Bone Joint Surg* 72A:550, 1990.

Heikkila E, Ryoppy S, Louchimo I: The management of primary acetabular dysplasia, *J Bone Joint Surg* 67B:25, 1985.

Heilman KM, Watson RT, Greer M: *Handbook for differential diagnosis of neurologic signs and symptoms,* New York, 1977, Appleton-Century-Crofts.

Heim HA: Scoliosis, *Clin Symp* 25:1, 1973.

Heinmann WG, Freiberger RH: Avascular necrosis of the femoral and humeral heads after high-dosage corticosteroid therapy, *N Engl J Med* 263:627, 1960.

Helfet AJ, Gruebel Lee DM: *Disorders of the lumbar spine,* Philadelphia, 1978, JB Lippincott.

Helfet AJ: *Disorder of the knee,* Philadelphia, 1974, JB Lippincott.

Helfet D, Schmeling G: Management of complex acetabular fractures through single nonextensile exposures, *Clin Orthop* 305:58, 1994.

Helliwell PS, Evans PF, Wright V: The straight cervical spine: does it indicate muscle spasm? *J Bone Joint Surg (Br)* 76:103, 1994.

Hellstrom M et al: Radiologic abnormalities of the thoracolumbar spine in patients, *Acta Radiol* 31:127, 1990.

Henderson RS: Osteotomy for unreduced congenital dislocation of the hip in adults, *J Bone Joint Surg* 52B:468, 1970.

Hendrix RW, Lin PJP, Kane WJ: Simplified aspiration or injection techniques for the sacroiliac joint, *J Bone Joint Surg* 64A:1249, 1982.

Henigan SP et al: The semimembranosus-tibial collateral ligament bursa, *J Bone Joint Surg* 76A:1322, 1994.

Henry JH: Conservative treatment of patellofemoral subluxation, *Clin Sports Med* 8:261, 1989.

Herkowitz HN, Kurz LT: Degenerative lumbar spondylolisthesis with spinal stenosis: a prospective study comparing decompression with decompression and intertransverse process arthrodesis *J Bone Joint Surg* 73A:802, 1991.

Herlin L: *Sciatic and pelvic pain due to lumbosacral nerve root compression,* Springfield, Ill, 1966, Charles C Thomas.

Hernandez RS, Cornell RG, Hensinger RN: Ultrasound diagnosis of neonatal congenital dislocation of the hip, *J Bone Joint Surg* 76A:539, 1994.

Herndon WA: Acute and chronic injury: its effect on growth in the young athlete. In Frana WA et al, editors: *Advances in sports medicine fitness,* vol 3, Chicago, 1990, Year-Book Medical.

Hernigou P et al: Deformities of the hip in adults who have sickle-cell disease and had avascular necrosis in childhood, *J Bone Joint Surg* 73:91, 1991.

Herno A et al: The predictive value of preoperative myelography in lumbar spinal stenosis, *Spine* 19:1335-8, 1994.

Heroux ME et al: Upper-extremity disability in essential tremor, *Arch Phys Med Rehabil* 87(5):661-670, 2006.

Herrera A et al: Management of types III and IV acetabular deficiencies with the longitudinal oblong revision cup, *J Arthroplasty* 21(6):857-864, 2006.

Herron LD, Pheasant HC: Prone knee-flexion provocative testing for lumbar disc protrusion, *Spine* 5:65, 1980.

Hertling D, Kessler R: *Management of common musculoskeletal disorders,* ed 2, Philadelphia, 1990, JB Lippincott.

Heuer F et al: Creep associated changes in intervertebral disc bulging obtained with a laser scanning device, *Clin Biomech* (in press, corrected proof).

Hiehle JF, Kneeland JB, Dalinka MK: Magnetic resonance imaging of the hip with emphasis on avascular necrosis, *Rheum Dis Clin North Am* 17:669, 1991.

Hijioka A et al: Degenerative change and rotator cuff tears: an anatomical study in 160 shoulders of 80 cadavers, *Arch Orthop Trauma Surg* 112:61, 1993.

Hillman TE et al: A practical posture for hand grip dynamometry in the clinical setting, *Clin Nutr* 24(2):224-248, 2005.

Hinkle CZ: *Fundamentals of anatomy & movement a workbook and guide,* St Louis, 1997, Mosby.

Hirsch C, Frankel VH: Analysis of forces producing fractures of the proximal end of the femur, *J Bone Joint Surg* 42B:633, 1960.

Hittner VJ: Episacroiliac lipomas, *Am J Surg* 78(3):382-383, 1949.

Ho CP, Sartoris DJ: Magnetic resonance imaging of the elbow, *Rheum Dis Clin North Am* 17:705, 1991.

Hochschuler SH, editor: *Spinal injuries in sports,* Spine 4, 1990.

Hoeksma HL et al: A comparison of the OARSI response criteria with patient's global assessment in patients with osteoarthritis of the hip treated with a non-pharmacological intervention, *Osteoarthr Cartil* 14(1):77-81, 2006.

Hofer M, Mahlaoui N, Prieur A-M: A child with a systemic febrile illness—differential diagnosis and management, *Best Pract Res Clin Rheumatol* 20(4):627-640, 2006.

Hoffman RM, Kent DL, Deyo RA: Diagnostic accuracy and clinical utility of thermography for lumbar radiculopathy: a meta-analysis, *Spine* 16:623, 1991.

Hollingshead WH, Jenkins DR: *Functional anatomy of the limbs and back,* Philadelphia, 1981, WB Saunders.

Hollinshead WH: *Anatomy for surgeons, vol 3, The back and limbs,* ed 2, New York, 1969, Harper & Row.

Holmquist LA, Wanlass RL: A multidimensional approach towards malingering detection, *Arch Clin Neuropsychol* 17(2):143-156, 2002.

Holtby R, Razmjou H: Accuracy of the Speed's and Yergason's tests in detecting biceps pathology and SLAP lesions: comparison with arthroscopic findings, *Arthroscopy* 20(3):231-236, 2004.

Holvey DN, Talbott JH: *The Merck manual of diagnosis and therapy,* ed 12, New Jersey, 1972, Merck.

Hopkinson WJ et al: Syndesmotic sprains of the ankle, *Foot Ankle* 10:325, 1990.

Hoppenfeld S: *Physical examination of the spine and extremities,* New York, 1976, Appleton-Century-Crofts.

Hopwood MB, Abram SE: Factors associated with failure of lumbar epidural steroids, *Reg Anesth Pain Med* 18:238, 1993.

Hori Y, Tamai S, Okuda H: Blood vessel transplantation to bone, *J Hand Surg* 4(1):23-33, 1979.

Hornberger JP: *Exercise physiology therapeutic exercise,* Sarasota, Fla, 1991, Joseph P Hornberger.

Howard RP et al: Head, neck, and mandible dynamics generated by `whiplash', *Accid Anal Prev* 30(4):525-534, 1998.

Howe JR, Taren JA: Foramen magnum tumors: pitfalls in diagnosis, *JAMA* 225:1060, 1973.

Hsu HC et al: Calcific tendinitis and rotator cuff tearing; a clinical and radiographic study, *J Shoulder Elbow Surg* 3:159, 1994.

Hubbard DR, Berkoff GM: Myofascial trigger points show spontaneous needle EMG activity, *Spine* 18:1803, 1993.

Huckell CB, Simmons ED, Zheng Y: The significance of annular tear of cervical disc for positive discography by age in discogenic pain, *Spine J* 5(4, suppl 1):S48-S49, 2005.

Hudgins WR: The crossed-straight-leg-raising test, *N Engl J Med* 297:1127, 1977.

Hudson ZL, Darthuy E: Iliotibial band tightness and patellofemoral pain syndrome a case-control study, *Phys Ther Sport* 7(4):173-271, 2006.

Hughes S, Benson MKD, Colton CL: *The principles and practice of musculoskeletal surgery,* Edinburgh, 1987, Churchill Livingstone.

Hughes S et al: Extrapelvic compression of the sciatic nerve, *J Bone Joint Surg* 74A:1533, 1992.

Hughston J: *Knee ligaments: injury and repair,* St Louis, 1993, Mosby.

Hughston JC et al: The classification of knee ligament instabilities: I. the medial compartment and cruciate ligaments, *J Bone Joint Surg* 58A:159, 1976.

Hughston JC, Norwood LA: The posterolateral drawer and external rotational recurvatum test for posterolateral rotary instability of the knee, *Clin Orthop* 147:82, 1980.

Hughston JC, Walsh WM, Puddu G: *Patellar subluxation and dislocation,* Philadelphia, 1984, WB Saunders.

Hunt AE, Smith RM: Mechanics and control of the flat versus normal foot during the stance phase of walking, *Clin Biomech* 19(4):391-397, 2004.

Hunt GC: Injuries of peripheral nerves of the leg, foot and ankle: an often unrecognized consequence of ankle sprains, *Foot* 13(1):14-18, 2003.

Hunter JM: Recurrent carpal tunnel syndrome, epineural fibrous fixation, and traction neuropathy, *Hand Clin* 7:491, 1991.

Huntoon MA: Anatomy of the cervical intervertebral foramina: vulnerable arteries and ischemic neurologic injuries after transforaminal epidural injections, *Pain* 117 (1-2):104-111, 2005.

Hurley J: Anatomy of the shoulder. In Nicholas J, Hershman E, editors: *The upper extremity in sports medicine,* St Louis, 1990, Mosby.

Hutton WC: The forces acting on a lumbar intervertebral joint, *J Manual Med* 5, 66, 1990.

Iannotti JP et al: Magnetic resonance imaging of the shoulder: sensitivity specificity and predictive value, *J Bone Joint Surg* 73A:17, 1991.

Ibrahim T et al: Displaced intra-articular calcaneal fractures: 15-Year follow-up of a randomised controlled trial of conservative versus operative treatment, *Injury* (in press, corrected proof).

Iczkovitz JM, Leek JC, Robbins DL: Pyogenic sacroiliitis, *J Rheumatol* 8:157, 1981.

Ido K et al: The validity of upright myelography for diagnosing lumbar disc herniation, *Clin Neurol Neurosurg* 104(1):30-35, 2002.

Imaeda T et al: Magnetic resonance imaging in scaphoid fractures, *J Hand Surg* 17B:20, 1992.

Inaba Y et al: Provoked anterior knee pain in medial osteoarthritis of the knee, *Knee* 10(4):351-355, 2003.

Indelicato PA et al: Clinical comparison of freeze-dried/fresh frozen patella tendon allografts for anterior cruciate ligament reconstruction of the knee, *Am J Sports Med* 18:335, 1990.

Indelicato PA, Hermansdorfer J, Huegel M: The nonoperative management of complete tears of the medial collateral ligament of the knee in intercollegiate football players, *Clin Orthop* 256:174, 1990.

Inerot S et al: Proteoglycan alterations during developing experimental osteoarthritis in a novel hip joint model, *J Orthop Res* 9:658, 1991.

Ingebretsen L et al: A prospective, randomized study of three surgical techniques for treatment of acute ruptures of the anterior cruciate ligament, *Am J Sports Med* 18: 585, 1990.

Inman VT: *The joints of the ankle*, Baltimore, 1976, Williams & Wilkins.

Insall J, Falvo KA, Wise DW: Chondromalacia patella, *J Bone Joint Surg* 58A:1, 1976.

Iowa Trial Lawyers Association: *Medical damages*, Des Moines, 1995, Iowa Trial Lawyers Association.

Isdale IC, Corrigan B: Backward luxation of the atlas, *Ann Rheum Dis* 29:6, 1970.

Isler B: Lumbosacral lesions associated with pelvic ring injuries, *J Orthop Trauma* 4:1, 1990.

Itamura J et al: Analysis of the bicipital groove as a landmark for humeral head replacement, *J Shoulder Elbow Surg* 11(4):322-326, 2002.

Itoi E et al: Dynamic anterior stabilizers of the shoulder with the arm in abduction, *J Bone Joint Surg* 76B:834, 1994.

Jabaley ME et al: Comparison of histologic and functional recovery after peripheral nerve repair, *J Hand Surg (Am)*1:119, 1976.

Jablonski S: *Dictionary of medical acronyms & abbreviations*, ed 3, Philadelphia, 1998, Hanley & Belfus.

Jackson BA, Schwane JA, Starcher BC: Effect of ultrasound therapy on the repair of Achilles tendon injuries in rats, *Med Sci Sports Exerc* 23:171, 1991.

Jackson HC, Winkelman KK, Bichel WH: Nerve endings in the human lumbar spine column and related structures, *J Bone Joint Surg* 48A:1272, 1966.

Jackson R: *The cervical syndrome*, ed 3, Springfield, Ill, 1966, Charles C Thomas.

Jackson RW, Kunkel SS, Taylor GJ: Lateral retinacular release for patellofemoral pain in the older patient, *Arthroscopy* 7:283, 1991.

Jacobs JW: Screening for organic mental syndromes in the medically ill, *Ann Intern Med* 86:40, 1977.

Jacobson T, Allen W: Surgical connection of the snapping iliopsoas tendon, *Am J Sports Med* 18:470, 1990.

Jafarnia K, Gabel GT, Morrey BF: Triceps tendinitis, *Oper Tech Sports Med* 9(4): 217-221, 2001.

Jagoda A, Riggio S: Mild traumatic brain injury and the postconcussive syndrome, *Emerg Med Clin North Am* 18(2):355-363, 2000.

Jahss MH: *Disorders of the foot*, Philadelphia, 1982, WB Saunders.

Jahss MH: Foot and ankle pain resulting from rheumatic conditions, *Curr Opin Rheumatol* 4:233, 1992.

Jakob RP, Hassler H, Staeubli HU: Observations on rotary instability of the lateral compartment of the knee, *Acta Orthop Scand Suppl* 191:1, 1981.

James JP: The etiology of scoliosis, *J Bone Joint Surg* 52B:410, 1970.

James SL: Running injuries to the knee, *J Am Acad Orthop Surg* 3:309, 1995.

Jarvik JG et al: Interreader reliability for a new classification of lumbar disk disease, *Acad Radiol* 3(7):537-544, 1996.

Jehl J, Crummy P: *Essentials of radiologic surgery*, ed 6, Philadelphia, 1993, JB Lippincott.

Jenis L et al: Complex cervical reconstruction: the effect of posterior cervical distraction on foraminal dimensions using a screw-rod system, *Spine J* 2(5, suppl 1):53, 2002.

Jenkins DH, Young MH: The operative treatment of sacroiliac subluxation and disruption of the symphysis pubis, *Injury* 10:139, 1978.

Jensen MC et al: Magnetic resonance imaging of the lumbar spine in people without back pain, *N Engl J Med* 331:69, 1994.

Jensen R et al: Quantitative sensory testing of patients with long lasting Patellofemoral pain syndrome, *Eur J Pain* (in press, corrected proof).

Jette AM: Using health-related quality of life measures in physical therapy outcomes research, *Phys Ther* 73:528, 1993.

Jobe C: Gross anatomy of the shoulder. In Rockwood C, Matsen F, editors: *The shoulder*, Philadelphia, 1990, WB Saunders.

Jobe FW et al: The shoulder in sports. In Rockwood CA Jr, Matsen FA III, editors: *The shoulder*, Philadelphia, 1992, WB Saunders.

Johansson H, Sjolander P, Sojka P: A sensory role for the cruciate ligaments, *Clin Orthop* 268:161, 1991.

Johnson DP, Eastwood DM, Witherow PJ: Symptomatic synovial plicae of the knee, *J Bone Joint Surg* 75A:1485, 1992.

Johnson I: Iliacus stretching for symptomatic relief of femoral mononeuropathy, *Clin Chiropr* 10(2):97-100, 2007.

Johnson KE: *Histology and cell biology*, ed 2, Baltimore, 1991, Williams & Wilkins.

Johnson MK: *The hand book*, Springfield, Ill, 1973, Charles C Thomas.

Johnson RJ: Low-back pain in sports: managing spondylolysis in young patients, *Phys Sports Med* 21:53, 1993.

Johnson RM, Murphy MJ, Southwick WO: Surgical approaches to the spine. In Rothman RH, Simeone FA, editors: *The spine*, ed 3, Philadelphia, 1992, WB Saunders.

Johnsson KE, Rosen I, Uden A: The natural course of lumbar spinal stenosis, *Clin Orthop* 279:82, 1992.

Jones DA: Irritable hip and campylobacter infection, *J Bone Joint Surg* 71B:227, 1989.

Jones DH, Kilgour RD, Comtois AS: Test-retest reliability of pressure pain threshold measurements of the upper limb and torso in young healthy women, *J Pain* (in press, corrected proof).

Jones JP Jr, Engelman EP: Osseous avascular necrosis associated with systemic abnormalities, *Arthritis Rheum* 5:728, 1966.

Jones MA: Clinical reasoning in manual therapy, *Phys Ther* 72:875, 1992.

Jonsson B, Stromquist B: Symptoms and signs in degeneration of the lumbar spine, a prospective consecutive study of 300 operated patients, *J Bone Joint Surg* 75B:272, 1993.

Jonsson B, Stromquist B: Symptoms and signs in degeneration of the lumbar spine, *J Bone Joint Surg* 75B:381, 1993.

Jonsson HJ, Cesarini K, Sahlstedt B, Rauschning W: Findings and outcome in whiplash-type neck distortions, *Spine* 19:2733, 1994.

Jonsson K: Nonunion of a fractured scaphoid tubercle, *J Hand Surg* 15A:283, 1990.

Jonsson T et al: Clinical diagnosis of ruptures of the anterior cruciate ligament: a comparative study of the Lachman test and the anterior drawer sign, *Am J Sports Med* 10:100, 1982.

Judge RD, Zuidema GD, Fitzgerald FT: *Clinical diagnosis: a physiologic approach*, Boston, 1982, Little, Brown.

Junqueira LC, Carneiro J, Kelly RO: *Basic histology*, ed 7, Norwalk, Conn, 1992, Appleton & Lange.

Jupiter JB: Current concepts review: fractures of the distal end of the radius, *J Bone Joint Surg* 73A:461, 1991.

Kadel NJ, Teitz CC, Kronmal RA: Stress fractures in ballet dancers, *Am J Sports Med* 20:445, 1992.

Kainberger FM et al: Injury of the Achilles tendon: diagnosis with sonography, *AMJ Am J Roentgenol* 155:1031, 1990.

Kakarla N, Boswell HB, Zurawin RK: A large pelvic mass in an adolescent patient with granulomatous nephritis: case report and discussion of treatment challenges, *J Pediatr Adolesc Gynecol* 19(3):223-229, 2006.

Kalebo P et al: Ultrasonography in the detection of partial patellar ligament ruptures (jumper's knee), *Skeletal Radiol* 20:285, 1991.

Kamkar A, Irrgang J, Whitney SL: Nonoperative management of secondary shoulder impingement syndrome, *J Orthop Sports Phys Ther* 17:21, 1993.

Kampa K: Mortality of hip fracture patients within one year of fracture, an overview, *Geritopics* 14:10, 1991.

Kang CH et al: MRI of paraspinal muscles in lumbar degenerative kyphosis patients and control patients with chronic low back pain, *Clin Radiol* 62(5):479-486, 2007.

Kang PB et al: Atypical presentations of spinal muscular atrophy type III (Kugelberg-Welander disease), *Neuromuscul Disord* 16(8):492-494, 2006.

Kanner R: *Pain management secrets,* Philadelphia, 1997, Hanley & Belfus.

Kannus P, Jozsa L: Histopathologic changes preceding spontaneous rupture of a tendon, *J Bone Joint Surg* 73A:1507, 1992.

Kannus P, Renstrom P: Current concepts review: treatment for acute tears of the lateral ligaments of the ankle, *J Bone Joint Surg* 73A:305, 1991.

Kapandji IA: *The physiology of the joints: the trunk and vertebral column,* vol 3, New York, 1974, Churchill Livingstone.

Kaplan EB: Treatment of tennis elbow (epicondylitis) by denervation, *J Bone Joint Surg* 41A:147, 1959.

Kapoor VK: Abdominal tuberculosis, *Medicine* 35(5):257-260, 2007.

Kapstad H et al: Changes in pain, stiffness and physical function in patients with osteoarthritis waiting for hip or knee joint replacement surgery, *Osteoarthr Cartil* (in press, corrected proof).

Karasick D, Schweitzer ME: Tear of the posterior tibial tendon causing asymmetric flatfoot: radiographic findings, *Am J Roentgenol* 161:1237, 1993.

Karasick D: Preoperative assessment of symptomatic bunionette deformity: radiologic findings, *AMJ Am J Roentgenol* 164:147, 1995.

Karkin-Tais A et al: 13-year study of pain in phantom limbs of amputees—victims of war in Sarajevo (period 1992-2005), *Eur J Pain* 10(Suppl 1):S98-S211, 2006.

Karlson J et al: Partial rupture of the patellar ligament, *Am J Sports Med* 19:403, 1992.

Karr SD: Subcalcaneal heel pain, *Orthop Clinic North Am* 25:161, 1994.

Kasch MC: Acute hand injuries. In Pedretti LW, Zolton B, editors: *Occupational therapy: practice skills for physical dysfunction,* ed 3, St Louis, 1990, Mosby.

Kasdan ML: *Occupational hand & upper extremity injuries & diseases,* ed 2, Philadelphia, 1998, Hanley & Belfus.

Kaspar S, Mandel S: Acromial impression fracture of the greater tuberosity with rotator cuff avulsion due to hyperabduction injury of the shoulder, *J Shoulder Elbow Surg* 13(1):112-114, 2004.

Kassarjian A, Brisson M, Palmer WE: Femoroacetabular impingement, *Eur J Radiol* (in press, corrected proof).

Katirji B, Weissman JD: The ankle jerk and the tibial H-reflex: a clinical and electrophysiological correlation, *Electromyogr Clin Neurophysiol* 34:331, 1994.

Katirji B: *Electromyography in clinical practice a case study approach,* St Louis, 1998, Mosby.

Katirji MB, Wilbourn AJ: High sciatic lesions mimicking peroneal neuropathy at the fibular head, *J Neurosci* 121:172, 1994.

Kato S et al: Glomus tumor beneath the plica synovialis in the knee: a case report, *Knee* 14(2):164-166, 2007.

Katz JN et al: Stability and responsiveness of utility measures, *Med Care* 32:183, 1994.

Katz WA: *Rheumatic diseases diagnosis and management,* Philadelphia, 1977, JB Lippincott.

Katznelson A, Nerubay J, Level A: Gluteal skyline (G.S.L.): a search for an objective sign in the diagnosis of disc lesions of the lower lumbar spine, *Spine* 7:74, 1982.

Kaufman RL: Popliteal aneurysm as a cause of leg pain in a geriatric patient, *J Manipulative Physiol Ther* 27(6):427-557, 2004.

Keats TE: *Atlas of normal roentgen variants that may simulate disease,* ed 6, St Louis, 1996, Mosby.

Kedroff L, Amis A, Newham D: Do patients with patellofemoral pain syndrome exhibit alterations in steadiness on hip and knee flexion? *Gait Posture* 24(suppl 2):S269-S270, 2006.

Keefe FJ: Behavioral assessment and treatment of chronic pain: current status and future directions, *J Consult Clin Psychol* 50:896, 1982.

Keene JA: Tendon injuries of the foot and ankle. In DeLee JD, Drez D, editors: *Orthopaedic sports medicine, principals and practice,* vol 2, Philadelphia, 1994, WB Saunders.

Keim HA: *The adolescent spine,* ed 2, New York, 1976, Springer-Verlag.

Keim HA: *The adolescent spine,* New York, 1982, Springer-Verlag.

Keiser RP, Grimes HA: Intervertebral disc space infections in children, *Clin Orthop* 30:163, 1963.

Kelikian H, Kelikian AS: *Disorders of the ankle,* Philadelphia, 1985, WB Saunders.

Keller TS et al: Influence of spine morphology on intervertebral disc loads and stresses in asymptomatic adults: implications for the ideal spine, *Spine J* 5(3):297-309, 2005.

Kelley WN et al: *Textbook of rheumatology,* vol 1, ed 4, Philadelphia, 1993, Saunders.

Kellgren JH: The anatomical source of back pain, *Rheumatol Rehab* 16:3, 1977.

Kelsey JL: An epidemiological study of acute herniated lumbar intervertebral disc, *Rheumatol Rehab* 14:144, 1975.

Kendall HO, Kendall FP, Wadsworth GE: *Muscle testing and function,* ed 2, Baltimore, 1971, Williams & Wilkins.

Kendall HO, Kendall FP, Wadsworth GE: *Muscles: testing and function,* ed 3, Baltimore, 1992, Williams & Wilkins.

Kendell FP, McCreary EK, Provance PG: *Muscles: testing and function,* ed 4, Baltimore, 1993, Williams & Wilkins.

Kennedy JC: *The injured adolescent knee,* Baltimore, 1979, Williams & Wilkins.

Kent DL et al: Diagnosis of lumbar spinal stenosis in adults: a meta-analysis of the accuracy of CT, MR, and myelography, *AJR Am J Roentgenol* 158:1135, 1992.

Kenter K et al: Dynamic and passive analysis of anterior capsular contractures of the glenohumeral joint, *J Shoulder Elbow Surg* 7(3):302-201, 1998.

Keret D et al: Coxa plana: the fate of the physis, *J Bone Joint Surg* 66A:870, 1984.

Kerimoglu S et al: Bucket-handle tear of medial plica, *Knee* 12(3):239-241, 2005.

Kerkhoffs GMMJ, Blankevoort L, van Dijk CN: A measurement device for anterior laxity of the ankle joint complex, *Clin Biomech* 20(2):218-222, 2005.

Kerkhoffs GMMJ et al: Anterior lateral ankle ligament damage and anterior talocrural-joint laxity: an overview of the in vitro reports in literature, *Clin Biomech* 16(8):635-643, 2001.

Kerluke L, McCabe SJ: Nonunion of the scaphoid: a critical analysis of recent natural history studies, *J Hand Surg* 18A:1, 1993.

Kernig W: Concerning a little noted sign of meningitis, *Arch Neurol* 21:216, 1969.

Kerr CD, Sybert DR, Albarracin NS: An analysis of flexor synovium in idiopathic carpal tunnel syndrome: report of 625 cases, *J Hand Surg* 17A:1028, 1992.

Kessel L, Watson M: The painful arc syndrome: clinical classification as a guide to management, *J Bone Joint Surg* 59B:166, 1977.

Kessler RM, Herling D: Assessment of musculoskeletal disorders. In Kessler RM, Herling D, editors: *Management of common musculoskeletal disorders,* ed. 2, Philadelphia, 1990, JB Lippincott.

Kessler RM, Hertling D: The hip. In Hertling D, Kessler RM, editors: *Management of common musculoskeletal disorders,* ed 2, Philadelphia, 1990, Lippincott.

Kettenbach G: *Writing S.O.A.P. notes,* Philadelphia, 1990, FA Davis.

Keuter EJW: Non-traumatic atlanto-axial dislocation associated with nasopharyngeal infections (Grisel's disease), *Acta Neurochirurg* 21:11, 1969.

Khan MA, Linder SM: Ankylosing spondylitis: clinical aspects, *Spine* 4:529, 1990.

Khoo LT, Fessler RG: Minimally invasive posterior cervical microendoscopic foraminotomy, *Spine J* 2(2, suppl 1):6, 2002.

Khurana R, Berney SM: Clinical aspects of rheumatoid arthritis, *Pathophysiology* 12(3):153-165, 2005.

Kiebhaber TR, Stern P: Upper extremity tendinitis and overuse syndrome in the athlete, *Clin Sports Med* 11:39, 1992.

Kim H-A, Lee S-R, Lee H: Acute peripheral vestibular syndrome of a vascular cause, *J Neurol Sci* 254(1-2):99-101, 2007.

Kim H-S et al: Comparison of the predictive value of computed tomography with myelography versus MRI using exercise treadmill exam in lumbar spinal stenosis, *Spine J* 3(5, suppl 1):84-85, 2003.

Kim JY et al: Non-traumatic peroneal nerve palsy: MRI findings, *Clin Radiol* 62(1):58-64, 2007.

Kim Y-W et al: Risk factors for leg length discrepancy in patients with congenital vascular malformation, *J Vasc Surg* 44(3):545-553, 2006.

Kimura J: *Electrodiagnosis in disease of nerve and muscle: principles and practice,* Philadelphia, 1983, FA Davis.

King JB et al: Lesions of the patellar ligament, *J Bone Joint Surg* 72B:46, 1990.

King L: Incidence of sacroiliac joint dysfunction and low back pain in fit college students, *J Manipulative Physiol Ther* 14:333, 1991.

Kingston RS: Radiology of the spine. In Watkins RG, editor: *The spine in sports,* St Louis, 1996, Mosby.

Kirby RL et al: Wheelchair-skill performance: controlled comparison between people with hemiplegia and able-bodied people simulating hemiplegia, *Arch Phys Med Rehabil* 86(3):387-393, 2005.

Kircher MT, Cappuccino A, Torpey BM: Muscular violence as a cause of humeral fractures in pitchers, *Contemp Orthop* 26:475, 1993.

Kirkaldy-Willis WH: *Managing low back pain,* New York, 1983, Churchill Livingstone.

Kisner C, Colby LA: *Therapeutic exercise; foundations and techniques,* ed 2, Philadelphia, 1990, FA Davis.

Kleiger B: Mechanisms of ankle injury, *Orthop Clin North Am* 5:127, 1974.

Kleinrensink GJ et al: Upper limb tension tests as tools in the diagnosis of nerve and plexus lesions: anatomical and biomechanical aspects, *Clin Biomech* 15(1):9-14, 2000.

Klenerman L: *The foot and its disorders,* ed 2, Boston, 1982, Blackwell Scientific.

Kline CR, Martin DP, Deyo RA: Health consequences of pregnancy and childbirth as perceived by women and clinicians, *Obstet Gynecol* 92(5):842-848, 1998.

Klippel JH, Dieppe PA: *Rheumatology,* vol 1-2, ed 2, London, 1998, Mosby.

Kloth LC, McCulloch JM, Feedar JA: *Wound healing: alternatives in management,* Philadelphia, 1990, FA Davis.

Knikou M et al: Pre- and post-alpha motoneuronal control of the soleus H-reflex during sinusoidal hip movements in human spinal cord injury, *Brain Res* 1103(1):123-139, 2006.

Knott R: A 14-year-old boy with metaphyseal dysplasia (Pyle's disease) and low back pain, *Clin Chiropr* 7(2):73-78, 2004.

Knutson GA: Examination of two subjects with severe, quantified anatomic leg length inequality using unloaded "functional" leg checks, *Clin Chiropr* 9(2):76-80, 2006.

Knutsson E, Martensson A: Isokinetic measurements of muscle strength in hysterical paresis, *Electroencephalogr Clin Neurophysiol* 61(5):370-374, 1985.

Koenigsberg R: *Churchill's illustrated medical dictionary,* New York, 1989, Churchill Livingstone.

Kolowich PA et al: Lateral release of the patella: indications and contraindications, *Am J Sports Med* 18:359, 1990.

Kono H et al: Lumbar juxta-facet cyst after trauma, *J Clin Neurosci* 13(6):694-696, 2006.

Konowitz KB: Reflex sympathy dystrophy syndrome sometimes misdiagnosed, often misunderstood, *J Am Chiro Assoc* 35:58, 1998.

Konradsen L, Halmer P, Sondergard L: Early mobilizing treatment for grade III ankle ligament injuries, *Foot Ankle* 12:69, 1991.

Kontos HA: Vascular diseases of the limbs. In Wyngaarden JB, Smith LH, Bennett JC, editors: *Cecil textbook of medicine,* ed 19, Philadelphia, 1992, WB Saunders.

Korovessis P, Sidiropoulos P, Dimas A: Complete fracture-dislocation of the thoracic spine without neurologic deficit: case report, *J Trauma* 36:122, 1994.

Koshino T: Changes in patellofemoral compressive force after anterior or anteromedial displacement of tibial tuberosity for chondromalacia patellae, *Clin Orthop* 266:133, 1991.

Koskinen SK, Hurme M, Kujala UM: Restoration of patellofemoral congruity by combined lateral release and tibial tuberosity transposition as assessed by MRI analysis, *Int Orthop* 15:363, 1991.

Kosteljanetz M, Bang F, Schmidt-Olsen S: The clinical significance of straight-leg raising (Lasègue's sign) in the diagnosis of prolapsed lumbar disc: interobserver variation and correlation with surgical findings, *Spine* 13:393, 1988.

Kostova V, Koleva M: Back disorders (low back pain, cervicobrachial and lumbosacral radicular syndromes) and some related risk factors, *J Neurol Sci* 192(1-2):17-25, 2001.

Kostuik JP: Adult scoliosis. In Weinstein J, Wiesel SW, editors: *The lumbar spine,* Philadelphia, 1990, WB Saunders.

Kottlors M, Muller K, Glocker FX: Muscle hypertrophy due to compression of the L5 nerve root, *Clin Neurophysiol* 118(4):e61-e62, 2007.

Kouchoukos NT et al: Operative therapy for femoral-popliteal arterial occlusive disease, *Circulation* 35(suppl 1):174, 1967.

Koval KJ, Zuckerman JD: Functional recovery after fracture of the hip, current concepts review, *J Bone Joint Surg* 76A:751, 1994.

Koyama Y et al: A study of the reality of daily life among patients with osteoarthritis of the hip undergoing conservative treatment, *J Orthop Nurs* (in press, corrected proof).

Kraemer BA, Young BL, Arfken S: Stenosing flexor tenosynovitis, *South Med J* 83:806, 1990.

Kramer J: *Intervertebral disc diseases,* Chicago, 1981, Mosby.

Kramer PA, Sarton-Miller I: The energetics of human walking: Is Froude number (Fr) useful for metabolic comparisons? *Gait Posture* (in press, corrected proof).

Krauspe R, Schmidt M, Schaible H: Sensory and innervation of the anterior cruciate ligament, *J Bone Joint Surg* 74A:390, 1992.

Krodel A, Sturtz H, Siebert CH: Indications for and results of operative treatment of spondylitis and spondylodiscitis, *Arch Orthop Trauma Surg* 110:78, 1991.

Kronberg M, Nemeth G, Brostrom LA: Muscle activity and coordination in the normal shoulder: an electromyographic study, *Clin Orthop Rel Res* 257:76, 1990.

Krumova EK et al: Diagnosing complex regional pain syndrome (CRPS) by a comprehensive analysis of long-term skin temperature changes, *Eur J Pain* 11(1, suppl 1):103-104, 2007.

Krupp MA, Chatton MJ: *Current diagnosis and treatment,* Los Altos, Calif, 1972, Lange Medical.

Kuan T-S et al: The spinal cord connections of the myofascial trigger spots, *Eur J Pain* 11(6):624-634, 2007.

Kujula UM et al: Scoring of patellofemoral disorders, *Arthroscopy* 9:159, 1993.

Kuklo T, Lehman R, Lenke L: Preoperative and postoperative computer tomography evaluation of structures at risk with anterior spinal fusion, *Spine J* 2(5, suppl 1):110-111, 2002.

Kuklo TR, Mackenzie WG, Keeler KA: Hip arthroscopy in Legg-Calve-Perthes disease, *Arthroscopy* 15(1):88-92, 1999.

Kumar R et al: Innervation of the spinal dura, myth or reality? *Spine* 21:18, 1996.

Kumar S, Narayan Y, Amell T: Analysis of low velocity frontal impacts, *Clin Biomech* 18(8):694-703, 2003.

Kuralay E et al: A quantitative approach to lower extremity vein repair, *J Vasc Surg* 36(6):1213-1218, 2002.

Kursuaogu-Brahme S, Gandry CR, Resnick D: Advanced imaging of the wrist, *Radiol Clin North Am* 228:307, 1990.

Kursunoglu-Brahme S, Resnick D: Magnetic resonance imaging of the knee, *Orthop Clin North Am* 21:561, 1990.

Kuruganti U et al: Strength and muscle coactivation in older adults after lower limb strength training, *Int J Ind Ergon* 36(9):761-766, 2006.

Kurutz M: Age-sensitivity of time-related in vivo deformability of human lumbar motion segments and discs in pure centric tension, *J Biomech* 39(1):147-157, 2006.

Kurutz M: In vivo age- and sex-related creep of human lumbar motion segments and discs in pure centric tension, *J Biomech* 39(7):1180-1190, 2006.

Lafforguw P et al: Early-stage avascular necrosis of the femoral head: MR imaging for prognosis in 31 cases with at least 2 years of follow-up, *Radiology* 187:199, 1993.

LaFreniere JG: *The low-back patient, procedures for treatment by physical therapy,* New York, 1985, Masson.

Lain TM: The military brace syndrome: a report of 16 cases of Erb's palsy occurring in military cadets, *J Bone Joint Surg* 51A:557, 1969.

Lakdawala A, El-Zebdeh M, Ireland J: Excision of a ganglion cyst from within the posterior septum of the knee--an arthroscopic technique, *Knee* 12(3):245-247, 2005.

Lally SJ: What tests are acceptable for use in forensic evaluations? A survey of experts, *Prof Psychol Res Pr* 34(5):491-498, 2003.

Lamas C et al: The anatomy and vascularity of the lunate: considerations applied to Kienbock's disease, *Chir Main* 26(1):13-20, 2007.

Lambert EH, Rooke ED: Myasthenic state and lung cancer. In Brain RL, Norris FH, editors: *The remote effects of cancer on the nervous system,* New York, 1965, Grune & Stratton.

Lancaster AR, Nyland J, Roberts CS: The validity of the motion palpation test for determining patellofemoral joint articular cartilage damage, *Phys Ther Sport* 8(2):59-65, 2007.

Lancourt J, Kettelhut M: Predicting return to work for lower back pain patients receiving worker's compensation, *Spine* 17:629, 1992.

Lander PH: Lumbar discography: current concepts and controversies, *Semin Ultrasound CT MRI* 26(2):81-88, 2005.

Landewe RBM, van der Heijde DMFM: Principles of assessment from a clinical perspective, *Best Pract Res Clin Rheumatol* 17(3):365-379, 2003.

Landsmeer JMF: *Atlas of anatomy of the hand,* Edinburgh, 1976, Churchill Livingstone.

Lange AK et al: Degenerative meniscus tears and mobility impairment in women with knee osteoarthritis, *Osteoarthr Cartil* 15(6):701-708, 2007.

Langlais F et al: Hip pain from impingement and dysplasia in patients aged 20-50 years. Workup and role for reconstruction, *Joint Bone Spine* 73(6):614-623, 2006.

Larkin J, Brage M: Ankle, hindfoot, and midfoot injuries. In Reider B, editor: *Sports medicine: the school aged athlete,* Philadelphia, 1991, WB Saunders.

Larsen CF, Brondum V, Skov O: Epidemiology of scaphoid fractures in Odense, Denmark, *Acta Orthop Scand* 63:216, 1992.

Larsen E, Angermann P: Association of ankle instability and foot deformity, *Acta Orthop Scand* 61:136, 1990.

Laskin RS: Total condylar knee replacement in patients who have rheumatoid arthritis, *J Bone Joint Surg* 72A:529, 1990.

Lassere M et al: Smallest detectable difference in radiological progression, *J Rheumatol* 26(3):731-739, 1999.

Latke PA: Soft tissue afflictions. In Steinberg ME, editor: *The hip and its disorders,* Philadelphia, 1992, WB Saunders.

Laude F, Boyer T, Nogier A: Anterior femoroacetabular impingement, *Joint Bone Spine* 74(2):127-132, 2007.

Lauder TD et al: Sports and physical training injury hospitalizations in the Army, *Am J Prevent Med* 18(3, suppl 1):118-128, 2000.

Laurin CA et al: The abnormal lateral patellofemoral angle: a diagnostic roentgenographic sign of recurrent patellar subluxation, *J Bone Joint Surg* 60A:55, 1978.

Lautenbacher S, Kundermann B, Krieg J-C: Sleep deprivation and pain perception, *Sleep Med Rev* 10(5):357-369, 2006.

Lavelle WF, Carl AL: Modern anterior scoliosis surgery, *Spine J* 5(5):581-582, 2005.

Lavy CBD, Barrett DS: *Questions and answers on Apley's concise system of orthopaedics and fractures,* Oxford, UK, 1991, Butterworth-Heinemann.

Lawrence DJ: Sacroiliac joint, part two, clinical considerations. In Cox JM, editor: *Low back pain: mechanism, diagnosis and treatment,* ed 5, Baltimore, 1990, Williams & Wilkins.

Lawrence JS: Generalized osteoarthrosis in a popular sample, *Am J Epidemiol* 90:381, 1969.

Leavitt F, Sweet JJ: Characteristics and frequency of malingering among patients with low back pain, *Pain* 25(3):357-364, 1986.

Leavitt F: Pain and deception: use of verbal pain measurement as a diagnostic aid in differentiating between clinical and simulated low-back pain, *J Psychosom Res* 29(5):495-505, 1985.

Lecuire J et al: 641 operations for sciatic neuralgia due to discal hernia, a computerized statistical study of the results, *Neurochirurgie (Stuttg)* 19:501, 1973.

Ledoux WR, Sangeorzan BJ: Clinical biomechanics of the peritalar joint, *Foot Ankle Clin North Am* 9(4):663-683, 2004.

Lee CC, Vainchenker U, Crupi RS: Ten-year-old boy with a swollen knee: unusual cause of knee pain, *J Emerg Med* 25(4):449-450, 2003.

Lee MLH: The intraosseous arterial pattern of the carpal lunate bone and its relation to avascular necrosis, *Acta Orthop Scand* 33:43, 1963.

Lee TH, Wapner KL, Hecht PJ: Plantar fibromatosis, current concepts review, *J Bone Joint Surg* 75A:1080, 1993.

Lee TMC et al: Neural correlates of feigned memory impairment, *Neuroimage* 28(2):305-313, 2005.

Lefevre-Colau MM et al: Reliability, validity, and responsiveness of the modified Kapandji index for assessment of functional mobility of the rheumatoid hand, *Arch Phys Med Rehabil* 84(7):1032-1038, 2003.

Leffert RD et al: Infra-clavicular brachial plexus injuries, *J Bone Joint Surg* 47B:9, 1965.

Leffert RD: Neurological problems. In Rockwood CA, Matsen FA, editors: *The shoulder,* vol 1, Philadelphia, 1990, WB Saunders.

Leffs M: *Back pain in the adolescent athlete,* Toronto, 1991, American Back Society.

Legan JM et al: Tears of the glenoid labrum: MR imaging of 88 arthroscopically confirmed cases, *Radiology* 179:241, 1991.

Lehner JT, Miller T, Mills A: Comparison of intermediate-term status in Legg-Calve-Perthes disease patients treated with varus derotational osteotomy with or without subsequent epiphysiodesis of the greater trochanter, *J Am Coll Surg* 199(3, suppl 1):50, 2004.

LeHuec JC et al: Epicondylitis after treatment with fluoroquinolone antibiotics, *J Bone Joint Surg* 77B:293, 1995.

Leibovitz A et al: Edema of the paretic hand in elderly post-stroke nursing patients, *Arch Gerontol Geriatr* 44(1):37-42, 2007.

Lenke L et al: Selection of the lowest instrumented vertebra in thoracic adolescent idiopathic scoliosis Lenke type 1 and 2 following segmental posterior spinal fusion, *Spine J* 4(5, suppl 1):S74-S75, 2004.

Lennox IA, McLauchlan J, Murali R: Failures of screening and management of congenital dislocation of the hip, *J Bone Joint Surg* 75B:72, 1993.

Leon HO et al: Intercondylar notch stenosis in degenerative arthritis of the knee, *Arthroscopy* 21(3):294-302, 2005.

Lephart SM, Henry TJ: Functional rehabilitation for the upper and lower extremity, *Orthop Clin North Am* 26:579, 1995.

Leppilahti J et al: Overuse injuries of the Achilles tendon, *Ann Chir Gynaecol* 80;202, 1991.

Lerner AJ: *The little black book of neurology,* ed 3, St Louis, 1995, Mosby.

Les RD, Gerhardt JJ: Range-of-motion measurements, *J Bone Joint Surg* 77A:784, 1995.

Lesher J et al: Hip joint pain referral patterns: a descriptive study, *Arch Phys Med Rehabil* 87(11):e23-e35, 2006.

Leslie BM, Ericson WB Jr, Morehead JR: Incidence of a septum within the first dorsal compartment of the wrist, *J Hand Surg* 15A:88, 1990.

Lestini WF, Bell GR: Spinal infections: patient evaluation. In *Seminars in spine surgery,* vol 2, Philadelphia, 1990, WB Saunders.

Letourmeau L, Dessureault M, Carette S: Rheumatoid iliopsoas bursitis presenting as unilateral femoral nerve palsy, *J Rheumatol* 18:462, 1991.

LeVeau B: Hip. In Richardson JK, Iglarsh JK, editors: *Clinical orthopaedic physical therapy,* Philadelphia, 1994, WB Saunders.

Levene DL: *Chest pain: an integrated diagnostic approach,* Philadelphia, 1977, Lea & Febiger.

Levick JR: An investigation into the validity of subatmospheric pressure recordings from synovial fluid and their dependence on joint angle, *J Physiol* 289:55, 1979.

Lewallen DG et al: Effects of retinacular release and tibial tubercle elevation in patellofemoral degenerative joint disease, *J Orthop Res* 8:856, 1990.

Lewis CB, Bottomley JM: Orthopaedic treatment considerations. In Lewis CB, Bottomley JM, editors: *Geriatric physical therapy: a clinical approach,* New York, 1994, Appleton & Lange.

Lewis CB, Knortz KA: *Orthopedic assessment and treatment of the geriatric patient,* St Louis, 1993, Mosby.

Lewis MH: Median nerve decompression after Colles' fracture, *J Bone Joint Surg* 60B:195, 1978.

Lewkonia RM, Kinsella TD: Pyogenic sacroiliitis: diagnosis and significance, *J Rheumatol* 8:153, 1981.

Lhermitte J, Bollak P, Nicholas M: Les douleurs a type de decharge electrique dans la sclerose en plaques, un cas e forme sensitive de la sclerose multiple, *Rev Neurol (Paris)* 2:56, 1924.

Lhermitte J: Etude de la commotion de la moelle, *Rev Neurol (Paris)* 1:210, 1932.

Licht PB, Christensen HW, Hoilund-Carlsen PF: Is there a role for premanipulative testing before cervical manipulation? *J Manipulative Physiol Ther* 23(3):175-179, 2000.

Liebenson C: Hip dysfunction and back pain, *J Bodywork Mov Ther* 11(2):111-115, 2007.

Lieou YC: *Syndrome sympathique cervical posterieur et arthrite cervicale chronique: etude clinique et radiologique,* Strasbourg, France,1928, Schuler and Minh.

Liesegang TJ: Ross syndrome plus: beyond Horner, Holmes-Adie, and Harlequin, *Neurology* 55:1841-1846, 2000; *Am J Ophthalmol* 131(6):826, 2001.

Lin JT, Stubblefield MD: De Quervain's tenosynovitis in patients with lymphedema: a report of 2 cases with management approach, *Arch Phys Med Rehabil* 84(10): 1554-1557, 2003.

Lindstrom G, Nystrom A: Incidence of post-traumatic arthrosis after primary healing of scaphoid fractures: a clinical and radiological study, *J Hand Surg* 15B:11, 1990.

Lindstrom G, Nystrom A: Natural history of scaphoid non-union, with special reference to "asymptomatic" cases, *J Hand Surg* 17B:697, 1992.

Linscheid RL, Dobyns JH: Rheumatoid arthritis of the wrist, *Ortho Clin North Am* 2:649, 1971.

Linscheid RL et al: Instability patterns of the wrist, *J Hand Surg* 8A:682, 1983.

Linscheid RL et al: Traumatic instability of the wrist, *J Bone Joint Surg* 54A:1612, 1972.

Linton RC, Indelicato PA: Medial ligament injuries. In DeLee JC, Drez D, editors: *Orthopedic sports medicine: principles and practice,* vol 1, Philadelphia, 1994, WB Saunders.

Lippitt S, Matsen F: Mechanisms of glenohumeral joint stability, *Clin Orthop* 291:20, 1993.

Lipscomb PR Jr., Lipscomb PR Sr., Bryan RS: Osteochondritis dissecans of the knee with loose fragments, *J Bone Joint Surg* 60A:235, 1978.

Lipson SJ: Fractures of the atlas associated with fractures of the odontoid process and transverse ligament ruptures, *J Bone Joint Surg* 59A:940, 1977.

Lisbona R, Rosenthall L: Observation on the sequential use of 99mTc-phosphate complex and 67Gd imaging in osteomyelitis and septic arthritis, *Radiology* 123:123, 1977.

Lister G: *The hand: diagnosis and indications,* Edinburgh, 1977, Churchill Livingstone.

Litchfield R et al: Rehabilitation of the overhead athlete, *J Orthop Sports Phys Ther* 18:433, 1993.

Liu P-C et al: Snapping knee symptoms caused by an intra-articular ganglion cyst, *Knee* 14(2):167-168, 2007.

Lloyd-Roberts GC, Clark RC: Ball and socket ankle joint in metatarsus adductus varus (S-shaped or serpentine foot), *J Bone Joint Surg* 55B:193, 1973.

Lloyd-Roberts GG: Suppurative arthritis in infancy, *J Bone Joint Surg* 42B:706, 1960.

Lluch AL: Thickening of the synovium of the digital flexor tendons: cause or consequence of the carpal tunnel syndrome? *J Hand Surg* 17B:209, 1992.

Lo YL et al: Superficial peroneal sensory and sural nerve conduction studies in peripheral neuropathy, *J Clin Neurosci* 13(5):547-549, 2006.

Locher S et al: Radiological anatomy of the obturator nerve and its articular branches: basis to develop a method of radiofrequency denervation for hip joint pain, *Eur J Pain* 10(suppl 1):s136-s137, 2006.

Long L, Huntley A, Ernst E: Which complementary and alternative therapies benefit which conditions? A survey of the opinions of 223 professional organizations, *Complement Ther Med* 9(3):178-185, 2001.

Longoria RK, Carpenter JL: Anaerobic phygenic sacroiliitis, *South Med J* 76:649, 1983.

Lonstein JE, Winter RB: Milwaukee brace treatment of adolescent idiopathic scoliosis—review of 1020 patients, *J Bone Joint Surg* 76A:1207, 1994.

Lorber J: Long-term follow-up of 100 children who recovered from tuberculous meningitis, *Pediatrics* 28:778, 1961.

Lorber J: Spina bifida cystica, *Arch Dis Child* 47:854, 1972.

Lorish DK et al: Disease and psychosocial factors related to physical functioning in rheumatoid arthritis, *J Rheumatol* 18:1150, 1991.

Losee RE, Ennis TRJ, Southwick WO: Anterior subluxation of the lateral tibial plateau: a diagnostic test and operative review, *J Bone Joint Surg* 60A:1015, 1978.

Loth TS: *Orthopedic boards review II a case study approach,* St Louis, 1996, Mosby.

Loth TS: *Orthopedic boards review,* St Louis, 1993, Mosby.

Lougher L, Southgate CRW, Holt MD: Coronary ligament rupture as a cause of medial knee pain, *Arthroscopy* 19(10):e157-e158, 2003.

Love BRT, Stevens PM, William PF: A long-term review of shelf arthroplasty. *J Bone Joint Surg* 62B:321, 1980.

Lovejoy CO: The natural history of human gait and posture. Part 3: the knee, *Gait Posture* 25(3):325-341, 2007.

Lovett AW: A contribution to the study of the mechanics of the spine, *Am J Anat* 2:457, 1983.

Lu T-W, Chen H-L, Wang T-M: Obstacle crossing in older adults with medial compartment knee osteoarthritis, *Gait Posture* (in press, corrected proof).

Lucas CE, Vlahos AL, Ledgerwood AM: Kindness kills: the negative impact of pain as the fifth vital sign, *J Am Coll Surg* (in press, corrected proof).

Lucas DB: Biomechanics of the shoulder joint, *Arch Surg* 107:425, 1973.

Lui TH, Ip K, Chow HT: Comparison of radiologic and arthroscopic diagnoses of distal tibiofibular syndesmosis disruption in acute ankle fracture, *Arthroscopy* 21(11):1370.e1-1370.e7, 2005.

Lui TH: Arthroscopy and endoscopy of the foot and ankle: indications for new techniques, *Arthroscopy* (in press, corrected proof).

Lynch AC, Lipscomb PR: The carpal-tunnel syndrome and Colles' fractures, *JAMA* 185:363, 1963.

Lynch AF: Tuberculosis of the greater trochanter, *J Bone Joint Surg* 64B:185, 1982.

Lynch GS, Schertzer JD, Ryall JG: Therapeutic approaches for muscle wasting disorders, *Pharmacol Ther* 113(3):461-487, 2007.

Lynch JM, Hennessy MJ: Third nerve palsy: harbinger of basilar artery thrombosis and locked-in syndrome? *J Stroke Cerebrovasc Dis* 14(1):42-43, 2005.

Mabin D: Compressions nerveuses distales du membre inferieur. Etude clinique et electrophysiologique, *Clin Neurophysiol* 27(1):9-24, 1997.

MacAusland WR, Mayo RA: *Orthopedics: a concise guide to clinical practices,* Boston, 1965, Little, Brown.

MacConaill MA, Basmajian JV: *Muscles and movements: a basis for human kinesiology,* Baltimore, 1969, Williams & Wilkins.

MacDermid JC, Michlovitz SL: Examination of the elbow: linking diagnosis, prognosis, and outcomes as a framework for maximizing therapy interventions, *J Hand Ther* 19(2):82-97, 2006.

MacEwen GD: Treatment of congenital dislocation of the hip in older children, *Clin Orthop* 225:86, 1987.

Macintosh JE, Pearcy MJ, Bogduk N: The axial torque of the lumbar back muscles; torsion strength of the back muscles, *Aust N Z J Surg* 63:205, 1993.

MacLean JJ, Owen JP, Iatridis JC: Role of endplates in contributing to compression behaviors of motion segments and intervertebral discs, *J Biomech* 40(1):55-63, 2007.

Macnab I: Acceleration extension injuries of the cervical spine. In Rothmann RH, Simeone FA, editors: *The spine,* vol 2, ed 2, Philadelphia, 1982, WB Saunders.

Macnab I: *Backache,* Baltimore, 1977, Williams & Wilkins.

Mader TJ, Ames A, Letourneau P: Pain management in paediatric trauma patients with long bone fracture, *Injury* 37(1):61-65, 2006.

Magee DJ: *Orthopedic physical assessment,* ed 3, Philadelphia, 1997, WB Saunders.

Magerl W, Treede R-D: Secondary tactile hypoesthesia: a novel type of pain-induced somatosensory plasticity in human subjects, *Neurosci Lett* 361(1-3):136-139, 2004.

Magora A: Investigation of the relation between low back pain and occupation: 4, physical requirements: bending, rotation, reaching and sudden maximal effort, *Scand J Rehabil Med* 5:186, 1973.

Maguire MF et al: A study exploring the role of intercostal nerve damage in chronic pain after thoracic surgery, *Eur J Cardiothorac Surg* 29(6):873-879, 2006.

Maher C, Adams R: Reliability of pain and stiffness assessments in clinical manual lumbar spine examination, *Phys Ther* 74:801, 1994.

Maigne JY, Maigne R, Guerin-Surville H: The lumbar mamillo-accessory foramen: a study of 203 lumbosacral spines, *Surg Radiol Anat* 13:29, 1991.

Maigne JY, Maigne R, Guerin-Surville H: Upper thoracic dorsal rami: anatomic study of their medial cutaneous branches, *Surg Radiol Anat* 13:190, 1991.

Maigne R: *Orthopaedic medicine: a new approach to vertebral manipulation,* Springfield, Ill, 1972, Charles C Thomas.

Maihofner C, DeCol R: Decreased perceptual learning ability in complex regional pain syndrome, *Eur J Pain* (in press, corrected proof).

Maiman DJ: Modern anterior scoliosis surgery, *Surg Neurol* 62(5):474-475, 2004.

Main WK, Scott WN: Knee anatomy. In Scott WN, editor: *Ligament and extensor mechanism injuries of the knee, diagnosis and treatment,* St Louis, 1991, Mosby.

Maitland GD: *Vertebral manipulation,* ed 5, London, 1986, Butterworth.

Maitland GD: *Vertebral manipulation,* London, 1973, Butterworths.

Majima M, Horii E, Nakamura R: Treatment of chronically dislocated elbows: a report of three cases, *J Shoulder Elbow Surg* (in press, corrected proof).

Makhsous M, Lin F, Zhang L-Q: Multi-axis passive and active stiffnesses of the glenohumeral joint, *Clin Biomech* 19(2):107-115, 2004.

Malanga GA et al: Physical examination of the knee: a review of the original test description and scientific validity of common orthopedic tests, *Arch Phys Med Rehabil* 84(4): 592-603, 2003.

Malen WJ, Bassett FH III, Goldner RD: Luxatio erecta: the inferior glenohumeral dislocation, *J Orthop Trauma* 4:19, 1990.

Malmivaara A et al: Rheumatoid factor and HLA antigens in wrist tenosynovitis and humeral epicondylitis, *Scand J Rheumatol* 24:154, 1995.

Malone TR, McPoil TG, Nitz AJ: *Orthopedic and sports physical therapy,* ed 3, St Louis, 1997, Mosby.

Manaster BJ: *Handbooks in radiology skeletal radiology,* Chicago, 1989, Year Book Medical Publishers.

Mandelbaum BR, Gross MC: Spondylolysis and spondylolisthesis. In Reider B, editor: *Sports medicine: the school-age athlete,* Philadelphia, 1991, WB Saunders.

Mann RA et al: Chronic rupture of the Achilles tendon; a new technique of repair, *J Bone Joint Surg* 73A:214, 1991.

Mann RA: *Surgery of the foot,* St Louis, 1986, Mosby.

Mannerfelt L et al: Rupture of the extensor pollicis longus tendon after Colles' fracture and by rheumatoid arthritis, *J Hand Surg* 15B:49, 1990.

Manniche C et al: Clinical trial of intensive muscle training for chronic low back pain, *Lancet* 24:1473, 1988.

Maquet PGJ: *Biomechanics of the knee: with application of the pathogenesis and the surgical treatment of osteoarthritis,* New York, 1976, Springer-Verlag.

Marcaud V et al: Vascularite restreinte au systeme nerveux peripherique: presentation clinique atypique vasculitis confined to peripheral nerves: an unusual clinical presentation, *Rev Med Intern* 23(6):558-562, 2002.

Marchand F, Ahmed A: Investigation of the laminate structure of lumbar disc anulus fibrosus, *Spine* 15:402, 1990.

Marchiori DM: *Clinical imaging with skeletal, chest, and abdomen pattern differentials,* St Louis, 1999, Mosby.

Mariani PP, Mauro CS, Margheritini F: Arthroscopic diagnosis of the snapping popliteus tendon, *Arthroscopy* 21(7):888-892, 2005.

Maritz NGJ et al: The rheumatoid wrist in black South African patients, *J Hand Surg* 28(4):373-375, 2003.

Markey KL, DiBenedetto M, Curl WW: Upper trunk brachial plexopathy, *Am J Sports Med* 21:650, 1993.

Markhashov AM: Variations in the arterial blood supply of the spine, *Vestn Khir* 94:64, 1965.

Marrero GH: Juvenile kyphosis, *Spine State Art Rev* 4:173, 1990.

Martel W: The occipito-atlanto-axial joints in rheumatoid arthritis and ankylosing spondylitis, *AJR Am J Roentgenol* 86:233, 1961.

Martens MA, Moeyersoons JP: Acute and recurrent effort-related compartment syndrome in sports, *Sports Med* 9:62, 1990.

Martin AF: The pathomechanics of the knee joint, *J Bone Joint Surg* 42A:13, 1960.

Martin DJ, Gardner ER: Transfer metatarsalgia after hallux valgus correction alleviated by 'auto-Helal' osteotomy of the second metatarsal, *Foot* 15(2):101-103, 2005.

Martin DR, Gaith WP: Results of orthoscopic debridement of glenoid labral tears, *Am J Sports Med* 23:4, 1995.

Martin JH: *Neuroanatomy text and atlas,* ed 2, Stamford, Conn, 1996, Appleton & Lange.

Martinez MA et al: Facial nerve neuropathy in congenital vascular and lymphatic malformations of the face, *Clin Neurophysiol* 117(suppl 1):1-2, 2006.

Martinez Maestre MA, Daza Manzano C, Martinez Lopez R: Postmenopausal endometrial tuberculosis, *Int J Gynecol Obstet* 86(3):405-406, 2004.

Martinoli C et al: Ultrasound of the elbow, *Eur J Ultrasound* 14(1):21-27, 2001.

Mason M, Currey HLF: *Clinical rheumatology,* Philadelphia, 1970, JB Lippincott.

Massie J et al: Antifibrotic gels versus a barrier sheet in the prevention of epidural fibrosis postlaminectomy, *Spine J* 2(2, suppl 1):35, 2002.

Mathers LH et al: *Clinical anatomy principles,* St Louis, 1996, Mosby.

Mathews DA, Suchman AL, Branch WT: Making "connexions": enhancing the therapeutic potential of patient-clinician relationships, *Ann Intern Med* 118:973, 1993.

Matsen F, Arntz C: Rotator cuff failure. In Rockwood C, Matsen F, editors: *The shoulder,* Philadelphia, 1990, WB Saunders.

Matsen F, Arntz C: Subacromial impingement. In Rockwood C, Matsen F, editors: *The shoulder,* Philadelphia, 1990, WB Saunders.

Matsen FA III, Arntz CT: Rotator cuff tendon failure in the shoulder. In Rockwood C, Matsen FA, editors: *The shoulder,* Philadelphia, 1990, WB Saunders.

Matsuo T et al: Application of thermography for evaluation of mechanical load on the muscles of upper limb during wheelchair driving, *J Biomech* 39(suppl 1):S537, 2006.

Maurissen JPJ et al: Factors affecting grip strength testing, *Neurotoxicol Teratol* 25(5): 543-553, 2003.

Maury AC, Southgate C, Owen T: Hypertrophic nonunion of the distal fibula after reduced triplane fracture of the distal tibia in a child, *Foot Ankle Surg* 9(4):229-232, 2003.

Maxted MJ, Jackson RK: Innominate osteotomy in Perthe's disease, *J Bone Joint Surg* 67B:399, 1985.

Mayer TG: A prospective two year study of functional restoration in industrial low back injury: an objective assessment procedure, *JAMA* 258:1763, 1987.

Mayfield JK et al: Biomechanical properties of human carpal ligaments, *Orthop Trans* 3:143, 1979.

Mayfield JK, Johnson RP, Kilcoyne RF: Carpal dislocations: pathomechanics and progressive perilunar instability, *J Hand Surg* 5:226, 1980.

Mayfield JK: Mechanism of carpal injuries, *Clin Orthop* 149:45, 1980.

Mayo Clinic & Mayo Foundation: *Clinical examination in neurology,* Philadelphia, 1981, WB Saunders.

Mayo Clinic: *Clinical examinations in neurology,* ed 3, Philadelphia, 1971, WB Saunders.

Mayrand N et al: Diagnosis and management of posttraumatic piriformis syndrome: a case study, *J Manipulative Physiol Ther* 29(6):486-491, 2006.

Mazion JM: *Illustrated manual of neurological reflexes/signs/tests, part I orthopedic signs/tests/maneuvers for office procedure, part II,* Orlando, 1980, Daniels.

McAndrew MP, Weinstein SL: A long-term follow-up of Legg-Calve-Perthes disease, *J Bone Joint Surg* 66A:860, 1984.

McBride ED: *Disability evaluation and principles of treatment of compensable injuries,* ed 6, Philadelphia, 1963, JB Lippincott.

McBryde A: Disorders of ankle and foot. In Grana WA, Kalenak A, editors: *Clinical sports medicine,* Philadelphia, 1991, WB Saunders.

McBryde A: Stress fractures of the foot and ankle. In DeLee JD, Drez D, editors: *Orthopaedic sport medicine, principles and practice,* vol 2, Philadelphia, 1994, WB Saunders.

McCarthy A, Vicenzino B: Treatment of osteitis pubis via the pelvic muscles, *Man Ther* 8(4):257-260, 2003.

McCarthy GM, McCarthy DJ: Intrasynovial corticosteroid therapy, *Bull Rheum Dis* 43:2, 1994.

McCarty DJ, Koopman WJ, editors: *Arthritis and allied conditions,* ed 12, Philadelphia, 1993, Lea & Febiger.

McDonald D et al: Total joint reconstruction. In *Orthopedic boards review,* St Louis, 1993, Mosby.

McDonnell MN et al: Impairments in precision grip correlate with functional measures in adult hemiplegia, *Clin Neurophysiol* 117(7):1474-1480, 2006.

McGann WA: History and physical examination. In Steinberg ME, editor: *The hip and its disorders,* Philadelphia, 1991, WB Saunders.

McGill S: Quantitative intramuscular myoelectric activity of the quadratus lumborum during a wide variety of tasks, *Clin Biomech* 11:170, 1996.

McGill SM: The influence of lordosis on axial trunk torque and trunk muscle myoelectric activity, *Spine* 17:1187, 1992.

McGoey BV et al: Effect of weight loss on musculoskeletal pain in the morbidly obese, *J Bone Joint Surg* 72B:322, 1990.

McKean KA et al: Gender differences exist in osteoarthritic gait, *Clin Biomech* 22(4): 400-409, 2007.

McKechnie B: Low back pain in the 1990's. In McKechnie B, McRae R, editors: *Clinical orthopaedic examination*, ed 3, Edinburgh, 1990, Churchill Livingstone.

McKee GK: Development of total prosthetic replacement of the hip, *Clin Orthop* 72:85, 1970.

McKenzie RA: *The lumbar spine mechanical diagnosis and therapy*, Wikanae, New Zealand, 1981, Spinal Publications.

McKibbin B, editor: *Recent advances in orthopaedics*, ed 4, Edinburgh, 1983, Churchill Livingstone.

McKibbin B: Anatomical factors in the stability of the hip joint in the newborn, *J Bone Joint Surg* 52B:148, 1970.

McKinnis LN: Fundamentals of radiology for physical therapists. In Richardson JK, Iglarsh ZA, editors: *Clinical orthopedic physical therapy*, Philadelphia, 1994, WB Saunders.

McLain RF, Steyer CM: Tendon ruptures with scaphoid nonunion, a case report, *Clin Orthop* 255:117, 1990.

McLaughlin HL: The "frozen" shoulder, *Clin Orthop* 20:126, 1961.

McMahon PJ et al: Glenohumeral translations are increased after a type II superior labrum anterior-posterior lesion: a cadaveric study of severity of passive stabilizer injury, *J Shoulder Elbow Surg* 13(1):39-44, 2004.

McMurray TP: *The Robert joint birthday volume*, London, 1928, Humphrey Milford.

McMurray TP: The semilunar cartilages, *Br J Surg* 29:407, 1942.

McNair PJ et al: Acute neck pain: Cervical spine range of motion and position sense prior to and after joint mobilization, *Man Ther* (in press, corrected proof).

McNeil et al: Trunk strengths in attempted flexion, extension, and lateral bending in healthy subjects and patients with low back disorders, *Spine* 5:529, 1980.

McNurty RY et al: Kinematics of the wrist, II, clinical applications, *J Bone Joint Surg* 600:955, 1978.

McPherson A et al: Imaging knee position using MRI, RSA/CT and 3D digitisation, *J Biomech* 38(2):263-268, 2005.

McPherson T: Benign tumors of fibrous tissue and adipose tissue of the hand, *J Hand Ther* 18(1):53-54, 2005.

McRae R: *Clinical orthopaedic examination*, ed 3, Edinburgh, 1990, Churchill Livingstone.

McRae R: *Practical fracture treatment*, ed 3, Edinburgh, 1994, Churchill-Livingstone.

Measured hip joint range of motion loss and its role in the pathogenesis of the athletic groin injury osteitis pubis, *J Sci Med Sport* 6(4, suppl 1):93-84, 2003.

Medical Economics Books: *Patient care flow chart manual*, ed 3, Ordell, NJ, 1982, Medical Economics Books.

Meenan RF, Gertman PM, Mason JH: Measuring health status in arthritis: the arthritis impact measurement scales, *Arthritis Rheum* 23(2):146-152, 1980.

Mehta JA, Bain GI: Elbow dislocations in adults and children, *Clin Sports Med* 23(4): 609-627, 2004.

Mellion MB: *Office sports medicine*, ed 2, St Louis, 1996, Mosby.

Mellion MB: *Sports medicine secrets,* Philadelphia, 1994, Hanley & Belfus.

Melloni P, Valls R: The use of MRI scanning for investigating soft-tissue abnormalities in the elbow, *Eur J Radiol* 54(2):303-313, 2005.

Melzack R: *The McGill pain questionnaire: pain measurement and assessment,* New York, 1983, Raven.

Mendez AA, Eyster RL: Displaced nonunion stress fracture of the femoral neck treated with internal fixation and bone graft, *Am J Sports Med* 20:230, 1992.

Mendoza RX, Nicholas JA, Sands A: Principals of shoulder rehabilitation in the athlete. In Nicholas JA, Hershman EB, editor: *The upper extremity in sports medicine,* St Louis, 1990, Mosby.

Menelaus MB: Lessons learned in the management of Legg-Calve-Perthes disease, *Clin Orthop* 209:41, 1986.

Mengel MB, Schwiebert LP: *Ambulatory medicine the primary care of families,* ed 2, Stamford, Conn, 1996, Appleton & Lange.

Mennell JM: *Back pain,* Boston, 1960, Little, Brown.

Mennell JM: *Foot pain,* Boston, 1969, Little, Brown.

Mennell JM: *The musculoskeletal system differential diagnosis from symptoms and physical signs,* Gaithersburg, Md, 1992, Aspen.

Mens J et al: Possible harmful effects of high intra-abdominal pressure on the pelvic girdle, *J Biomech* 39(4):627-635, 2006.

Merchant AC: Patellofemoral disorders, biomechanics, diagnosis, and non-operative treatment. In McGinty JB, editor: *Operative arthroscopy,* New York, 1991, Raven.

Merchant AC: Patellofemoral malalignment and instabilities. In Ewing JW, editor: *Articular cartilage and knee joint function: basic science and arthroscopy,* New York, 1990, Raven.

Merchant AC: Radiologic evaluation of the patellofemoral joint. In Aichroth PM, Cannon WD, editors: *Knee surgery,* London, 1992, Martin Dunitz.

Mercier LR, Pettid FJ: *Practical orthopedics,* ed 4, St Louis, 1995, Mosby.

Mercier LR, Pettid FJ: *Practical orthopedics,* ed 5, St Louis, 2000, Mosby.

Merkow RL, Lane JM: Paget's disease of bone, *Orthop Clin North Am* 21:171, 1990.

Merle D'Aubigne R: Nerve injuries in fractures and dislocations of the shoulder, *Surg Clin North Am* 43:1685, 1963.

Merle H et al: Natural history of the visual impairment of relapsing neuromyelitis optica, *Ophthalmology* 114(4):810-815, 2007.

Merskey H: *Pain and psychological medicine, textbook of pain,* Edinburgh, 1984, Churchill Livingstone.

Mester AR et al: Enteropathic arthritis in the sacroiliac joint. Imaging and differential diagnosis, *Eur J Radiol* 35(3):199-208, 2000.

Meyer HM Jr et al: Central nervous system syndromes of viral etiology: a study of 713 cases, *Am J Med* 29:334, 1960.

Meyers JE, Millis SR, Volkert K: A validity index for the MMPI-2, *Arch Clin Neuropsychol* 17(2):157-169, 2002.

Meyers JE, Volbrecht ME: A validation of multiple malingering detection methods in a large clinical sample, *Arch Clin Neuropsychol* 18(3):261-276, 2003.

Meyers JF: Elbow arthroscopy. In Shahriaree H, editor: *O'Connor's textbook of arthroscopic surgery,* Philadelphia, 1992, JB Lippincott.

Micheli LJ, Trapman E: Spinal deformities. In Torg S, Welsh RP, Shephard RJ, editors: *Current therapy in sports medicine,* ed 2, St Louis, 1990, Mosby.

Micheli LJ: Reflex sympathetic dystrophy may stem from sports (news brief), *Physician Sports Med* 18:35, 1990.

Michelow BJ et al: The natural history of obstetrical brachial plexus palsy, *Plast Reconstr Surg* 93:675, 1994.

Michelson JD et al: Examination of the pathologic anatomy of ankle fractures, *J Trauma* 32:65, 1992.

Middleton GD, McFarlin JE, Lipsky PE: Prevalence and clinical impact of fibromyalgia in systemic lupus erythematous, *Arthritis Rheum* 8:1181, 1994.

Miles KA, Lamont AC: Ultrasonic demonstration of the elbow fat pads, *Clin Radiol* 40(6):602-604, 1989.

Milgram JE: Office measures for relief of painful foot, *J Bone Joint Surg* 46A:1095, 1964.

Milgram JW et al: Resection arthroplasty for septic arthritis of the hip in ambulatory and nonambulatory adult patients, *Clin Orthop* 272:181, 1991.

Millender LH, Nalebuff EA, Feldon PG: Rheumatoid arthritis, In Green D, editor: *Operative hand surgery,* New York, 1982, Churchill Livingstone.

Miller B: Manual therapy treatment of myofascial pain and dysfunction. In Rachlin ES, editor: *Myofascial pain and fibromyalgia,* St Louis, 1994, Mosby.

Miller JH, Beggs I: Detection of intraarticular bodies of the elbow with saline arthrosonography, *Clin Radiol* 56(3):231-234, 2001.

Miller M: Adult reconstruction and sports medicine. In Miller M, editor: *Review of orthopaedics,* Philadelphia, 1992, WB Saunders.

Miller MD: *Review of orthopaedics,* Philadelphia, 1992, WB Saunders.

Million T, Green CJ, Meagher RB: *Million behavioral health inventory,* ed 3, Minneapolis, 1982, Interpretive Scoring System.

Mills GP: The treatment of tennis elbow, *Dr Med J* 1:12, 1928.

Minamikawa Y et al: de Quervain's syndrome: surgical and anatomical studies of the fibroosseous canal, *Orthopedics* 14:545, 1991.

Minns RJ: The role of gait analysis in the management of the knee, *Knee* 12(3):157-162, 2005.

Mino DE, Palmer AK, Levinsohn EM: The role of radiography and computerized tomography in the diagnosis of subluxation and dislocation of the distal radioulnar joint, *J Hand Surg* 8A:23, 1983.

Mirkopulos N, Myer TJ: Isolated avulsion of the popliteus tendon, *Am J Sports Med* 19:417, 1991.

Mirvis SE, Young JWR: *Imaging in trauma and critical care,* Baltimore, 1991, Williams & Wilkins.

Misamore GW, Woodward C: Evaluation of degenerative lesions of the rotator cuff: a comparison of arthrography and ultrasonography, *J Bone Joint Surg* 73A:704, 1991.

Mishra S: A new test for demonstrating the action of flexor digitorum superficialis (FDS) tendon, *J Plastic Reconstr Aesthet Surg* 59(12):1342-1344, 2006.

Mitchell S et al: The need for a falls prevention programme for patients undergoing hip and knee replacement surgery, *J Orthop Nurs* (in press, corrected proof).

Mitchell SW: *Injuries of nerves and their consequences,* Philadelphia, 1972, JB Lippincott.

Moberg E: Criticism and study of methods for examining sensibility of the hand, *Neurology* 12:8, 1962.

Moberg E: Relation of touch and deep sensation to hand reconstruction, *Am J Surg* 109:353, 1965.

Modic MT, Masaryk TJ, Ross JS: *Magnetic resonance imaging of the spine,* ed 2, St Louis, 1994, Mosby.

Mody BS et al: Nonunion of fractures of the scaphoid tuberosity, *J Bone Joint Surg* 75B:423, 1993.

Moe JH, Kettleson DN: Idiopathic scoliosis, *J Bone Joint Surg* 52A:1509, 1970.

Moe JH et al: *Scoliosis and other spinal deformities,* Philadelphia, 1978, WB Saunders.

Mohagheghi AA et al: Differences in gastrocnemius muscle architecture between the paretic and non-paretic legs in children with hemiplegic cerebral palsy, *Clin Biomech* (in press, corrected proof).

Moldaver J: Tinel's sign: its characteristics and significance, *J Bone Joint Surg* 60A:412, 1978.

Moldofsky H: Chronobiological influences on fibromyalgia syndrome: theoretical and therapeutic implications, *Baillieres Clin Rheumatol* 8:801, 1994.

Moll JH, Wright V: Measurement of spinal movement. In Jayson M, editor: *Lumbar spine and back pain,* New York, 1976, Grune & Stratton.

Moll JMH, Wright V: An objective clinical study of chest expansion, *Ann Rheum Dis* 31:1, 1972.

Moll JMH: *Manual of rheumatology,* Edinburgh, 1987, Churchill Livingstone.

Momeni M, Baele P, Lavand'Homme P: Postoperative mapping of sensitive dysesthesia and residual pain after sternotomy for cardiac surgery, *J Pain* 8(4, suppl 1):S30, 2007.

Montgomery SP, Erwin WE: Scheuermann's kyphosis: long-term results of Milwaukee brace treatment, *Spine* 6:5, 1981.

Monzon DG, Iserson KV, Vazquez JA: Single fascia iliaca compartment block for post-hip fracture pain relief, *J Emerg Med* 32(3):257-262, 2007.

Mooney V, Robertson J: The facet syndrome, *Clin Orthop* 115:149, 1976.

Mooney V: Differential diagnosis of low back disorders. In Frymoyer JW, editor: *The adult spine: principles and practice,* New York, 1991, Raven.

Moore FH: Examination of infant's hips: can it do harm? *J Bone Joint Surg* 71B:4, 1989.

Moore FJ et al: The relationship between head-neck-shaft angle, calcar width, articular cartilage and bone volume in arthrosis of the hip, *Br J Rheumatol* 35:432, 1994.

Moore KL: *Clinically oriented anatomy,* ed 3, Baltimore, 1992, Williams & Wilkins.

Moosabhoy MA, Gard SA: Methodology for determining the sensitivity of swing leg toe clearance and leg length to swing leg joint angles during gait, *Gait Posture* 24(4): 493-501, 2006.

Moran SL et al: The use of the 4 + 5 extensor compartmental vascularized bone graft for the treatment of Kienböck's disease, *J Hand Surg* 30(1):50-58, 2005.

Moreau JF: Re: "Ultrasound: is there a future in diagnostic imaging?" *J Am Coll Radiol* 4(1):78-79, 2007.

Mori Y et al: Lateral retinaculum release in adolescent patellofemoral disorders: its relationship to peripheral nerve injury in the lateral retinaculum, *Bull Hosp J Dis Orthop* 51:218, 1991.

Moriwaki K et al: Neuropathic pain and prolonged regional inflammation as two distinct symptomatological components in complex regional pain syndrome with patchy osteoporosis—a pilot study, *Pain* 72(1-2):277-282, 1997.

Morrey BF, An K: *Biomechanics of the shoulder,* Philadelphia, 1990, WB Saunders.

Morris JM, Lucas DB, Bresler B: Role of the trunk in stability of the spine, *J Bone Joint Surg* 43A:327, 1961.

Morrisey RT et al: Measurement of Cobb angle on radiographs of patients who have scoliosis: evaluation of intrinsic error, *J Bone Joint Surg* 72A:320, 1990.

Morse JL et al: Maximal dynamic grip force and wrist torque: the effects of gender, exertion direction, angular velocity, and wrist angle, *Appl Ergon* 37(6):737-742, 2006.

Morton DJ: *Biomechanics of the human foot, American Academy of Orthopaedic Surgeons Instructional Course Lectures,* vol 2, Ann Arbor, Mich, 1944, JW Edwards.

Mosby-Year Book, Inc: *Expert 10-minute physical examination,* St Louis, 1997, Mosby-Year Book.

Moseley HF: *Shoulder lesions,* ed 3, Baltimore, 1969, Williams & Wilkins.

Moseley JB et al: EMG analysis of the scapular muscles during a shoulder rehabilitation program, *Am J Sports Med* 10:128, 1992.

Mosler AB, Blanch PD, Hiskins BC: The effect of manual therapy on hip joint range of motion, pain and eggbeater kick performance in water polo players, *Phys Ther Sport* 7(3):128-136, 2006.

Mountcastle VB: The view from within: pathways to the study of perception, *Johns Hopkins Med J* 136:109, 1975.

Mourad LA: *Orthopedic disorders,* St Louis, 1991, Mosby.

Mower WR et al: Use of plain radiography to screen for cervical spine injuries, *Ann Emerg Med* 38(1):1-7, 2001.

Mubarak SJ et al: The medial tibial stress syndrome: a cause of shin splints, *Am J Sports Med* 10:201, 1992.

Mubarak SJ, Hargens AR: *Compartment syndromes and Volkmann's contracture,* vol 3, Philadelphia, 1981, WB Saunders.

Muirhead-Allwood W, Catterall A: The treatment of Perthes disease, *J Bone Joint Surg* 64B:282, 1982.

Mulford K: Greater trochanteric bursitis, *J Nurse Pract* 3(5):328-332, 2007.

Mullark RE: *The anatomy of varicose veins,* Springfield, Ill, 1965, Charles C Thomas.

Mulleman D et al: Pathophysiology of disk-related sciatica. I. Evidence supporting a chemical component, *Joint Bone Spine* 73(2):151-158, 2006.

Muller W: *The knee: form, function and ligament reconstruction,* New York, 1983, Springer-Verlag.

Mulliken JB: Cutaneous vascular anomalies. In McCarthy JG, editor: *Plastic surgery, vol 5, tumors of the head and neck and skin,* Philadelphia, 1990, WB Saunders.

Munetea T et al: Computerized tomographic analysis of tibial tubercle position in the painful female patellofemoral joint, *Am J Sports Med* 22:67, 1994.

Munuera L, Reinoso F, Martinez-Moreno E: *The innervation of the anterior cruciate ligament and the patellar ligament of the knee, thesis,* Madrid, 1992, Universidad Autonoma.

Murnaghan JP: Frozen shoulder. In Rockwood C, Matsen F, editors: *The shoulder,* Philadelphia, 1990, WB Saunders.

Murphy AJ et al: Reliability of a test of musculotendinous stiffness for the triceps-surae, *Phys Ther Sport* 4(4):175-181, 2003.

Murphy BJ: MR imaging of the elbow, *Radiology* 184:525, 1992.

Murphy DR et al: Interexaminer reliability of the hip extension test for suspected impaired motor control of the lumbar spine, *J Manipulative Physiol Ther* 29(5):374-377, 2006.

Murphy ME: Primary pyogenic infection of sacroiliac joint, *N Y State J Med* 77:1309, 1977.

Murray AW, Robb JE: Pelvic osteotomy for the management of hip displacement in neuromuscular disorders, *Curr Orthop* (in press, corrected proof).

Murray KJ: Hypermobility disorders in children and adolescents, *Best Pract Res Clin Rheumatol* 20(2):329-351, 2006.

Musette P et al: Determinants of severity for superficial cellulitis (erysipelas) of the leg: a retrospective study, *Eur J Intern Med* 15(7):446-450, 2004.

Myerson MS, Quill GE: Late complications of fractures of the calcaneus, *J Bone Joint Surg* 75A:331, 1993.

Myerson MS: Injuries to the forefoot and toes. In Jahss MH, editor: *Disorders of the foot and ankle: medical and surgical management,* vol 2, ed 2, Philadelphia, 1991, WB Saunders.

Myllymaki T et al: Ultrasonography of jumper's knee, *Acta Radiol* 31:47, 1990.

Nabhan A et al: Simple decompression or subcutaneous anterior transposition of the ulnar nerve for cubital tunnel syndrome, *J Hand* 30(5):521-524, 2005.

Nachemson A: The lumbar spine-an orthopaedic challenge, *Spine* 1:59, 1976.

Nachemson AL: Newest knowledge on low back pain, *Clin Orthop* 2279:8, 1992.

Naidu SH, Heppenstall RB: Compartment syndrome of the forearm and hand, *Hand Clin* 10:13, 1994.

Nakagawa H et al: Microendoscopic discectomy (MED) for lumbar disc prolapse, *J Clin Neurosci* 10(2):231-235, 2003.

Nakamura P, Imaeda T, Miura T: Scaphoid malunion, *J Bone Joint Surg* 73B:134, 1991.

Nakamura R et al: Analysis of scaphoid fracture displacement by three dimensional computed tomography, *J Hand Surg* 16A:485, 1991.

Nakamura R et al: Scaphoid non-union with D.I.S.I. deformity, a survey of clinical cases with special reference to ligamentous injury, *J Hand Surg* 16B:156, 1991.

Nakamura SI: Afferent pathways of discogenic low back pain: evaluation of L2 spinal nerve infiltration, *J Bone Joint Surg* 78B:606, 1996.

Nardone DA et al: A model for the diagnostic medical interview: nonverbal, verbal and cognitive assessments, *J Gen Intern Med* 7:437, 1992.

Nash CL, Moe JH: A study of vertebral rotation, *J Bone Joint Surg* 52A:223, 1969.

Nash CL: Scoliosis bracing, *J Bone Joint Surg* 62A:848, 1980.

Neblett R et al: Quantifying lumbar flexion-relaxation phenomenon: theory and clinical applications, *Spine J* 2(5, suppl 1):97, 2002.

Neer CS II: *Shoulder reconstruction,* Philadelphia, 1990, WB Saunders.

Neer CS: Anterior acromioplasty for the chronic impingement syndrome in the shoulder, *J Bone Joint Surg* 54A:41, 1972.

Nelson EC: Using outcome measures to improve care delivered by physicians and hospitals. In Heithoff KA, Lohr KN, editors: *Effectiveness and outcomes in healthcare,* Washington DC, 1990, Institute of Medicine, National Academy Press.

Netter F: *The Ciba collection of medical illustration, vol 8: the musculoskeletal system,* Summitt, NJ, 1990, Ciba Geigy.

Nettina SM: *The Lippincott manual of nursing practice,* ed 6, Philadelphia, 1996, Lippincott.

Neumann DA et al: An electromyographic analysis of hip abductor muscle activity when subjects are carrying loads in one or both hands, *Phys Ther* 72:207, 1992.

Neumann DA, Hase AD: The electromyographic analysis of the hip abductors during load carriage: implications for hip joint protection, *J Orthop Sports Phys Ther* 19:296, 1994.

Neumann G et al: Prevalence of labral tears and cartilage loss in patients with mechanical symptoms of the hip: evaluation using MR arthrography, *Osteoarthr Cartil* (in press, corrected proof).

Neumann RD: Traumatic knee injuries. In Mellion MB, editor: *Sports medicine secrets,* Philadelphia, 1994, Hanley & Belfus.

Neumann WP et al: Trunk posture: reliability, accuracy, and risk estimates for low back pain from a video based assessment method, *Int J Ind Ergon* 28(6):355-365, 2001.

Neuschwander D, Drez D, Finney T: Lateral meniscal variant with absence of the posterior coronary ligament, *J Bone Joint Surg* 74A:1186, 1992.

Neviaser JS: Musculoskeletal disorders of the shoulder region causing cervicobrachial pain: differential diagnosis and treatment, *Surg Clin North Am* 43:1703, 1963.

Newman JS et al: Detection of soft-tissue hyperemia: value of power Doppler sonography, *AJR Am J Roentgenol* 163:385, 1994.

Newman JS et al: Power Doppler sonography of synovitis: assessment of therapeutic response—preliminary observations, *Radiology* 198:582, 1996.

Newton RW: *Color atlas of pediatric neurology,* St Louis, 1995, Mosby-Wolfe.

Ng GYF, Fan ACC: Does elbow position affect strength and reproducibility of power grip measurements? *Physiotherapy* 87(2):68-72, 2001.

Nicholas JA, Hershman EB: *The Lower extremity & spine in sports medicine,* ed 2, St Louis, 1995, Mosby.

Nicholas JA, Hershman EB: *The upper extremity in sports medicine,* ed 2, St Louis, 1995, Mosby.

Nicholas JA: The five-one reconstruction for anteromedial instability of the knee, *J Bone Joint Surg* 55A:899, 1973.

Nielsen KD, Wester JU, Lorensten A: The shoulder impingement syndrome: the results of surgical decompression, *J Shoulder Elbow Surg* 3:12, 1994.

Niere KR, Torney SKSK: Clinicians' perceptions of minor cervical instability, *Man Ther* 9(3):144-150, 2004.

Niitsu M: Moving knee joint: technique for kinematic MR imaging, *Radiology* 174:569, 1990.

Niranjan NS, Price RD, Govilkar P: Fascial feeder and perforator-based V-Y advancement flaps in the reconstruction of lower limb defects, *Br J Plast Surg* 53(8):679-689, 2000.

Nirschi RP: Elbow tendinosis/tennis elbow, *Clin Sports Med* 4:851, 1992.

Nirschi RP: Muscle and tendon trauma. In Morrey BF, editor: *The elbow and its disorders,* Philadelphia, 1993, Saunders.

Nirschi RP: Patterns of failed healing in tendon injury. In Buckwalter J, Leadbetter W, Goodwin P, editors: *Sports induced soft tissue inflammation,* Chicago, 1991, American Academy of Orthopedic Surgeons.

Nishada T et al: H reflex in S-1 radiculopathy: latency versus amplitude controversy revisited, *Muscle Nerve* 19:915, 1996.

Nitta H et al: Study on dermatomes by means of selective lumbar spinal nerve block, *Spine* 18:1782, 1993.

Nobel J, Galasko CSB: *Recent developments in orthopaedic surgery,* Manchester, UK, 1987, Manchester University Press.

Noble HB, Hajek MR, Porter M: Diagnosis and treatment of iliotibial band tightness in runners, *Sports Med* 10:67, 1984.

Nogradi A, Vrbova G: The use of a neurotoxic lectin, volkensin, to induce loss of identified motoneuron pools, *Neuroscience* 50(4):975-986, 1992.

Nolan WV III et al: Results of treatment of severe carpal tunnel syndrome, *J Hand Surg* 17A:1020, 1992.

Noonan KJ et al: Use of the Milwaukee brace for progressive idiopathic scoliosis, *J Bone Joint Surg* 78A;557, 1996.

Nordin M, Anderson GBJ, Pope MH: *Musculoskeletal disorders in the workplace: principles and practice,* St Louis, 1997, Mosby.

Nordin M, Frankel VH: *Basic biomechanics of the musculoskeletal system,* ed 2, Philadelphia, 1989, Lea & Febiger.

Nordt WE, Garretson RB, Plotkin E: The measurement of subacromial contact pressure in patients with impingement syndrome, *Arthroscopy* 15(2):121-125, 1999.

Noriyasu S et al: On the morphology and frequency of Weitbrecht's retinacula in the hip joint, *Okajimas Folia Anat Jpn* 70:87, 1993.

Norman GF: Sacroiliac disease and its relationship to lower abdominal pain, *Am J Surg* 116:54, 1968.

Norris SH, Watt I: The prognosis of neck injuries resulting from rear-end vehicle collisions, *J Bone Joint Surg* 65B:608, 1983.

Norris T: Treatment and physical examination of the shoulder. In Nicholas J, Hershman E, editors: *The upper extremity in sports medicine,* St Louis, 1990, Mosby.

Nourissat G, Kakuda C, Dumontier C: Arthroscopic excision of osteoid osteoma of the elbow, *Arthroscopy* (in press, corrected proof).

Noyes FR et al: Clinical paradoxes of anterior cruciate instability and a new test to detect its instability, *Orthop Trans* 2:36, 1978.

Noyes FR et al: Posterior subluxations of the medial and lateral tibiofemoral compartments: an in vitro ligament sectioning study in cadaveric knees, *Am J Sports Med* 21:407, 1993.

Noyes FR et al: The anterior cruciate ligament-deficient knee with varus alignment, *Am J Sports Med* 20:707, 1992.

Numaguci Y: Osteitis condensans ilii, including its resolution, *Radiology* 98:1, 1971.

Nunn D: The ring uncemented plastic-on-metal total hip replacement, *J Bone Joint Surg* 70B:40, 1988.

Nyland J et al: Wrist circumference is related to patellar tendon thickness in healthy men and women, *Clin Imaging* 30(5):335-338, 2006.

Oaklander AL et al: Evidence of focal small-fiber axonal degeneration in complex regional pain syndrome-I (reflex sympathetic dystrophy), *Pain* 120(3):235-243, 2006.

Ober FB: The role of the iliotibial and fascia lata as a factor in the causation of low-back disabilities and sciatic, *J Bone Joint Surg* 18:105, 1936.

O'Brien SJ, Miller AN, Drakos MC: Arthroscopic subdeltoid approach to the biceps transfer, *Oper Tech Sports Med* 15(1):20-26, 2007.

O'Brien SJ et al: The anatomy and histology of the inferior glenohumeral ligament complex of the shoulder, *Am J Sport Med* 18:449, 1990.

O'Connor CE, Pekow PS, Klingersmith MT: Brachial plexus injury (burners) incidence and risk factors in collegiate football players: a prospective study, *J Athletic Training* 33(suppl):5, 1998.

O'Connor J et al: Geometry of the knee. In Daniel D, editor: *Knee ligaments: structure, function, injury and repair,* New York, 1990, Raven.

O'Connor MI, Carrier BI: Metastatic disease of the spine, *Orthopedics* 15:611, 1992.

O'Donoghue DH: *Treatment of injuries to athletes,* ed 3, Philadelphia, 1976, WB Saunders.

O'Donoghue DH: *Treatment of injuries to athletes,* ed 4, Philadelphia, 1984, WB Saunders.

O'Drsicoll SW, Ball DF, Morrey BF: Posterolateral rotary instability of the elbow, *J Bone Joint Surg* 73A:440, 1991.

O'Drsicoll SW et al: The anatomy of the lateral ulnar collateral ligament, *Clin Anat* 5:296, 1992.

O'Dwyer KJ, Howie CR: Medial epicondylitis of the elbow, *Int Orthop* 19:69, 1995.

Ogilvie-Harris DJ, Basinski A: Arthroscopic synovectomy of the knee for rheumatoid arthritis, *Arthroscopy* 7:91, 1991.

Ogilvie-Harris DJ, Saleh K: Generalized synovial chondromatosis of the knee: a comparison of removal of the loose bodies alone with arthroscopic synovectomy, *Arthroscopy* 10:166, 1994.

Oh VMS: Brain infarction and neck calisthenics, *Lancet* 342:739, 1993.

Oka Y, Umeda K, Ikeda M: Cyst-like lesions of the lunate resembling Kienbock's disease: a case report, *J Hand Surg* 26(1):130-134, 2001.

Olden KW, Drossman DA: Psychologic and psychiatric aspects of gastrointestinal disease, *Med Clin North Am* 84(5):1313-1327, 2000.

Oleson M, Adler D, Goldsmith P: A comparison of forefoot stiffness in running and running shoe bending stiffness, *J Biomech* 38(9):1886-1894, 2005.

Olivieri L et al: Differential diagnosis between osteitis condensans ilii and sacroiliitis, *J Rheumatol* 17:1504, 1990.

Olmarker K, Rydevik B: Pathophysiology of sciatica, *Orthop Clin North Am* 22:223, 1991.

Olson WH et al: *Handbook of symptom-oriented neurology,* ed 2, St Louis, 1994, Mosby.

Olson WH, Brumback RA: *Handbook of symptom-oriented neurology,* Chicago, 1989, Mosby.

Olson WH et al: *Handbook of symptom-oriented neurology,* ed 2, St Louis, 1994, Mosby.

Omer GE Jr et al: The neurovascular cutaneous island pedicles for deficient median nerve sensibility: new technique and results of serial functional tests, *J Bone Joint Surg* 52A:1181, 1970.

Omer GE Jr, Vogel JA: Determination of physiological length of a reconstructed muscle tendon unit through muscle stimulation, *J Bone Joint Surg* 47A:304, 1965.

Omer GE Jr: Evaluation and reconstruction of the forearm and hand after acute traumatic peripheral nerve injuries, *J Bone Joint Surg* 50A:1454, 1968.

Omer GE Jr: Sensation and sensibility in the upper extremity, *Clin Orthop* 104:30, 1974.

Omer GE, Spinner M: *Management of peripheral nerve problems,* Philadelphia, 1981, WB Saunders.

Orava S et al: Diagnosis and treatment of stress fractures located at the mid-tibial shaft in athletes, *Int J Sports Med* 12:419, 1991.

O'Reilly MAR, Massouh H: Pictorial review: the sonographic diagnosis of pathology in the Achilles tendon, *Clin Radiol* 48:202, 1993.

O'Riain S: New and simple test of nerve function in hand, *BMJ* 3(5881):615-616, 1973.

O'Riain S: Shrivel test: a new and simple test of nerve function in the hand, *BMJ* 3:615, 1973.

Osborne G: Compression neuritis of the ulnar nerve at the elbow, *Hand Clin* 2:10, 1970.

Osterweis M, Kleinman A, Mechanic D: *Pain and disability: clinical, behavioral and public policy perspectives, report of the Institute of Medicine Committee on Pain, Disability and Chronic Illness Behavior,* Washington, DC, 1987, National Academy Press.

O'Sullivan M et al: Iliopsoas tendonitis: a complication after total hip arthroplasty, *J Arthroplasty* 22(2):166-170, 2007.

O'Sullivan PB et al: The relationship between posture and back muscle endurance in industrial workers with flexion-related low back pain, *Man Ther* 11(4):264-271, 2006.

Otcenasek M et al: New approach to the urogynecological ultrasound examination, *Eur J Obstet Gynecol Reprod Biol* 103(1):72-74, 2002.

Owen R, Goodfellow J, Bullough P, editors: *Scientific foundations of orthopaedics and traumatology,* London, 1980, Heinemann.

O'Young B, Young MA, Stiens SA: *PM&R secrets,* Philadelphia, 1997, Hanley & Belfus.

Ozel SK, Kazez A: Horner syndrome due to first rib fracture after major thoracic trauma, *J Pediatr Surg* 40(10):e17-e19, 2005.

Padley S et al: Assessment of a single spine radiograph in low back pain, *Br J Radiol* 63:535, 1990.

Pagana KD, Pagana TJ: *Mosby's manual of diagnostic and laboratory tests,* St Louis, 1998, Mosby.

Pagnanelli DM, Barrer SJ: Bilateral carpal tunnel release at one operation: report of 228 patients, *Neurosurgery* 31:1030, 1992.

Pagnani M, Cooper D, Warren R: Extrusion of the medial meniscus: case report, *Arthroscopy* 7:297, 1991.

Pagnani MJ, Galinat BJ, Warren RF: Glenohumeral instability. In Nicholas JA, Hershman EB, editors: *The upper extremity in sports medicine,* St Louis, 1990, Mosby.

Pahle JA, Raunio P: The influence of wrist position on finger deviation in the rheumatoid hand: a clinical and radiological study, *J Bone Joint Surg* 51B:664, 1969.

Paley D, Hall H: Intra-articular fractures of the calcaneus, *J Bone Joint Surg* 75A: 342, 1993.

Palmer AK, Glisson RR, Werner FW: Ulnar variance determination, *J Hand Surg* 7:376, 1982.

Palmer AK, Livensohn EM, Kuzma GR: Arthrography of the wrist, *J Hand Surg* 8:15, 1983.

Palmer AK: Fractures of the distal radius. In Green DP, editor: *Operative hand surgery,* ed 2, New York, 1993, Churchill Livingstone.

Palmer DH et al: Endoscopic carpal tunnel release, *Arthroscopy* 9:498, 1993.

Palmgren PJ et al: Improvement after chiropractic care in cervicocephalic kinesthetic sensibility and subjective pain intensity in patients with nontraumatic chronic neck pain, *J Manipulative Physiol Ther* 29(2):100-106, 2006.

Palumbo RC et al: Ligamentous injuries to the knee: a retrospective analysis, *Orthop Trans* 16:321, 1992.

Panjabi MM et al: Thoracolumbar burst fracture: a biomechanical investigation of its multidirectional flexibility, *Spine* 19:578, 1994.

Panjabi MM, White AA: *Clinical biomechanics of the spine,* ed 2, Philadelphia, 1990, JB Lippincott.

Panjabi MM: The stabilizing system of the spine, part II, neutral zone and instability hypothesis, *J Spinal Disord* 5:390, 1992.

Panzer DM, Gatterman MI: Sacroiliac subluxation syndrome. In Gatterman MI, editor: *Foundations of chiropractic: subluxation,* St Louis, 1995, Mosby.

Paoloni JA, Appleyard RC, Murrell GAC: The Orthopaedic Research Institute-Tennis Elbow Testing System: a modified chair pick-up test—interrater and intrarater reliability testing and validity for monitoring lateral epicondylosis, *J Shoulder Elbow Surg* 13(1):72-77, 2004.

Pap G et al: Evaluation of wrist and hand handicap and postoperative outcome in rheumatoid arthritis, *Hand Clinics* 19(3):471-481, 2003.

Papacharalampous X et al: The effect of contrast media on the synovial membrane, *Eur J Radiol* 55(3):426-430, 2005.

Papaioannu T, Stokes I, Kenwright J: Scoliosis associated with limb length inequality, *J Bone Joint Surg* 64A:59, 1982.

Papakonstantinou DK et al: Unilateral pulmonary edema due to lung re-expansion following pleurocentesis for spontaneous pneumothorax. The role of non-invasive continuous positive airway pressure ventilation, *Int J Cardiol* 114(3):398-400, 2007.

Pardiwala DN, Nagda TV: Arthroscopic chondral cyst excision in a stiff Perthes' hip, *Arthroscopy* (in press, corrected proof).

Parker JC, Wright GE: The implications of depression for pain and disability in rheumatoid arthritis, *Arthritis Care Res* 8:279, 1995.

Parker MJ, Pryor GA: *Hip fracture management,* Boston, 1993, Blackwell.

Parkes JC: Overuse injuries of the elbow. In Nicholas JA, Hershman EB, editors: *The upper extremity in sports medicine,* St Louis, 1990, Mosby.

Parmar HV, Triffitt PD, Gregg PJ: Intra-articular fractures of the calcaneum treated operatively or conservatively, *J Bone Joint Surg* 75B: 932, 1993.

Parsons TA: The snapping scapula and subscapular exostosis, *J Bone Joint Surg* 55B:345, 1963.

Partheni M et al: Radiculopathy after lumbar discectomy due to intraspinal retained Surgicel: clinical and magnetic resonance imaging evaluation, *Spine J* 6(4):455-458, 2006.

Pascual E, Jovani V: Synovial fluid analysis, *Best Pract Res Clin Rheumatol* 19(3): 371-386, 2005.

Paterson D, Salvage JP: The nuclide bone scan in the diagnosis of Perthes disease, *Clin Orthop* 209:23, 1986.

Patin JR, Hamot HB, Singer JM: Replicated evidence on the construct validity of the SCAG (Sandoz Clinical Assessment-Geriatric) scale, *Prog Neuropsychopharmacol Biol Psychiatry* 8(2):293-306, 1984.

Patten J: *Neurological differential diagnosis,* ed 2, London, 1996, Springer.

Patterson RJ, Bickel WH, Dahlin DC: Idiopathic avascular necrosis of the head of the femur: a study of fifty-two cases, *J Bone Joint Surg* 42A:267, 1964.

Patton K: *Student survival guide for anatomy and physiology,* St Louis, 1999, Mosby.

Payne EE et al: The cervical spine, *Brain* 80:571, 1957.

Peace KAL, Lee JC, Healy J: Imaging the infrapatellar tendon in the elite athlete, *Clin Radiol* 61(7):570-578, 2006.

Peat G et al: How reliable is structured clinical history-taking older adults with knee problems? Inter- and intraobserver variability of the KNE-SCI, *J Clin Epidemiol* 56(11):1030-1037, 2003.

Pecina MM, Krmpotic-Nemanic J, Markiewitz AD: *Tunnel syndromes,* Boca Raton, Fla, 1991, CRC Press.

Pedowitz RA et al: Modified criteria for the objective diagnosis of chronic compartment syndrome of the leg, *Am J Sports Med* 18:35, 1990.

Pegoli L et al: The ishiguro extension block technique for the treatment of mallet finger fracture: indications and clinical results, *J Hand Surg* 28(1):15-17, 2003.

Pereira CE et al: Meta-analysis of femoropopliteal bypass grafts for lower extremity arterial insufficiency, *J Vasc Surg* 44(3):510, 2006.

Perhala RS et al: Local infectious complications following large joint replacement in rheumatoid arthritis patients treated with methotrexate versus those not treated with methotrexate, *Arthritis Rheum* 34:146, 1991.

Perkin, GD: *Mosby's color atlas and text of neurology,* London, 1998, Mosby-Wolfe.

Perleik PC, Guilford WB: Magnetic resonance imaging to assess vascularity of scaphoid nonunions, *J Hand Surg* 16A:479, 1991.

Perrone C et al: Pyogenic and tuberculous spondylodiscitis (vertebral osteomyelitis) in 80 adult patients, *Clin Infect Dis* 19:746, 1994.

Persselin JE: Diagnosis of rheumatoid arthritis, medial and laboratory aspects, *Clin Orthop* 265:73, 1991.

Peterfy CG et al: MR imaging of the arthritic knee: improved discrimination of cartilage, synovium and effusion with pulsed saturation transfer and fat-suppressed T1-weighted sequences, *Radiology* 191:413, 1994.

Peterfy CG, Genant HK: Emerging applications of magnetic resonance imaging for evaluating the articular cartilage, *Radiol Clin North Am* 34:195, 1996.

Peters JW, Trevino SG, Renstrom PA: Chronic lateral ankle instability, *Foot Ankle* 12:182, 1991.

Peterson AR et al: Variations in dorsomedial hand innervation, electrodiagnostic implications, *Arch Neurol* 49:870, 1992.

Peterson CK et al: Prevalence of hyperplastic articular pillars in the cervical spine and relationship with cervical lordosis, *J Manipulative Physiol Ther* 22(6):390-394, 1999.

Petrek JA, Heelan MC: Incidence of breast carcinoma-related lymphedema, *Cancer* 83(12 suppl II):2776-81, 1998.

Pfeiffer WH, Cracchiolo A: Clinical results after tarsal tunnel decompression, *J Bone Joint Surg* 76A:1222, 1994.

Pfeiffer WH, Gross JL, Seeger LL: Osteochondritis dissecans of the patella, *Clin Orthop* 271:207, 1991.

Phalen GS: The carpal-tunnel syndrome: seventeen years' experience in diagnosis and treatment of six hundred fifty-four hands, *J Bone Joint Surg* 48A:211, 1966.

Pheasant S: *Ergonomics, work and health,* Gaithersburg, Md, 1991, Aspen.

Philippon MJ, Schenker ML: Arthroscopy for the treatment of femoroacetabular impingement in the athlete, *Clin Sports Med* 25(2):299-308, 2006.

Phillips LH, Parks TS: Electrophysiologic mapping of the segmental anatomy of the muscles of the lower extremity, *Muscle Nerve* 14:1213, 1991.

Pilling LF, Brannick TL, Swenson WM: Psychological characteristics of patients having pain as a presenting symptom, *Can Med Assoc J* 97:287, 1967.

Pincus T et al: Persistent back pain—why do physical therapy clinicians continue treatment? A mixed methods study of chiropractors, osteopaths and physiotherapists, *Eur J Pain* 10(1):67-76, 2006.

Pitner MA: Pathophysiology of overuse injuries in the hand and wrist, *Hand Clin* 6:355, 1990.

Planner AC, Donaghy M, Moore NR: Causes of lumbosacral plexopathy, *Clin Radiol* 61(12):987-995, 2006.

Polley HF, Hunder GG: *Rheumatologic interviewing and physical examination of the joints,* ed 2, Philadelphia, 1978, WB Saunders.

Pollock RG et al: The use of arthroscopy in the treatment of resistant frozen shoulder, *Clin Orthop* 304:30, 1994.

Pomeranz SJ, Pretorius HT, Ramsingh PS: Bone scintigraphy and multimodality imaging in bone neoplasia: strategies for imaging in the new health care climate, *Semin Nucl Med* 24:188, 1994.

Pomianowski S et al: The effect of forearm rotation on laxity and stability of the elbow, *Clin Biomech* 16(5):401-407, 2001.

Poole G, Ward E: Causes of mortality in patients with pelvic fractures, *Orthopedics* 17:691, 1994.

Pool-Goudzwaard AL et al: Insufficient lumbopelvic stability: a clinical, anatomical and biomechanical approach to 'a-specific' low back pain, *Man Ther* 3(1):12-20, 1998.

Pope AM, Tarlov AR: *Disability in America: toward a national agenda for prevention,* Washington, DC, 1991, National Academy Press.

Pope CF: Radiologic evaluation of tendon injuries, *Clin Sports Med* 11:579, 1992.

Pope MH et al: *Occupational low back pain assessment, treatment and prevention,* St Louis, 1991, Mosby.

Pope MH, Frymoyer JW, Krag MH: Diagnosing instability, *Clin Orthop* 279:60, 1992.

Porta M: A comparative trial of botulinum toxin type A and methylprednisolone for the treatment of myofascial pain syndrome and pain from chronic muscle spasm, *Pain* 85(1-2):101-105, 2000.

Porter JN: Raynaud's syndrome. In Sabiston DC Jr, editor: *Davis Christopher textbook of surgery,* Philadelphia, 1977, WB Saunders.

Porterfield JA, DeRosa C: *Mechanical low back pain: perspectives in functional anatomy,* Philadelphia, 1991, WB Saunders.

Post M: *Physical examination of the musculoskeletal system,* Chicago, 1987, Mosby.

Postacchini F, Cinotti G: Bone regrowth after surgical decompression for lumbar spinal stenosis, *J Bone Joint Surg* 74B:862, 1992.

Potter HG et al: Lateral epicondylitis: correlation of MR imaging, surgical, and histophysiologic findings, *Radiology* 196:43, 1995.

Poul J et al: Early diagnosis of congenital dislocation of the hip, *J Bone Joint Surg* 53B:56, 1971.

Powell MR et al: Detecting symptom- and test-coached simulators with the test of memory malingering, *Arch Clin Neuropsychol* 19(5):693-702, 2004.

Pradhan S: Shank sign in myotonic dystrophy type-1 (DM-1), *J Clin Neurosci* 14(1):27-32, 2007.

Pratt NE: *Clinical musculoskeletal anatomy,* Philadelphia, 1991, JB Lippincott.

Prescott E et al: Fibromyalgia in the adult Danish population: I. A prevalence study, *Scand J Rheumatol* 22:233, 1993.

Preston DC et al: The median-ulnar latency difference studies are comparable in mild carpal tunnel syndrome, *Muscle Nerve* 17:1469, 1994.

Prichasuk S, Subhadrabandhu T: The relationship of pes planus and calcaneal spur to plantar heel pain, *Clin Orthop* 306:192, 1994.

Prichasuk S: The heel pad in plantar heel pain, *J Bone Joint Surg* 76B:140, 1994.

Prineas J: Polyneuropathies of undetermined cause, *Acta Neurol Scand* 46(suppl 44):1, 1970.

Pronsati MP: Treatment of thoracic outlet syndrome comes under scrutiny, *Adv Physical Therapists* Sept:14, 1991.

Protas JM, Jackson WT: Evaluating carpal instabilities with fluoroscopy, *AJR Am J Roentgenol* 135:137, 1980.

Prystowsky JB et al: Prospective analysis of the incidence of deep venous thrombosis in bariatric surgery patients, *Surgery* 138(4):759-765, 2005.

Przybyla A et al: Outer annulus tears have less effect than endplate fracture on stress distributions inside intervertebral discs: relevance to disc degeneration, *Clin Biomech* 21(10):1013-1019, 2006.

Przybylski G, Marion DW: Injury to the vertebrae and spinal cord. In Moore EE, Mattox KL, Feliziano DV, editors: *Trauma,* ed 3, Stanford, Conn, 1996, Appleton & Lange.

Puno R et al: Treatment recommendations for idiopathic scoliosis: an assessment of the Lenke classification, *Spine J* 2(5, suppl 1):61, 2002.

Puno R et al: A comparison of the King and the Lenke classification systems of adolescent idiopathic scoliosis, *Spine J* 2(5, suppl 1):60-61, 2002.

Puranen J: The medial tibial syndrome, *Ann Chir Gynecol* 80:215, 1991.

Qin C, Farber JP, Foreman RD: Gastrocardiac afferent convergence in upper thoracic spinal neurons: a central mechanism of postprandial angina pectoris, *J Pain* (in press, corrected proof).

Quigley TB: The nonoperative treatment of symptomatic calcareous deposits in the shoulder, *Surg Clin North Am* 43:1495, 1963.

Quirk R: Common foot and ankle injuries in dance, *Orthop Clin North Am* 25:123, 1994.

Qureshi F, Stanley D: The painful elbow, *Surgery (Oxford)* 24(11):368-372, 2006.

Raatikainen T, Mikko P, Puranen J: Arthrography, clinical examination, and stress radiograph in the diagnosis of acute injury to the lateral ligaments of the ankle, *Am J Sports Med* 20:2, 1992.

Rachlin ES: *Myofascial pain and fibromyalgia trigger point management,* St Louis, 1994, Mosby.

Radin EL: The physiology and degeneration of joints, *Arthritis Rheum* 2:245, 1972.

Radnovc BP, Sturzenegger M, Stefano GD: Long-term outcome after whiplash injury: a two-year follow-up considering features of injury mechanism and somatic, radiologic, and psychosocial factors, *Medicine* 74:281, 1995.

Raffetto JD et al: Differences in risk factors for lower extremity arterial occlusive disease, *J Am Coll Surg* 201(6):918-924, 2005.

Raja SN: Workshop Summary: CRPS—a disease with many faces, *Eur J Pain* 11(1, suppl 1):30-31, 2007.

Rajadhyaksha AD, Mont MA, Becker L: An unusual cause of knee pain 10 years after arthroscopy, *Arthroscopy* 22(11):1253.e1-1253.e3, 2006.

Ramsey M: Results From grade II, III, and IV spondylolisthesis with open reduction and posterior lumbar interbody fusion, *Spine J* 6(5, suppl 1):140S, 2006.

Ramsey RG: *Neuroradiology,* Philadelphia, 1987, WB Saunders.

Rana NA et al: Upward translocation of the dens in rheumatoid arthritis, *J Bone Joint Surg* 55B:471, 1973.

Ranawat CS et al: Cervical spine fusion in rheumatoid arthritis, *J Bone Joint Surg* 61A:1003, 1979.

Ranawat CS, Figgie MP: Early complications of total hip replacement. In Steinberg ME, editor: *The hip and its disorders,* Philadelphia, 1991, WB Saunders.

Ranawat CS: Surgery for rheumatoid arthritis: the hip, *Curr Orthop* 3:146, 1989.

Ranawat VS, Dowell JK, Heywood-Waddington MB: Stress fractures of the lumbar pars interarticularis in athletes: a review based on long-term results of 18 professional cricketers, *Injury* 34(12):915-919, 2003.

Rang M, editor: *The growth plate and its disorders,* Edinburgh, 1969, Livingstone.

Rantanen J, Hurme M, Falck B: The lumbar multifidus muscle five years after surgery for a lumbar intervertebral disc herniation, *Spine* 18:568, 1993.

Rao JP, Bronstein R: Dislocation following arthroplasties of the hip: incidence, prevention and treatment, *Orthop Rev* 20:261, 1991.

Rao UB, Joseph B: The influence of footwear on the prevalence of flatfoot, *J Bone Joint Surg* 74B:525, 1992.

Raphael BA et al: Validation and test characteristics of a 10-item neuro-ophthalmic supplement to the NEI-VFQ-25, *Am J Ophthalmol* 142(6):1026.e2-1035.e2, 2006.

Rasmussen O, Tovberg-Jansen I: Anterolateral rotational instability in the ankle joint, *Acta Orthop Scand* 52:99, 1981.

Raspe HH: Back pain. In Silman AJ, Hochberg M, editors: *Epidemiology of the rheumatic diseases,* Oxford, UK, 1993, Oxford University Press.

Rat A-C et al: Development and testing of a specific quality-of-life questionnaire for knee and hip osteoarthritis: OAKHQOL (osteoarthritis of knee hip quality of life), *Joint Bone Spine* 73(6):697-704, 2006.

Ratliff AHC: Perthes disease: a study of thirty-four hips observed for thirty years, *J Bone Joint Surg* 49B:102, 1967.

Ravaud P et al: Assessing smallest detectable change over time in continuous structural outcome measures: application to radiological change in knee osteoarthritis, *J Clin Epidemiol* 52(12):1225-1230, 1999.

Ravel R: *Clinical laboratory medicine clinical application of laboratory data,* ed 6, St Louis, 1995, Mosby.

Rayan G, Jensen C: Thoracic outlet syndrome: provocative examination maneuvers in a typical population, *J Shoulder Elbow Surg* 4(2):113-117, 1995.

Reed R: *Malingering, symposium papers,* Los Angeles, 1986, American College of Chiropractic Orthopedists.

Regan W, Korinek S, Morrey B, An K-N: biomechanical study of ligaments around the elbow joint, *Clin Orthop* 271:170, 1991.

Regan W, Lapner PC: Prospective evaluation of two diagnostic apprehension signs for posterolateral instability of the elbow, *J Shoulder Elbow Surg* 15(3):344-346, 2006.

Regan W et al: Microscopic histopathology of chronic refractory lateral epicondylitis, *Am J Sports Med* 20:746, 1992.

Regan WD, Morrey BF: Physical examination of the elbow. In Morrey BF, editor: *The elbow and its disorders,* Philadelphia, 1993, WB Saunders.

Reginster J-Y: Managing the osteoporotic patient today, *Bone* 40(5, suppl 1):S12-S18, 2007.

Reid DC: *Problems of the hip, pelvis, and sacroiliac joint, sports injury assessment and rehabilitation,* New York, 1992, Churchill Livingstone.

Reid DC: *Sports injury assessment and rehabilitation,* New York, 1992, Churchill Livingstone.

Reikeras O: Is there a relationship between femoral anteversion and leg torsion? *Skeletal Radiol* 10:409, 1991.

Reilly PJ, Torg JS: Athletic injury to the cervical nerve roots and brachial plexus, *Op Tech Sports Med* 1:231, 1993.

Relwani JG et al: Luxatio erecta in an adolescent with axillary artery and brachial plexus injury, *Injury Extra* (in press, corrected proof).

Renne JW: The iliotibial band friction syndrome, *J Bone Joint Surg* 57A:1110, 1975.

Renshaw TS: *Pediatric orthopaedics,* Philadelphia, 1987, Saunders.

Renstrom AFH, Kannus P: Injuries of the foot and ankle. In DeLee JD, Drez D, editors: *Orthopaedic sports medicine, principles and practice,* vol 2, Philadelphia, 1994, WB Saunders.

Renstrom AFH: Persistently painful sprained ankle, *J Am Acad Orthop Surg* 2:270, 1994.

Resnick D, Niwayama G: *Diagnosis of bone and joint disorders,* Philadelphia, ed 3, 1995, WB Saunders.

Resnick D, Niwayama G: *Diagnosis of bone and joint disorders,* Philadelphia, 1981, WB Saunders.

Resnick NW, Greenspan SL: Senile osteoporosis reconsidered, *JAMA* 261:1025, 1989.

Rethnam U, Sinha A: Instability of the proximal tibiofibular joint, an unusual cause for knee pain, *Injury Extra* 37(5):190-192, 2006.

Rhodes I, Matzinger F, Matzinger MA: Transient osteoporosis of the hip, *Can Assoc Radiol J* 44:399, 1993.

Rich K: Effects of leg and body position on transcutaneous oxygen measurements in healthy subjects and subjects with peripheral artery disease after lower-extremity arterial revascularization: a pilot study, *J Vasc Nurs* 20(4):125-135, 2002.

Ricklin P, Ruttiman A, Del Buono MA: *Meniscus lesions: practical problems of clinical diagnosis, arthrography and therapy,* New York, 1971, Grune & Stratton.

Riddle DL: Foot and ankle. In Richardson JK, Iglarsh ZA, editors: *Clinical orthopaedic physical therapy,* Philadelphia, 1994, WB Saunders.

Ridehalgh C, Greening J, Petty NJ: Effect of straight leg raise examination and treatment on vibration thresholds in the lower limb: a pilot study in asymptomatic subjects, *Man Ther* 10(2):136-143, 2005.

Riehl R: Rehabilitation of lower leg injuries. In Prentice WE, editor: *Rehabilitation techniques in sports medicine,* ed 2, St Louis, 1994, Mosby.

Riggs BL, Melton LJ III: *Osteoporosis: etiology, diagnosis and management,* New York, 1988, Raven.

Riley GP et al: Glycosaminoglycans of human rotator cuff tendons: changes with age and in chronic rotator cuff tendinitis, *Ann Rheum Dis* 53:367, 1994.

Riley GP et al: Tendon degeneration and chronic shoulder pain; changes in the collagen composition of the human rotator cuff tendons in rotator cuff tendinitis, *Ann Rheum Dis* 53:359, 1994.

Ring PA: Complete replacement arthroplasty of the hip by the ring prosthesis, *J Bone Joint Surg* 50B:720, 1968.

Rizk TE, Pinals RS, Talaiver AS: Corticosteroid injections in adhesive capsulitis; investigation of their value and site, *Arch Phys Med Rehabil* 72:20, 1991.

Rizzello G et al: Para-articular osteochondroma of the knee, *Arthroscopy* (in press, corrected proof).

Rizzo PF et al: Diagnosis of occult fractures about the hip, magnetic resonance imaging compared with bone scanning, *J Bone Joint Surg* 75A:395, 1993.

Ro CS: Sacroiliac joint. In Cox JM, editor: *Low back pain: mechanism, diagnosis and treatment,* ed 5, Baltimore, 1990, Williams & Wilkins.

Roach HI, Shearer JR, Archer C: The choice of an experimental model: a guide for research workers, *J Bone Joint Surg* 71B:549, 1989.

Roach KE, Miles T: Normal hip and knee active range of motion: the relationship to age, *Phys Ther* 71:656, 1991.

Robb CA et al: Comparison of non-operative and surgical treatment of displaced calcaneal fractures, *Foot* (in press, corrected proof).

Robbins SL: Blood vessels. In Robbins SL, editor: *Pathologic basis of disease,* Philadelphia, 1974, WB Saunders.

Roberts DK, Pomeranz SJ: Current status of magnetic resonance in radiologic diagnosis of foot and ankle injuries, *Orthop Clin North Am* 25:61, 1994.

Roberts JM et al: Comparison of unrepaired, primarily repaired, and polygalactin mesh-reinforced Achilles tendon lacerations in rabbits, *Clin Orthop* 181:244, 1993.

Robertson A et al: The fabella: a forgotten source of knee pain? *Knee* 11(3):243-245, 2004.

Robertson CM, Coopersmith CM: The systemic inflammatory response syndrome, *Microbes Infect* 8(5):1382-1389, 2006.

Robinson D, On E, Halperin N: Anterior compartment syndrome of the thigh in athletes: indications for conservative treatment, *J Trauma* 32:183, 1992.

Rockwood CA Jr, Eilbert RE: Camptocormia, *J Bone Joint Surg* 51A:533, 1969.

Rockwood CA, Green DP, Bucholz RW, editors: *Rockwood and Green's fractures in adults,* vol II, ed 3, Philadelphia, 1991, JB Lippincott.

Rockwood CA, Young DC: Disorders of the acromioclavicular joint. In Rockwood CA, Matsen FA, editors: *The shoulder,* vol 2, Philadelphia, 1990, WB Saunders.

Rode S et al: Health anxiety levels in chronic pain clinic attenders, *J Psychosom Res* 60(2):155-161, 2006.

Rodnitzky RL: *Van Allen's pictorial manual of neurologic tests,* St Louis, 1988, Mosby.

Rodnitzky RL: *Van Allen's pictorial manual of neurologic tests: a guide to the performance and interpretation of the neurologic examination,* ed 3, Chicago, 1969, Mosby.

Rodosky MW, Harner CD, Fu FH: The role of the long head of the biceps muscle and superior glenoid labrum in anterior stability of the shoulder, *Am J Sport Med* 22:121, 1994.

Roetert EP et al: The biomechanics of tennis elbow, an integrated approach, *Clin Sports Med* 14:47, 1995.

Rogers AW: *Textbook of anatomy,* New York, 1992, Churchill-Livingstone.

Rogers LF, Hendrix RW: Evaluating the multiple injured patients radiographically, *Orthop Clin North Am* 21:437, 1990.

Rogers LR: *Radiology of skeletal trauma,* ed 2, London, 1992, Churchill Livingstone.

Rolak LA: *Neurology secrets,* ed 2, Philadelphia, 1998, Hanley & Belfus.

Rompe JD et al: Chronic lateral epicondylitis of the elbow: a prospective study of low-energy shockwave therapy and low-energy shockwave therapy plus manual therapy of the cervical spine, *Arch Phys Med Rehabil* 82(5):578-582, 2001.

Roos DB et al: Thoracic outlet syndrome, *Arch Surg* 93:71, 1966.

Rooser B, Bengtson S, Hagglund G: Acute compartment syndrome from anterior thigh muscle contusion: a report of eight cases, *J Orthop Trauma* 5:57, 1991.

Rose KA, Kim WS: The effect of chiropractic care for a 30-year-old male with advanced ankylosing spondylitis: a time series case report, *J Manipulative Physiol Ther* 26(8):524-532, 2003.

Rosenbaum RB, Ochoa JL: *Carpal tunnel syndrome and other disorders of the median nerve,* Boston, 1993, Butterworth-Heinemann.

Rosenberg ZS et al: The elbow: MR features of nerve disorders, *Radiology* 188:235, 1993.

Ross JS: Diagnostic imaging. In *Spine,* Salt Lake City, 2004, Amirsys.

Rossi P et al: Magnetic resonance imaging findings in piriformis syndrome: a case report, *Arch Phys Med Rehabil* 82(4):519-521, 2001.

Rossignol M, Suissa S, Abenhaim L: The evolution of compensated occupational spinal injuries: a three-year follow-up study, *Spine* 17:1043, 1992.

Rotes-Querol J: The syndrome of psychogenic rheumatism, *Clin Rheum Dis* 5:797, 1979.

Rothman RH, Simeone FA, editors: *The spine,* vol 1-2, Philadelphia, 1975, WB Saunders.

Rothman RH, Simeone FA: *The spine,* Philadelphia, 1982, WB Saunders.

Rowell RM, Stites J, Stone-Hall K: A case report of an unstable cervical spine fracture: parallels to the thoracolumbar chance fracture, *J Manipulative Physiol Ther* 29(7):586-589, 2006.

Rowland LP: *Merritt's textbook of neurology,* ed 7, Philadelphia, 1984, Lea & Febiger.

Royle SC et al: The significance of chondromalacic changes on the patella, *Arthroscopy* 7:158, 1991.

Royle SG: Compartment syndrome following forearm fracture in children, *Injury* 21:73, 1990.

Rubens DJ et al: Rheumatoid arthritis: evaluation of wrist extensor tendons with clinical examination versus MR imaging—a preliminary report, *Radiology* 187:831, 1993.

Ruch DS, Papadonikolakis A, Campolattaro RM: The posterolateral plica: a cause of refractory lateral elbow pain, *J Shoulder Elbow Surg* 15(3):367-370, 2006.

Ruge D, Wiltse LL: *Spinal disorders: diagnosis and treatment,* Philadelphia, 1977, Lea & Febiger.

Rumack CM, Wilson SR, Charboneau JW: *Diagnostic ultrasound,* vol 1-2, ed 2, St Louis, 1998, Mosby.

Rumball K, Jarvis J: Seat-belt injuries of the spine in young children, *J Bone Joint Surg* 74B:572, 1992.

Russotti GM, Conventry MB, Stauffer RN: Cemented total hip arthroplasty with contemporary techniques, *Clin Orthop* 235:141, 1988.

Rust M: Achilles tendon injuries in athletes, *Ann Chir Gynaecol* 80:188, 1991.

Ruwe PA et al: Can MR imaging effectively replace diagnostic arthroscopy? *Radiology* 183:335, 1992.

Saal JA, Dillingham MF: Nonoperative treatment and rehabilitation of disc, facet, and soft tissue injuries. In Nicholas JA, Hershman EB, editors: *The lower extremity and spine in sports medicine,* vol 2, St Louis, 1995, Mosby.

Saal JA, Saal JS, Herzog RJ: The natural history of lumbar intervertebral disc extrusions treated nonoperatively, *Spine* 15:683, 1990.

Sacsh BL et al: Primary osseous neoplasms of the thoracic and lumbar spine, *Orthop Trans* 8:422, 1984.

Safran M, Ahmad CS, Elattrache NS: Ulnar collateral ligament of the elbow, *Arthroscopy* 21(11):1381-1395, 2005.

Sahin G, Demirtas M: An overview of MR arthrography with emphasis on the current technique and applicational hints and tips, *Eur J Radiol* 58(3):416-430, 2006.

Saidoff DC, McDonough AL: Critical pathways in therapeutic intervention: lower extremity, St Louis, 1997, Mosby.

Saidoff DC, McDonough AL: *Critical pathways in therapeutic intervention,* St Louis, 1997, Mosby.

Saito Y et al: Facioscapulohumeral muscular dystrophy with severe mental retardation and epilepsy, *Brain Dev* 29(4):231-233, 2007.

Saji MJ, Upakhyay SS, Leong JCY: Increased femoral neck-shaft angles in adolescent idiopathic scoliosis, *Spine* 20:303, 1995.

Salovey P et al: Reporting chronic pain episodes on health surveys. In *Vital health statistics,* vol 6, Hyattsville, Md, 1992, National Center for Health Statistics.

Salter RB, Harris WR: Injuries involving the epiphyseal plate, *J Bone Joint Surg* 45A:587, 1963.

Salter RB: *Textbook of disorders and injuries of the musculoskeletal system,* Baltimore, 1970, Williams & Wilkins.

Sammarco GJ, Stephens MM: Neuropraxia of the femoral nerve in a modern dancer, *Am J Sports Med* 19:413, 1991.

Sampson SP, Wisch D, Badalamente MA: Complications of conservative and surgical treatment of de Quervain's disease and trigger fingers, *Hand Clin* 10:73, 1994.

Sanada H et al: Vascular function in patients with lower extremity peripheral arterial disease: a comparison of functions in upper and lower extremities, *Atherosclerosis* 178(1):179-185, 2005.

Sandifer PH: *Neurology in orthopaedics,* London, 1967, Butterworths.

Sano H, Wakabayashi I, Itoi E: Stress distribution in the supraspinatus tendon with partial-thickness tears: an analysis using two-dimensional finite element model, *J Shoulder Elbow Surg* 15(1):100-105, 2006.

Saro C et al: Plantar pressure distribution and pain after distal osteotomy for hallux valgus: a prospective study of 22 patients with 12-month follow-up: *Foot* 17(2):84-93, 2007.

Sarris I, Sotereanos DG: Distal biceps tendon ruptures, *J Am Soc Surg Hand* 2(3):121-128, 2002.

Sasai K et al: Two-level disc herniation in the cervical and thoracic spine presenting with spastic paresis in the lower extremities without clinical symptoms or signs in the upper extremities, *Spine J* 6(4):464-467, 2006.

Sasaki H et al: Grip strength predicts cause-specific mortality in middle-aged and elderly persons, *Am J Med* 120(4):337-342, 2007.

Satterfield WH, Johnson DL: Arthroscopic patellar "Bankart" repair after acute dislocation, *Arthroscopy* 21(5):627.e1-627.e5, 2005.

Saudek CE: The hip. In Gould JA, editor: *Orthopaedic and sports physical therapy,* ed 2, St Louis, 1990, Mosby.

Sauser DD, Thodorson SH, Fahr LM: Imaging of the elbow, *Radiol Clin North Am* 28:923, 1990.

Savoie Iii FH, Field LD, Ramsey JR: Posterolateral rotatory instability of the elbow: diagnosis and management, *Oper Tech Sports Med* 14(2):81-85, 2006.

Saxena K, Stavas J: Inferior glenohumeral dislocation, *Ann Emerg Med* 12(11):718-720, 1983.

Schadt DC et al: Chronic atherosclerotic occlusion of the femoral artery, *JAMA* 175:937, 1961.

Schafer RC: *Clinical biomechanics,* ed 2, Baltimore, 1987, Williams & Wilkins.

Scham SM, Taylor TKF: Tension signs in lumbar disc prolapse, *Clin Orthop* 75:195, 1971.

Schamblin ML, Safran MR: Injury of the distal biceps at the musculotendinous junction, *J Shoulder Elbow Surg* 16(2):208-212, 2007.

Schapira D: Transient osteoporosis of the hip, *Semin Arthritis Rheum* 22:98, 1992.

Scheck M: Long-term follow up of treatment of comminuted fractures of the distal end of the radius by transfixation with Kirschner wires and cast, *J Bone Joint Surg* 44A:337, 1962.

Schenck RC, Heckman JD: Injuries of the knee, *Clin Symp* 45:1, 1993.

Schepsis AA, Leach RE, Gorzyca J: Plantar fasciitis: etiology, treatment, surgical results and review of the literature, *Clin Orthop* 266:185, 1991.

Schiltenwolf M, Martini AK, Mau H: Measurement of intraosseous pressure in lunate necrosis, *J Hand Surg* 19(suppl 1):28-29, 1994.

Schindler OS: Synovial plicae of the knee, *Curr Orthop* 18(3):210-219, 2004.

Schlosstein L et al: High association of an HL-A antigen W 27 with ankylosing spondylitis and rheumatoid arthritis, *Ann Rheum Dis* 20:47, 1961.

Schmalziried TP, Amstutz HC, Dorey FJ: Nerve palsy associated with total hip replacement, risk factors and prognosis, *J Bone Joint Surg* 73A:1074, 1991.

Schmalzried TP: The infected hip: telltale signs and treatment options, *J Arthroplasty* 21(4, suppl 1):97-100, 2006.

Schmorl G, Junghanns H: *The human spine in health and disease,* Am ed 2, New York, 1971, Grune & Stratton (Translated by EF Bessmann).

Schneck CD: Mesgarzadeh M, Bonakdarpour A: MR imaging of the most commonly injured ankle ligaments, *Radiology* 184:507, 1992.

Schneider RC, Livingston KE, Cave AJE: "Hangman's fracture" of the cervical spine, *J Meirpsirg* 22:141, 1965.

Schofferman J et al: Childhood psychological trauma and chronic refractory low back pain, *Clin J Pain* 9:260, 1993.

Schofferman J, Wassermann S: Successful treatment of low back pain and/or neck pain due to a motor vehicle accident, *Spine* 19:1007, 1994.

Schon LC, Glennon TP, Baxter DE: Heel pain syndrome, electrodiagnostic support for nerve entrapment, *Root Ankle* 14:129, 1993.

Schon LC: Nerve entrapment, neuropathy and nerve dysfunction in athletes, *Orthop Clin North Am* 25:47, 1994.

Schram S, Taylor T: Tension signs in lumber disc prolapse, *Clin Orthop* 75:195, 1971.

Schreuders TAR et al: Strength measurements of the intrinsic hand muscles: a review of the development and evaluation of the Rotterdam intrinsic hand myometer, *J Hand Ther* 19(4):393-402, 2006.

Schueller G: MRI atlas of orthopedics and traumatology of the knee, *Eur J Radiol* 51(3):293-238, 2004.

Schulte KR et al: The outcome of Charnley total hip arthroplasty with cement after a minimum of twenty year follow-up, *J Bone Joint Surg* 75A:961, 1993.

Schulz BW, Ashton-Miller JA, Alexander NB: Maximum step length: relationships to age and knee and hip extensor capacities, *Clin Biomech* (in press, corrected proof).

Schumacher HR, Bomalski JS: *Case studies in rheumatology for the house officer,* Baltimore, 1990, Williams & Wilkins.

Schumacher HR, Klippel JH, Koopman WJ: *Primer on the rheumatic diseases,* ed 10, Atlanta, 1993, Arthritis Foundation.

Schurch B: The predictive value of plantar flexion of the toes in the assessment of neuropathic voiding disorders in patients with spine lesions at the thoracolumbar level, *Arch Phys Med Rehabil* 80(6):681-686, 1999.

Schwartz ML, Al-Zahrani S: Diagnostic imaging of elbow injuries in the throwing athlete, *Oper Tech Sports Med* 4(2):84-90, 1996.

Schwarzer AC et al: Prevalence and clinical features of lumbar zygapophyseal joint pain: a study in an Australian population with chronic low back pain, *Ann Rheum Dis* 54:100, 1995.

Scioli MW: Achilles tendinitis, *Orthop Clin North Am* 25:177, 1994.

Scott JT, editor: *Copeman's textbook of the rheumatic diseases,* ed 6, Edinburgh, 1986, Churchill Livingstone.

Scott NW: *Office orthopedic practice: the orthopedic clinics of North America,* vol 13, Philadelphia, 1982, WB Saunders.

Scott WN: *The knee,* vol 1-2, St Louis, 1994, Mosby.

Scranton PE et al: Mucoid degeneration of the patellar ligament in athletes, *J Bone Joint Surg* 74A:435, 1992.

Scrivani SJ et al: Taste perception after lingual nerve repair, *J Oral Maxillofac Surg* 58(1):3-5, 2000.

Scuderi GR, McCann PD, Bruno PJ: *Sports medicine: principles of primary care,* St Louis, 1997, Mosby.

Scutellari PN, Orzincolo C: Rheumatoid arthritis: sequences, *Eur J Radiol* 27(suppl 1): S31-S38, 1998.

Sebast C, Denelli WJ: Osteochondrosis. In DeLee JC, Drez D, editors: *Orthopedic sports medicine: principles and practice,* vol 1, Philadelphia, 1994, WB Saunders.

Sebastianelli WJ et al: Isolated avulsion of the biceps femoris insertion, *Clin Orthop* 259:200, 1990.

Secher Jensen T et al: Magnetic resonance imaging findings as predictors of clinical outcome in patients with sciatica receiving active conservative treatment, *J Manipulative Physiol Ther* 30(2):98-108, 2007.

Seddon H: *Surgical disorders of the peripheral nerves,* Baltimore, 1968, Williams & Wilkins.

Segal A, Krauss ES: Infected total hip arthroplasty after intravesical bacillus Calmette Guérin therapy, *J Arthroplasty* (in press, corrected proof).

Seidel HM et al: *Mosby's guide to physical examination,* ed 4, St Louis, 1999, Mosby.

Seikaly H et al: The clavipectoral osteomyocutaneous free flap, *Otolaryngol Head Neck Surg* 117(5):547-554, 1997.

Sells LL, German DC: An update on gout, *Bull Rheum Dis* 43:4, 1994.

Selye H: The experimental production of calcified deposits in the rotator cuff, *Surg Clin North Am* 43:1483, 1963.

Sennwald G: *The wrist,* New York, 1990, Springer-Verlag.

Seo K-S et al: In vitro measurement of pressure differences using manometry at various injection speeds during discography, *Spine J* 7(1):68-73, 2007.

Seror P: Symptoms of thoracic outlet syndrome in women with carpal tunnel syndrome, *Clin Neurophysiol* 116(10):2324-2329, 2005.

Seror P: The long thoracic nerve conduction study revisited in 2006, *Clin Neurophysiol* 117(11):2446-2450, 2006.

Seto JL, Brewster CE: Rehabilitation of meniscal injuries. In Greenfield BH, editor: *Rehabilitation of the knee: a problem-solving approach,* Philadelphia, 1993, FA Davis.

Shankman GA: *Fundamental orthopedic management for the examiner,* St Louis, 1997, Mosby.

Shankman GA: *Fundamental orthopedic management for the physical therapist assistant,* St Louis, 1997, Mosby.

Sharma JB et al: High prevalence of Fitz-Hugh-Curtis syndrome in genital tuberculosis, *Int J Gynecol Obstet* (in press, corrected proof).

Sharp J, Purser DW: Spontaneous atlanto-axial dislocation in ankylosing spondylitis and rheumatoid arthritis, *Ann Rheum Dis* 20:47, 1961.

Shea KG, Nilsson K, Belzer J: Patellar dislocation in skeletally immature athletes, *Oper Tech Sports Med* 14(3):188-196, 2006.

Shechtman O, Taylor C: How do therapists administer the rapid exchange grip test? A survey, *J Hand Ther* 15(1):53-61, 2002.

Sheehan DV, Harnett-Sheehan K, Raj BA: The measurement of disability, *Int Clin Psychopharmacol* 11:S89-S95, 1996.

Shehata SMK, Shabaan BS: Diaphragmatic injuries in children after blunt abdominal trauma, *J Pediatr Surg* 41(10):1727-1731, 2006.

Shelbourne KD et al: Arthrofibrosis in acute anterior cruciate ligament reconstructions, *Am J Sports Med* 19:332, 1991.

Shelbourne KD, Nitz PA: The O'Donoghue triad revisited, *Am J Sports Med* 19: 474, 1991.

Shelbourne KD, Porter DA: Anterior cruciate ligament-medial collateral ligament injury: non-operative management of medial collateral ligament tears with anterior cruciate reconstruction, *Am J Sports Med* 20:283, 1992.

Shellock FG et al: Evaluation of patients with persistent symptoms after lateral retinacular release by kinematic magnetic resonance imaging of the patellofemoral joint, *Arthroscopy* 6:226, 1990.

Shelton GL, Thigpen LK: Rehabilitation of patellofemoral dysfunction: a review of literature, *J Orthop Sports Phys Ther* 14:243, 1991.

Sherbondy PS, Sebastianelli WJ: Stress fractures of the medial malleolus and distal fibula, *Clin Sports Med* 25(1):129-137, 2006.

Sherlock DA, Gibson PH, Benson MKD: Congenital subluxation of the hip, *J Bone Joint Surg* 67B:390, 1985.

Sherman MS: The nerves of bones, *J Bone Joint Surg* 45A:522, 1963.

Sherr VT: Human babesiosis—an unrecorded reality: absence of formal registry undermines its detection, diagnosis and treatment, suggesting need for immediate mandatory reporting, *Med Hypotheses* 63(4):609-615, 2004.

Shin DS, Lee K, Kim D: Biomechanical study of lumbar spine with dynamic stabilization device using finite element method, *Comput Aided Des* 39(7):559-567, 2007.

Shino K et al: Reconstruction of the anterior cruciate ligament using allogenic tendon, *Am J Sports Med* 18:457, 1990.

Sieper J et al: Diagnosing reactive arthritis: role of clinical setting in the value of serologic and microbiologic assays, *Arthritis Rheum* 46(2):319-327, 2002.

Silberstein SD, Lipton RB, Goadsby PJ: *Headache in clinical practice,* Oxford, UK, 1998, ISIS Medical Media.

Silliman JF, Dean MT: Neurovascular injuries to the shoulder complex, *J Orthop Sports Phys Ther* 18:442, 1993.

Silliman JF, Hawkins RJ: Classification and physical diagnosis of instability of the shoulder, *Clin Orthop* 291:7, 1993.

Silliman JF, Hawkins RJ: Current concepts and recent advances in the athlete's shoulder, *Clin Sports Med* 10:693, 1991.

Silver D: Circulatory problems of the upper extremity. In Sabiston DC Jr, editor: *Davis Christopher textbook of surgery,* Philadelphia, 1985, WB Saunders.

Simmons E, Cameron JC: Patella alta and recurrent dislocation of the patella, *Clin Orthop* 274:265, 1992.

Simmons EH, Bernstein AJ: Fractures of the spine in ankylosing spondylitis. In Floman Y, Farcy JP, Argenson C, editors: *Thoracolumbar spine fractures,* New York, 1993, Raven.

Simmons EH, Graziano GP, Heffner R Jr: Muscle disease as a cause of kyphotic deformity in ankylosing spondylitis, *Spine* 16:S351, 1991.

Simmons EH: Kyphotic deformity of the spine in ankylosing spondylitis, *Clin Orthop* 128:65, 1977.

Simon D et al: Recognition and discrimination of prototypical dynamic expressions of pain and emotions, *Pain* (in press, corrected proof).

Simons DG: Clinical and etiological update of myofascial pain from trigger points, *J Musculoskel Pain* 4:93, 1996.

Simons DG: Muscle pain syndromes, *J Manual Med* 6:3, 1991.

Simons GW, Sty JR, Storkshak RJ: Retroperitoneal and retrofascial abscesses, *J Bone Joint Surg* 65A:1041, 1983.

Singal DP et al: HLA antigens in osteitis condensans ilii and ankylosing spondylitis, *J Rheumatol* 4(suppl 3):105, 1977.

Singh SK, Ioli JP, Chiodo CP: The surgical treatment of Morton's neuroma, *Curr Orthop* 19(5):379-384, 2005.

Sisk TD: Knee realignment and replacement in the recreational athlete. In DeLee JC, Drez D, editors: *Orthopedic sports medicine: principals and practice,* vol 2, Philadelphia, 1994, WB Saunders.

Skoff HD: "Postpartum/newborn" de Quervain's tenosynovitis of the wrist, *Am J Orthop (Belle Mead, NJ)* 30(5):428-430, 2001.

Skyhar MJ, Warren RF, Altchek DW: Instability of the shoulder. In Nicholas JA, Hershman EB, editors: *The upper extremity in sports medicine,* St Louis, 1990, Mosby.

Sledge CB, Poss R: *The year book of orthopedics 1997,* St Louis, 1997, Mosby.

Slick DJ et al: Detecting malingering: a survey of experts' practices, *Arch Clin Neuropsychol* 19(4):465-473, 2004.

Slipman CW et al: Provocative cervical discography symptom mapping, *Spine J* 5(4): 381-388, 2005.

Slocum DB et al: A clinical test for anterolateral rotary instability of the knee, *Clin Orthop* 118:63, 1976.

Slocum DB, Larson RL: Rotary instability of the knee, *J Bone Joint Surg* 50A:211, 1968.

Smart K, Doody C: The clinical reasoning of pain by experienced musculoskeletal physiotherapists, *Man Ther* 12(1):40-49, 2007.

Smillie IS: *Diseases of the knee joint,* New York, 1974, Longmans.

Smillie IS: *Injuries of the knee joint,* Edinburgh, 1970, E & S Livingstone.

Smith ET, Pevey JK, Shindler TO: The erector spinae transplant: a misnomer, *Clin Orthop* 20:144, 1963.

Smith FM: *Surgery of the elbow,* ed 2, Philadelphia, 1972, WB Saunders.

Smith G et al: Hip pain caused by buttock claudication: relief of symptoms by transluminal angioplasty, *Clin Orthop* 284:176, 1992.

Smith KL, Harvey FJ, Stalley PD: Nonunion of a pathologic juvenile scaphoid fracture after osteomyelitis, *J Hand Surg* 16A:493, 1991.

Smith MD, Bohlman HH: Spondylolisthesis treated by a single-stage operation combining decompression with in situ posterolateral and anterior fusion, *J Bone Joint Surg* 72:415, 1990.

Smith PH, Benn RT, Sharp J: Natural history of rheumatoid cervical luxations, *Ann Rheum Dis* 31:431, 1972.

Smith RC, Hoppe RB: The patient's story: integrating the patient and physician centered approaches to interviewing, *Ann Intern Med* 115:470, 1991.

Smith SA et al: Straight leg raising: anatomical effects on the spinal nerve root without and with fusion, *Spine* 18:992, 1993.

Smith TC et al: Reliability of standard health assessment instruments in a large, population-based cohort study, *Ann Epidemiol* 17(7):525-532, 2007.

Smith-Petersen MN: Painful affections of lower back. In Christopher F: *Textbook of surgery,* ed 5, Philadelphia, 1949, WB Saunders.

Smorto MP, Basmajian JV: *Clinical electroneurography: an introduction to nerve conduction tests,* Baltimore, 1972, William & Wilkins.

Snijders CJ et al: Effects of slouching and muscle contraction on the strain of the iliolumbar ligament, *Man Ther* (in press, corrected proof).

Snijders CJ, Vleeming A, Stoeckart R: Transfer of lumbosacral load to iliac bones and legs. Part 1: biomechanics of self-bracing of the sacroiliac joints and its significance for treatment and exercise, *Clin Biomech* 8(6):285-294, 1993.

Snyder SJ et al: Partial thickness rotator cuff tears: results of arthroscopic treatment, *Arthroscopy* 7:1, 1991.

Snyder SJ, Karzel RP, Del Pizzo W: SLAP lesions of the shoulder, *Arthroscopy* 6:274, 1990.

Sobel J, Pettrone F, Nirschl R: Prevention and treatment of upper extremity sports injuries. In Nicholas J, Hershman E, editors: *The extremity in sports medicine,* St Louis 1990, Mosby.

Solomon L: Patterns of osteoarthritis of the hip, *J Bone Joint Surg* 58B:176, 1976.

Solomonow M, D'Ambrosia R: Neural reflex arcs and muscle control of knee stability and motion. In Scott NW, editor: *Ligament and extensor mechanism injuries of the knee, diagnosis and treatment,* St Louis, 1991, Mosby.

Somerville EW: A long-term follow-up of congenital dislocation of the hip, *J Bone Joint Surg* 60B:25, 1978.

Soslowsky LJ et al: Articular geometry of the glenohumeral joint, *Clin Orthop* 285:181, 1992.

Southmayd WW, Millender LH, Nalebuff EA: Rupture of the flexor tendons in the index finger after Colles' fracture case report, *J Bone Joint Surg* 57A:562, 1975.

Spacek E et al: Disability induced by hand osteoarthritis: are patients with more symptoms at digits 2-5 interphalangeal joints different from those with more symptoms at the base of the thumb? *Osteoarthr Cartil* 12(5):366-373, 2004.

Spangfort E: Lasègue's sign in patients with lumbar disc herniation, *Acta Orthop* 42:459, 1971.

Spapen HD et al: The straight back syndrome, *Neth J Med* 36:29, 1990.

Specht NT, Russo RD: *Practical guide to diagnostic imaging,* St Louis, 1998, Mosby.

Spencer PS: The traumatic neuroma and proximal stump, *Bull Hosp Joint Dis* 35: 85, 1974.

Spengler DM, Szpalski M: Newer assessment approaches for the patient with low back pain, *Contemp Orthop* 21, 1990.

Spinner M, Spencer PS: Nerve compression lesions of the upper extremity: a clinical and experimental review, *Clin Orthop* 104:46, 1974.

Spinner M: *Injuries of the major branches of peripheral nerves of the forearm,* Philadelphia, 1972, WB Saunders.

Spinner RJ, Morgenlander JC, Nunley JA: Ulnar nerve function following total elbow arthroplasty: a prospective study comparing preoperative and postoperative clinical and electrophysiologic evaluation in patients with rheumatoid arthritis, *J Hand Surg* 25(2):360-364, 2000.

Spittell JA Jr et al: Arteriovenous fistula complicating lumbar disc surgery, *N Engl J Med* 268:1162, 1963.

Spivak JM, Vaccaro AR, Cotler JM: Thoracolumbar spine trauma. I: evaluation and classification, *J Am Acad Orthop Surg* 3:345, 1995.

Spring H et al: *Stretching and strengthening exercises,* New York, 1991, Thieme.

Sprou G: Basilar artery insufficiency secondary to obstruction of left subclavian artery, *Circulation* 28:259, 1963.

Spurling RG, Scoville WB: Lateral rupture of the cervical intervertebral discs, *Syn Gyn Obstet* 78:350, 1944.

St. Claire SM: Diagnosis and treatment of fibromyalgia syndrome, *J Neuromusc Syst* 2:3, 1994.

Staheli LT: Medial femoral torsion, *Orthop Clin North Am* 11:39, 1980.

Stamford JA: Descending control of pain, *Br J Anaesth* 75:217, 1995.

Stanitski CL: Anterior knee pain syndromes in the adolescent, *J Bone Joint Surg* 75A:1407, 1993.

Stanley J: Radial tunnel syndrome: a surgeon's perspective, *J Hand Ther* 19(2):180-185, 2006.

Stanley K: Ankle sprains are always more than "just a sprain," *Postgrad Med* 89:251, 1991.

Starlanyl D, Copeland ME: *Fibromyalgia & chronic myofascial pain syndrome: a survival manual,* Oakland, Calif, 1996, New Harbinger.

Staubli HU, Birrer S: The popliteus tendon and its fascicles at the popliteal hiatus: gross anatomy and functional arthroscopic evaluation with and without anterior cruciate ligament deficiency, *Arthroscopy* 6:209, 1990.

Stauffer ES et al: Fractures and dislocations of the spine. Part II, the thoracolumbar spine. In Rockwood CA, Green DP, Bucholz RW, editors: *Fractures in adults,* ed 3, Philadelphia, 1991, JB Lippincott.

Stedman TL: *Stedman's medical dictionary,* ed 25, Baltimore, 1990, Williams & Wilkins.

Steensen RN, Dopirak RM, Maurus PB: Minimally invasive "crescentic" imbrication of the medial patellofemoral ligament for chronic patellar subluxation, *Arthroscopy* 21(3):371-375, 2005.

Stein C: The control of pain in peripheral tissue by opioids, *N Engl J Med* 332:1685, 1995.

Steinberg ME, Steinberg DR: Avascular necrosis of the femoral head. In Steinberg ME, editor: *The hip and its disorders,* Philadelphia, 1991, WB Saunders.

Steinbert ME, Steinberg DR: Evaluation and staging of avascular necrosis, *Semin Arthroplasty* 2:175, 1991.

Steinbrocher O: The painful shoulder. In Hollander JL, McCarty DJ, editors: *Arthritis and allied conditions,* ed 8, Philadelphia, 1972, Lea & Febiger.

Steinkamp LA et al: Biomechanical consideration in patellofemoral joint rehabilitation, *Am J Sports Med* 21:438, 1993.

Steinmann SP: Elbow arthroscopy, *J Am Soc Surg Hand* 3(4):199-207, 2003.

Stephens MM: Haglund's deformity and retrocalcaneal bursitis, *Orthop Clinic North Am* 25:41, 1994.

Stern PJ: Tendinitis, overuse syndromes, and tendon injuries, *Hand Clin* 6:467, 1990.

Stevens A, Lowe J: *Histology,* New York, 1992, Gower Medical.

Stevens JC et al: Conditions associated with carpal tunnel syndrome, *Mayo Clin Proc* 67:541, 1992.

Stevenson J: When the trauma patient is elderly, *J Perianesth Nurs* 19(6):392-400, 2004.

Stewart DL, Abeln SH: *Documenting functional outcomes in physical therapy,* St Louis, 1993, Mosby.

Stewart JDM, Hallett JP: *Traction and orthopaedic appliances,* Edinburgh, 1983, Churchill Livingstone.

Stiell IG et al: Implementation of the Ottawa ankle rules, *JAMA* 271:827, 1994.

Stiles RG, Otte MT: Imaging of the shoulder, *Radiology* 188:603, 1993.

Stillerman C, Weiss M: Management of thoracic disc disease, *Clin Neurosurg* 38:325, 1992.

Stinson JT: Spondylolysis and spondylolisthesis in the athlete, *Clin Sports Med* 12:517, 1993.

Stith WJ: Exercise and the intervertebral disc, *Spine* 4:259, 1990.

Stochkendahl MJ et al: Manual examination of the spine: a systematic critical literature review of reproducibility, *J Manipulative Physiol Ther* 29(6):475-462, 2006.

Stock G: *The book of questions,* New York, 1985, Workman Publishing.

Stojilovic N et al: Analysis of prosthetic knee wear debris extracted from synovial fluid, *Appl Surf Sci* 252(10):3760-3766, 2006.

Stoller DW: *Magnetic resonance imaging in orthopaedics & sports medicine,* Philadelphia, 1993, JB Lippincott.

Stone JA: MR myelography of the spine and MR peripheral nerve imaging, *Magn Reson Imaging Clin North Am* 11(4):543-558, 2003.

Storen G: The radiocapitellar relationship, *Acta Chir Scand* 116:144, 1995.

Storm S et al: Compliance with electrodiagnostic guidelines for patients undergoing carpal tunnel release, *Arch Phys Med Rehabil* 86(1):8-11, 2005.

Strange FGS: The prognosis in sacro-iliac tuberculosis, *Br J Surg* 50:561, 1963.

Stratford PW et al: Measurement properties of the WOMAC LK 3.1 pain scale, *Osteoarthr Cartil* 15(3):266-272, 2007.

Strauss E et al: Intraindividual variability as an indicator of malingering in head injury, *Arch Clin Neuropsychol* 17(5):423-444, 2002.

Strege D: Upper extremity. In Loth T, editor: *Orthopaedic boards review,* St Louis, 1993, Mosby.

Strickland E et al: In vivo contact pressures during rehabilitation. Part 1: acute phase, *Phys Ther* 72:691, 1992.

Strum GM et al: Acute anterior cruciate reconstructions, *Clin Orthop* 253;184, 1990.

Strunk J et al: Three-dimensional Doppler sonographic vascular imaging in regions with increased MR enhancement in inflamed wrists of patients with rheumatoid arthritis, *Joint Bone Spine* 73(5):518-522, 2006.

Stubbs MJ, Field LD, Savoie Iii FH: Osteochondritis dissecans of the elbow, *Clin Sports Med* 20(1):1-9, 2001.

Sugden P et al: Dermal dendrocytes in Dupuytren's disease: a link between the skin and pathogenesis? *J Hand Surg* 18B:662, 1993.

Sugimoto H et al: Early-stage rheumatoid arthritis: diagnostic accuracy of MR imaging, *Radiology* 198:185, 1996.

Suh J-T, Cheon S-J, Choi S-J: Synovial hemangioma of the knee, *Arthroscopy* 19(7): e77-e80, 2003.

Sun F, Tauchi P, Stark L: Binocular alternating pulse stimuli: experimental and modeling studies of the pupil reflex to light, *Math Biosci* 67(2):225-245, 1983.

Sunderland S: *Nerves and nerve injuries,* Baltimore, 1968, Williams & Wilkins.

Sunderland S: *Nerves and nerve injuries,* ed 2, New York, 1979, Churchill Livingstone.

Susuke S et al: Diagnosis by ultrasound of congenital dislocation of the hip joint, *Clin Orthop* 217:171, 1987.

Sutton D, Young JWR: *A concise textbook of clinical imaging,* ed 2, St Louis, 1995, Mosby.

Sutton D: *A textbook of radiology and imaging,* ed 5, London, 1993, Churchill Livingstone.

Swanson AB et al: Pathogenesis of rheumatoid deformities in the hand. In Cruess RL, Mitchell NS, editors: *Surgery of rheumatoid arthritis,* Philadelphia, 1971, JB Lippincott.

Swanson AB: Disabling arthritis at the base of the thumb: treatment by resection of the trapezium and flexible (silicone) implant arthroplasty, *J Bone Joint Surg* 54(3):456-471, 1972.

Sward L et al: Anthropometric characteristics, passive hip flexion, and spinal mobility in relation to back pain in patients, *Spine* 15:376, 1990.

Sward L et al: Disc degeneration and associated abnormalities of the spine in elite patients: a magnetic resonance imaging study, *Spine* 16:437, 1991.

Sward L: The thoracolumbar spine in young elite patients, *Sports Med* 13:357, 1992.

Swartout R, Compere EL: Ischiogluteal bursitis: the pain in the arse, *JAMA* 227:551, 1974.

Swartz MN, Dodge PR: Bacterial meningitis: general clinical features, special problems and unusual meningeal reactions mimicking bacterial meningitis, *N Engl J Med* 272:725, 1965.

Sweere JJ: *Chiropractic family practice: a clinical manual,* Gaithersburg, Md, 1992, Aspen.

Swezey RI: Non-fibrositic lumbar subcutaneous nodules: prevalence and clinical significance, *Br J Rheumatol* 30:376, 1991.

Swointkowski MF: Intracapsular fractures of the hip, *J Bone Joint Surg* 76A:129, 1994.

Szlachter BN et al: Relaxin in normal and pathologenic pregnancies, *Obstet Gynecol* 59:167, 1982.

Tachdjian MO: *Pediatric orthopedics,* Philadelphia, 1972, WB Saunders.

Tachdjian MO: *The child's foot,* Philadelphia, 1985, WB Saunders.

Takao M et al: A case of superficial peroneal nerve injury during ankle arthroscopy, *Arthroscopy* 17(4):403-404, 2001.

Taleisnik J: The ligaments of the wrist, *J Hand Surg* 1(2):110-118, 1976.

Taleisnik J: Rheumatoid arthritis of the wrist. In Strickland JW, Steichen JB, editors: *Difficult problems in hand surgery,* St Louis, 1982, Mosby.

Tamai K et al: Dynamic magnetic resonance imaging for the evaluation of synovitis in patients with rheumatoid arthritis, *Arthritis Rheum* 37:1151, 1994.

Tamea CD, Henning CD: Pathomechanics of the pivot shift maneuver, *Am J Sports Med* 9:31, 1981.

Tan JC, Horn SE: *Practical manual of physical medicine and rehabilitation,* St Louis, 1998, Mosby.

Tan JC, Nordin M: The role of physical therapy in the treatment of cervical disc disease, *Orthop Clin North Am* 23:435, 1992.

Tashjian RZ et al: Functional outcomes and general health status after ulnohumeral arthroplasty for primary degenerative arthritis of the elbow, *J Shoulder Elbow Surg* 15(3):357-366, 2006.

Tatarek NE: Variation in the human cervical neural canal, *Spine J* 5(6):623-631, 2005.

Tavakkolizadeh A, Klinke M, Davies MS: Bilateral distal fibular stress fractures, *Foot Ankle Surg* 11(3):171-173, 2005.

Taybi H, Lachman RS: *Radiology of syndromes, metabolic disorders, and skeletal dysplasias,* ed 4, St Louis, 1996, Mosby.

Taylor CJ, Bansal R, Pimpalnerkar A: Acute distal biceps tendon rupture—a new surgical technique using a de-tensioning suture to brachialis, *Injury* 37(9):838-842, 2006.

Taylor JC: Fractures of the lower extremity. In Crenshaw AH, editor: *Campbell's operative orthopedics,* ed 8, St Louis, 1992, Mosby.

Taylor JR: The development and adult structure of lumbar intervertebral discs, *J Manual Med* 5:43, 1990.

Taylor RW, Sonson RD: Separation of the pubic symphysis, an underrecognized peripartum complication, *J Reprod Med* 31:203, 1986.

Tehranzadeh J, Palmer S: Imaging of cervical spine trauma, *Semin Ultrasound CT MRI* 17(2):93-104, 1996.

Teichner G, Wagner MT: The Test of Memory Malingering (TOMM): normative data from cognitively intact, cognitively impaired, and elderly patients with dementia, *Arch Clin Neuropsychol* 19(3):455-464, 2004.

Tenuta JJ, Arciero RA: Arthroscopic evaluation of meniscal repairs: factors that affect healing, *Am J Sports Med* 22:797, 1994.

Terjesen T, Berdland T, Berg V: Ultrasound for hip assessment in the newborn, *J Bone Joint Surg* 71B:767, 1989.

Terjesen T: Ultrasonography in the primary evaluation of Perthe's disease, *J Pediatr Orthop* 13:437, 1993.

Terrett AGJ: *Malpractice avoidance for chiropractors,* West Des Moines, Iowa, 1996, National Chiropractic Mutual Insurance Company.

Teshima R, Otsuka T, Yamamoto K: Effects of nonweight bearing on the hip, *Clin Orthop* 279:149, 1992.

Tetsworth K, Paley D: Malalignment and degenerative arthropathy, *Orthop Clin North Am* 25:367, 1994.

Tettenborn B et al: Postoperative brainstem and cerebellar infarcts, *Neurology* 43:471, 1993.

Thein LA: Rehabilitation of shoulder injuries. In Prentice WE, editor: *Rehabilitation techniques in sports medicine,* ed 2, St Louis, 1994, Mosby.

Theisler CW: *Migraine headache disease diagnostic and management strategies,* Gaithersburg, Md, 1990, Aspen.

Thelander U et al: Straight leg raising test versus radiologic size, shape, and position of lumbar disc hernias, *Spine* 17:395, 1992.

Theruvil B et al: Vascular malformations in muscles around the knee presenting as knee pain, *Knee* 11(2):155-158, 2004.

Thibodeau G, Patton K: *Pocket reference to accompany anatomy & physiology,* ed 3, St Louis, 1996, Mosby.

Thibodeau GA, Patton KT: *Anatomy & physiology,* ed 3, St Louis, 1996, Mosby.

Thibodeau GA, Patton KT: *Anatomy & physiology,* ed 4, St Louis, 1999, Mosby.

Thibodeau GA, Patton KT: *Pocket reference to accompany anatomy & physiology,* ed 3, St Louis, 1996, Mosby.

Thomas LC, Rivett DA, Bolton PS: Pre-manipulative testing and the use of the velocimeter, *Man Ther* (in press, corrected proof).

Thomas NWM: Low back pain, sciatica, cervical and lumbar spondylosis, *Surgery (Oxford)* 25(4):155-159, 2007.

Thompson AJ, Polman C, Hohlfeld R: *Multiple sclerosis: clinical challenges and controversies,* St Louis, 1997, Mosby.

Thompson GH: Back pain in children, *J Bone Joint Surg* 75A:928, 1993.

Thompson JM: *Clinical outlines for health assessment,* St Louis, 1997, Mosby.

Thompson JS, Phelph TH: Repetitive strain injuries, how to deal with the epidemic of the 1990's, *Postgrad Med* 88:143, 1990.

Thompson RE, Pearcy MJ, Barker TM: The mechanical effects of intervertebral disc lesions, *Clin Biomech* 19(5):448-455, 2004.

Thompson T, Doherty J: Spontaneous rupture of the tendon of Achilles: a new clinical diagnostic test, *Anat Rec* 158:126, 1967.

Thompson TC, Doherty JH: Spontaneous rupture of the tendon of Achilles: a nonclinical diagnostic test, *J Trauma* 2:126, 1962.

Thompson TC: A test for rupture of the tendon of Achilles, *Acta Orthop Scand* 32:461, 1992.

Thorson E, Szabo RM: Common tendinitis problems in the hand and forearm, *Orthop Clin North Am* 23:65, 1992.

Thurston SE: *The little black book of neurology,* Chicago, 1987, Mosby.

Ticker J, Beam G, and Warner JJP: Recognition and treatment of refractory posterior capsular contracture of the shoulder, *Arthroscopy* 12(3):353-354, 1996.

Tiel-van Buul MM et al: Radiography and scintigraphy of suspected scaphoid fracture, a long-term study in 160 patients, *J Bone Joint Surg* 75B:61, 1993.

Tiel-van Buul MM et al: Radiography of the carpal scaphoid, experimental evaluation of "the carpal box" and first clinical results, *Invest Radiol* 27:954, 1992.

Timgren J, Soinila S: Reversible pelvic asymmetry: an overlooked syndrome manifesting as scoliosis, apparent leg-length difference, and neurologic symptoms, *J Manipulative Physiol Ther* 29(7):561-565, 2006.

Timm K: Knee. In Richardson JK, Iglarsh ZA, editors: *Clinical orthopaedic physical therapy,* Philadelphia, 1994, WB Saunders.

Timmerman LA, Andrews JR: Undersurface tear of the ulnar collateral ligament in baseball players, *Am J Sports Med* 22:33, 1994.

Tinel J: *Nerve wounds: symptomatology of peripheral nerve lesions caused by war wounds (translated by F Rothwell; edited by CA Joll),* New York, 1918, William Wood.

Toalt V et al: Evidence for viral etiology of transient synovitis of the hip, *J Bone Joint Surg* 75B:973, 1993.

Toghill PJ: *Examining patients an introduction to clinical medicine,* London, 1990, Edward Arnold.

Tollison CD, Satterthwaite JR, Tollison JW: *Handbook of pain management,* ed 2, Baltimore, 1994, Williams & Wilkins.

Toohey AK et al: Iliopsoas bursitis; clinical features, radiographic findings, and disease associations, *Semin Arthritis Rheum* 10:41, 1990.

Torg JS et al: The relationship of development narrowing of the cervical spinal canal to reversible and irreversible injury of the cervical spinal cord in football players, *J Bone Joint Surg (Am)* 78:1308, 1996.

Torg JS, Shepard RJ: *Current therapy in sports medicine,* ed 3, St Louis, 1995, Mosby.

Torres L et al: The relationship between specific tissue lesions and pain severity in persons with knee osteoarthritis, *Osteoarthr Cartil* 14(10):1033-1040, 2006.

Townsend H et al: Electromyographic analysis of the glenohumeral muscles during a baseball rehabilitation program, *Am J Sports Med* 19:264, 1991.

Traill Z, Richards MA, Moore NR: Magnetic resonance imaging of metastatic bone disease, *Clin Orthop* 312:76, 1995.

Tranier S et al: Value of somatosensory evoked potentials in saphenous entrapment neuropathy, *J Neurol Neurosurg Psychiatry* 55:461, 1992.

Traub M et al: The use of chest computed tomography versus chest X-ray in patients with major blunt trauma, *Injury* 38(1):43-47, 2007.

Tredgett MW, Davis TRC: Rapid repeat testing of grip strength for detection of faked hand weakness, *J Hand Surg* 25(4):372-375, 2000.

Tronzo RG, editor: *Surgery of the hip joint,* Philadelphia, 1973, Lea & Febiger.

Truex RC, Carpenter MB: *Human neuroanatomy,* ed 6, Baltimore, 1969, Williams & Wilkins.

Trumble TE, Benirschke SK, Vedder NB: Ipsilateral fractures of the scaphoid and radius, *J Hand Surg* 18A:8, 1993.

Tsou PM, Yau A, Hodgson AR: Embryogenesis and prenatal development of congenital vertebral anomalies and their classification, *Clin Orthop* 152:211, 1980.

Tsou PM: Embryology of congenital kyphosis, *Clin Orthop* 128:18, 1977.

Tsuritani I et al: Impact of obesity on musculoskeletal pain and difficulty of daily movements in Japanese middle-aged women, *Maturitas* 42(1):23-30, 2002.

Tsuruike M et al: Age comparison of H-reflex modulation with the Jendrassik maneuver and postural complexity, *Clin Neurophysiol* 114(5):945-953, 2003.

Tubiana R: *The hand,* Philadelphia, 1981, WB Saunders.

Tullos HS, King JW: Lesions of the pitching arm in adolescents, *JAMA* 220:264, 1972.

Tumeh SS, Tohmeh AG: Nuclear medicine techniques in septic arthritis and osteomyelitis, *Rheum Dis Clin North Am* 17:559, 1991.

Turek SL: *Orthopaedics principles and their application,* ed 3, Philadelphia, 1977, JB Lippincott.

Turk DC et al: Effects of type of symptom onset on psychological distress and disability in fibromyalgia syndrome patients, *Pain* 68(2-3):423-430, 1996.

Turk N et al: Discriminatory ability of calcaneal quantitative ultrasound in the assessment of bone status in patients with inflammatory bowel disease, *Ultrasound Med Biol* 33(6):863-869, 2007.

Turkcapar N et al: Late onset rheumatoid arthritis: clinical and laboratory comparisons with younger onset patients, *Arch Gerontol Geriatr* 42(2):225-231, 2006.

Turnbull TJ, Dymowski JJ: Emergency department use of hand-held Doppler ultrasonography, *Am J Emerg Med* 7(2):209-215, 1989.

Turner PG, Green JH, Galasko CS: Back pain in childhood, *Spine* 14:812, 1989.

Turnipseed WD, Pozniak M: Popliteal entrapment as a result of neurovascular compression by the soleus and plantaris muscles, *J Vasc Surg* 15:284, 1992.

Twomey L, Taylor JR: Structural and mechanical disc changes with age, *J Manual Med* 5:58, 1990.

Ubbink DT, Vermeulen H: Spinal cord stimulation for critical leg ischemia: a review of effectiveness and optimal patient selection, *J Pain Symptom Manage* 31(4, suppl 1): S30-S35, 2006.

Uhthoff H, Sarkar K: Calcifying tendinitis. In Rockwood C, Matsen F, editors: *The shoulder,* Philadelphia, 1990, WB Saunders.

Uhthoff J: Prenatal development of the iliolumbar ligament, *J Bone Joint Surg* 75:93, 1993.

Urban LM: The straight-leg-raising test: a review, *J Orthop Sports Phys Ther* 2:117, 1981.

Urbaniak JR: Complication of treatment of carpal tunnel syndrome. In Gelberman RH, editor: *Operative nerve repair and reconstruction,* vol 2, Philadelphia, 1991, JB Lippincott.

Ursavas A et al: Breast and osteoarticular tuberculosis in a male patient, *Diagn Microbiol Infect Dis* (in press, corrected proof).

U.S. Preventative Services Task Force: *Guide to clinical preventive services,* ed 2, Alexandria, Va, 1996, International Medical Publishing.

Vail TP, Malone TR, Basset FH: Long-term functional results in patients with anterolateral rotatory instability treated by iliotibial band transfer, *Am J Sports Med* 20:274, 1992.

Vallejo MC et al: Piriformis syndrome in a patient after cesarean section under spinal anesthesia, *Reg Anesth Pain Med* 29(4):364-367, 2004.

Van Beusekom GT: The neurological syndrome associated with cervical luxations in rheumatoid arthritis, *Acta Orthop Belg* 58:38, 1972.

Van De Kar THJ et al: Clinical value of electrodiagnostic testing following repair of peripheral nerve lesions: a prospective study, *J Hand Surg* 27(4):345-349, 2002.

Van Dillen LR et al: Symmetry of timing of hip and lumbopelvic rotation motion in 2 different subgroups of people with low back pain, *Arch Phys Med Rehabil* 88(3): 351-360, 2007.

Van Holsbeeck M, Introcaso JH: *Musculoskeletal ultrasound,* St Louis, 1991, Mosby.

Van Kampen A, Huiskes R: The three-dimensional tracking pattern of the human patella, *J Orthop Res* 8:372, 1990.

Vance RM, Gelberman RH: Acute ulnar neuropathy with fractures at the wrist, *J Bone Joint Surg* 60A:962, 1978.

Vanderpool DW et al: Peripheral compression lesions of the ulnar nerve, *J Bone Joint Surg* 50B:792, 1968.

Vanderstraeten G, Ozcakar L, Verstraete K: Thoracic outlet syndrome portending Klippel-Feil syndrome, *Joint Bone Spine* 73(6):763-764, 2006.

Vasquez MA et al: The utility of the venous clinical severity score in 682 limbs treated by radiofrequency saphenous vein ablation, *J Vasc Surg* 45(5):1008.e2-1015.e2, 2007.

Vayssairat M et al: A new cold test for the diagnosis of Raynaud's phenomenon, *Ann Vasc Surg* 1(4):474-478, 1987.

Veeming A et al: The posterior layer of the thoracolumbar fascia, its function in load transfer from spine to legs, *Spine* 20:753, 1995.

Verhaven EFC et al: The accuracy of three-dimensional magnetic resonance imaging in the diagnosis of ruptures of the lateral ligaments of the ankle, *Am J Sports Med* 19:583, 1991.

Verma NN, Drakos M, O'Brien SJ: Arthroscopic transfer of the long head biceps to the conjoint tendon, *Arthroscopy* 21(6):764.e1-764.e5, 2005.

Vernon L, Dooley J, Acusta A: Upper lumbar and thoracic disc pathology: a magnetic resonance imaging analysis, *J Neuromusculoskel Syst* 59:63, 1993.

Vernon-Roberts B, Perie CJ: Degenerative changes in the intervertebral disc of the lumbar spine and their sequela, *Rheum Rehab* 16:13, 1977.

Verrall GM et al: Hip joint range of motion reduction in sports-related chronic groin injury diagnosed as pubic bone stress injury, *J Sci Med Sport* 8(1):77-84, 2005.

Verrall GM et al: Hip joint range of motion restriction precedes athletic chronic groin injury, *J Sci Med Sport* (in press, corrected proof).

Veys EM et al: HLA and infective sacroiliitis, *Lancet* 2:349, 1974.

Vicenzino B: Lateral epicondylalgia: a musculoskeletal physiotherapy perspective, *Man Ther* 8(2):66-79, 2003.

Vidal MA et al: Preiser's disease, *Ann Chir Main Memb Super* 10:227, 1991.

Viere RG et al: Use of the Pavlik harness in congenital dislocation of the hip, an analysis of failures of treatment, *J Bone Joint Surg* 72A:238, 1990.

Vignon E et al: Osteoarthritis of the knee and hip and activity: a systematic international review and synthesis (OASIS), *Joint Bone Spine* 73(4):442-455, 2006.

Vingard E et al: Sports and osteoarthritis of the hip: an epidemiologic study, *Am J Sports Med* 21:195, 1993.

Vleeming A et al: The posterior layer of the thoracolumbar fascia. Its function in load transfer from spine to legs, *Spine* 20:753, 1995.

Vleeming A et al: Mobility in the sacroiliac joints in the elderly: a kinematic and radiological study, *Clin Biomech* 7(3):170-176, 1992.

Voche P, Merle M: Wartenberg's sign: a new method of surgical correction, *J Hand Surg* 20(1):49-52, 1995.

Voight ML, Wieder DL: Comparative reflex response times of vastus medialis obliquus and vastus lateralis in normal subjects and subjects with extensor mechanism dysfunction: an electromyographic study, *Am J Sports Med* 19:131, 1991.

von Prince K, Butler B: Measuring sensory function of the hand in peripheral nerve injuries, *Am J Occup Ther* 21:385, 1967.

von Prince K: Occupational therapy's interest in function following peripheral nerve injury, *Med Bull US Army Eur* 23:143, 1966.

Voorhies RM, Jiang X, Thomas N: Predicting outcome in the surgical treatment of lumbar radiculopathy using the Pain Drawing Score, McGill Short Form Pain Questionnaire, and risk factors including psychosocial issues and axial joint pain, *Spine J* (in press, corrected proof).

Vrahas MS et al: Contribution of passive tissues to the intersegmental moments at the hip, *J Biomech* 23:357, 1990.

Waddell G et al: Nonorganic physical signs in low back pain, *Spine* 5:177, 1980.

Waddell G et al: Objective clinical evaluation of physical impairment in chronic low back pain, *Spine* 17:617, 1992.

Waddell G: A new clinical model for the treatment of low back pain, *Spine* 12:632, 1987.

Waddell G: An approach to backache, *Br J Hosp Med* 28:187, 1982.

Wadsworth TG: *The elbow,* New York, 1982, Churchill Livingstone.

Wagner FW Jr: The dysvascular foot: a system for diagnosis and treatment, *Foot Ankle* 2:64, 1981.

Wainwright D: The shelf operation for hip dysplasia in adolescence, *J Bone Joint Surg* 58B:159, 1976.

Wakefield TS, Frank RG: *The clinician's guide to neuro musculoskeletal practice,* Abbotsford, Wis, 1995, Allied Health of Wisconsin.

Waldron VD: A test for chondromalacia patella, *Orthop Rev* 12:103, 1983.

Wall JR, Millis SR: Can motor measures tell us if someone is trying? An assessment of sincerity of effort in simulated malingering, *Arch Clin Neuropsychol* 14(1):40-41, 1999.

Wallace R, Cohen AS: Tuberculous arthritis: a report of two cases with review of biopsy and synovial fluid findings, *Am J Med* 61:277, 1976.

Walsh MJ: Evaluation of orthopedic testing of the low back for non-specific low back pain, *J Manipulative Physiol Ther* 21:232, 1998.

Walsh TR et al: Lumbar discography in normal subjects, a controlled, prospective study, *J Bone Joint Surg* 72A:1081, 1990.

Walsh WM, Helzer-Julin MJ: Patellar tracking problems in athletes, *Prim Care* 19:303, 1992.

Walsh WM: Patellofemoral joint. In DeLee JC, Drez D, editors: *Orthopaedic sports medicine: principles and practice,* vol 2, Philadelphia, 1994, WB Saunders.

Walshe FMR: *Diseases of the nervous system,* ed 11, Baltimore, 1970, Williams & Wilkins.

Walter F, Haynes MB, Markel DC: A randomized prospective study evaluating the effect of patellar eversion on the early functional outcomes in primary total knee arthroplasty, *J Arthroplasty* (in press, corrected proof).

Walters A: Psychogenic regional pain alias-hysterical pain, *Brain* 84:1, 1961.

Wang M, Dumas GA: Mechanical behavior of the female sacroiliac joint and influence of the anterior and posterior sacroiliac ligaments under sagittal loads, *Clin Biomech* 13(4-5):293-29, 1998.

Wang T-G et al: Assessment of stretching of the iliotibial tract with Ober and modified Ober tests: an ultrasonographic study, *Arch Phys Med Rehabil* 87(10):1407-1411, 2006.

Wang Z et al: Treatment of spinal tuberculosis with ultrashort-course chemotherapy in conjunction with partial excision of pathologic vertebrae, *Spine J* (in press, corrected proof).

Ward WL, Belhobek GH, Anderson TE: Arthroscopic elbow findings: correlation with preoperative radiographic studies, *Arthroscopy* 8:498, 1992.

Warner JJP et al: Arthroscopic release of chronic, refractory capsular contracture of the shoulder, *J Bone Joint Surg Am* 78(12):1808-1816, 1996.

Warner JP, Ticker JB, Beim GM: Recognition and treatment of refractory posterior capsular contracture of the shoulder, *Arthroscopy* 16(6):673-674, 2000.

Warwick R, Williams PL: *Gray's anatomy,* ed 35, Philadelphia, 1973, WB Saunders.

Waseem M, Jari S, Paton RW: Glomus tumour, a rare cause of knee pain: a case report, *Knee* 9(2):161-163, 2002.

Wasilewski SA, Frankel U: Rotator cuff pathology, *Clin Orthop* 267:65, 1991.

Watanabe Y et al: Functional anatomy of the posterolateral structures of the knee, *Arthroscopy* 9:57, 1993.

Watchmaker GP, Lee G, Mackinnon SE: Intraneural topography of the ulnar nerve in the cubital tunnel facilitates anterior transposition, *J Hand Surg Am* 19:915, 1994.

Waters P, Kasser J: Infection of the infrapatellar bursa, *J Bone Joint Surg* 72A:1095, 1990.

Watkins RG: *The spine in sports,* St Louis, 1996, Mosby.

Watson HK, Makhlouf MV: Examination of scaphoid, *J Hand Surg (Am)* 13(5):657-660, 1988.

Watt I: Magnetic resonance imaging in orthopaedics, *J Bone Joint Surg* 73:534, 1991.

Wavreille G et al: Anatomical bases of the second toe composite dorsal flap for simultaneous skin defect coverage and tendinous reconstruction of the dorsal aspect of the fingers, *J Plast Reconst Aesth Surg* (in press, corrected proof).

Wedgewood RJ, Schaller JG: The pediatric arthritides, *Hosp Pract (Off Ed)* 12:83, 1977.

Wehbe MA, Schneider LH: Mallet fractures, *J Bone Joint Surg* 66(5):658-669, 1984.

Weigang E et al: Incidence of neurological complications following overstenting of the left subclavian artery, *Eur J Cardiothorac Surg* 31(4):628-636, 2007.

Weiler PJ, King GJ, Geertzbein SD: Analysis of sagittal plane instability of the lumbar spine in vivo, *Spine* 12:1300, 1990.

Weineck J: *Functional anatomy in sports,* ed 2, St Louis, 1990, Mosby.

Weinerman SA, Bockman RS: Medical therapy of osteoporosis, *Orthop Clin North Am* 21:109, 1990.

Weinstein S: Tactile sensitivity of the phalanges, *Percept Mot Skills* 14:351, 1962.

Weinstein SL, Buckwalter JA: *Turek's orthopaedics principles and their application,* ed 5, Philadelphia, 1994, JB Lippincott.

Weinstein SL: Adolescent idiopathic scoliosis: prevalence and natural history, *Am Acad Orthop Surg Lect* 38:115, 1989.

Weinstein SM, Assessment and rehabilitation of the athlete with a "stinger": a model for the management of noncatastrophic athletic cervical spine injury, *Clin Sports Med* 17(1):127-135, 1998.

Weir J, Abrahams PH: *Imaging atlas of human anatomy,* CD-ROM, version 2.0, London, 1997, Mosby.

Weisl H: Intertrochanteric osteotomy for osteoarthritis, *J Bone Joint Surg* 62B:37, 1980.

Weiss AP, Steichen JB: Synovial sarcoma causing carpal tunnel syndrome, *J Hand Surg* 17A:1024, 1992.

Weiss A-PC, Akelman E, Tabatabai M: Treatment of de Quervain's disease, *J Hand Surg* 19A:595, 1994.

Weiss JM, Ramachandran M: Hip and pelvic injuries in the young athlete, *Oper Tech Sports Med* 14(3):212-217, 2006.

Weiss W, Flippen HJ: The changing incidence and prognosis of tuberculous meningitis, *Am J Med Sci* 250:46, 1965.

Weller IMR, Kunz M: Physical activity and pain following total hip arthroplasty, *Physiotherapy* 93(1):23-29, 2007.

Wenger DR, Ward WT, Herring JA: Legg-Calve-Perthes disease, *J Bone Joint Surg* 73A:778, 1991.

Werner JL, Omer GE Jr: Evaluating cutaneous pressure sensation of the hand, *Am J Occup Ther* 24:247, 1970.

Westkaemper JG, Varitimidis SE, Sotereanos DG, Posterior interosseous nerve palsy in a patient with rheumatoid synovitis of the elbow: a case report and review of the literature, *J Hand Surg* 24(4):727-731, 1999.

Westmark KD, Weissman BN: Complications of axial arthropathies, *Orthop Clin North Am* 21:427, 1990.

White A: Biomechanical stability of the cervical spine, *Clin Orthop* 109:85, 1975.

White AA III, Panjabi MM: *Clinical biomechanics of the spine,* Philadelphia, 1978, JB Lippincott.

White AA III, Panjabi MM: The basic kinematics of the human spine, a review of past and current knowledge, *Spine* 3:12, 1978.

White AA, Panjabi MM: *Clinical biomechanics of the spine,* ed 2, Philadelphia, 1990, Lippincott.

White AA: Kinematics of the normal spine as related to scoliosis, *J Biomech* 4:405, 1971.

White AH, Schofferman JA: *Spine care,* vol 1-2, St Louis, 1995, Mosby.

White G: *Levene's color atlas of dermatology,* ed 2, London, 1997, Mosby-Wolfe.

White G: *Regional dermatology,* London, 1994, Mosby-Wolfe.

White KP, Nielson WR: Cognitive behavioral treatment of fibromyalgia syndrome: a follow-up assessment, *J Rheumatol* 22:717, 1995.

White KP, Speechley M, Harth M, Ostbye T: Fibromyalgia in rheumatology practice: a survey of Canadian rheumatologists, *J Rheumatol* 22:722, 1995.

Whitenack SH et al: Thoracic outlet syndrome complex: diagnoses and treatment. In Hunter JM et al, editors: *Rehabilitation of the hand: surgery and therapy,* ed 3, St Louis, 1990, Mosby.

Whiteside TE: Traumatic kyphosis of the thoracolumbar spine, *Clin Orthop* 128:78, 1977.

Whitmore I, Willan PLT: *Multiple choice questions in human anatomy,* London, 1995, Mosby.

Whitmore RG et al: Bow hunter's syndrome caused by accessory cervical ossification: posterolateral decompression and the use of intraoperative Doppler ultrasonography, *Surg Neurol* 67(2):169-171, 2007.

Whyte Ferguson L: Knee pain: addressing the interrelationships between muscle and joint dysfunction in the hip and pelvis and the lower extremity, *J Bodywork Mov Ther* 10(4):287-296, 2006.

Wicke L: *Atlas of radiographic anatomy,* ed 5, Philadelphia, 1994, Lea & Febiger.

Wickstrom J, LaRocca H: Trauma: head and neck injuries from acceleration-deceleration forces. In Ruge D, Wiltse LL, editors: *Spinal disorders: diagnosis and treatment,* Philadelphia, 1977, Lea & Febiger.

Wiegand R et al: Cervical spine geometry correlated to cervical degenerative disease in a symptomatic group, *J Manipulative Physiol Ther* 26(6):341-346, 2003.

Wiener E et al: Contrast enhanced cartilage imaging: comparison of ionic and non-ionic contrast agents, *Eur J Radiol* (in press, corrected proof).

Wiens E, Lane S: The anterior interosseous nerve syndrome, *Can J Surg* 21:354, 1978.

Wiesel SW, Bernini P, Rothman RH: *The aging lumbar spine,* Philadelphia, 1982, WB Saunders.

Wiesel SW, editor: *The lumbar spine,* Philadelphia, 1990, WB Saunders.

Wiesler ER et al: Ultrasound in the diagnosis of ulnar neuropathy at the cubital tunnel, *J Hand Surg* 31(7):1088-1093, 2006.

Wijnhoven HAH, de Vet HCW, Picavet HSJ: Explaining sex differences in chronic musculoskeletal pain in a general population, *Pain* 124(1-2):158-166, 2006.

Wilder DG: The biomechanics of vibration and low back pain, *Am J Ind Med* 23:577, 1993.

Wiles P, Sweetnam R: *Essentials of orthopaedics,* London, 1965, JA Churchill.

Wilk KE: Rehabilitation of medial capsular injuries. In Greenfield BH, editor: *Rehabilitation of the knee: a problem solving approach,* Philadelphia, 1993, FA Davis.

Wilkerson LA: Ankle injuries in athletes, *Prim Care* 19:337, 1992.

Wilkins RH, Brody IA: Lasègue's sign, *Arch Neurol* 21:219, 1969.

Wilkins RW, Coffman JD: Tests of peripheral vascular efficiency, *Practitioner* 188:346, 1962.

Wilkinson M: The anatomy and pathology of cervical spondylosis, *Proc Roy Soc Lond (Belg)* 57:159, 1964.

Willeford G: *Medical word finder,* West Nyack, NY, 1967, Parker Publishing.

Williams GR, Rockwood CA: Fractures of the scapula. In DeLee JC, Drez D, editors: *Orthopaedic sports medicine: principals and practice,* vol 1, Philadelphia, 1994, WB Saunders.

Williams GR, Rockwood CA: Injuries to the acromioclavicular joint. In DeLee JC, Drez D, editors: *Orthopaedic sports medicine: principals and practice,* vol 1, St Louis, 1994, WB Saunders.

Williams MM, Snyder SJ, Buford D Jr: The Buford complex, the cord-like middle glenohumeral ligament and absent anterosuperior labrum complex; a normal anatomic capsulolabral variant, *Arthroscopy* 10:2417, 1994.

Williams P, Warwick R: *Gray's anatomy,* ed 36, Philadelphia, 1980, WB Saunders.

Williams PF, editor: *Orthopaedic management in childhood,* Oxford, UK, 1982, Blackwell.

Williams TM et al: Verification of the pressure provocative test in carpal tunnel syndrome, *Ann Plast Surg* 19:8, 1992.

Willis Jr WD, Coggeshall RE: *Sensory mechanisms of the spinal cord,* ed 2, New York, 1991, Plenum.

Wilson FC: *The musculoskeletal system,* Philadelphia, 1975, JB Lippincott.

Wilson RM, Fowler P: Arthroscopic anatomy. In Scott WN, editor: *Arthroscopy of the knee: diagnosis and treatment,* Philadelphia, 1990, WB Saunders.

Windsor RE, Lox DM: *Soft tissue injuries: diagnosis and treatment,* Philadelphia, 1998, Hanley & Belfus.

Wing PC, Wilfling FJ, Kokan PJ: *Comprehensive analysis of disability following lumbar intervertebral fusion: medical diagnosis and management,* Philadelphia, 1987, WB Saunders.

Wingstrand H, Wingstrand A, Krantz P: Intracapsular and atmospheric pressure in the dynamics and stability of the hip, *Acta Orthop Scand* 61:231, 1990.

Winter D: *Biomechanics and motor control of human movement,* ed 2, New York, 1990, Wiley-Interscience.

Winternitz WA et al: Acute compartment syndrome of the thigh in sports related injuries not associated with femoral fractures, *Am J Sports Med* 20:476, 1992.

Wiss DA: Supracondylar and intercondylar fractures of the femur. In Rockwood CA, Green DP, Bucholz RW, editors: *Rockwood and Green's fractures in adults,* ed 3, Philadelphia, 1991, JB Lippincott.

Witczak JW, Masear VR, Meyer RD: Triggering of the thumb with de Quervain's stenosing tendovaginitis, *J Hand Surg* 15A:265, 1990.

Withrington RH, Sturge RA, Mitchell N: Osteitis condensans ilii or sacro-iliitis? *Scand J Rheumatol* 14:163, 1985.

Witt J, Pess G, Gelberman RH: Treatment of de Quervain's tenosynovitis: a prospect study of the results of injection of steroids and immobilization in a splint, *J Bone Joint Surg* 73A:219, 1991.

Woerman AL, Binder-Macleod SA: Leg-length discrepancy assessment: accuracy and precision in five clinical methods of evaluation, *J Orthop Sports Phys Ther* 5:230, 1984.

Wolfe F et al: The prevalence and characteristics of fibromyalgia in the general population, *Arthritis Rheum* 38:19, 1995.

Wollin M, Lovell G: Osteitis pubis in four young football players: a case series demonstrating successful rehabilitation, *Phys Ther Sport* 7(4):173-174, 2006.

Wood JE: *The veins,* Boston, 1965, Little, Brown.

Woodhall R, Hayes GJ: The well-leg-raising test, *N Engl J Med* 297:1127, 1977.

Woodland LH, Francis RS: Parameters and comparisons of the quadriceps angle of college-aged men and women in the supine and standing positions, *Am J Sports Med* 20:209, 1992.

Woolf CJ: Somatic pain-pathogenesis and prevention, *Br J Anaesth* 75:169, 1995.

Wray CC, Eason S, Huskinson J: Coccygodynia, aetiology and treatment, *J Bone Joint Surg* 73B:335, 1991.

Wright IS et al: The subclavian steal and other shoulder girdle syndromes, *Trans Am Clin Climatol Assoc* 76:13, 1964.

Wright IS: Neurovascular syndrome produced by hyperabduction of the arms, *Am Heart J* 29:1, 1945.

Wright IS: *Vascular diseases in clinical practice,* Chicago, 1948, Mosby.

Wright V: The shoulder-hand syndrome, *Rep Rheum Dis* 24:1, 1966.

Wu WC, Wong TC, Yip TH: Chronic finger joint instability reconstructed with bone-ligament-bone graft from the iliac crest, *J Hand Surg* 29(5):494-501, 2004.

Wuelker N, Plitz W, Roetman B: Biomechanical data concerning the shoulder impingement syndrome, *Clin Orthop* 303:242, 1994.

Wyke B: Morphological and functional features of the innervation of the costovertebral joints, *Folia Morphol* 23:296, 1975.

Wynne-Davis R: Acetabular dysplasia and familial joint laxity: two etiological factors in congenital dislocation of the hip, *J Bone Joint Surg* 52B:704, 1970.

Wynn-Parry CB: *Rehabilitation of the hand,* ed 3, London, 1973, Butterworths.

Xiao Y, Zhang G, Zuo X: Diagnostic value of high-resolution ultrasonography for imaging of the knee, elbow and wrist joints in rheumatoid arthritis, *Ultrasound Med Biol* 32(5, suppl 1):P253-P268, 2006.

Xu GL et al: Normal variation of the lumbar facet joint capsules, *Clin Anat* 4:11122, 1991.

Xu GL, Haughton VM, Carrera GF: Lumbar facet joint capsule: appearance at MR imaging and CT, *Radiology* 177:415, 1990.

Yacoe ME et al: Dupuytren's contracture: MR imaging findings and correlation between MR signal intensity and cellularity of lesions, *AJR Am J Roentgenol* 160:813, 1993.

Yagci N et al: Relationship between balance performance and musculoskeletal pain in lower body comparison healthy middle aged and older adults, *Arch Gerontol Geriatr* 45(1):109-119, 2007.

Yahara ML: Shoulder. In Richardson JK, Iglarsh ZA, editors: *Clinical orthopaedic physical therapy,* Philadelphia, 1994, WB Saunders.

Yamada K et al: Scoliosis associated with Prader-Willi syndrome, *Spine J* 7(3):345-348, 2007.

Yamamoto M et al: Psychological aspects of psychogenic deafness in children, *Int J Pediatric Otorhinolaryngol* 21(2):113-120, 1991.

Yamazaki H et al: The two locations of ganglions causing radial nerve palsy, *J Hand Surg* (in press, corrected proof).

Yang RS, Tsuang YH, Liu TK: Traumatic dislocation of the hip, *Clin Orthop* 265:218, 1991.

Yao L et al: Plantar plate of the foot: findings on conventional arthrography and MR imaging, *AMJ Am J Roentgenol* 163:641, 1994.

Yashon D: *Spinal injury,* New York, 1978, Appleton-Century-Crofts.

Yates PJ et al: Early MRI diagnosis and non-surgical management of spontaneous osteonecrosis of the knee, *Knee* 14(2):112-116, 2007.

Yazaki N et al: Bilateral Kienbock's disease, *J Hand Surg* 30(2):133-136, 2005.

Yeamans DC et al: Pain, management of. In *Encyclopedia of the Social & Behavioral Sciences,* Oxford, UK, 2001, Pergamon.

Yelin E: Musculoskeletal conditions and employment, *Arthritis Care Res* 8:311, 1995.

Yergason RM: Supination sign, *J Bone Joint Surg* 12:160, 1931.

Yochum T, Rowe L: *Essentials of skeletal radiology,* ed 2, Baltimore, 1996, Williams & Wilkins.

Yochum TR, Rowe LJ: Measurements in skeletal radiology. In Yochum TR, Rowe LJ, editors: *Essentials of skeletal radiology,* vol 1, Baltimore, 1987, Williams & Wilkins.

Yochum TR: *A closer look at spondylolisthesis,* East Rutherford, NJ, 1990, NYCC Second Multidisciplinary Symposium.

Yogasakaran S, Menezes F: Acute neuropathic pain after surgery: are we treating them early/late? *Acute Pain* 7(3):145-149, 2005.

Yokoyama T et al: Neurological findings for screening thoracic myelopathy, *Spine J* 4(5, suppl 1):S30, 2004.

Yorgancigil H, Karahan N, Baydar ML: Multiple loose bodies in the joints: from snowstorm to hailstones, *Arthroscopy* 20(8):e113-e116, 2004.

Yoshizawa H, Kobayashi S, Hachiya Y: Blood supply of nerve roots and dorsal root ganglia, *Orthop Clin North Am* 22:195, 1991.

Yosipovitch G et al: Trigger finger in young patients with insulin dependent diabetes, *J Rheumatol* 17:951, 1990.

Young D, Zimmerman G, Toomey M: Osteitis pubis, *J Sci Med Sport* 2(1, suppl 1): 94-260, 1999.

Young DC, Rockwood CA: Fractures of the clavicle. In DeLee JC, Drez D, editors: *Orthopaedic sports medicine: principals and practice,* vol 1, Philadelphia, 1994, WB Saunders.

Young JWR, Mirvis SE, editors: *Imaging in trauma and critical care,* Baltimore, 1991, Williams & Wilkins.

Younger CP, DeFiore JC: Rupture of the flexor tendons to the fingers after a Colles' fracture: a case report, *J Bone Joint Surg* 59A:828, 1977.

Yousem DM: *Case review head and neck imaging,* St Louis, 1998, Mosby.

Yuen EC, Olney RK, So YT: Sciatic neuropathy: clinical and prognostic features in 73 patients, *Neurology* 44:1669, 1994.

Yuen EC, So YT, Olney RK: The electrophysiologic features of sciatic neuropathy in 100 patients, *Muscle Nerve* 18:414, 1995.

Yunus M et al: Primary fibromyalgia (fibrositis): clinical study of 50 patients with matched normal controls, *Semin Arthritis Rheum* 11(1):151-171, 1981.

Zacher J, Gursche A: 'Hip' pain, *Best Pract Res Clin Rheumatol* 17(1):71-85, 2003.

Zamir E, Read RW, Rao NA: Self-inflicted anterior scleritis, *Ophthalmology* 108(1): 192-195, 2001.

Zangger P et al: Assessing damage in individual joints in rheumatoid arthritis: a new method based on the Larsen system, *Joint Bone Spine* 71(5):389-396, 2004.

Zatouroff M: *Diagnosis in color physical signs in general medicine,* ed 2, London, 1996, Mosby-Wolfe.

Zeitz K, McCutcheon H: Observations and vital signs: ritual or vital for the monitoring of postoperative patients? *Appl Nurs Res* 19(4):204-211, 2006.

Zembsch A et al: Positioning device for optimal active kinematic real-time magnetic resonance imaging of the knee joint: a technical note, *Clin Biomech* 13(4-5): 308-313, 1998.

Ziadeh MJ, Richardson JK: Arnold-Chiari malformation with syrinx presenting as carpal tunnel syndrome: a case report, *Arch Phys Med Rehabil* 85(1):158-161, 2004.

Zitelli BJ, Davis HW: *Atlas of pediatric physical diagnosis,* ed 2, London, 1992, Wolfe.

Zoega H: Fracture of the lower end of the radius with ulnar nerve palsy, *J Bone Joint Surg* 48V:514, 1966.

Zsoter T, Cronin RFP: Venous distensibility in patients with varicose veins, *Can Med Assoc J* 94:1293, 1966.

Zwierska I et al: Upper- vs lower-limb aerobic exercise rehabilitation in patients with symptomatic peripheral arterial disease: a randomized controlled trial, *J Vasc Surg* 42(6):1122-1123, 2005.

INDEX

Note: Entries followed by "b" indicate boxes; "f" figures; "t" tables.

A

Abbott-Saunders test,
174-175, 175f
Abduction
relief sign, 83-86, 84t, 86f
stress test, 574-575, 575f
Abductor
system insufficiency,
562-563, 563f
weakness, generalized,
505-507, 506f
Ability depreciation
assessment, 42b
Abnormal sacroiliac joint
movement
rotational shifting,
504, 504f
torsion, 502-503, 502f
Abscess, gluteal,
457-458, 458f
Acceleration-deceleration
injury, 126, 127t-128t
syndrome, 119-121,
119t-120t, 121f
Acetabular syndromes
dysplasia, 536
fracture, 485
Achilles tendon
rupture, 657-658, 658f
swelling, 624
Acromion change types, 216
Active straight-leg-raise
(ASLR) test, 438
Activities of daily living
(ADL), 43-45
Actual leg-length test,
534-535, 535f.
See also Leg-length.
Acute inflammatory spine
lesion, 337-340, 340f
Acute whiplash associated
disorder (WAD),
112-115, 112t-114t, 115f
AD. *See* Alzheimer
disease (AD).
Adams positions, 312-317,
313t-314t, 315f
Adams test, supported,
483-484, 483f

Adduction stress test,
576-577, 577f
Adhesion
dura matter-fibrous tissue,
135-137, 137f
dural sleeve, 367-368,
368f, 385-386, 386f,
415-417, 416f
ischiotrochanteric groove,
406-407, 407f
shoulder capsulitis,
135-137, 137t
ADL. *See* Activities of daily
living (ADL).
Adson procedures
Adson test, 176-177, 177f
modified Adson
maneuver, 97
Adult-onset osteonecrosis,
546-548, 548f
Adventitial cystic disease,
637
Allen test, 268-271,
269b-270b, 271f
Allis sign, 536-538, 538f
Altman Classification,
modified, 403
Alzheimer disease (AD), 339t
Amoss sign, 316-317,
316t, 317f
Anatomic leg-length
difference, 541. *See also*
Leg-length.
Anatomy essentials
elbow, 232-233
forearm, wrist, and hand,
259-261
knee, 571
lower leg, ankle, and foot,
624-625
pelvis and sacroiliac joint,
477-478
spine
cervical, 11, 70-72
lumbar, 356
thoracic, 332t
Anderson/
D'Alonzo odontoid
process fracture
classification, 131

Anesthesia
face, 718-719, 719f
feigned, 732-733, 733f
regional test, 732-733, 733f
simulated, 722, 722f
Anghelescu sign, 318-320,
320f
Ankle, foot, and lower leg
assessments
anatomy essentials for,
624-625
cross-reference tables for
ankle-foot differentiation
by onset, 623t
by procedure, 619t-621t
by syndrome or tissue,
622t
fundamentals of, 617-625
procedures
anterior drawer sign,
ankle, 631-632, 632f
Buerger test, 633-634,
634f
circumference test, calf,
635-636, 636f
claudication test,
637-638, 638f
Duchenne sign,
639-640, 640f
foot tourniquet test,
641-642, 642f
Helbings sign, 643, 643f
Hoffa sign, 644, 644f
Homans sign, 645, 645f
imaging studies, 630-631
Keen sign, 646-647, 647f
Morton test, 648-649,
648t, 649f
Moses test, 652, 652f
Moszkowicz test,
650-651, 651f
motion assessments,
625-627, 626f-627f
muscle function
assessments,
627-629, 628f-629f
Perthes test, 653-654,
654f
Strunsky sign, 655-656,
656f

Ankle, foot, and lower leg
assessments—cont'd
Thompson test, 657-658,
658f
Tinel sign, foot,
659-660, 660f
of syndromes and tissues
adventitial cystic
disease, 637
anterolateral
compartment
syndrome,
639-640, 640f
arterial insufficiency,
641-642, 642f
arterial occlusive disease,
637-638, 638f
arteriosclerosis
obliterans, 652, 652f
atrophy, 635-636, 636f
collateral circulation
inadequacy, 650-
651, 651f
compartment syndrome,
641-642, 642f
fistula, arteriovenous,
650-651, 651f
forefoot disorders,
655-656, 656f
fracture, calcaneus,
644, 644f
fracture, distal fibular
vs. distal tibular,
646-647, 647f
hypertrophy, 635-636,
636f
ischemia, Volkmann,
635-636, 636f
Klippel Trenaunay
syndrome,
650-651, 651f
metatarsalgia, 648-649,
648t, 649f
Morton neuroma,
648-649, 648t, 649f
peripheral vascular
disease (PVD),
633-634, 634f
pes planus, 643, 643f
popliteal artery
entrapment
syndrome, 637
rupture, Achilles tendon,
657-658, 658f
saphenous vein valve
incompetencies,
653-654, 654f
sprain, anterior
talofibular ligament,
631-632, 632f
superficial varicosities,
653-654, 654f

Ankle, foot, and lower leg
assessments—cont'd
swelling, Achilles
tendon, 624
tarsal tunnel syndrome,
659-660, 660f
thrombophlebitis,
645, 645f
vascular compromise,
633-634, 634f
Ankylosing spondylitis
(AS), 24-26, 316-317,
316t, 317f, 324, 324f,
328-329, 329f
Anosmia, feigned, 712-713,
713f
Antalgia sign, 362-366,
363t, 364f-366f
Anterior cruciate ligament
injury, 589-592, 591f-
592f, 597-600, 598f,
600f, 610-611, 610f
Anterior drawer sign, ankle,
631-632, 632f
Anterior drawer test,
positive, 590
Anterior innominate test,
480-482, 482f
Anterior interosseous nerve
syndrome, 288
Anterior sacroiliac ligament
injury, 514-515, 514f
sprain, 489-490, 490f
Anterior shoulder dislocation
trauma, 182-183,
182f-183f
Anterior vertebral
compression fracture,
462
Anterolateral syndromes
compartment, 639-640,
640f
rotary instability, 601,
601f, 610-611, 610f
Anteromedial bundle injury,
589-592, 591f-592f
Anteversion, femoral, 608-
609, 609f
Anvil test, 539-540, 540f
Apex test, 504, 504f
Apley compression test,
578-579, 579f
Apparent leg-length test,
541-542, 542f.
See also Leg-length.
Apprehension test
patella, 580-581, 581f
shoulder dislocation
trauma, 182-183,
182f-183f
Arc measurements, 229t
Arc of movement, 53-54

Arcuate-popliteus complex
injury, 589-592,
591f-592f, 597-600,
598f, 600f, 610-611, 610f
Arnold international
classification, modified,
383
Arterial insufficiency,
641-642, 642f
Arterial occlusive disease,
637-638, 638f
Arteriosclerosis obliterans,
652, 652f
Arteriovenous fistula,
650-651, 651f
Arthritis
ankylosing spondylitis,
(AS), 24-26, 316-317,
316t, 317f, 324, 324f,
328-329, 329f
basal thumb joint, 274, 274f
imaging studies and, 24-26
Larsen rheumatoid
arthritis grading
system, 424t-425t,
424t-426t
lumbar, 423-427, 424t-
426t, 427f
osteoarthritis (OA), 26
psoriatic arthritis (PA), 25
rheumatoid arthritis (RA),
24-26
spondyloarthropathies,
352t-353t
tuberculosis (TB), hip,
546-548, 548f
Arthrography, contrast, 31
Arthrosis, 423-427,
424t-426t, 427f
AS. *See* Ankylosing
spondylitis (AS).
ASLR test. *See* Active
straight-leg-raise
(ASLR) test.
Assessments
cardinal symptoms and
signs and, 37-62
elbow, 226-252
forearm, wrist, and hand,
253-301
fundamentals of, 1-36
hip, 516-563
knee, 564-616
lower leg, ankle, and foot,
617-660
malingering, 661-762
pelvis and sacroiliac joint,
473-515
shoulder, 157-225
spine
cervical, 63-156
lumbar, 344-472

Assessments—cont'd
  thoracic, 302-343
Ataxia, 732-733, 733f
Atlantoaxial injury, 133,
  140-142, 141t, 142f
Atonic bladder, 62
Atrophy
  lower extremity,
    635-636, 636f
  muscular, 59-60, 60t
Avascular necrosis, 230,
  246, 544
Axial trunk-loading test,
  691-693, 692t, 693f
Axillary artery neurovascular
  compromise, 222-223,
  223f
Axillary pseudoaneurysm,
  184

B

B test, 662
Back screening, 451-452,
  452f
Bakody procedures
  Bakody sign, 83-86,
    84t, 86f
  reverse Bakody maneuver,
    209-210, 210f
Ballottement test, 606, 606f
Barlow test, 536
Barré-Liéou sign, 87-89, 89f
Barthel index, 743-744
Basal thumb joint arthritis,
  274, 274f
Basilar artery stenosis,
  153-156, 156f
Bayes theorem, 3
Bechterew sitting test,
  367-368, 368f
Beevor sign, 321-323, 323f
Beighton criteria, 56-58, 58b
Belt test, 483-484, 483f
Bench test, 694-695, 695f
Benign soft-tissue
  tumors, 457
Biceps tendon
  long head
    injury, 220-221, 221f
    instability, 187
    rupture, 206, 206f
  overuse injury, 203-205,
    205f
  tendinitis, 174-175, 175f,
    215, 215f
Bikele sign, 91-92, 91f
Bilateral foot drop, 759t
Bilateral hamstring spasms,
  421-422, 422f
Bilateral hand activity
  index, 753

Bilateral leg-lowering test,
  369-370, 370f
Bilateral limb-dropping test,
  742-745, 745f
Bilateral straight-leg-raise
  test, 380-381, 381f
Bimalleolar fracture, 646
Binocular blindness, 716.
  See also Blindness.
Bipolar disorders, 760b
Bladder control, 62
Blindness
  feigned, 712-713, 713f
  feigned color blindness,
    735-737, 736t, 737f
  simulated, 716-717, 717f
  total binocular, 716
Blinking, reflex, 720-721
Blond McIndoe cold
  intolerance symptom
  severity (CISS)
  questionnaire, 294t-295t
Bony pelvis fracture,
  511-513, 512f
Boot-top fracture, 646
Borg pain scales, 673
Bounce home test, 582-583,
  583f
Bowstring procedures
  bowstring sign, 371-372,
    372f
  Forestier bowstring sign,
    328-329, 329f
Boxer's elbow, 230-231
Bracelet test, 272-273, 273f
Brachial plexus
  neurovascular
    compression,
    174-175, 175f
  plexopathy, 232t
  tension test, 93-94, 94f
Bragard sign, 373, 373f
Brainstem
  ischemia, 148
  syndromes, 155
Brudzinski/Kernig sign,
  139, 400-402, 402f
Bryant sign, 184-185, 185f
Buerger test, 633-634, 634f
Bundle injury, 589-592,
  591f-592f
Burns bench test, 694-695,
  695f
Bursitis
  gluteal, 457-458, 458f
  radiohumeral, 240-242,
    240t-241t, 242f
  subacromial, 192-193,
    193f, 232t
Buttock, sign of the,
  457-458, 458f

C

Calcaneus fracture, 644, 644f
Calf circumference test,
  635-636, 636f
Can test, 224
Capital epiphysis, 551
Capitellum avascular
  necrosis, 230, 246
Capsular sprain, lumbosacral,
  483-484, 483f
Capsule injury
  posterolateral, 599-600,
    600f, 610-611, 610f
  posteromedial, 589-592,
    591f-592f
Capsulitis
  facet, 100-104, 101t-102t,
    103f
  shoulder adhesion,
    135-137, 137t
Caput ulnae syndrome,
  272-273, 273f
Cardinal symptoms and
  signs, 37-62
  cardinal presenting
    symptoms, 39-45
    ability depreciation
      assessment, 42b
    activities of daily living
      (ADL) assessment,
      43-45
    disability and handicap,
      42-45
    disability PILS, 5b, 42b
    function assessments,
      12-14, 45. *See also*
      Function assessments.
    pain and sensibility,
      39-40
    peripheral nociceptors, 41
    regional periarticular
      syndromes, 40t-41t
    stiffness, 41-42
    weakness, 41
  cardinal signs, 47-62
    arc of movement, 53-54
    Beighton criteria,
      56-58, 58b
    bladder control, 62
    circulation, decreased,
      47-48
    cramps, 61
    crepitation, 58-59, 59t
    edema, joint *vs.* soft-
      tissue, 48, 48t
    erythema, 49, 49t-51t
    fasciculations, 60-61
    fixed deformity, 54-55,
      54t-55t
    gait impairment, 62
    impaired micturition, 62

Cardinal symptoms and signs—cont'd
joint plane motion, 56t
Leeds Assessment of Neuropathic Symptoms and Signs (LANSS) Pain Scale, 52b-53b
movement, 56-58, 56t, 58b
muscular atrophy, 59-60, 60t
part dimension changes, 47
posture, 47
range-of-motion (ROM), 56
skin changes, 48-49
spasm, 61
stability, 58, 58t
swelling sites, diffuse, 48, 48t
systemic lupus erythematosus (SLE), 49, 49t-51t
tenderness, 51
tetany, 61-62
tremor classification, 61t
warmth, 51
fundamentals of, 37-39
palpation and, 39
system illness, 45-47
emotional liability, 45-46
fatigue, 45
referred symptoms, 46-47, 46t-47t
sleep disturbance, 45
visual inspection and, 37-38
Carotid artery stenosis, 153-156, 156f
Carpal lift sign, 275, 275f
Carpal system injury, 257
Carpal tunnel syndrome (CPS), 232t, 286-287, 286f-287f
Carpometacarpal articulation internal derangement, 276, 276f
Cascade sign, 276, 276f
Castellvi classification, 374t
Cauda equina syndrome, 459-460, 460f
Cerebellar injury, 155
Cerebral palsy (CP)
hemiplegic movement patterns, 746
Cervical collapse sign, 106, 115, 146

Cervical compression test
foraminal, 83-86, 84t, 86f, 105-106, 106f, 209-210, 210f
maximum, 119-121, 119t-120t, 121f
Cervical rib thoracic outlet syndrome (TOS), 174-177, 175f, 177f, 189. *See also* Thoracic outlet syndrome (TOS).
Cervical spine assessments, 63-156
anatomy essentials for, 11, 70-72
cross reference tables for
by procedure, 65t-66t
by syndrome or tissue, 67t-68t
fundamentals of, 63-72
procedures
Bakody sign, 83-86, 84t, 86f
Barré-Liéou sign, 87-89, 89f
Bikele sign, 91-92, 91f
brachial plexus tension test, 93-94, 94f
cervical collapse sign, 106, 115, 146
compression test, foraminal, 83-86, 84t, 86f, 105-106, 106f
compression test, Jackson, 112-115, 112t-114t, 115f
compression test, maximum cervical, 119-121, 119t-120t, 121f
compression test, Naffziger, 122-123, 123f
concave *vs.* convex test, 119-121, 119t-120t, 121f
cramp test, 120
Dejerine sign, 95-96, 95f
DeKleyn test, 97-99, 99f
distraction test, 100-104, 101t, 103f
doorbell sign, 94
extension rotation test, 97
finger-flexion test, 120
Hallpike maneuver, 107-109, 108f
Hautant test, 110-111, 111f
Houle test, 97
imaging studies, 80-82, 81b, 82t

Cervical compression test—cont'd
Kernig/Brudzinski sign, 139
Lhermitte sign, 116-118, 117t, 118f
Maigne test, 97-98
modified Adson maneuver, 97
motion assessments, 72-76, 73f-77f
muscle function assessments, 77-80, 77f-80f
O'Donoghue maneuver, 124-130, 127t-128t, 129f-130f
provocative tests, common, 69t-70t
reclination test, sitting, 97-98
Rust sign, 131-134, 132t, 133f-134f
scalene relief test, 120
shoulder abduction relief sign, 83-86, 84t, 86f
shoulder depression test, 135-137, 137f
Smith and Estridge maneuver, 97-98
Soto-Hall sign, 138-139, 139f
spinal percussion test, 140-142, 141t, 142f
Spurling test, 143-146, 143t-144t, 145f-146f
swallowing test, 147, 147f
triad of Dejerine, 95-96, 95f
Underburg test, 148-150, 150f
Valsalva maneuver, neuro-orthopedic application, 151-152, 152f
vertebral artery patency tests, 97
vertebrobasilar artery functional maneuver, 153-156, 156f
Wallenberg test, 97
of syndromes or tissues
acceleration-deceleration syndromes, 119-121, 119t-120t, 121f, 126, 127t-128t
acute whiplash associated disorders (WAD), 112-115, 112t-114t, 115f

Cervical compression
test—cont'd
adhesion, dura matter-
fibrous tissue
adhesion degrees,
135-137, 137f
atlantoaxial injury, 133,
140-141, 141t, 142,
142f
capsulitis, shoulder
adhesion, 135-137,
137f
cervical disc syndromes,
101t, 143t-144t
compression, C5 nerve
root, 93-94, 94f
compression, carotid
artery, 153-156, 156f
compression, cervical
nerve root
compression
syndrome, 143-146,
143t-144t, 145f-146f
compression, nerve root,
83-86, 84t, 86f,
93-94, 94f, 100-104,
101t-102t, 103f,
112-115, 112t-114t,
115f
encroachment,
intervertebral
foraminal, 100-104,
101t-102t, 103f
encroachment, nerve
root, 105-106, 106f
epidural fibrosis, 136
exostosis, cervical spine,
138-139, 139f
exostosis, degenerative
joint disease, 112-
115, 112t-114t, 115f
facet capsulitis, 100-
104, 101t-102t, 103f
facet syndrome, 119-
121, 119t-120t, 121f
facial purpura, 153
fracture, odontoid
process, 131-134,
132t, 133f-134f
fracture, spinal
compression, 95-96,
95f
fracture, upper cervical
spine, 131-134, 132t,
133f-134f
fracture, vertebral, 138-
139, 139f
herniation, intervertebral
disc, 95-96, 95f,
112-115, 112t-114t,
115f, 151-152, 152f

Cervical compression
test—cont'd
Horner syndrome, 110
inflammatory edema,
112-115, 112t-114t,
115f
intimal arterial wall
damage, 148
irritation, febrile
meningeal, 138-139,
139f
ischemia, brainstem, 148
ischemia,
vertebrobasilar, 154
ischemic symptoms,
vertebrobasilar
arterial, 107
lesion, intervertebral
disc, 138-139, 139f,
147, 147f
locked-in syndrome
(LIS), 88
meningitis, brachial
plexus, 91-92, 91f
meningitis, nosocomial,
138-139, 139f
muscular strain,
119-121, 119t-120t,
121f
myelopathy, cervical
spine, 116-118, 117t,
118f
myofascial pain
syndrome, 119-121,
119t-120t, 121f, 141t
nerve root compression
syndrome, 119-121,
119t-120t, 121f
neuritis, brachial plexus,
91-92, 91f
neuropathies, 117
osseous injury,
140-141, 141t, 142,
142f
osteophyte, cervical
spine anterior
portion, 147, 147f
osteophytes, 151-152,
152f
progressive degenerative
cervical spinal canal
narrowing, 116-118,
117t, 118f
protrusion, intervertebral
disc, 95-96, 95f
radiculopathies, 101t-102t
rheumatoid arthritis
(RA), upper cervical,
131-134, 132t, 133f-
134f
sleep palsy, 93

Cervical compression
test—cont'd
soft-tissue injury,
140-141, 141t,
142f
space-occupying lesion,
112-115, 112t-114t,
115f
space-occupying mass,
122-123, 123f, 147,
147f, 151-152, 152f
spondylosis, 151-152,
152f
sprain, ligamentous,
126, 138-139, 139f,
147, 147f
sprain, severe cervical
spine, 131-134, 132t,
133f-134f
stenosis, basilar/carotid/
vertebral artery,
153-156, 156f
strain, isometric
muscular, 124-130,
124t, 127t-128t,
129f-130f
strain, muscular, 138-
139, 139f, 147, 147f
subluxation, cervical
spine, 138-139, 139f
subluxation, nerve root,
112-115, 112t-114t,
115f
subluxation, severe
upper cervical spine,
131-134, 132t, 133f-
134f
tumor, intervertebral,
147, 147f
tumor, spinal cord,
95-96, 95f
vasospasm, 149
vertebral artery
syndrome, 87-90,
89f, 97-99, 99f,
110-111, 111f
vertebrobasilar artery
(VBA) insufficiency,
107-109, 108f,
153-156, 156f, 156t
vertebrobasilar artery
(VBA) syndrome,
148-150, 150f
Wallenberg syndrome,
110
Chest expansion test, 324,
324f
Chief complaint, 6
Chiene test, 543-545, 545f
Childress duck waddle test,
584-585, 585f

Chondromalacia patellae, 586-588, 588f

Chronic syndromes
arterial occlusive disease, 637-638, 638f
lateral epicondylitis, 240-242, 240t-241t, 242f
lumbar strain, 480t
recurrent shoulder dislocation, 194

Circulation, decreased, 47-48

Circumference test
calf, 635-636, 636f
thigh, 614, 614f

CISS questionnaire.
See Cold intolerance symptom severity (CISS) questionnaire.

Clarke sign, 586-588, 588f

Claudication test, 637-638, 638f

Clinical laboratory tests, 14-20
interpretation of, 14
listing of, 16b-19b
for low back pain diagnoses, 15t
synovial fluid tests, 19-20, 19b-20b

Clinical reasoning, pain-based, 6

Codman sign, 187-188, 188f

Cold intolerance symptom severity (CISS) questionnaire, 294t-295t

Collapse sign, cervical, 106, 115, 146

Collateral circulation inadequacy, 650-651, 651f

Collateral ligament
injury, lateral, 576-577, 577f, 599-600, 600f, 610-611, 610f
instability, lateral *vs.* medial, 243-244, 244f, 248-249, 248f-249f

Colles fracture, 285, 285f

Color blindness, feigned, 735-737, 736t, 737f

Coma, Glasgow outcome scale, 138-139, 139f, 723-724

Compartment syndrome
anterolateral, 639-640, 640f
lower extremity, 641-642, 642f

Complex regional pain syndrome type I (CRPS-I) diagnostic criteria, 383

Compression tests
Apley, 578-579, 579f
cervical foraminal, 83-86, 84t, 86f, 105-106, 106f, 209-210, 210f
fracture
anterior vertebral, 462
spinal, 95-96, 95f
iliac, 495-496, 495f
interscalene, 209-210, 210f
Jackson, 112-115, 112t-114t, 115f
knee, 578-579, 579f, 604-605, 605f
maximum cervical, 119-121, 119t-120t, 121f
Naffziger, 122-123, 123f
nerve, 294-296, 294t-295t, 296f
neurovascular, subclavian artery, 176-177, 177f
Noble, 604-605, 605f
shoulder, 213-214, 214f
sternal, 341-343, 342t, 343f
vertebral deformities, 311

Computed tomography (CT), 27-28, 29t-31t.
See also Tomography.

Concave *vs.* convex test, 119-121, 119t-120t, 121f

Congenital syndromes
hip articulation dislocation, 551-552, 552f
hip dysplasia, 536
pain insensitivity, 738, 738f
subluxation, 536

Contracture
Dupuytren, 232t
flexion, 560, 560f
gracilis muscle, 560, 560f
iliotibial band, 556-557, 557f
interphalangeal capsular, 274, 274f

Contrast arthrography, 31

Conventional radiography, 21-27, 21t

Convex *vs.* concave test, 119-121, 119t-120t, 121f

Coordination-disturbance testing, 714-715, 715f

Coordination loss, nonorganic, 714-715, 715f

Costal structures
fracture, 341-343, 342t, 343f
hypermobile *vs.* hypomobile, 331, 331f

Costal structures—cont'd
tissue integrity, 332-333, 333f

Costochondritis, 341-343, 342t, 343f

Costoclavicular conditions
costoclavicular maneuver, 189-191, 190f-191f
costoclavicular syndrome, 189
neurovascular space narrowing, 211

Costovertebral syndrome, 342t

Cotton fracture, 646

Cox sign, 374-375, 374t, 375f

Coxa vara, 533

Cozen test, 240-242, 240t-241t, 242f

CPS. *See* Carpal tunnel syndrome (CPS).

Cramps
as cardinal sign, 61
cramp test, 120

Cranial nerves, 10

Crepitation, 58-59, 59t

Crescendo transient ischemic attacks (TIAs), 154

Cross-over sign, 385-386, 386f

Cross-reference tables
by procedure
elbow, 277t
forearm, wrist, and hand, 254t-255t
knee, 565t-567t
lower leg, ankle, and foot, 619t-621t
malingering, 667t-669t
pelvis and sacroiliac joint, 474t-475t
shoulder, 158t-159t
spine, cervical, 65t-66t
spine, lumbar, 345t-349t
spine, thoracic, 303t-304t
by syndrome or tissue
elbow, 277t
forearm, wrist, and hand, 256t
knee, 568t-569t
lower leg, ankle, and foot, 622t-623t
malingering, 670t
pelvis and sacroiliac joint, 476t
shoulder, 160t-161t
spine, cervical, 67t-68t
spine, lumbar, 350t-352t
spine, thoracic, 305t

CRPS-I criteria.
See Complex Regional
Pain Syndrome Type I
(CRPS-I) diagnostic
criteria.
Cruciate ligament injury,
589-592, 591f-592f,
597-600, 598f, 600f,
610-611, 610f
CT. *See* Computed
tomography (CT).
Cubital tunnel syndrome,
243-244, 244f
Cuignet test, 716-717, 717f
Cysts, ganglion, 294

D

Dallas pain
questionnaire, 673
Dawbarn sign, 192-193, 193f
De Quervain tenosynovitis,
232t
Deafness, simulated,
710-721, 721f
Decreased circulation, 47-48
Deep-tendon reflexes, 9-10
Deficiency
leg-length, 534-535, 535f
structural, femoral *vs.*
tibial portion,
536-538, 538f
Deformity, fixed, 54-55,
54t-55t
Degenerative syndromes
disc disease, 363-366,
363t-364t, 365f-366f
joint disease exostosis,
112-115, 112t-114t,
115f
rotator cuff tendinitis,
180-181, 180f-181f
scapholunate advance
collapse (SLAC), 265
wrist articulation,
272-273, 273f
Dejerine sign, 95-96, 95f
Dejour's classification, 595
DeKleyn test, 97-99, 99f
Dellon moving two-point
discrimination test,
277-278, 278f
Demianoff sign, 376-377,
377f
Denervation
hypersensitivity, 431-433,
432t
peripheral, 290, 290f
Depression and depressive
disorders, 663b, 760b
Depression test, shoulder,
135-137, 137f

Derangement
carpometacarpal
articulations, 276, 276f
elbow, 301. 301f
hand, 301. 301f
phalanges internal
derangement, 276, 276f
wrist derangement, 301.
301f
Dermatographism, 339
Dermatologic changes, 48-49
Dermatome sensory
disturbances, 277-278,
278f
Destructive processes, spine,
318-320, 320f
Deyerle sign, 378-379, 379f
Diagnostic imaging
modalities. *See* Imaging
studies.
Diagnostic laboratory tests,
14-20
interpretation of, 14
listing of, 16b-19b
for low back pain
diagnoses, 15t
synovial fluid tests,
19-20, 19b-20b
Differential sign, Lasègue,
403-405, 404t, 405f
Diffuse joint swelling, 48, 48t
DII. *See* Disease Impact
Index (DII).
Dimension changes, 47
Diminished peripheral nerve
sensibility, 298-300,
299f
Disability PILS, 5b, 42b
Disc syndromes
extrusion, 364
fragmentation, 455
lesion, 367-370, 368f, 370f,
373, 373f, 415-417,
416f, 454
protrusion, 364, 418-419,
418f
rupture, 420, 420f
Discography, 28
Discoid meniscus, 582
Discrepancy
leg-length, apparent,
541-542, 542f
leg-length, true, 534-535,
535f
Disease Impact Index (DII),
673b
Disease repercussion profile,
672-673
Dislocation
hip, 543-545, 545f,
551-552, 552f

Dislocation—cont'd
proximal interphalangeal,
291, 291f
shoulder, 194-195, 201-
202, 202f
anterior, 174-175, 175f,
182-183, 182f-183f
chronic recurrent,
194-195
glenohumeral
articulation,
184-185, 185f
posterior humerus,
182-183, 182f-183f
Displacement test, 612-613,
613f
Disputed neurogenic
thoracic outlet syndrome
(dnTOS), 178. *See also*
Thoracic outlet
syndrome (TOS).
Distal fibular fracture,
646-647, 647f
Distal tingling on percussion
(DTP) sign, 251-252,
252f, 292-293, 293f
Distraction test
Apley, 578-579, 579f
cervical spine, 100-104,
101t, 103f
knee, 578-579, 579f
dnTOS. *See* Disputed
neurogenic thoracic
outlet syndrome
(dnTOS).
Doorbell sign, 94
Doppler ultrasonic vascular
testing, 36
Double-leg-raise test,
380-381, 381f
Draftsman's elbow, 231
Drawer test, 589-592,
591f-592f
ankle, 631-632, 632f
Gerber and Ganz, 182-
183, 182f-183f
knee, 589-592, 591f-592f
positive anterior, 590
positive posterior, 581
Drop arm test, 187-188,
188f
Dryer sign, 593-594, 594f
DSM-III-R, mood disorders,
760b
DTP sign. *See* Distal
tingling on percussion
(DTP) sign.
Duchenne sign, 639-640,
640f
Duck waddle test, 584-585,
585f

Dugas test, 194-195, 195f
Dupuytren contracture, 232t
Dura matter-fibrous tissue
   adhesion, 135-137, 137f
Dural sleeve adhesion, 367-
   368, 368f, 385-386,
   386f, 415-417, 416f
Dysplasia, hip, 536
Dystonia, 440-442, 441f

E

Early pondyloarthropathy,
   339t
Edema
   inflammatory, 112-115,
      112t-114t, 115f
   joint vs. soft-tissue, 48, 48t
Effort thrombosis, 196
Elbow assessments, 226-252
   anatomy essentials for,
      232-233
   cross-reference tables for
      by procedure, 277t
      by syndrome and tissue,
         277t
   fundamentals of, 226-233
   procedures
      Cozen test, 240-242,
         240t-241t, 242f
      functional arc
         measurements, 229t
      Golfer elbow test, 245,
         245f
      imaging studies, 239, 246
      Kaplan sign, 246-247,
         247f
      ligamentous instability
         test, 248-249,
         248f-249f
      motion assessments,
         233-235, 233f-235f
      muscle function
         assessments,
         236-239, 236f-238f
      Tinel sign, 251-252, 252f
      Wadsworth elbow
         flexion test, 243-244,
         244f
   of syndromes or tissues
      boxer's elbow, 230-231
      bursitis, radiohumeral,
         240-242, 240t-241t,
         242f
      collateral ligament
         instability, lateral vs.
         medial, 248-249,
         248f-249f
      cubital tunnel syndrome,
         243-244, 244f
      derangement, 301, 301f
      draftsman's elbow, 231

Elbow assessments—cont'd
   epicondylitis, lateral,
      240-242, 240t-241t,
      242f, 246-247, 247f,
      250, 250f
   epicondylitis, medial,
      245, 245f
   hyperextension overload
      syndrome, 230-231
   little leaguer's elbow, 230
   miner's elbow, 231
   monarticular syndrome,
      232t
   necrosis, capitellum
      avascular, 230, 246
   neuropathy, ulnar,
      251-252, 252f
   olecranon impingement
      syndrome, 230-231
   osteochondritis
      dissecans, 230
   palsy, ulnar, 243-244,
      244f
   Panner disease, 230
   pushed vs. pulled
      elbow, 232
   student's elbow, 231
   swelling sites, 246
   tennis elbow, 250, 250f
   upper extremity
      periarticular
      syndrome, 232t
Electrodiagnostic testing,
   34-35, 34t-35t
Electromyography
   (EMG), 36
Electronic patient records
   (EPRs), 5
Elvey test, 222
Ely sign, 382-384, 384f
EMG. See Electromyography
   (EMG).
Emotional liability, 45-46
Empty can test, 224
Encroachment
   cervical nerve root,
      105-106, 106f
   intervertebral foramen,
      100-104, 101t-102t,
      103f, 415-417, 416f
Entrapment
   popliteal artery, 637
   ulnar nerve, 232t
Epicondylitis
   lateral, 240-242, 240t-
      241t, 242f, 246-247,
      247f, 250, 250f
   medial, 245, 245f
Epidural fibrosis, 136
Epilepsy aura, 712
Epiphysis, capital, 551

EPRs. See Electronic patient
   records (EPRs).
Erector muscle strain,
   spinal, 480t
Erichsen sign, 485-486, 486f
Erythema, 49, 49t-51t
Essential assessments
   fundamentals of, 12-14
   motion
      elbow, 233-235,
         233f-235f
      forearm, wrist, and hand,
         261-264, 261f-264f
      hip, 525-529, 526f-529f
      knee, 571-572, 572f
      lower leg, ankle, and foot,
         625-627, 626f-627f
      pelvis and sacroiliac
         joint, 478
      shoulder, 163-168,
         164t-168t
      spine, cervical, 72-76,
         73f-77f
      spine, lumbar, 356-358,
         356f-358f, 360t-361t
      spine, thoracic, 306-310,
         307f-310f
   muscle function
      elbow, 236-239,
         236f-238f
      forearm, wrist, and hand,
         265-267, 265f-267f
      hip, 530-533, 530f-532f
      knee, 572-573, 572f-573f
      lower leg, ankle, and foot,
         627-629, 628f-629f
      pelvis and sacroiliac
         joint, 478-479
      shoulder, 169-172,
         170f-172f
      spine, cervical, 77-80,
         77f-80f
      spine, lumbar, 358-362,
         362f
      spine, thoracic, 310-311,
         311f
Essential tremor (ET), 715
Estridge and Smith
   maneuver, 97-98
ET. See Essential tremor
   (ET).
EuroQual thermometer, 672
Evaluations
   cardinal symptoms and
      signs, 37-62
   elbow, 226-252
   forearm, wrist, and hand,
      253-301
   fundamentals of, 1-36
   hip, 516-563
   knee, 564-616

Evaluations—cont'd
lower leg, ankle, and foot,
617-660
malingering, 661-762
pelvis and sacroiliac joint,
473-515
shoulder, 157-225
spine
cervical, 63-156
lumbar, 344-472
thoracic, 302-343
Exostosis
degenerative joint disease,
112-115, 112t-114t,
115f
vertebral, 367-368, 368f
Extension rotation test, 97
Extensor syndromes
mechanisms
malalignment, 595
tendinitis, 232t
Extinction tactile
discrimination, 298
Extremity assessments
forearm, wrist, and hand,
253-301
screenings, 451-452, 452f
Extremity screening,
451-452, 452f
Extrusion, disc, 364

F

FABERE sign, 558-559, 559f
Face
anesthesia, hysterical vs.
simulated, 718-719,
719f
anesthesia testing,
718-719, 719f
facial purpura, 153
pain, hysterical, 707, 707f
Facet conditions
capsulitis, 100-104,
101t-102t, 103f
facet syndrome, 119-121,
119t-120t, 121f
Fajersztajn test, 385-386,
386f
Fasciculations, 60-61
Fasciitis, palmar, 232t
Fatigue, 45
Fatty acid muscle
degeneration, 216
Febrile meningeal irritation,
138-139, 139f
Feigned syndrome
assessments. See
Malingering assessments.
Femoral syndromes
anteversion, increased,
608-609, 609f

Femoral syndromes—cont'd
capital epiphysis, 551
fracture
femoral head, 539-540,
540f
femoral neck, 539-540,
540f, 543-545, 545f
nerve
inflammation, 382-384,
384f, 448-450, 450f
traction test, 387-389,
388f
structural deficiency,
536-538, 538f
Fibrocartilage complex
injury, 260t
Fibromyalgia
impact questionnaire, 672
syndrome, 337-340, 339t,
340f
tender point examination
protocol, 337-340, 340f
Fibrosis
epidural, 136
fibrositic infiltration,
459-460, 460f
lumbar, 423-427,
424t-426t, 427f
Finger-flexion test, 120
Finkelstein test, 279, 279f
Finsterer sign, 280-281, 281f
Fistula, arteriovenous,
650-651, 651f
Fixed deformity, 54-55,
54t-55t
Flexed-hip test, 696, 696f
Flexibility test,
lumbopelvic, 479
Flexion procedures
contracture, iliopsoas,
560, 560f
elbow, 243-244, 244f
finger-flexion test, 120
flexion-abduction-external
rotation-extension
(FABERE) sign,
558-559, 559f
plantar, 704-705, 705f
Flip sign, 697, 697f
Foot, ankle, and lower leg
assessments
anatomy essentials for,
624-625
cross-reference tables for
ankle-foot differentiation
by onset, 623t
by procedure, 619t-621t
by syndrome or tissue,
622t
fundamentals of, 617-625
procedures

Foot, ankle, and lower leg
assessments—cont'd
anterior drawer sign,
ankle, 631-632, 632f
Buerger test, 633-634,
634f
circumference test, calf,
635-636, 636f
claudication test,
637-638, 638f
Duchenne sign,
639-640, 640f
foot tourniquet test,
641-642, 642f
Helbings sign, 643, 643f
Hoffa sign, 644, 644f
Homans sign, 645, 645f
imaging studies, 630-631
Keen sign, 646-647, 647f
Morton test, 648-649,
648t, 649f
Moses test, 652, 652f
Moszkowicz test,
650-651, 651f
motion assessments,
625-627, 626f-627f
muscle function
assessments,
627-629, 628f-629f
Perthes test, 653-654,
654f
Strunsky sign, 655-656,
656f
Thompson test, 657-658,
658f
Tinel sign, foot, 659-
660, 660f
of syndromes and tissues
adventitial cystic
disease, 637
anterolateral compartment
syndrome, 639-640,
640f
arterial insufficiency,
641-642, 642f
arterial occlusive disease,
637-638, 638f
arteriosclerosis
obliterans, 652, 652f
atrophy, 635-636, 636f
collateral circulation
inadequacy,
650-651, 651f
compartment syndrome,
641-642, 642f
fistula, arteriovenous,
650-651, 651f
forefoot disorders,
655-656, 656f
fracture, calcaneus,
644, 644f

Foot, ankle, and lower leg
assessments—cont'd
fracture, distal fibular
vs. distal tibular,
646-647, 647f
hypertrophy, 635-636,
636f
Klippel Trenaunay
syndrome, 650-651,
651f
metatarsalgia, 648-649,
648t, 649f
Morton neuroma,
648-649, 648t, 649f
peripheral vascular
disease, 633-634,
634f
pes planus, 643, 643f
popliteal artery
entrapment
syndrome, 637
rupture, Achilles tendon,
657-658, 658f
saphenous vein valve
incompetencies,
653-654, 654f
sprain, anterior
talofibular ligament,
631-632, 632f
superficial varicosities,
653-654, 654f
swelling, Achilles
tendon, 624
tarsal tunnel syndrome,
659-660, 660f
thrombophlebitis,
645, 645f
vascular compromise,
633-634, 634f
Volkmann ischemia,
635-636, 636f
Foot-drop
feigned, 751-752, 752f
unilateral *vs.* bilateral, 759t
Foramen syndromes
cervical, 83-86, 84t, 86f,
105-106, 106f
compression test, 83-86,
84t, 86f, 105-106, 106f
encroachment,
intervertebral,
100-104, 101t-102t,
103f
occlusion, intervertebral,
415-417, 416f
Forearm, wrist, and hand
assessments, 253-301
anatomy essentials for,
259-261
cross-reference tables
by procedure, 254t-255t

Forearm, wrist, and hand
assessments—cont'd
by syndrome or tissue,
256t
fundamentals of, 253-259
malingering and, 753-754,
754f. *See also*
Malingering
assessments.
procedures
Allen test, 268-271,
269b-270b, 271f
bracelet test, 272-273,
273f
Bunnel-Littler test,
274, 274f
carpal lift sign, 275, 275f
cascade sign, 276, 276f
Dellon moving two-
point discrimination
test, 277-278, 278f
distal tingling on
percussion (DTP)
sign, 292-293, 293f
Finkelstein test, 279, 279f
Finsterer sign, 280-281,
281f
forearm-and-wrist-
weakness test,
753-754, 754f
formication sign,
292-293, 293f
Froment paper sign,
282-283, 282f
Hoffman-Tinel sign,
292-293, 293f
interphalangeal neuroma
test, 284, 284f
Janet test, 278
Maisonneuve sign,
285, 285f
motion assessments,
261-264, 261f-264f
muscle function
assessments,
265-267, 265f-267f
O'Riain sign, 290, 290f
Phalen sign, 286-287,
286f-287f
pinch grip test, 288-289,
289f
prayer sign, 286-287,
286f-287f
shrivel test, 290, 290f
tight retinacular
ligaments test, 291,
291f
Tinel sign (wrist),
292-293, 293f
tourniquet test, 294-296,
294t-295t, 296f

Forearm, wrist, and hand
assessments—cont'd
Wartenberg sign, 297,
297f
Weber two-point
discrimination test,
298-300, 299f
wringing test, 301. 301f
of syndromes and tissues
anterior interosseous
nerve syndrome, 288
arthritis, basal thumb
joint, 274, 274f
arthritis, rheumatoid,
272-273, 273f
caput ulnae syndrome,
272-273, 273f
carpal tunnel syndrome
(CPS), 286-287,
286f-287f
compression, median
nerve, 294-296,
294t-295t, 296f
compression, posterior
interosseous nerve,
294-296, 294t-295t,
296f
contracture,
interphalangeal
capsular, 274, 274f
degenerative changes,
scapholunate
advance collapse
(SLAC), 265
degenerative changes,
wrist articulations,
272-273, 273f
de Quervain disease,
279, 279f
derangement,
carpometacarpal
articulation, 276, 276f
derangement, elbow,
301, 301f
derangement, hand, 301,
301f
derangement, phalanges
internal, 276, 276f
derangement, wrist, 301,
301f
dermatome sensory
disturbances,
277-278, 278f
dislocation, proximal
interphalangeal,
291, 291f
fixation, phalangeal
retinacular ligament,
291, 291f
fracture, carpal, 275,
275f

Forearm, wrist, and hand assessments—cont'd
fracture, colles, 285, 285f
ganglion cysts, 294
Hoffman disease, 279, 279f
interdigital neuroma, 284, 284f
Kienböck disease, 280-281, 281f
lunate carpal septic necrosis, 280-281, 281f
median nerve distribution, 292-293, 293f
obstruction, peripheral vascular, 268-271, 269b-270b, 271f
palsy, medial nerve, 286-287, 286f-287f
palsy, ulnar, 297, 297f
palsy, ulnar nerve, 282-283, 282f
peripheral nerve denervation, 290, 290f
peripheral nerve sensibility, 298-300, 299f
peripheral neuropathy, 292-293, 293f
reflex sympathetic dystrophy-complex regional pain syndrome (RDS-CRS), 268-271, 269b-270b, 271f
rheumatoid deformity, 272
sprain, carpal, 275, 275f
tenosynovitis, thumb, 279, 279f
triangular fibrocartilage complex injury, 260t
ulnar nerve distribution, 292-293, 293f
wrist carpal system injury, 257
Forefoot disorders, 655-656, 656f
Forestier bowstring sign, 328-329, 329f
Formication sign, 251-252, 252f, 292-293, 293f
Foster-Kennedy syndrome, 712
Fouchet sign, 595
Fracture
acetabular, 485
Anderson/D'Alonzo classification, 131

Fracture—cont'd
anterior vertebral compression, 462
bimalleolar, 646
bony pelvis, 511-513, 512f
boot-top/skier, 646
calcaneus, 644, 644f
carpal, 275, 275f
colles, 285, 285f
costal structure, 341-343, 342t, 343f
cotton, 646
distal fibular vs. distal tibular, 646-647, 647f
femoral head, 539-540, 540f
femoral neck, 539-540, 540f, 543-545, 545f
hip, 543-544
insufficiency, 511-513, 512f
lumbopelvic, 440-442, 441f
Maisonneuve, 646
odontoid process, 131-134, 132t, 133f-134f
patella, 593-594, 594f
pelvic ring, 511-513, 512f
periprosthetic patella, 593
Pott, 646
proximal femur, 544
sacroiliac, 495-496, 495f
spinal, 95-96, 95f, 334, 462
subtrochanteric, 543
thoracolumbar, 334
toddler, 646
trimalleolar, 646
upper cervical spine, 131-134, 132t, 133f-134f
vertebral, 138-139, 139f
Fragmentation, intervertebral disc, 455
Frank degeneration of facets, 448
Friction syndrome, 604-605, 605f
Froment paper sign, 282-283, 282f
Function assessments
elbow, 236-239, 236f-238f
forearm, wrist, and hand, 265-267, 265f-267f
fundamentals of, 12-14, 45
hip, 530-533, 530f-532f
knee, 572-573, 572f-573f
lower leg, ankle, and foot, 627-629, 628f-629f
pelvis and sacroiliac joint, 478-479
shoulder, 169-172, 170f-172f
spine

Function assessments—cont'd
cervical, 77-80, 77f-80f
lumbar, 358-362, 362f
thoracic, 310-311, 311f
Functional ambulation classification, 742
Functional arc measurements, 229t
Functional leg-length difference, 541. See also Leg-length.
Functional vision loss, 716-717, 717f
Fundamentals
background perspectives of, 1-5
Bayes theorem, 3
cardinal signs and symptoms, 37-62. See also Cardinal symptoms and signs.
chief complaint, 6
clinical assessments, 2
clinical laboratory tests, 14-20
interpretation of, 14
listing of, 16b-19b
for low back pain diagnoses, 15t
synovial fluid tests, 19-20, 19b-20b
clinical reasoning, pain-based, 6
diagnoses, 5, 5b
electronic patient records (EPRs), 5
evaluation process phases, 2
histories, 5
imaging studies, 21-36
abilities vs. limitations of, 26-28, 31-36, 33b, 34t-35t
arthritides and, 24-26
contrast arthrography, 31
diagnostic ultrasound, 32-33
discography, 28
Doppler ultrasonic vascular testing, 36
electrodiagnostic testing, 34-35, 34t-35t
electromyography (EMG), 36
magnetic resonance imaging (MRI), 28-31, 29f-30t
myelography, 33
nerve conduction velocity (NCV) tests, 35

Fundamentals—cont'd
plain-film (conventional)
radiography, 21-27,
21t
preferred views for,
22t-23t
radionuclide scans, 31
skeletal trauma and,
22t-24t
thermography, 34
tomography,
conventional *vs.* CT,
27-28, 29t-31t
tomography, PET
scans, 31
tomography, SPECT
scans, 31
video fluoroscopy, 32
joint end-feel categories, 12
muscular assessments,
12-14
neurologic evaluations, 9-11
observation and
inspection, 6-7, 7b
orthopedic tests, 20
pain and pain patterns,
local *vs.* referred, 11
palpation, 7-9, 8t
physical examination
précis, 4
range-of-motion (ROM), 12
stability tests, 12, 13t
vital signs, 11

G

Gaenslen test, 487-488, 488f
Gaenslen-Lewin test,
500-501, 501f
Gait observations, 500
Galeazzi sign, 536-538, 538f
Ganglion cysts, 294
Gapping test, 489-490, 490f
Gault test, 720-721, 721f
Gauvin sign, 546-548, 547f
GBS. *See* Guillian-Barré
syndrome (GBS).
Generalized abductor
muscular weakness,
505-507, 506f
Generalized spinal lesions,
418-419, 418f
Genu valgum, 608-609, 609f
George screening procedure,
196-198, 197f-198f
Glasgow-Leige scale, 725
Glasgow outcome scale,
138-139, 139f, 723-724
Glenohumeral articulation
dislocation, 184-185, 185f
Gluteal abscess, bursitis, and
tumors, 457-458, 458f

Gluteus syndromes, 480t
Goldthwait sign, 491-492,
491f
Golfer elbow test, 245, 245f
Gonococcal tenosynovitis,
232t
Goutallier grading system,
216
Gracilis muscle contracture,
560, 560f
Graphesthesia, 298
Grasp stages, 288
Grinding test, 578-579, 579f
Grip-strength-loss test, 755-
756, 756f
Groove adhesion, 406-407,
407f
Guilland sign, 549-550, 549f
Guillian-Barré syndrome
(GBS), 321-323, 323f

H

HAD scale. *See* Hospital
Anxiety and Depression
(HAD) scale.
Hallpike maneuver,
107-109, 108f
Halstead maneuver,
199-200, 200f
Hamilton test, 201-202, 202f
Hamstring spasms, 421-422,
422f
Hand, wrist, and forearm
assessments, 253-301
anatomy essentials for,
259-261
cross-reference tables
by procedure, 254t-255t
by syndrome or tissue,
256t
fundamentals of, 253-259
procedures
Allen test, 268-271,
269b-270b, 271f
bracelet test, 272-273,
273f
carpal lift sign, 275, 275f
cascade sign, 276, 276f
Dellon moving two-
point discrimination
test, 277-278, 278f
Finkelstein test, 279, 279f
Finsterer sign, 280-281,
281f
formication sign,
292-293, 293f
Froment paper sign,
282-283, 282f
hand activity index, 753
Hoffman-Tinel sign,
292-293, 293f

Hamstring spasms—cont'd
interphalangeal neuroma
test, 284, 284f
Janet test, 278
Maisonneuve sign, 285,
285f
O'Riain sign, 290, 290f
Phalen sign, 286-287,
286f-287f
pinch grip test, 288-289,
289f
prayer sign, 286-287,
286f-287f
shrivel test, 290, 290f
tight retinacular ligaments
test, 291, 291f
Tinel sign, 292-293, 293f
tourniquet test, 294-296,
294t-295t, 296f
wringing test, 301. 301f
of syndromes and tissues
anterior interosseous
nerve syndrome, 288
arthritis, basal thumb
joint, 274, 274f
arthritis, rheumatoid,
272-273, 273f
caput ulnae syndrome,
272-273, 273f
carpal tunnel syndrome
(CPS), 286-287,
286f-287f
compression, median
nerve, 294-296,
294t-295t, 296f
compression, posterior
interosseous
nerve, 294-296,
294t-295t, 296f
contracture,
interphalangeal
capsular, 274, 274f
degenerative changes,
scapholunate
advance collapse
(SLAC), 265
degenerative changes,
wrist articulations,
272-273, 273f
de Quervain disease,
279, 279f
derangement,
carpometacarpal
articulation, 276,
276f
derangement, elbow,
301, 301f
derangement, hand, 301,
301f
derangement, phalanges
internal, 276, 276f

Hamstring spasms—cont'd
derangement, wrist, 301,
301f
dermatome sensory
disturbances,
277-278, 278f
fixation, phalangeal
retinacular ligament,
291, 291f
fracture, carpal, 275, 275f
fracture, colles, 285, 285f
ganglion cysts, 294
Hoffman disease, 279,
279f
interdigital neuroma,
284, 284f
Kienböck disease,
280-281, 281f
lunate carpal septic
necrosis, 280-281,
281f
median nerve
distribution,
292-293, 293f
obstruction, peripheral
vascular, 268-271,
269b-270b, 271f
palsy, medial nerve,
286-287, 286f-287f
palsy, ulnar, 297, 297f
palsy, ulnar nerve,
282-283, 282f
peripheral nerve
denervation, 290,
290f
peripheral nerve
sensibility, 298-300,
299f
peripheral neuropathy,
292-293, 293f
proximal interphalangeal
dislocation, 291, 291f
reflex sympathetic
dystrophy-complex
regional pain
syndrome (RDS-
CRS), 268-271,
269b-270b, 271f
rheumatoid deformity,
272
sprain, carpal, 275, 275f
tenosynovitis, thumb,
279, 279f
triangular fibrocartilage
complex injury, 260t
ulnar nerve distribution,
292-293, 293f
wrist carpal system
injury, 257
HAQ. *See* Health Assessment
Questionnaire (HAQ).

Hautant test, 110-111, 111f
Hawkin impingement
test, 224
Health assessment
questionnaire (HAQ), 672
Hearing loss, simulated,
710-721, 721f
Heel
Ely heel-to-buttock test,
382-384, 384f
heel/toe walk test, 390-
393, 390t-392t, 393f
Helbings sign, 643, 643f
Hemiplegic posturing,
746-747, 747f
Herniation
lumbar nucleus pulposus,
363-366, 363t-364t,
365f-366f
thoracic intervertebral
disc, 325
Hibbs test, 493-494, 494f
Hip assessments, 516-563
anatomy essentials,
524-525
cross-reference
tables for
by procedure, 517t-519t
by syndrome or tissue,
520t
fundamentals of, 516-525
procedures
Allis sign, 536-538, 538f
anvil test, 539-540, 540f
Barlow test, 536
Chiene test, 543-545,
545f
FABERE sign, 558-559,
559f
Galeazzi sign, 536-538,
538f
Gauvin sign, 546-548,
547f
Guilland sign, 549-550,
549f
hip telescoping test,
551-552, 552f
imaging studies, 533
Jansen test, 553, 553f
leg-length
measurements, 541
leg-length test, actual,
534-535, 535f
leg-length test, apparent,
541-542, 542f
Ludloff sign, 554-555,
555f
male simple calculated
osteoporosis risk
estimation
(MSCORE), 539

Hip assessments—cont'd
motion assessments,
525-529, 526f-529f
muscle function
assessments,
530-533, 530f-532f
Ober test, 556-557, 557f
Ortolani test, 536
Patrick test, 558-559,
559f
Phelps test, 560, 560f
range-of-motion (ROM)
tests, 525, 526f
telescoping test,
551-552, 552f
Thomas test, 561, 561f
Trendelenburg test,
562-563, 563f
of syndromes or tissues
abductor system
insufficiency,
562-563, 563f
avascular necrosis, 544
contracture, gracilis
muscle, 560, 560f
contracture, iliopsoas
flexion, 560, 560f
contracture, iliotibial
band, 556-557, 557f
coxa vara, 533
dislocation, 543-545,
545f
dislocation, congenital,
551-552, 552f
dysplasia, congenital,
536
fracture, 543-545, 545f
fracture, femoral head,
539-540, 540f
fracture, femoral neck,
539-540, 540f,
543-545, 545f
fracture, malunion *vs.*
non-union,
543-544
fracture, proximal
femur, 544
fracture, subtrochanteric
complications, 543
irritation, meningeal,
549-550, 549f
joint disease *vs.*
intervertebral
radiculopathy,
403-405, 404t,
405f
leg-length deficiency,
534-535, 535f
leg-length difference,
anatomic *vs.*
functional, 541

Hip assessments—cont'd
  leg-length discrepancy, apparent, 541-542, 542f
  leg-length discrepancy, true, 534-535, 535f
  osseous deformities, proximal femur, 533
  osteoarthritis (OA), 553, 553f, 558-559, 559f
  osteonecrosis, adult-onset, 546-548, 548f
  osteoporosis, 524
  pathologic conditions, hip joint, 560, 560f
  pathologic conditions, intracapsular coxa, 558-559, 559f
  pathologic conditions vs. sacroiliac disease, 485-486, 486f
  piriformis syndrome, 553, 553f
  slipped femoral capital epiphysis, 551
  structural deficiency, femoral portion, 536-538, 538f
  structural deficiency, tibial portion, 536-538, 538f
  transient synovitis, 557
  traumatic separation, lesser trochanter, 554-555, 555f
  tuberculosis (TB) arthritis, 546-548, 548f
Histories, 5
Hoffa sign, 644, 644f
Hoffman disease, 279, 279f
Hoffman-Tinel sign, 251-252, 252f, 292-293, 293f
Homans sign, 645, 645f
Hoover sign, 748-750, 749t, 750f
Horner syndrome, 110
Hospital anxiety and depression (HAD) scale, 672
Houle test, 97
Hughston knee instability index, 590
Humeral ligament involvement, 224-225, 225f
  transverse test, 220-221, 221f
Humerus, posterior, 174-175, 175f
Hyndman sign vs. Bragard sign, 371

Hyperabduction
  maneuver, 222-223, 223f
  thoracic outlet syndrome (TOS), 213-214, 214f, 222-223, 223f. See also Thoracic outlet syndrome (TOS).
Hyperextension
  overload syndrome, 230-231
  test, 394-396, 396f
Hypermobility
  costal structures, 331, 331f
  syndrome, 56-58, 58b
Hypersensitivity
  denervation, 431-433, 432t
  mastoid process, 698-699, 699f
Hypertonicity, knee vs. thigh, 614, 614f
Hypertrophy, 635-636, 636f
Hypochondriasis, 339t
Hypokalemic paralysis, 749t
Hypothyroidism, 339t
Hysterical syndrome assessments. See Malingering assessments.

I

Ilia on sacrum unilateral forward displacement, 480-482, 482f
Iliac compression test, 495-496, 495f
Iliocostalis lumborum musculature spasm, 376-377, 377f
Iliopsoas flexion contracture, 560, 560f
Iliotibial band
  contracture, 556-557, 557f
  friction syndrome, 604-605, 605f
  injury, 589-592, 591f-592f, 599-600, 600f, 610-611, 610f
Imaging studies
  abilities vs. limitations of, 26-28, 31-36, 33b, 34t-35t
  contrast arthrography, 31
  discography, 28
  Doppler ultrasonic vascular testing, 36
  electrodiagnostic testing, 34-35, 34t-35t
  electromyography (EMG), 36
  fundamentals of, 21-36
  magnetic resonance imaging (MRI), 28-31, 29t-30t

Imaging studies—cont'd
  myelography, 33
  nerve conduction velocity (NCV) tests, 35
  plain-film (conventional) radiography, 21-27, 21t
    preferred views for, 22t-23t
  radionuclide scanning, 31
  of syndromes or tissues
    arthritides, 24-26
    elbow, 239, 246
    hip, 533
    knee, 573
    lower leg, ankle, and foot, 630-631
    pelvis and sacroiliac joint, 479
    shoulder, 173
    skeletal trauma, 22t-24t
    spine, cervical, 80-82, 81b, 82t
    spine, lumbar, 362
    spine, thoracic, 311
  thermography, 34
  tomography, 27-31
    conventional vs. computed (CT), 27-28, 29t-31t
    positron emission tomography (PET) scans, 31
    single-photon emission computed tomography (SPECT) scans, 31
Imai sensory recovery classification, 299t
Impingement
  sign, 203-205, 205f
  syndrome, 204
  test, 224
Infective pathogens. See Pathogens.
Infiltration, fibrositic, 459-460, 460f
Inflammation
  meningeal, 400-402, 402f
  nerve
    femoral, 448-450, 450f
    lumbar, 382-384, 384f
    sciatic, 408-414, 412t, 413f
  nerve root
    L3-L4, 394-396, 396f
    lumbar, 428-430, 430f
    pericapsular, 397-399, 399f
    sacroiliac, 465-467, 466f, 495-496, 495f
Inflammatory syndromes
  edema, 112-115, 112t-114t, 115f

Inflammatory
    syndromes—cont'd
    inflammatory bowel
        disease (IBD), 339t
    myopathy, 339t
    spine lesions, acute,
        337-340, 340f
Innominate test, 480-482,
    482f
Insensitivity to pain, 738,
    738f
Inspection and observation,
    6-7, 7b, 37-38
Instability test, 248-249,
    248f-249f
Insufficiency fracture,
    511-513, 512f
Intercostal syndromes
    neuralgia, 342t
    strain, 342t
    tissue integrity, 332-333,
        333f
Interdigital neuroma, 284,
    284f
Internal derangement
    carpometacarpal
        articulation, 276, 276f
    knee, 579
    phalanges, 276, 276f
Interosseous nerve
    compression, posterior,
        294-296, 294t-295t,
        296f
    syndrome, anterior, 288
Interphalangeal syndromes
    capsular contracture,
        274, 274f
    dislocation, proximal, 291,
        291f
    neuroma test, 284, 284f
Interscalene compression,
    209-210, 210f
Interstitial cystitis, 339t
Intervertebral conditions
    disc
        fragmentation, 455
        herniation, thoracic, 325
        lesion, 272f, 367-373,
            368f, 370f, 415-417,
            416f, 454
        nucleus prolapse,
            374-375, 374t, 375f
        protrusion, 95-96, 95f,
            362-366, 418-419,
            418f
        rupture, 420, 420f
        syndrome, 316-317,
            316t, 317f, 385-386,
            386f, 406-407,
            407f, 438-439,
            439f, 440-442, 441f

Intervertebral
    conditions—cont'd
    syndrome, lower,
        445-447, 447f
    encroachment
        foraminal, 100-104,
            101t-102t, 103f
        nerve root, 397-399, 399f
    lesions, nerve root,
        406-407, 407f
    occlusion, foramen,
        415-417, 416f
    radiculopathy, 403-405,
        404t, 405f
    space-occupying mass, 420,
        420f, 437-439, 439f
    tumors, 147, 147f
Intraarticular abnormality,
    499, 499f
Intracapsular coxa
    pathologic conditions,
        558-559, 559f
Intradiscal pressure, 462
Irritation
    meningeal, 138-139, 139f,
        400-402, 402f
    nerve
        sciatic, 378-379, 379f
        spinal, 373, 373f
    nerve root, lumbar,
        428-430, 430f
Ischemia
    brainstem, 148
    vertebrobasilar, 154
    Volkmann, 635-636, 636f
Isosceles triangle, elbow, 228

J

Jackson compression test,
    112-115, 112t-114t, 115f
Janet test, 278, 300, 722, 722f
Jansen test, 553, 553f
Joint edema, 48, 48t
Joint end-feel categories, 12
Joint motion test, 706, 706f
Joint pathologic conditions,
    hip, 560, 560f
Joint plane motion, 56t
Jump sign, 339
Jumper's knee, 588

K

Kaplan sign, 246-247, 247f
Keen sign, 646-647, 647f
Kemp test, 397-399, 399f
Kernig/Brudzinski sign,
    139, 400-402, 402f, 549
Kienböck disease staging,
    280-281, 281f
Klippel Trenaunay
    syndrome, 650-651, 651f

Knee assessments, 564-616
    anatomy essentials for, 571
    cross-reference tables for
        by procedure, 565t-567t
        by syndrome or tissue,
            568t-569t
    fundamentals of, 564-571
    procedures
        apprehension test, patella,
            580-581, 581f
        bounce home test,
            582-583, 583f
        Childress duck waddle
            test, 584-585, 585f
        Clarke sign, 586-588,
            588f
        compression test, Apley,
            578-579, 579f
        compression test, Noble,
            604-605, 605f
        distraction test, 578-579,
            579f
        drawer test, 589-592,
            591f-592f
        drawer test, positive
            anterior, 590
        drawer test, positive
            posterior, 581
        Dryer sign, 593-594, 594f
        Fouchet sign, 595
        grinding test, 578-579,
            579f
        imaging studies, 573
        knee-bending test,
            prone, 448-450, 450f
        knee-to-shoulder test,
            497-498, 498f
        Lachman test, 597-598,
            598f
        lateral pivot shaft
            maneuver, 599-600,
            600f
        Losee test, 601, 601f
        McIntosh test, 599-600,
            600f
        McMurray sign,
            602-603, 602f
        motion assessments,
            571-572, 572f
        muscle function
            assessments,
            572-573, 572f-573f
        patella ballottement test,
            606, 606f
        Payr sign, 607, 607f
        Q-angle test, 606-609,
            609f
        Slocum test, 610-611,
            611f
        Steinmann sign,
            612-613, 613f

Knee assessments—cont'd
stress test, abduction,
574-575, 575f
stress test, adduction,
576-577, 577f
tenderness displacement
test, 612-613, 613f
thigh circumference test,
614, 614f
Wilson sign, 615-616,
616f
of syndromes or tissues
anterolateral rotary
instability, 601,
601f, 610-611, 610f
arcuate-popliteus
complex injury,
589-592, 591f-592f,
597-600, 598f, 600f,
610-611, 610f
bundle injury,
anteromedial,
589-592, 591f-592f
bundle injury,
posterolateral,
597-598, 598f
capsule injury,
posterolateral,
599-600, 600f,
610-611, 610f
capsule injury,
posterolateral vs.
posteromedial,
589-592, 591f-592f
chondromalacia patellae,
586-588, 588f
collateral ligament
injury, 578-579, 579f
collateral ligament
injury, lateral,
576-577, 577f,
599-600, 600f,
610-611, 610f
collateral ligament
injury, medial,
574-575, 575f,
589-592, 591f-592f
cruciate ligament injury,
anterior, 589-592,
591f-592f, 597-600,
598f, 600f, 610-611,
610f
cruciate ligament injury,
posterior, 589-592,
591f-592f, 610-611,
610f
extensor mechanism
malalignment,
595-596, 596f
femoral anteversion,
increased, 608-609,
609f

Knee assessments—cont'd
fracture, patella,
593-594, 594f
genu valgum, 608-609,
609f
hypertonicity, thigh,
614, 614f
iliotibial band friction
syndrome, 604-605,
605f
iliotibial band injury,
589-592, 591f-592f,
599-600, 600f,
610-611, 610f
internal derangement of
knee (IDK), 579
joint effusion, 606, 606f
lateral tibial torsion,
increased, 608-609,
609f
locking, 613
loose body in knee,
615-616, 616f
meniscus injury, lateral,
602-603, 602f
meniscus injury, medial,
607, 607f
meniscus tear, 578-579,
579f, 582-583, 583f
meniscus tear, lateral vs.
medial, 584-585,
585f, 610-611, 610f
oblique ligament injury,
posterior, 589-592,
591f-592f, 597-598,
598f
osteochondritis dissecans,
615-616, 616f
patella alta, 608-609, 609f
patella dislocation,
580-581, 581f
patellofemoral
dysfunction, 595-596,
596f, 608-609, 609f
pathologic conditions,
meniscus, 578
peripatellar syndrome,
595-596, 596f
posteromedial capsule
injury, 589-592,
591f-592f
proximal tibiofibular joint
dysfunction, 576
subluxation, patella,
608-609, 609f
tensor fascia lata,
610-611, 610f
tracking disorder,
patellar, 595-596,
596f
Kyphosis, thoracic,
328-329, 329f

L

L2–L3-L4 mid-lumbar
nerve root involvement,
387-389, 388f
L2–L3 nerve root lesions,
448-450, 450f
L3–L4 nerve root
inflammation, 394-396,
396f
L5–S1 nerve root motor
deficiency, 390-393,
390t-392t, 393f
Laboratory tests, 14-20
interpretation of, 14
listing of, 16b-19b
for low back pain
diagnoses, 15t
synovial fluid tests, 19-20,
19b-20b
Lachman test, 597-598, 598f
Laguerre test, 499, 499f
Lamb bilateral hand activity
index, 753
LANSS. See Leeds
Assessment of
Neuropathic Symptoms
and Signs (LANSS)
Pain Scale.
Larsen-Johansson
disease, 588
Larsen rheumatoid arthritis
grading system, 424t-
425t, 424t-426t
Lasègue tests
Lasègue differential sign,
403-405, 404t, 405f
Lasègue sign, 415-417,
416f
rebound, 406-407, 407f
sitting, 408-414, 412t, 413f
Lateral collateral ligament
instability, 243-244,
244f, 248-249, 248f-249f
Lateral epicondylitis,
240-242, 240t-241t,
242f, 246-247, 247f,
250, 250f
Lateral meniscus injury,
602-603, 602f
Lateral meniscus tear,
584-585, 585f, 610-611,
610f
Lateral pivot shaft
maneuver, 599-600,
600f
Lateral tibial torsion,
increased, 608-609, 609f
Leeds assessment of
neuropathic symptoms
and signs (LANSS)
pain scale, 52b-53b

Leg-length
actual, 534-535, 535f
deficiency, 534-535, 535f
difference, anatomic *vs.*
functional, 541
discrepancy
apparent, 541-542, 542f
true, 534-535, 535f
measurements, 541
Leg-lowering test, 369-370,
370f
Leg paresis, feigned,
748-750, 749t, 750f
Lenke scoliosis
classification, 314t
Lesion
disc, intervertebral,
367-373, 368f, 370f,
373f, 415-417, 416f,
454
lumbosacral, 369-370,
370f, 415-417, 416f
nerve root
intervertebral, 406-407,
407f
L2-L3, 448-450, 450f
lumbar, 385-386, 386f
mixed motor
peripheral, 432
sacroiliac, 415-417, 416f,
440-442, 441f,
495-496, 495f
spine
acute inflammatory,
337-340, 340f
generalized, 418-419,
418f
trigeminal, 718-719, 719f
Lesser trochanter, traumatic
separation, 554-555, 555f
Lewin-Gaenslen test,
500-501, 501f
Lewin tests
punch, 418-419, 418f
snuff, 420, 420f
standing, 421-422, 422f
supine, 423-427, 424t-
426t, 427f
Lhermitte sign, 116-118,
117t, 118f
Libman sign, 698-699,
699f
Lift sign, 275, 275f
Ligament syndromes
collateral, 578-579, 579f
instability, 248-249,
248f-249f
lateral, 576-577, 577f,
599-600, 600f,
610-611, 610f
cruciate

Ligament
syndromes—cont'd
anterior, 589-592,
591f-592f, 597-600,
598f, 600f, 610-611,
610f
posterior, 589-592,
591f-592f, 610-611,
610f
fixation, phalangeal
retinacular, 291, 291f
humeral, transverse,
224-225, 225f
instability test, 248-249,
248f-249f
oblique, posterior,
589-592, 591f-592f,
597-598, 598f
residual function of, 13f
retinacular test, 291, 291f
sacroiliac
anterior, 514-515, 514f
posterior, 511-513, 512f
sprain
ligamentous, 397-399,
399f
sacroiliac, 483-484, 483f
talofibular, anterior,
631-632, 632f
Limb-dropping test
bilateral, 742-745, 745f
upper extremity, 723-725,
725f
Limping categories, 537
Lindner sign, 428-430, 430f
LIS. See Locked-in
syndrome (LIS).
Listeria monocytogenes, 376
Little leaguer's elbow, 230
Loading forces, hip, 523
Locked-in syndrome (LIS),
88, 155
Locking, knee, 613
Lombard test, 726, 726f
Long head
injury, 220-221, 221f
rupture, 206, 206f
Loose body in knee,
615-616, 616f
Low back pain
characteristics of, 355t
differential red flags in, 442
feigned, 697, 697f
gender prevalence
in, 353t
nonorganic, 708-709, 709f
screening, 451-452, 452f
symptom durations of, 443t
three headings for, 451
working status
classification, 443t

Lower extremity. *See also*
Lower leg, ankle, and
foot assessments.
paresis, feigned, 742-745,
745f
screening, 451-452, 452f
Lower intervertebral disc
syndrome, 445-447, 447f
Lower leg, ankle, and foot
assessments, 617-660
cross-reference tables for
ankle-foot differentiation
by onset, 623t
by procedure, 619t-621t
by syndrome or tissue,
622t
fundamentals of, 617-625
anatomy essentials,
624-625
shoe design features, 618
procedures
anterior drawer sign,
ankle, 631-632, 632f
Buerger test, 633-634,
634f
circumference test, calf,
635-636, 636f
claudication test,
637-638, 638f
Duchenne sign,
639-640, 640f
foot tourniquet test,
641-642, 642f
Helbings sign, 643, 643f
Hoffa sign, 644, 644f
Homans sign, 645, 645f
imaging studies,
630-631
Keen sign, 646-647, 647f
Morton test, 648-649,
648t, 649f
Moses test, 652, 652f
Moszkowicz test,
650-651, 651f
motion assessments,
625-627, 626f-627f
muscle function
assessments,
627-629, 628f-629f
Perthes test, 653-654,
654f
Strunsky sign, 655-656,
656f
Thompson test,
657-658, 658f
Tinel sign, foot,
659-660, 660f
of syndromes
and tissues
adventitial cystic
disease, 637

Lower leg, ankle, and foot
assessments—cont'd
anterolateral
compartment
syndrome, 639-640,
640f
arterial insufficiency,
641-642, 642f
arterial occlusive disease,
637-638, 638f
arteriosclerosis
obliterans, 652, 652f
atrophy, 635-636, 636f
collateral circulation
inadequacy, 650-651,
651f
compartment syndrome,
641-642, 642f
fistula, arteriovenous,
650-651, 651f
forefoot disorders,
655-656, 656f
fracture, calcaneus, 644,
644f
fracture, distal fibular vs.
distal tibular,
646-647, 647f
hypertrophy, 635-636,
636f
ischemia, Volkmann,
635-636, 636f
Klippel Trenaunay
syndrome, 650-651,
651f
lesion, superficial
peroneal nerve,
639-640, 640f
metatarsalgia, 648-649,
648t, 649f, 655-656,
656f
Morton neuroma,
648-649, 648t, 649f
peripheral vascular
disease, 633-634,
634f
pes planus, 643, 643f
popliteal artery
entrapment
syndrome, 637
rupture, Achilles tendon,
657-658, 658f
saphenous vein valve
incompetencies,
653-654, 654f
sprain, anterior
talofibular ligament,
631-632, 632f
superficial varicosities,
653-654, 654f
swelling, Achilles
tendon, 624

Lower leg, ankle, and foot
assessments—cont'd
tarsal tunnel syndrome,
659-660, 660f
thrombophlebitis, 645,
645f, 650-651, 651f
vascular compromise,
633-634, 634f
Ludington test, 206, 206f
Ludloff sign, 554-555, 555f
Lumbar spine assessments,
344-472
anatomy essentials for, 356
cross-reference tables for
by procedure, 345t-349t
by syndrome or tissue,
350t-352t
fundamentals of, 344-355
malingering, 691-696,
692t, 693f, 695f, 696f
procedures for
active straight-leg-raise
(ASLR) test, 438
antalgia sign, 362-366,
363t, 364f-366f
Bechterew sitting test,
367-368, 368f
bilateral leg-lowering
test, 369-370, 370f
bilateral straight-leg-
raise test, 380-381,
381f
bowstring sign, 371-372,
372f
Bragard sign, 373,
373f
Cox sign, 374-375, 374t,
375f
Demianoff sign,
376-377, 377f
Deyerle sign, 378-379,
379f
double-leg-raise test,
380-381, 381f
Ely sign, 382-384, 384f
Fajersztajn test,
385-386, 386f
femoral nerve traction
test, 387-389, 388f
heel/toe walk test,
390-393, 390t-392t,
393f
hyperextension test,
394-396, 396f
imaging studies, 362
Kemp test, 397-399, 399f
Kernig/Brudzinski sign,
400-402, 402f
Lasègue differential
sign, 403-405,
404t, 405f

Lumbar spine
assessments—cont'd
Lasègue rebound test,
406-407, 407f
Lasègue sign, 415-417,
416f
Lasègue sitting test,
408-414, 412t, 413f
Lewin punch test,
418-419, 418f
Lewin snuff test,
420, 420f
Lewin standing test,
421-422, 422f
Lewin supine test,
423-427, 424t-426t,
427f
Lindner sign, 428-430,
430f
matchstick test,
431-433, 432t
Mennell sign, 434-436,
436f
Milgram test, 437-439,
439f
Minor sign, 440-442,
441f
motion assessments,
356-358, 356f-358f,
359t-361t, 360t-361t
muscle function
assessments,
358-362, 362f
Nachlas test, 442-444,
443t, 444f
Neri sign, 445-447, 447f
prone knee-bending test,
448-450, 450f
Quick test, 451-452,
452f
Schober test, 453, 453f
Sicard sign, 454-456,
456f
sign of the buttock,
457-458, 458f
skin pinch test,
459-460, 460f
spinal percussion test,
461-464, 464f
straight-leg-raise test,
465-467, 466f
Turyn sign,
468-470, 470f
Vanzetti sign, 471-472,
472f
of syndromes and tissues
arthrosis, lumbosacral,
423-427, 424t-426t,
427f
flexibility, lumbopelvic,
479

Lumbar spine
assessments—cont'd
fracture, lumbopelvic,
440-442, 441f
lesions, lumbosacral,
415-417, 416f
lesions, lumbosacral
mechanical,
369-370, 370f
lumbopelvic spine
muscular syndromes,
481
lumbopelvic syndromes,
480t
lumbosacral disorders,
442-444, 443t, 444f
lumbosacral
involvement,
465-467, 466f
lumbosacral joint
involvement,
380-381, 381f,
508-510, 509f
motion, spine, 453, 453f
spine abnormality,
491-492, 491f
sprain, lumbosacral,
440-442, 441f
sprain, lumbosacral
capsular, 483-484,
483f
strain, chronic, 480t
strains, lumbosacral,
440-442, 441f,
445-447, 447f
subluxation syndrome,
415-417, 416f,
445-447, 447f
Lunate carpal septic
necrosis, 280-281, 281f
Lupus erythematosus.
See Systemic lupus
erythematosus (SLE).

M

Magnetic resonance
imaging (MRI), 28-31,
29t-30t
Magnuson test, 700, 700f
Maigne test, 97-98
Maisonneuve fracture, 646
Maisonneuve sign,
285, 285f
Major depression, 760b
Malalignment, extensor
mechanisms, 595
Male Simple Calculated
Osteoporosis Risk
Estimation (MSCORE),
539
Malignant tissue lesions, 554

Malingering assessments,
661-762
cross-reference tables
by procedure, 667t-669t
by syndrome or tissue,
670t
fundamentals of, 661-672
outcomes and other
assessments, 662,
672-675
b test, 662
Borg pain scales, 673
Dallas pain
questionnaire, 673
Disease Impact Index
(DII), 673b
disease repercussion
profile, 672-673
EuroQual thermometer,
672
fibromyalgia impact
questionnaire, 672
health assessment
questionnaire
(HAQ), 672
hospital anxiety and
depression (HAD)
scale, 672
Millennium Cohort
study and, 675
neuroorthostatic
malingering tests, 673
Oswestry disability
indices, 673
symptom magnification
indexing, 673
test of memory
malingering
(TOMM), 662
Victoria Symptom
Validity Test
(VSVT), 662
Waddell indexing, 673,
674t
procedures (pain
qualification and
quantification),
683-709
axial trunk-loading test,
691-693, 692t, 693f
Burns bench test,
694-695, 695f
flexed-hip test, 696, 696f
flip sign, 697, 697f
Libman sign, 698-699,
699f
Magnuson test, 700, 700f
Mannkopf sign, 701, 701f
marked part pain-
suggestibility test,
702-703, 702f

Malingering
assessments—cont'd
plantar flexion test,
704-705, 705f
Quebec classification
system, 691, 692t
related joint motion test,
706, 706f
Seeligmuller sign,
707, 707f
trunk rotational test,
708-709, 709f
procedures (paralysis
qualification and
quantification),
739-762
Barthel index, 743-744
bilateral limb-dropping
test, lower
extremities,
742-745, 745f
hemiplegic posturing,
746-747, 747f
Hoover sign, 748-750,
749t, 750f
Lamb bilateral hand
activity index, 753
simulated foot-drop test,
751-752, 752f
simulated forearm-and-
wrist-weakness test,
753-754, 754f
simulated grip-strength-
loss test, 755-756,
756f
tripod test, 757-758,
757f-758f
procedures (sensory deficit
qualification and
quantification),
709-738
anosmia testing,
712-713, 713f
coordination-disturbance
testing, 714-715,
715f
Cuignet test, 716-717,
717f
facial anesthesia testing,
718-719, 719f
Gault test, 720-721,
721f
Janet test, 722, 722f
limb-dropping test,
upper extremities,
723-725, 725f
Lombard test, 726, 726f
Marcus Gunn sign, 727,
727f
midline tuning-fork test,
728, 728f

Malingering
assessments—cont'd
optokinetic nystagmus
test, 712-713, 713f
position-sense testing,
731, 731f
regional anesthesia
testing, 732-733,
733f
Romberg sign, 734, 734f
Snellen test, 735-737,
736t, 737f
station test, 734, 734f
Stoicism indexing, 738,
738f
of syndromes and tissues
anesthesia, feigned,
732-733, 733f
anesthesia, simulated,
722, 722f, 728, 728f
anosmia, feigned,
712-713, 713f
ataxia, nonorganic,
732-733, 733f
blindness, feigned,
712-713, 713f
blindness, simulated,
716-717, 717f
color blindness, feigned,
735-737, 736t, 737f
coordination loss,
nonorganic,
714-715, 715f
deafness, simulated,
710-721, 721f, 726,
726f
depression symptoms,
663b
essential tremor (ET), 715
face anesthesia,
hysterical vs.
simulated, 718-719,
719f
face pain, hysterical,
707, 707f
fibromyalgia syndrome
vs. malingering, 339t
foot drop, feigned,
751-752, 752f
foot drop, unilateral vs.
bilateral, 759t
forearm weakness,
simulated, 753-754,
754f
grip strength loss,
simulated, 755-756,
756f
hypokalemic paralysis,
749t
insensitivity to pain,
congenital, 738, 738f

Malingering
assessments—cont'd
leg paresis, feigned,
748-750, 749t, 750f
lesions, trigeminal,
718-719, 719f
low back pain, feigned,
697, 697f, 700, 700f,
704-705, 705f
low back pain,
nonorganic,
708-709, 709f
lower extremity paresis,
feigned, 742-745,
745f
lumbar pain, simulated,
757-758, 757f-758f
lumbar spine
malingering,
691-696, 692t,
693f, 694-695,
695f, 696, 696f
mastoid process
hypersensitivity,
698-699, 699f
mood disorders, 760b
movement disorders,
organic vs.
psychogenic,
739-741, 740t
optic neural function,
normal, 727, 727f
pain, feigned, 706, 706f
pain exaggeration,
702-703, 702f
position sense loss,
feigned, 731, 731f
simulated pain, 701, 701f
steppage gait, feigned,
751-752, 752f
thalamic pain, 733
unconsciousness,
feigned, 723-725,
725f
vision loss, functional,
716-717, 717f
wrist weakness,
simulated, 753-754,
754f
Malunion vs. non-union, hip
fracture, 543-544
Mannkopf sign, 701, 701f
Marcus Gunn sign, 727, 727f
Marked part
pain-suggestibility test,
702-703, 702f
Mastoid process
hypersensitivity,
698-699, 699f
Matchstick test, 431-433,
432t

Maximum cervical
compression test,
119-121, 119t-120t,
121f
Mazion procedures
cuff maneuver, 216-217,
217f
pelvic maneuver, 480-482,
482f
shoulder maneuver,
207-208, 207f
McIntosh test, 599-600, 600f
McMurray sign, 602-603,
602f
MD. See Muscular
dystrophy (MD).
Mechanical dysfunction,
sacoliliac, 497-498, 498f
Mechanical lumbosacral
lesions, 369-370, 370f
Mechanical spine
syndrome, 305
Medial collateral ligament
instability, 243-244,
244f
Medial epicondylitis, 245,
245f
Medial meniscus
injury, 602-603, 602f, 607,
607f
tear, 584-585, 585f,
610-611, 610f
Median nerve
compression, 294-296,
294t-295t, 296f
distribution, peripheral
neuropathy, 292-293,
293f
palsy, 286-287, 286f-287f
Medical Research council
(MRC) sum score, 322
Meningeal irritation or
inflammation, 400-402,
402f
Meningitis, tuberculosis
(TB), 318-320, 320f
Meniscus injury
lateral, 602-603, 602f
medial, 602-603, 602f,
607, 607f
pathologic conditions, 578
posterior horn, 607, 607f
tear, 578-579, 579f,
582-583, 583f
tear, lateral vs. medial,
584-585, 585f,
610-611, 610f
Mennell sign, 434-436, 436f
Mensuration common
areas, 10
Meralgia paresthetica, 449

Metatarsalgia, 648-649, 648t, 649f
Mid-lumbar nerve root involvement, 387-389, 388f
Midline tuning-fork test, 728, 728f
Milgram test, 437-439, 439f
Millennium Cohort study, 675
Miner's elbow, 231
Minnesota Multiphasic Personality Inventory, 2nd edition (MMPI-2), 761b-762b
Minor sign, 440-442, 441f
Mixed motor peripheral nerve lesion, 432
MMPI-2. *See* Minnesota Multiphasic Personality Inventory, 2nd edition (MMPI-2).
Mobile units, wrist, 259
Modalities, imaging. *See* Imaging studies.
Modified Adson maneuver, 97
Modified Altman classification, 403
Modified Arnold international classification, 383
Modified Beighton mobility index, 58b
Modified Larsen rheumatoid arthritis grading system, 424t-425t, 424t-426t
Modified New York criteria, 316t
Modified Wiltse classification, 394-395
Monarticular syndrome, 232t
Monocular blindness, 716. *See also* Blindness.
Mood disorders, 760b
Morning numbness, 191
Morton neuroma, 648-649, 648t, 649f
Morton test, 648-649, 648t, 649f
Moschcowitz test, 650-651, 651f
Moses test, 652, 652f
Moszkowicz test, 650-651, 651f
Motion assessments
elbow, 233-235, 233f-235f
forearm, wrist, and hand, 261-264, 261f-264f
fundamentals of, 12-14
hip, 525-529, 526f-529f

Motion assessments—cont'd
knee, 571-572, 572f
lower leg, ankle, and foot, 625-627, 626f-627f
pelvis and sacroiliac joint assessments, 478
related joint, 706, 706f
shoulder, 163-168, 164t-168t
spine
cervical, 72-76, 73f-77f
lumbar, 356-358, 356f-358f, 360t-361t
thoracic, 306-310, 307f-310f
Motor deficiency, 390-393, 390t-392t, 393f
Movement arc, 53-54
Movement disorders, organic *vs.* psychogenic, 739-741, 740t
Moving two-point discrimination test, 277-278, 278f
MRC sun score. *See* Medical Research council (MRC) sum score.
MRI. *See* Magnetic resonance imaging (MRI).
MS. *See* Multiple sclerosis (MS).
MSCORE. *See* Male Simple Calculated Osteoporosis Risk Estimation (MSCORE).
Multiple-level spinal fractures, 334
Multiple sclerosis (MS), 339t
Muscle function assessments
elbow, 236-239, 236f-238f
forearm, wrist, and hand, 265-267, 265f-267f
fundamentals of, 12-14, 45
hip, 530-533, 530f-532f
knee, 572-573, 572f-573f
lower leg, ankle, and foot, 627-629, 628f-629f
pelvis and sacroiliac joint, 478-479
shoulder, 169-172, 170f-172f
spine
cervical, 77-80, 77f-80f
lumbar, 358-362, 362f
thoracic, 310-311, 311f
Muscular atrophy, 59-60, 60t

Muscular dystrophy (MD), 440-442, 441f
Muscular spasm
piriformis, 406-407, 407f
sacrolumbalis, 367-368, 368f, 376-377, 377f
Musculoskeletal disorder assessments
cardinal symptoms and signs and, 37-62
elbow, 226-252
forearm, wrist, and hand, 253-301
fundamentals of, 1-36
hip, 516-563
knee, 564-616
lower leg, ankle, and foot, 617-660
malingering, 661-762
pelvis and sacroiliac joint, 473-515
shoulder, 157-225
spine
cervical, 63-156
lumbar, 344-472
thoracic, 302-343
Myelography, 33
Myelopathy
disability grades, 132t
T10 spinal level-associated, 321-323, 323f
Myofascial conditions
pain syndrome, 119-121, 119t-120t, 121f, 141t, 339
trigger points, 431t
Myopathy, inflammatory, 339t

N

Nachlas test, 442-444, 443t, 444f
Naffziger compression test, 122-123, 123f
NCV tests. *See* Nerve conduction velocity (NCV) tests.
Neck flexion movement, 371
Necrosis
avascular, 230, 246, 544
lunate carpal septic, 280-281, 281f
Neer impingement test, 224
Neisseria gonorrhoeae, 376
Neisseria meningitidis, 376
Neri sign, 445-447, 447f
Nerve conduction velocity (NCV) tests, 35
Nerve denervation, peripheral, 290, 290f

Nerve inflammation
femoral, 382-384, 384f,
448-450, 450f
lumbar radicular, 382-384,
384f
sciatic, 408-414, 412t, 413f
Nerve irritation
sciatic, 378-379, 379f
spinal, 373, 373f
Nerve palsy
medial, 286-287, 286f-287f
ulnar, 282-283, 282f
Nerve root
compression, lumbar,
371-372, 372f
encroachment,
intervertebral,
397-399, 399f
inflammation
L3–L4, 394-396, 396f
lumbar, 428-430, 430f
mid-lumbar, 387-389,
388f
irritation, lumbar,
428-430, 430f
lesion
intervertebral, 406-407,
407f
L2–L3, 448-450, 450f
lumbar, 385-386, 386f
motor deficiency, 390-393,
390f-392t, 393f
subluxation, cervical,
112-115, 112t-114t,
115f
T1–T2, 325-327, 327f,
330-331, 330f
T1 test, 325-327, 327f
Nerve traction test,
387-389, 388f
Neural sensory unit, 298
Neuralgia, intercostal, 342t
Neuritis, sciatic, 373, 373f,
504, 504f
Neurogenic thoracic outlet
(nTOS), 178, 208
Neurologic evaluations, 9-11
Neuroma
interdigital, 284, 284f
interphalangeal,
284, 284f
Neuroorthostatic
malingering tests, 673
Neuropathy
differential diagnoses,
755
vs. fibromyalgia
syndrome, 339t
posterior interosseous,
251-252, 252f
ulnar, 251-252, 252f

Neurovascular
compression
brachial plexus, 174-175,
175f
subclavian artery,
176-177, 177f
Neurovascular space
narrowing, 211
New York criteria, 316t
Noble compression tests,
604-605, 605f
Nociceptors, peripheral, 41
Nocturnal dysesthesia, 191
Nocturnal palsy, 191
Non-union vs. malunion, hip
fracture, 543-544
Nonorganic syndromes
ataxia, 732-733, 733f
coordination loss,
714-715, 715f
low back pain, 708-709,
709f
Nontraumatic osteoarthritis
(OA), shoulder, 201
nTOS. See Neurogenic
thoracic outlet (nTOS).
Nurick myelopathic
disability grade, 132t
Nystagmus test, 712-713,
713f

O

OA. See Osteoarthritis
(OA).
Ober test, 556-557, 557f
Oblique ligament injury,
589-592, 591f-592f,
597-598, 598f
Observation and inspection,
6-7, 7b, 37-38
Obstruction, subclavian
venous, 189
Occipital lobe injury, 155
Occlusion
arterial occlusive disease,
637-638, 638f
carotid, 155
intervertebral foramen,
415-417, 416f
O'Donoghue maneuver,
124-130, 127t-128t,
129f-130f
Odontoid process
fracture, 131-134,
132t, 133f-134f
Olecranon impingement
syndrome, 230-231
Olfactory nerve
syndromes, 712
Optic neural function, 727,
727f

Optokinetic nystagmus test,
712-713, 713f
Organic vs. psychogenic
movement disorders,
739-741, 740t
Organisms, infective.
See Pathogens.
O'Riain sign, 290, 290f
Orthopedic physical
assessments
cardinal symptoms and
signs and, 37-62
elbow, 226-252
forearm, wrist, and hand,
253-301
fundamentals of, 1-36
hip, 516-563
knee, 564-616
lower leg, ankle, and foot,
617-660
lumbar spine, 344-472
malingering, 661-762
pelvis and sacroiliac joint,
473-515
shoulder, 157-225
spine
cervical, 63-156
lumbar, 344-472
thoracic, 302-343
Ortiguera and Berry
classification, 593
Ortolani test, 536
Osseous syndromes
lumbar spine injury,
461-464, 464f
proximal femur
deformities, 533
spinal integrity, 334-336,
335f-336f
Osteoarthritis (OA)
hip joint, 553, 553f, 558-
559, 559f
imaging studies and, 26
shoulder, nontraumatic vs.
posttraumatic, 201
Osteochondritis dissecans,
230, 615-616, 616f
Osteonecrosis,
546-548, 548f
Osteoporosis, 524
Ostitis pubis classification,
489
Oswestry disability
indices, 673
Ottawa ankle rules, 631
Outcomes and other
malingering
assessments, 662,
672-675. See also
Malingering
assessments.

Outcomes and other malingering assessments—cont'd
b test, 662
Borg pain scales, 673
Dallas pain questionnaire, 673
Disease Impact Index (DII), 673b
disease repercussion profile, 672-673
EuroQual thermometer, 672
fibromyalgia impact questionnaire, 672
health assessment questionnaire (HAQ), 672
hospital anxiety and depression (HAD) scale, 672
Millennium Cohort study and, 675
neuroorthostatic malingering tests, 673
Oswestry disability indices, 673
symptom magnification indexing, 673
test of memory malingering (TOMM), 662
Victoria Symptom Validity Test (VSVT), 662
Waddell indexing, 673, 674t
Overload syndrome, 230-231
Overuse injury, 203-205, 205f

P

PA. *See* Psoriatic arthritis (PA).
Paget-Schroetter syndrome, 178, 196
Pain qualification and quantification, 683-709. *See also* Malingering assessments.
axial trunk-loading test, 691-693, 692t, 693f
Burns bench test, 694-695, 695f
flexed-hip test, 696, 696f
flip sign, 697, 697f
Libman sign, 698-699, 699f
Magnuson test, 700, 700f
Mannkopf sign, 701, 701f
marked part pain-suggestibility test, 702-703, 702f

Pain qualification and quantification—cont'd
plantar flexion test, 704-705, 705f
Quebec classification system, 691, 692t
related joint motion test, 706, 706f
Seeligmuller sign, 707, 707f
trunk rotational test, 708-709, 709f
Painful arc syndrome, 219
Palmar fasciitis, 232t
Palpation, 7-9, 8t
Palsy
nocturnal, 191
sleep, 93
ulnar, 243-244, 244f
Panner disease, 230
Paralysis qualification and quantification, 739-762. *See also* Malingering assessments.
Barthel index, 743-744
bilateral limb-dropping test, lower extremities, 742-745, 745f
hemiplegic posturing, 746-747, 747f
Hoover test, 748-750, 749t, 750f
Lamb bilateral hand activity index, 753
simulated foot-drop testing, 751-752, 752f
simulated forearm-and-wrist-weakness testing, 753-754, 754f
simulated grip-strength-loss test, 755-756, 756f
tripod test, 757-758, 757f-758f
Paraspinal soft-tissue integrity, 334-336, 335f-336f
Paresis
leg, feigned, 748-750, 749t, 750f
lower extremity, feigned, 742-745, 745f
Part dimension changes, 47
Passive scapular approximation test, 330, 330f
Patellar syndromes
apprehension test, 580-581, 581f
ballottement test, 606, 606f

Patellar syndromes—cont'd
fracture, 593-594, 594f
patella alta, 608-609, 609f
patellar malacia, 586-587
patellofemoral dysfunction, 595-596, 596f, 608-609, 609f
subluxation, 608-609, 609f
tracking disorder, 595-596, 596f
Patency tests, 97
Pathogens
enteric gram-negative bacilli, 400
Haemophilus influenzae type b, 401
Listeria monocytogenes, 376, 400
Neisseria gonorrhoeae, 376
Neisseria meningitidis, 376, 400
Staphylococcus, 401
Streptococcus agalactiae, 401
Streptococcus pneumoniae, 400
Ureaplasma urealyticum, 376
Pathologic conditions
hip, 485-486, 486f
hip joint, 560, 560f
intracapsular coxa, 558-559, 559f
meniscus, 578
reflexes, 10
sacroiliac joint, 434-436, 436f
scoliosis, 312-317, 313t-314t, 315f
shoulder, 207-208, 207f
Patient histories, 5
Patrick test, 558-559, 559f
Patterns, pain, 11
Payr sign, 607, 607f
Pectoralis strain, 342t
Pediatric limping categories, 537
Pelvis and sacroiliac joint assessments, 473-515
anatomy essentials for, 477-478
cross-reference tables for
by procedure, 474t-475t
by syndrome or tissue, 476t
fundamentals of, 473-478
procedures
belt test, 483-484, 483f

Pelvis and sacroiliac joint assessments—cont'd
Erichsen sign, 485-486, 486f
Gaenslen test, 487-488, 488f
gait observations, 500
gapping test, 489-490, 490f
Goldthwait sign, 491-492, 491f
Hibbs test, 493-494, 494f
hip-abduction stress test, 505-507, 506f
iliac compression test, 495-496, 495f
iliac crests compression test, 495-496, 495f
imaging studies, 479
innominate test, anterior, 480-482, 482f
knee-to-shoulder test, 497-498, 498f
Laguerre test, 499, 499f
Lewin-Gaenslen test, 500-501, 501f
lumbopelvic flexibility tests, 479
Mazion pelvic maneuver, 480-482, 482f
motion assessments, 478
muscle function assessments, 478-479
Piedallu sign, 502-503, 502f
sacral apex test, 504, 504f
sacroiliac resisted-abduction test, 505-507, 506f
sacroiliac stretch test, 489-490, 490f
Smith-Petersen test, 508-510, 509f
squish test, 511-513, 512f
supported Adams test, 483-484, 483f
Yeoman test, 514-515, 514f
of syndromes or tissues
abductor weakness, 505-507, 506f
anterior sacroiliac ligament injury, 514-515, 514f
chronic lumbar strain, 480t

Pelvis and sacroiliac joint assessments—cont'd
fracture, acetabular, 485
fracture, bony pelvis, 511-513, 512f
fracture, insufficiency, 511-513, 512f
fracture, pelvic ring, 511-513, 512f
fracture, sacroiliac, 495-496, 495f
gluteus maximus/medius/minimus syndrome, 480t
inflammation, sacroiliac, 495-496, 495f
lesion, sacroiliac, 495-496, 495f
lumbopelvic spine muscular syndromes, 481
lumbopelvic syndromes, 480t
ostitis pubis, 489
piriformis syndrome, 480t, 505-507, 506f
posterior sacroiliac ligament damage, 511-513, 512f
pyogenic sacroiliitis, 497-498, 498f
quadratus lumborum syndrome, 480t
sacroiliac disease, 487-488, 488f, 493-494, 494f
sacroiliac disease vs. hip joint pathologic conditions, 485-486, 486f
sacroiliac intraarticular abnormality, 499, 499f
sacroiliac joint abnormal rotational shifting, 504, 504f
sacroiliac joint abnormal torsion movement, 502-503, 502f
sacroiliac joint abnormality, 500-501, 501f
sacroiliac joint vs. lumbosacral joint involvement, 508-510, 509f
sacroiliac mechanical dysfunction, 497-498, 498f
sciatic neuritis, 504, 504f

Pelvis and sacroiliac joint assessments—cont'd
spinal erector muscle strain, 480t
sprain, anterior sacroiliac ligament, 489-490, 490f
sprain, lumbosacral capsular, 483-484, 483f
sprain, sacroiliac, 495-496, 495f
sprain, sacroiliac joint, 491-492, 491f, 505-507, 506f
sprain, sacroiliac ligament, 483-484, 483f
subluxation, sacroiliac, 495-496, 495f
subluxation, sacroiliac joint, 505-507, 506f
unilateral forward displacement, 480-482, 482f
Percussion test, 140-142, 141t, 142f, 334-336, 335f-336f, 461-464, 464f
Periarticular region syndromes, 40t-41t, 232t
Pericapsular inflammation, 397-399, 399f
Peripatellar syndrome, 595-596, 596f
Peripheral nerve denervation, 290, 290f
neuropathy, 292-293, 293f
sensibility, diminished, 298-300, 299f
Peripheral nociceptors, 41
Peripheral vascular syndromes
disease, lower extremity, 633-634, 634f
obstruction, wrist, 268-271, 269b-270b, 271f
Periprosthetic patella fracture, 593
Perthes test, 653-654, 654f
Pes planus, 643, 643f
PET scans. See Positron emission tomography (PET) scans.
Petersen-Smith test, 508-510, 509f
Phalangeal retinacular ligaments fixation, 291, 291f
Phalanges internal derangement, 276, 276f

Phalen sign, 286-287, 286f-287f
Physical assessments
  cardinal symptoms and signs and, 37-62
  elbow, 226-252
  forearm, wrist, and hand, 253-301
  fundamentals, 1-36
  hip, 516-563
  knee, 564-616
  lower leg, ankle, and foot, 617-660
  malingering, 661-762
  pelvis and sacroiliac joint, 473-515
  shoulder, 157-225
  spine
    cervical, 63-156
    lumbar, 344-472
    thoracic, 302-343
Piedallu sign, 502-503, 502f
Pinch grip test, 288-289, 289f
Pinch test, skin, 459-460, 460f
Piriformis muscular spasm, 406-407, 407f
Piriformis syndrome, 406, 480t, 553, 553f
Pivot shaft maneuver, lateral, 599-600, 600f
Plain-film (conventional) radiography, 21-27, 21t
Plantar flexion test, 704-705, 705f
Plexopathy, brachial, 232t
Polymyalgia rheumatica, 339t
Popliteal artery, 637
Position-sense testing, 731, 731f
Positive drawer test
  anterior, 590
  posterior, 581
Positron emission tomography (PET) scans, 31
Posterior cruciate ligament injury, 589-592, 591f-592f, 610-611, 610f
Posterior dislocation of humerus, 174-175, 175f
Posterior drawer test, positive, 581
Posterior horn injury, 607, 607f
Posterior humerus shoulder dislocation, 182-183, 182f-183f

Posterior interosseous nerve compression, 294-296, 294t-295t, 296f
Posterior interossous neuropathy, 251-252, 252f
Posterior oblique ligament injury, 589-592, 591f-592f, 597-598, 598f
Posterior sacroiliac ligament damage, 511-513, 512f
Posterolateral bundle injury, 597-598, 598f
Posterolateral capsule injury, 589-592, 591f-592f, 599-600, 600f, 610-611, 610f
Posterolateral intervertebral disc protrusion, 362-366
Posteromedial capsule injury, 589-592, 591f-592f
Posteromedial intervertebral disc protrusion, 362-366
Posttraumatic neurovascular compression, 178
Posttraumatic osteoarthritis (OA), shoulder, 201
Posture, 47
Posturing, hemiplegic, 746-747, 747f
Pott fracture, 646
Prayer sign, 286-287, 286f-287f
Preferred views, imaging studies, 22t-23t. *See also* Imaging studies.
Presenting symptoms, 39-45. *See also* Cardinal symptoms and signs.
  ability depreciation assessment, 42b
  activities of daily living (ADL) assessment, 43-45
  disability and handicap, 42-45
  disability PILS, 5b, 42b
  function assessments, 12-14, 45
  functional assessments, 45. *See also* Function assessments.
  pain and sensibility, 39-40
  peripheral nociceptors, 41
  regional periarticular syndromes, 40t-41t
  stiffness, 41-42
  weakness, 41
Pressure, intra discal, 462
Procedures

cardinal symptoms and signs and, 37-62
elbow, 226-252
forearm, wrist, and hand, 253-301
fundamentals of, 1-36
hip, 516-563
knee, 564-616
lower leg, ankle, and foot, 617-660
malingering, 661-762
pelvis and sacroiliac joint, 473-515
shoulder, 157-225
spine
  cervical, 63-156
  lumbar, 344-472
  thoracic, 302-343
Prolapse
  disc, 398
  disc nucleus, 374-375, 374t, 375f
Prone knee-bending test, 448-450, 450f
Prostrate leg-raise test, 385-386, 386f
Protrusion, disc, 95-96, 95f, 364, 418-419, 418f
Provocative tests, cervical spine, 69t-70t
Proximal femur
  fracture, 544
  osseous deformities, 533
Proximal interphalangeal dislocation, 291, 291f
Proximal tibiofibular joint dysfunction, 576
Pseudoaneurysm, axillary, 184
Psoriatic arthritis (PA), 25
Psychogenic *vs.* organic movement disorders, 739-741, 740t
Pulled *vs.* pushed elbow, 232
Pulses, wrist, 270
Punch test, Lewin, 418-419, 418f
Pushed *vs.* pulled elbow, 232
Pyogenic sacroiliitis, 497-498, 498f

Q

Q-angle test, 606-609, 609f
Quadriceps muscular strain, 448-450, 450f
Qualification and quantification assessments. *See also* Malingering assessments.

Qualification and
  quantification
  assessments—cont'd
  pain, 683-709
  paralysis, 739-762
  sensory deficit, 709-738
Quebec classification
  system, 691, 692t
Quebec Task Force on
  Spinal Disorders, 709
Quervain disease, 279, 279f
Quick test, 451-452, 452f

R

RA. *See* Rheumatoid
  arthritis (RA).
Radial neuropathy,
  251-252, 252f
Radiculopathy
  cervical spine, 101t-102t
  chronic S1-S2, 412t
  dorsal patterns, 390t
  lumbar, upper, 387t, 388
  lumbosacral, 409
  vs. peroneal neuropathy,
    391t-392t
  sciatic, 454-456, 456f,
    468-470, 470f
Radiocarpal joint, 261
Radiography, plain-film,
  21-27, 21t
Radiohumeral bursitis,
  240-242, 240t-241t,
  242f
Radionuclide scans, 31
Range-of-motion (ROM)
  tests, 12, 56, 525-526,
  526f
Rebound test, 406-407, 407f
Reclination test, 97-98
Recurrent dislocation
  patella, 580-581, 581f
  shoulder, 194
Reduced visual acuity, 716
Referred symptoms, 11,
  46-47, 46t-47t
Reflex
  blinking, 720-721
  fundamentals of, 9-10
  reflex sympathetic
    dystrophy-complex
    regional pain
    syndrome
    (RDS-CRS), 268-271,
    269b-270b, 271f
Regional anesthesia testing,
  732-733, 733f
Regional periarticular
  syndromes, 40t-41t
Related joint motion test,
  706, 706f

Repercussion profile,
  672-673
Resisted-abduction test,
  505-507, 506f
Restless leg syndrome
  (RLS), 410-411
Retinacular ligament test,
  291, 291f
Reverse Bakody maneuver,
  209-210, 210f
Reversible ischemia
  neurologic deficits
  (RINDs), 154
Rheumatoid arthritis (RA),
  272-273, 273f
  vs. fibromyalgia
    syndrome, 339t
  imaging studies and,
    24-26
  rheumatoid deformity, 272
  upper cervical, 131-134,
    132t, 133f-134f
Rib
  motion test, 331, 331f
  syndromes, 342t
  thoracic outlet, 174-175,
    175f. *See also*
    Thoracic outlet
    syndrome (TOS).
RINDs. *See* Reversible
  ischemia neurologic
  deficits (RINDs).
RLS. *See* Restless leg
  syndrome (RLS).
Rock test, 207-208, 207f
ROM tests. *See*
  Range-of-motion
  (ROM) tests.
Romberg sign, 734, 734f
Roos test, 211-212, 211f
Root, nerve. *See* Nerve root.
Rotary instability, 601,
  601f, 610-611, 610f
Rotation
  extension test, 97
  shifting, sacroiliac
    joint, 504, 504f
  test, trunk, 708-709, 709f
Rotator cuff
  degenerative tendinitis,
    180-181, 180f-181f
  tear, 216-217, 217f
  complex, 187-188, 188f
  supraspinatus, 216-217,
    217f
Rupture
  Achilles tendon, 657-658,
    658f
  biceps long head, 206, 206f
  intervertebral disc, 420,
    420f

Rust sign, 131-134, 132t,
  133f-134f

S

Sacral apex test, 504, 504f
Sacroiliac joint and pelvis
  assessments, 473-515
  anatomy essentials for,
    477-478
  cross-reference tables for
    by procedure, 474t-475t
    by syndrome or tissue,
      476t
  fundamentals of, 473-478
  procedures
    belt test, 483-484, 483f
    Erichsen sign, 485-486,
      486f
    Gaenslen test, 487-488,
      488f
    gait observations, 500
    gapping test, 489-490,
      490f
    Goldthwait sign,
      491-492, 491f
    Hibbs test, 493-494,
      494f
    hip-abduction stress test,
      505-507, 506f
    iliac compression test,
      495-496, 495f
    imaging studies, 479
    innominate test, anterior,
      480-482, 482f
    knee-to-shoulder test,
      497-498, 498f
    Laguerre test, 499, 499f
    Lewin-Gaenslen test,
      500-501, 501f
    lumbopelvic flexibility
      tests, 479
    Mazion pelvic maneuver,
      480-482, 482f
    motion assessments, 478
    muscle function
      assessments, 478-479
    Piedallu sign, 502-503,
      502f
    sacral apex test, 504,
      504f
    sacroiliac resisted-
      abduction test, 505-
      507, 506f
    sacroiliac stretch test,
      489-490, 490f
    Smith-Petersen test,
      508-510, 509f
    squish test, 511-513,
      512f
    supported Adams test,
      483-484, 483f

Sacroiliac joint and pelvis assessments—cont'd
of syndromes and tissues
abductor muscular weakness, 505-507, 506f
anterior ligament injury, 514-515, 514f
fracture, acetabular, 485
fracture, bony pelvis, 511-513, 512f
fracture, insufficiency, 511-513, 512f
fracture, pelvic ring, 511-513, 512f
fracture, sacroiliac, 495-496, 495f
gluteus maximus/medius/minimus syndrome, 480t
inflammation, sacroiliac, 495-496, 495f
lesions, sacroiliac, 495-496, 495f
lumbopelvic spine muscular syndromes, 481
lumbopelvic syndromes, 480t
ostetis pubis, 489
pathologic conditions, 485-486, 486f
piriformis syndrome, 480t
posterior sacroiliac ligament damage, 511-513, 512f
pyogenic sacroiliitis, 497-498, 498f
sacroiliac disease, 487-488, 488f, 493-494, 494f
sacroiliac intraarticular abnormality, 499, 499f
sacroiliac joint abnormal rotational shifting, 504, 504f
sacroiliac joint abnormal torsion movement, 502-503, 502f
sacroiliac joint abnormality, 500-501, 501f
sacroiliac joint sprain vs. lumbosacral spine abnormality, 491-492, 491f
sacroiliac joint vs. lumbosacral joint

Sacroiliac joint and pelvis assessments—cont'd
involvement, 508-510, 509f
sacroiliac mechanical dysfunction, 497-498, 498f
sciatic neuritis, 504, 504f
sprain, anterior ligament, 489-490, 490f
sprain, lumbosacral capsular, 483-484, 483f
sprain, sacroiliac, 495-496, 495f
sprain, sacroiliac joint, 505-507, 506f
sprain, sacroiliac ligament, 483-484, 483f
strain, chronic lumbar, 480t
strain, spinal erector muscle, 480t
subluxation, sacroiliac, 495-496, 495f
subluxation, sacroiliac joint, 505-507, 506f
unilateral forward displacement, 480-482, 482f
Saphenous vein valve incompetencies, 653-654, 654f
Scalene
maneuver, 176-177, 177f
relief test, 120
scalenus-anticus syndrome, 174-175, 175f, 189
scalenus-anticus test, 176-177, 177f
Scans. See Imaging studies.
Scapholunate advance collapse (SLAC), 265
Scapular approximation test, passive, 330, 330f
Schelelmann sign, 332-333, 333f
Schober test, 453, 453f
Sciatic nerve
inflammation, 408-414, 412t, 413f
irritation, 378-379, 379f
neuritis, 373, 373f, 504, 504f
phenomenon, 385-386, 386f
radiculopathy, 454-456, 456f, 468-470, 470f

Sciatic scoliosis, 471-472, 472f
Sciatica, 339t, 367-368, 368f, 415-417, 416f, 423-427, 424t-426t, 427f, 468-470, 470f
Scoliosis
pathologic vs. structural, 312-317, 313t-314t, 315f
sciatic, 471-472, 472f
Screening procedure, George, 196-198, 197f-198f
Seeligmuller sign, 707, 707f
Sensibility qualities, 39-40, 298
Sensory deficit qualification and quantification, 709-738. See also Malingering assessments.
anosmia testing, 712-713, 713f
coordination-disturbance testing, 714-715, 715f
Cuignet test, 716-717, 717f
facial anesthesia testing, 718-719, 719f
Gault test, 720-721, 721f
Janet test, 722, 722f
limb-dropping test, upper extremities, 723-725, 725f
Lombard test, 726, 726f
Marcus Gunn sign, 727, 727f
midline tuning-fork test, 728, 728f
optokinetic nystagmus test, 712-713, 713f
position-sense testing, 731, 731f
regional anesthesia testing, 732-733, 733f
Romberg sign, 734, 734f
Snellen test, 735-737, 736t, 737f
station test, 734, 734f
Stoicism indexing, 738, 738f
Sensory recovery classification, 299t
Separation, trochanter, 554-555, 555f
Septic necrosis, 280-281, 281f
Sequestered discs, 364
Severe sprain, thoracic, 316-317, 316t, 317f

Severe upper cervical spine subluxation, 131-134, 132t, 133f-134f
Shoe design features, 618
Shoulder assessments, 157-225
  anatomy essentials for, 163
  cross-reference tables for
    by procedure, 158t-159t
    by syndrome or tissue, 160t-161t
  fundamentals of, 157-163
  procedures
    Abbott-Saunders test, 174-175, 175f
    Adson test, 176-177, 177f
    Allen maneuver, 178-179, 179f
    Apley scratch test, 180-181, 180f-181f
    apprehension test, 182-183, 182f-183f
    Bryant sign, 184-185, 185f
    Calloway test, 186, 186f
    Codman sign, 187-188, 188f
    costoclavicular maneuver, 189-191, 190f-191f
    Dawbarn sign, 192-193, 193f
    drawer tests of Gerber and Ganz, 182-183, 182f-183f
    drop arm test, 187-188, 188f
    Dugas test, 194-195, 195f
    Elvey test, 222
    empty can test, 224
    George screening procedure, 196-198, 197f-198f
    Halstead maneuver, 199-200, 200f
    Hamilton test, 201-202, 202f
    Hawkin impingement test, 224
    hyperabduction maneuver, 222-223, 223f
    imaging studies, 173
    impingement sign, 203-205, 205f
    Ludington test, 206, 206f
    Mazion cuff maneuver, 216-217, 217f

Shoulder
  assessments—cont'd
    Mazion shoulder maneuver, 207-208, 207f
    motion assessments, 163-168, 164t-168t
    muscle function assessments, 169-172, 170f-172f
    Neer impingement test, 224
    reverse Bakody maneuver, 209-210, 210f
    Roos test, 211-212, 211f
    shoulder compression test, 213-214, 214f
    shoulder rock test, 207-208, 207f
    speed test, 215, 215f
    subacromial push-button sign, 216-217, 217f
    supraspinatus press test, 218-219, 219f
    supraspinatus test, 224
    transverse humeral ligament test, 220-221, 221f
    Wright test, 222-223, 223f
    Yergason test, 224-225, 225f
  of syndromes or tissues
    axillary artery neurovascular compromise, 222-223, 223f
    axillary pseudoaneurysm, 184
    biceps long head injury, 220-221, 221f
    biceps long head rupture, 206, 206f
    biceps overuse injury, 203-205, 205f
    biceps tendinitis, 174-175, 175f, 215, 215f
    bursitis, subacromial, 192-193, 193f
    cervical rib thoracic outlet, 174-175, 175f
    compression, cervical foraminal, 209-210, 210f
    compression, interscalene, 209-210, 210f
    costoclavicular neurovascular space narrowing, 211

Shoulder
  assessments—cont'd
    degenerative tendinitis of rotator cuff tendons, 180-181, 180f-181f
    dislocation, 184, 194-195, 195f, 201-202, 202f
    dislocation, anterior, 182-183, 182f-183f, 194
    dislocation, chronic recurrent, 194
    dislocation, glenohumeral articulation, 184-185, 185f
    dislocation, posterior humerus, 182-183, 182f-183f
    effort thrombosis, 196
    glenohumeral articulation dislocation, 184-185, 185f
    humerus dislocation, 186, 186f
    impingement syndrome, 204
    neurovascular compress of subclavian artery and brachial plexus, 174-175, 175f
    obstruction, subclavian venous, 189
    osteoarthritis (OA), nontraumatic vs. posttraumatic, 201
    Paget-Schroetter syndrome, 196
    painful arc syndrome, 219
    pathologic process, 207-208, 207f
    rotator cuff tear, 216-217, 217f
    rotator cuff tear, complex, 187-188, 188f
    scalenus anticus, 174-175, 175f
    subclavian artery stenosis or occlusion, 196-198, 197f-198f
    supraspinatus syndrome, 218
    supraspinatus tendon/muscle tear, 218-219, 219f
    supraspinatus tendon overuse injury, 203-205, 205f

Shoulder
assessments—cont'd
supraspinatus tendon
rotator cuff tear,
216-217, 217f
tenosynovitis, 215, 215f,
224-225, 225f
thoracic outlet syndrome
(TOS), 176-179,
177f, 179f, 189-191,
190f-191f, 199-200,
200f, 211-212, 211f
thoracic outlet
syndrome (TOS),
hyperabduction
type, 213-214, 214f,
222-223, 223f
transverse humeral
ligament
involvement,
224-225, 225f
upper-extremity
neurogenic
syndromes, 209
Shrivel test, 290, 290f
Sicard sign, 454-456, 456f
Sign of the buttock,
457-458, 458f
Significant pathologic
process, shoulder,
207-208, 207f
Signs and symptoms.
See Cardinal symptoms
and signs.
Simulated foot-drop testing,
751-752, 752f
Simulated forearm-
and-wrist-weakness test,
753-754, 754f
Simulated grip-strength-loss
test, 755-756, 756f
Simulated syndrome
assessments. *See*
Malingering assessments.
Single-photon emission
computed tomography
(SPECT) scans, 31
Sitting reclination test, 97-98
Sitting test
Bechterew, 367-368, 368f
Lasègue, 408-414, 412t,
413f
Skeletal trauma, imaging
studies and, 22t-24t
Skier fracture, 646
Skin changes, 48-49
Skin pinch test, 459-460,
460f
SLAC. *See* Scapholunate
advance collapse
(SLAC).

SLE. *See* Systemic lupus
erythematosus (SLE).
Sleep
disturbance, 45
palsy, 93
tetany, 61-62, 191
Slipped femoral capital
epiphysis, 551
Slocum test, 610-611, 611f
Smith and Estridge
maneuver, 97-98
Smith-Petersen test,
508-510, 509f
Snellen test, 735-737, 736t,
737f
Soft-tissue
edema, 48, 48t
injury, lumbar spine,
461-464, 464f
integrity, paraspinal,
334-336, 335f-336f
Somatoform pain disorder,
339t
Soto-Hall sign, 138-139,
139f
Space-occupying mass
intervertebral, 420, 420f,
437-439, 439f
in nerve root path,
465-467, 466f
Spasm
fundamentals of, 61
hamstring, 421-422, 422f
muscular, 367-368, 368f
piriformis, 406-407, 407f
sacrolumbalis
musculature, 376-377,
377f
Spastic bladder, 62
SPECT scans. *See* Single-
photon emission
computed tomography
(SPECT) scans.
Speed test, 215, 215f
Spine assessments
cervical spine, 63-156
lumbar, 344-472
thoracic spine, 302-343
Spondylitis, ankylosing,
24-26, 316-317, 316t,
317f, 328-329, 329f
Spondyloarthropathy,
339t, 352t-353t
Spondylolisthesis, 415-417,
416f
Spondylosis
cervical spine, 151-152,
152f
Lewin supine test,
423-427, 424t-426t,
427f

Sponge test, 337-340, 340f
Sprain
carpal, 275, 275f
ligament
ligamentous, 397-399,
399f
lumbosacral, 440-442,
441f
lumbosacral capsular,
483-484, 483f
sacroiliac, 483-484,
483f, 495-496, 495f
sacroiliac, anterior,
489-490, 490f
sacroiliac joint, 491-492,
491f
talofibular, anterior,
631-632, 632f
thoracic, severe, 316-317,
316t, 317f
Spurling test, 143-146,
143t-144t, 145f-146f
Squish test, 511-513, 512f
Stability tests, 12, 13t, 58,
58f
Standing test, 421-422, 422f
Station test, 734, 734f
Steinmann sign, 612-613,
613f
Stenosis, arterial, 153-156,
156f
Stereognosis, 298
Sternal compression test,
341-343, 342t, 343f
Stiffness, 41-42
Stoicism indexing, 738,
738f
Straight-leg-raise test,
380-381, 381f, 465-467,
466f
Strain
chronic lumbar strain, 480t
intercostal, 342t
knee, 448-450, 450f
lumbosacral, 440-442,
441f, 445-447, 447f
muscular, 397-399, 399f,
448-450, 450f
pectoralis, 342t
sacroiliac, 445-447, 447f
spinal erector muscle
strain, 480t
Stress test
abduction, 574-575, 575f
adduction, 576-577, 577f
hip-abduction, 505-507,
506f
Stretch test, 489-490, 490f
Stroke in evolution, 154
Strunsky sign, 655-656,
656f

Student's elbow, 231
Subacromial syndromes
  bursitis, 192-193, 193f,
    232t
  push-button sign, 216-217,
    217f
Subclavian syndromes
  neurovascular
    compression, 176-177,
    177f
  venous obstruction, 189
Subluxation
  cervical nerve root,
    112-115, 112t-114t,
    115f
  cervical spine, 138-139,
    139f
  lumbopelvic, 445-447,
    447f
  patella, 608-609, 609f
  sacroiliac, 495-496, 495f
  sacroiliac joint, 505-507,
    506f
  severe upper cervical
    spine, 131-134, 132t,
    133f-134f
  vertebral, 367-368, 368f
Subtrochanteric fracture,
    543
Superficial reflexes, 9
Superficial varicosities,
    653-654, 654f
Supine test, 423-427,
    424t-426t, 427f
Supported Adams test,
    483-484, 483f
Supraspinatus tendon
  degenerative tendinitis,
    180-181, 180f-181f
  overuse injury, 203-205,
    205f
  press test, 218-219, 219f
  rotator cuff tear, 216-217,
    217f
  syndrome, 218
  tear, 218-219, 219f
  test, 224
Swallowing test, 147, 147f
Swelling sites
  diffuse, 48, 48t
  elbow, 246
Symptoms and signs.
  See Cardinal symptoms
    and signs.
Syndrome or tissue
  assessments
  cardinal symptoms and
    signs and, 37-62
  elbow, 226-252
  forearm, wrist, and hand,
    253-301

Syndrome or tissue
  assessments—cont'd
  fundamentals of, 1-36
  hip, 516-563
  knee, 564-616
  lower leg, ankle, and foot,
    617-660
  malingering, 661-762
  pelvis and sacroiliac joint,
    473-515
  shoulder, 157-225
  spine
    cervical, 63-156
    lumbar, 344-472
    thoracic, 302-343
Synovial fluid tests, 19-20,
    19b-20b
Synovitis, transient, 557
System illness, 45-47
Systemic lupus
  erythematosus (SLE),
    49, 49t-51t, 339t

T

T1–T2 nerve root problems,
    330-331, 330f
T10 spinal level-associated
    myelopathy, 321-323,
    323f
Tactile discrimination, 298
Tarsal tunnel syndrome,
    659-660, 660f
TB. *See* Tuberculosis (TB).
Telescoping test, 551-552,
    552f
Tender point examination
    protocol, 337-340, 340f
Tenderness
  as cardinal sign, 51
  Steinmann displacement
    test, 612-613, 613f
Tendinitis
  biceps, 174-175, 175f,
    215, 215f
  rotator cuff, 180-181,
    180f-181f
Tennis elbow, 250, 250f
Tenosynovitis
  de Quervain, 232t
  gonococcal, 232t
  procedures, 215, 215f,
    224-225, 225f
  thumb, 279, 279f
Tension test, brachial
  plexus, 93-94, 94f
Tensor fascia lata, 610-611,
    610f
Test of memory malingering
    (TOMM), 662
Tetany, 61-62, 191
Thalamic pain, 733

Thalamus injury, 155
Thermography, 34
Thigh circumference test,
    614, 614f
Thomas test, 561, 561f
Thompson test, 657-658,
    658f
Thoracic outlet syndrome
    (TOS)
  Adson test, 176-177, 177f
  Allen maneuver, 178-179,
    179f
  anatomopathologic
    causes, 208
  assessments for, 174-179,
    175f, 177f, 179f,
    189-191, 190f-191f,
    199-200, 200f,
    211-212, 211f
  classification of, 178, 189
  disputed neurogenic
    (dnTOS), 178
  hyperabduction type,
    213-214, 214f,
    222-223, 223f
  neurogenic (nTOS), 178,
    208
  vascular (vTOS), 178
Thoracic spine
  assessments, 302-343
  anatomy essentials
    for, 311
  cross-reference tables for
    by procedure, 303t-304t
    by syndrome or tissue,
    305t
  fundamentals of, 302-310
  procedures
    Adams positions,
    312-317, 313t-314t,
    315f
    Amoss sign, 316-317,
    316t, 317f
    Anghelescu sign,
    318-320, 320f
    Beevor sign, 321-323,
    323f
    chest expansion test,
    324, 324f
    fibromyalgia tender
    point examination
    protocol, 337-340,
    339t, 340f
    first thoracic nerve root
    test, 325-327, 327f
    Forestier bowstring sign,
    328-329, 329f
    imaging studies, 311
    motion assessments,
    306-310,
    307f-310f

Thoracic spine
assessments—cont'd
muscle function
assessments,
310-311, 311f
passive scapular
approximation test,
330, 330f
rib motion test, 331, 331f
Schelelmann sign,
332-333, 332t, 333f
spinal percussion test,
334-336, 335f-336f
sponge test, 337-340,
340f
sternal compression
test, 341-343,
342t, 343f
of syndromes or tissues
ankylosing spondylitis
(AS), 316-317, 316t,
317f, 328-329, 329f
compression, vertebral
deformities, 311
costal structures,
hypermobile vs.
hypomobile, 331,
331f
costal tissue integrity,
332-333, 332t, 333f
costochondritis,
341-343, 342t, 343f
costovertebral
syndrome, 342t
fibromyalgia syndrome,
337-340, 339t, 340f
fractures, costal
structure, 341-343,
342t, 343f
fractures, multiple-level
spinal, 334
fractures,
thoracolumbar, 334
Guillian-Barré
syndrome (GBS),
321-323, 323f
herniation, intervertebral
disc, 325
intercostal neuralgia,
342t
intercostal strain, 342t
intercostal tissue
integrity, 332-333,
332t, 333f
intervertebral disc
syndrome, 316-317,
316t, 317f
kyphosis, 328-329, 329f
lesions, acute
inflammatory, 337-
340, 340f

Thoracic spine
assessments—cont'd
mechanical spine
syndrome, 305
myelopathy, 321-323,
323f
nerve root involvement,
325-327, 327f
nerve root problems,
T1-T2, 330-331,
330f
paraspinal soft-tissue
integrity, 334-336,
335f-336f
pectoralis strain, 342t
referred pain, 325-326
rib syndromes, 342t
scoliosis, pathologic vs.
structural, 312-317,
313t-314t, 315f
spinal ankylosis, 324,
324f
spinal osseous integrity,
334-336, 335f-336f
spine destructive
processes,
318-320, 320f
sprain, severe, 316-317,
316t, 317f
thoracic spine
syndromes, 313t
thorax syndromes, 342t
Tietze syndrome,
341-343, 342t, 343f
tuberculosis (TB),
meningitis, 318-320,
320f
tuberculosis (TB),
vertebrae,
318-320, 320f
Thoracolumbar
fractures, 334
Thorax syndromes, 342t
Thrombophlebitis,
645, 645f
Thrombosis, effort, 196
Thumb
joint arthritis, 274, 274f
tenosynovitis, 279, 279f
TIAs. See Transient
ischemic attacks (TIAs).
Tibia
lateral torsion, 608-609,
609f
tibial portion structural
deficiency, 536-538,
538f
tibiofibular joint
dysfunction, 576
Tietze syndrome, 341-343,
342t, 343f

Tight retinacular ligaments
test, 291, 291f
Tinel sign
elbow, 251-252, 252f
foot, 659-660, 660f
wrist, 292-293, 293f
Tissue or syndrome
assessments
cardinal symptoms and
signs and, 37-62
elbow, 226-252
forearm, wrist, and hand,
253-301
fundamentals of, 1-36
hip, 516-563
knee, 564-616
lower leg, ankle,
and foot, 617-660
malingering, 661-762
pelvis and sacroiliac joint,
473-515
shoulder, 157-225
spine
cervical, 63-156
lumbar, 344-472
thoracic, 302-343
Toddler fracture, 646
TOMM. See Test
of memory
malingering (TOMM).
Tomography
conventional vs. computed
(CT), 27-28, 29t-31t
positron emission
tomography (PET)
scans, 31
single-photon emission
computed tomography
(SPECT) scans, 31
Torsion movement,
sacroiliac joint, 502-503,
502f
TOS. See Thoracic
outlet syndrome
(TOS).
Total binocular blindness,
716
Tourniquet test, 294-296,
294t-295t, 296f,
641-642, 642f
Tracking disorder, patellar,
595-596, 596f
Transient ischemic attacks
(TIAs), 154
Transient synovitis, 557
Transverse humeral
ligament test, 220-221,
221f, 224-225, 225f
Trauma, imaging studies
and, 22t-24t
Tremor classification, 61t

Trendelenburg test, 562-563, 563f
Triad of Dejerine, 95-96, 95f
Triangular fibrocartilage complex injury, 260t
Trigeminal lesions, 718-719, 719f
Trimalleolar fracture, 646
Tripod test, 757-758, 757f-758f
Trochanter, lesser, 554-555, 555f
True leg-length discrepancy, 534-535, 535f. *See also* Leg-length.
Trunk rotational test, 708-709, 709f
Tuberculosis (TB)
  arthritis, 546-548, 548f
  meningitis, 318-320, 320f
  vertebrae, 318-320, 320f
Tumors
  gluteal, 457-458, 458f
  intervertebral, 147, 147f
  spinal cord, 95-96, 95f, 373, 373f
Tuning-fork test, 728, 728f
Turyn sign, 468-470, 470f
Twitch response, 339
Two-point discrimination test, 277-278, 278f

U

Ulnar nerve
  compression, 243-244, 244f
  distribution, 292-293, 293f
  entrapment, 232t
  neuropathy, 251-252, 252f
  neuropathy, peripheral, 292-293, 293f
  palsy, 243-244, 244f, 282-283, 282f
Unconsciousness, feigned, 723-725, 725f
Underburg test, 148-150, 150f
Unilateral disc herniation
  L3-L4, 428
  L4-L5, 429
  L5-S1, 429
Unilateral syndromes
  foot drop, 509t
  forward displacement, 480-482, 482f
  hamstring spasms, 421-422, 422f
Upper cervical spine syndromes, 131-134, 132t, 133f-134f. *See also* Cervical spine assessments.

Upper-extremity assessments. *See* Forearm, wrist, and hand assessments.
Ureaplasma urealyticum, 376

V

Valgus stress test, 574-575, 575f
Valsalva maneuver, 151-152, 152f, 420, 420f
Vanzetti sign, 471-472, 472f
Varicosities, superficial, 653-654, 654f
Varus stress test, 576-577, 577f
Vascular compromise, 633-634, 634f
Vascular thoracic outlet syndrome (vTOS), 178. *See also* Thoracic outlet syndrome (TOS).
Vasospasm, 149
VBA. *See* Vertebrobasilar artery (VBA).
Venous obstruction, subclavian, 189
Vertebrae tuberculosis (TB), 318-320, 320f
Vertebral artery
  patency tests, 97
  stenosis, 153-156, 156f
  syndrome, 87-90, 89f, 97-99, 99f, 110-111, 111f
Vertebral compression
  deformities, 311
  fractures, anterior, 462
Vertebral exostosis, 367-368, 368f
Vertebral fracture, 138-139, 139f
Vertebral subluxation, 367-368, 368f
Vertebrobasilar artery (VBA)
  functional maneuver, 153-156, 156f
  insufficiency, 107-109, 108f, 153-156, 156t
  ischemia, 154
  syndrome, 148-150, 150f
Victoria Symptom Validity Test (VSVT), 662
Vision loss, functional, 716-717, 717f
Visual acuity and field, reduced, 716
Visual inspection, 37-38
Vital signs, 11
Volkmann ischemia, 635-636, 636f

VSVT. *See* Victoria Symptom Validity Test (VSVT).
vTOS. *See* Vascular thoracic outlet syndrome (vTOS).
Vulnerability, patellar dislocation, 580-581, 581f

W

WAD. *See* Whiplash associated disorder (WAD).
Waddell indexing, 673, 674t
Waddle test, 584-585, 585f
Wadsworth elbow flexion test, 243-244, 244f
Waking numbness, 191
Walk test, 390-393, 390t-392t, 393f
Wallenberg syndrome, 110, 155
Wallenberg test, 97
Wallerian degeneration sequence, 371
Warmth, 51
Wartenberg nocturnal dysesthesia, 191
Weakness, 41
Well-leg raise test of Fajersztajn, 385-386, 386f
Whiplash associated disorder (WAD), 112-115, 112t-114t, 115f
Wilson sign, 615-616, 616f
Wiltse Classification, modified, 394-395
Wright hyperabduction syndrome, 189
Wright test, 222-223, 223f
Wringing test, 301. 301f
Wrist, hand, and forearm assessments, 253-301
  anatomy essentials for, 259-261
  cross-reference tables
    by procedure, 254t-255t
    by syndrome or tissue, 256t
  fundamentals of, 253-259
  malingering and, 753-754, 754f
  procedures
    Allen test, 268-271, 269b-270b, 271f
    bracelet test, 272-273, 273f
    carpal lift sign, 275, 275f
    cascade sign, 276, 276f

Wrist, hand, and forearm
  assessments—cont'd
  Dellon moving
    two-point
    discrimination test,
    277-278, 278f
  distal tingling on
    percussion
    (DTP) sign,
    292-293, 293f
  Finkelstein test, 279, 279f
  Finsterer sign, 280-281,
    281f
  formication sign,
    292-293, 293f
  Froment paper sign,
    282-283, 282f
  Hoffman-Tinel sign,
    292-293, 293f
  interphalangeal neuroma
    test, 284, 284f
  Janet test, 278
  Maisonneuve sign, 285,
    285f
  O'Riain sign, 290, 290f
  Phalen sign, 286-287,
    286f-287f
  pinch grip test, 288-289,
    289f
  prayer sign, 286-287,
    286f-287f
  shrivel test, 290, 290f
  tight retinacular
    ligaments test, 291,
    291f
  Tinel sign, 292-293, 293f
  tourniquet test, 294-296,
    294t-295t, 296f
  wringing test, 301, 301f
  of syndromes and tissues
    anterior interosseous
      nerve syndrome, 288
    basal thumb joint
      arthritis, 274, 274f
    caput ulnae syndrome,
      272-273, 273f
    carpal tunnel syndrome
      (CPS), 286-287,
      286f-287f
    carpometacarpal
      articulations internal
      derangement, 276,
      276f

Wrist, hand, and forearm
  assessments—cont'd
  degenerative changes,
    scapholunate
    advance collapse
    (SLAC), 265
  degenerative changes,
    wrist articulations,
    272-273, 273f
  de Quervain disease,
    279, 279f
  dermatome sensory
    disturbances,
    277-278, 278f
  elbow derangement,
    301, 301f
  fracture, carpal, 275, 275f
  fracture, colles, 285, 285f
  ganglion cysts, 294
  hand derangement, 301,
    301f
  Hoffman disease, 279,
    279f
  interdigital neuroma,
    284, 284f
  interphalangeal capsular
    contractures, 274,
    274f
  Kienböck disease,
    280-281, 281f
  lunate carpal septic
    necrosis, 280-281,
    281f
  medial nerve palsy,
    286-287, 286f-287f
  median nerve
    compression, 294-296,
    294t-295t, 296f
  median nerve distribution,
    peripheral
    neuropathy, 292-293,
    293f
  peripheral nerve
    denervation, 290,
    290f
  peripheral nerve
    sensibility,
    diminished,
    298-300, 299f
  peripheral vascular
    obstruction, wrist,
    268-271, 269b-270b,
    271f

Wrist, hand, and forearm
  assessments—cont'd
  phalangeal retinacular
    ligaments fixation,
    291, 291f
  phalanges internal
    derangement, 276,
    276f
  posterior interosseous
    nerve compression,
    294-296, 294t-295t,
    296f
  proximal interphalangeal
    dislocation, 291, 291f
  reflex sympathetic
    dystrophy-complex
    regional pain
    syndrome (RDS-
    CRS), 268-271,
    269b-270b, 271f
  rheumatoid arthritis
    (RA), 272-273, 273f
  rheumatoid deformity,
    272
  sprain, carpal, 275, 275f
  tenosynovitis, thumb,
    279, 279f
  triangular fibrocartilage
    complex injury, 260t
  ulnar nerve distribution,
    peripheral
    neuropathy,
    292-293, 293f
  ulnar nerve palsy,
    282-283, 282f
  wrist carpal system
    injury, 257
  wrist derangement, 301,
    301f
  wrist weakness,
    simulated, 753-754,
    754f

Y

Yeoman test, 514-515, 514f
Yergason test, 224-225, 225f

Z

Ziedman and Ducker
  modification, 132t
Zygapophyseal joint menisci
  types, 100

LISTING OF TESTS ALPHABETICALLY AND ANATOMICALLY

Chapter 3 — Cervical Spine

Bakody sign, 83
Barre-Lieou sign, 87
Bikele sign, 91
Brachial plexus tension test, 93
Dejerine sign, 95
DeKleyn test, 97
Distraction test, 100
Foraminal compression test, 105
Hallpike maneuver, 107
Hautant test, 110
Jackson compression test, 112
Lhermitte sign, 116
Maximum cervical compression test, 119
Naffziger test, 122
O'Donoghue maneuver, 124
Rust sign, 131
Shoulder depression test, 135
Soto-Hall sign, 138
Spinal percussion test, 140
Spurling test, 143
Swallowing test, 147
Underburg test, 148
Valsalva maneuver, 151
Vertebrobasilar artery functional maneuver, 153

Chapter 4 — Shoulder

Abbott-Saunders test, 174
Adson test, 176
Allen maneuver, 178
Apley test, 180
Apprehension test, 182
Bryant sign, 184
Calloway test, 186
Codman sign, 187
Costoclaviclar maneuver, 189
Dawbarn sign, 192
Dugas test, 194
George screening procedure, 196

Halstead maneuver, 199
Hamilton test, 201
Impingement sign, 203
Ludington test, 206
Mazion shoulder maneuver, 207
Reverse Bakody maneuver, 209
Roos test, 211
Shoulder compression test, 213
Speed test, 215
Subacromial push-button sign, 216
Supraspinatus press test, 218
Transverse humeral ligament test, 220
Wright test, 222
Yergason test, 224

Chapter 5 — Elbow

Cozen test, 240
Elbow flexion test, 243
Golfer elbow test, 245
Kaplan test, 246
Ligamentous instability test, 248
Mills test, 250
Tinel sign at the elbow, 251

Chapter 6 — Forearm, Wrist, and Hand

Allen test, 268
Bracelet test, 272
Bunnel-Littler test, 274
Carpal lift sign, 275
Cascade sign, 276
Dellon moving two-point discrimination test, 277
Finkelstein test, 279
Finsterer sign, 280
Froment paper sign, 282
Interphalangeal neuroma test, 284
Maisonneuve sign, 285

Phalen sign, 286
Pinch grip test, 288
Shrivel test, 290
Test for tight retinacular ligaments, 291
Tinel sign at the wrist, 292
Tourniquet test, 294
Wartenberg sign, 297
Weber two-point discrimination test, 298
Wringing test, 301

Chapter 7 — Thoracic Spine

Adams positions, 312
Amoss sign, 316
Anghelescu sign, 318
Beevor sign, 321
Chest expansion test, 324
First thoracic nerve root test, 325
Forestier bowstring sign, 328
Passive scapular approximation test, 330
Rib motion test, 331
Schepelmann sign, 332
Spinal percussion test, 334
Sponge test, 337
Sternal compression test, 341

Chapter 8 — Lumbar Spine

Antalgia sign, 363
Bechterew sitting test, 367
Bilateral leg-lowering test, 369
Bowstring sign, 371
Bragard sign, 373
Cox sign, 374
Demianoff sign, 376
Deyerle sign, 378
Double leg-raise test, 380
Ely sign, 382
Fajersztajn test, 385

Femoral nerve traction test, 387
Heel/toe walk test, 390
Hyperextension test, 394
Kemp test, 397
Kernig/Brudzinski sign, 400
Lasègue differential sign, 403
Lasègue rebound test, 406
Lasègue sitting test, 408
Lasègue test, 415
Lewin punch test, 418
Lewin snuff test, 420
Lewin standing test, 421
Lewin supine test, 423
Lindner sign, 428
Matchstick test, 431
Mennell sign, 434
Milgram test, 437
Minor sign, 440
Nachlas test, 442
Neri sign, 445
Prone knee-bending test, 448
Quick test, 451
Schober test, 453
Sicard sign, 454
Sign of the buttock, 457
Skin pinch test, 459
Spinal percussion test, 461
Straight-leg-raising test, 465
Turyn sign, 468
Vanzetti sign, 471

Chapter 9 — Pelvis and Sacroiliac Joint

Anterior innominate test, 480
Belt test, 483
Erichsen sign, 485
Gaenslen test, 487
Gapping test, 489
Goldthwait sign, 491
Hibbs test, 493
Iliac compression test, 495
Knee-to-shoulder test, 497
Laguerre test, 499
Lewin-Gaenslen test, 500
Piedallu sign, 502
Sacral apex test, 504
Sacroiliac resisted-abduction test, 505
Smith-Petersen test, 508
Squish test, 511
Yeoman test, 514

Chapter 10 — Hip

Actual leg-length test, 534
Allis sign, 536

Anvil test, 539
Apparent leg-length test, 541
Chiene test, 543
Gauvain sign, 546
Guilland sign, 549
Hip telescoping test, 551
Jansen test, 553
Ludloff sign, 554
Ober test, 556
Patrick test, 558
Phelps test, 560
Thomas test, 561
Trendelenburg test, 562

Chapter 11 — Knee

Abduction stress test, 574
Adduction stress test, 576
Apley compression test, 578
Apprehension test for the patella, 580
Bounce home test, 582
Childress duck waddle test, 584
Clarke sign, 586
Drawer test, 589
Dreyer sign, 593
Fouchet sign, 595
Lachman test, 597
Lateral pivot shift maneuver, 599
Losee test, 601
McMurray sign, 602
Noble compression test, 604
Patella ballottement test, 606
Payr sign, 607
Q-angle test, 608
Slocum test, 610
Steinmann sign, 612
Thigh circumference test, 614
Wilson sign, 615

Chapter 12 — Leg, Ankle, and Foot

Anterior drawer sign of the ankle, 631
Buerger test, 633
Calf circumference test, 635
Claudication test, 637
Duchenne sign, 639
Foot tourniquet test, 641
Helbings sign, 643
Hoffa test, 644
Homans sign, 645
Keen sign, 646
Morton test, 648

Moszkowicz test, 650
Moses test, 652
Perthes test, 653
Strunsky sign, 655
Thompson test, 657
Tinel foot sign, 659

Chapter 13 — Malingering

Axial trunk-loading test, 691
Burns bench test, 694
Flexed-hip test, 696
Flip test, 697
Libman sign, 698
Magnuson test, 700
Mannkopf sign, 701
Marked part pain-suggestibility test, 702
Plantar flexion test, 704
Related joint motion test, 706
Seeligmuller sign, 707
Trunk rotational test, 708
Anosmia testing, 712
Coordination-disturbance testing, 714
Cuignet test, 716
Facial anesthesia testing, 718
Gault test, 720
Janet test, 722
Limb-dropping test (upper extremities), 723
Lombard test, 726
Marcus Gunn sign, 727
Midline tuning-fork test, 728
Optokinetic nystagmus test, 729
Position-sense testing, 731
Regional anesthesia testing, 732
Romberg sign, 734
Snellen test, 735
Stoicism indexing, 738
Bilateral limb-dropping test (lower extremities), 742
Hemiplegic posturing, 746
Hoover sign, 748
Simulated foot-drop testing, 751
Simulated forearm-and-wrist-weakness testing, 753
Simulated grip-strength-loss testing, 755
Tripod test (bilateral leg-fluttering test), 757

LISTING OF TESTS ACCORDING TO THE POSITION OF THE PATIENT

The Standing Examination

Adams positions, 312
Antalgia sign, 363
Anterior innominate test, 480
Axial trunk-loading test, 691
Belt test, 483
Burns bench test, 694
Chest expansion test, 324
Childress duck waddle test, 584
Claudication test, 637
Dejerine sign, 95
Forestier bowstring sign, 328
Heel/toe walk test, 390
Helbings sign, 643
Hemiplegic posturing, 746
Kemp test, 397
Lewin punch test, 418
Lewin snuff test, 420
Lewin standing test, 421
Magnuson test, 700
Mazion shoulder maneuver, 207
Mennell sign, 434
Neri sign, 445
Passive scapular approximation test, 330
Perthes test, 653
Q-angle test, 608
Quick test, 451
Romberg sign, 734
Schepelmann sign, 332
Schober test, 453
Simulated foot-drop testing, 751
Spinal percussion test, 140, 334, 461
Trendelenberg test, 562
Trunk rotational test, 708
Underburg test, 148
Valsalva maneuver, 151
Vanzetti sign, 471

The Sitting Examination

Abbott-Saunders test, 174
Adson test, 176
Allen maneuver, 178
Allen test, 268
Anosmia testing, 712
Apley test, 180
Apprehension test, 182
Apprehension test for the patella, 580
Bakody sign, 83
Barre-Lieou sign, 87
Bechterew sitting test, 367
Bikele sign, 91
Bracelet test, 272
Brachial plexus tension test, 93
Bryant sign, 184
Bunnel-Littler test, 274
Calloway test, 186
Carpal lift sign, 275
Cascade sign, 276
Codman sign, 187
Coordination-disturbance testing, 714
Costoclavicular maneuver, 189
Cozen test, 240
Cuignet test, 714
Dawbarn sign, 192
Dellon moving two-point discrimination test, 277
Deyerle sign, 378
Distraction test, 100
Dugas test, 194
Elbow flexion test, 243
Facial anesthesia testing, 718
Finkelstein test, 279
Finsterer sign, 280
First thoracic nerve root test, 325
Flip sign, 697

Foraminal compression test, 105
Froment paper sign, 282
Gault test, 720
George screening procedure, 196
Golfer elbow test, 245
Halstead maneuver, 199
Hamilton test, 201
Hautant test, 110
Impingement sign, 203
Interphalangeal neuroma test, 284
Jackson compression test, 112
Janet test, 722
Kaplan sign, 246
Lasègue sitting test, 408
Lhermitte sign, 116
Libman sign, 698
Ligamentous instability test, 248
Lindner sign, 428
Lombard test, 726
Ludington test, 206
Ludloff sign, 554
Maisonneuve sign, 285
Marcus Gunn sign, 727
Marked part pain-suggestibility test, 702
Maximum cervical compression test, 119
Midline tuning-fork test, 728
Mills test, 250
Minor sign, 440
Naffziger test, 122
Optokinetic nystagmus test, 729
O'Donoghue maneuver, 124
Payr sign, 607
Phalen sign, 286
Piedallu sign, 502
Pinch grip test, 288

Position-sense testing, 731
Regional anesthesia testing, 732
Related joint motion test, 706
Reverse Bakody maneuver, 209
Roos test, 211
Rust sign, 131
Seeligmuller sign, 707
Shoulder compression test, 213
Shoulder depression test, 135
Shrivel test, 290
Simulated forearm-and-wrist-weakness testing, 753
Simulated grip-strength-loss testing, 755
Slocum test, 610
Snellen test, 735
Speed test, 215
Spurling test, 143
Stoicism indexing, 738
Subacromial push-button sign, 216
Supraspinatus press test, 218
Swallowing test, 147
Test for tight retinacular ligaments, 291
Tinel sign at the elbow, 251
Tinel sign at the wrist, 292
Tourniquet test, 294
Transverse humeral ligament test, 220
Tripod test (bilateral leg-fluttering test), 757
Vertebrobasilar artery functional maneuver, 153
Wartenberg sign, 297
Weber two-point discrimination test, 298
Wright test, 222
Wringing test, 301
Yergason test, 224

The Supine Examination

Abduction stress test, 574
Actual leg-length test, 534
Adduction stress test, 576
Allis sign, 536
Amoss sign, 316
Anghelescu sign, 318
Anterior drawer sign of the ankle, 631

Anvil test, 539
Apparent leg-length test, 541
Beevor sign, 321
Bilateral leg-lowering test, 369
Bilateral limb-dropping test (lower extremities), 742
Bounce home test, 582
Bowstring sign, 371
Bragard sign, 373
Buerger test, 633
Calf circumference test, 635
Chiene test, 543
Clarke sign, 586
Cox sign, 374
DeKleyn test, 97
Demianoff sign, 376
Deyerle sign, 378
Double leg-raise test, 380
Drawer test, 589
Dreyer sign, 593
Duchenne sign, 639
Fajersztajn test, 385
Flexed-hip test, 696
Foot tourniquet test, 641
Fouchet sign, 595
Gapping test, 489
Goldthwait sign, 491
Guilland sign, 549
Hallpike maneuver, 107
Hip telescoping test, 551
Homans sign, 645
Hoover sign, 748
Jansen test, 553
Keen sign, 646
Kernig/Brudzinski sign, 400
Knee-to-shoulder test, 497
Lachman test, 597
Laguerre test, 499
Lasègue differential sign, 403
Lasègue rebound test, 406
Lasègue test, 415
Lateral pivot shift maneuver, 599
Lewin supine test, 423
Limb-dropping test (upper extremities), 723
Losee test, 601
McMurray sign, 602
Milgram test, 437
Morton test, 648
Moszkowicz test, 650
Noble compression test, 604

Patella ballottement test, 606
Patrick test, 558
Plantar flexion test, 704
Rib motion test, 331
Sicard sign, 454
Sign of the buttock, 457
Smith-Petersen sign, 508
Soto-Hall sign, 138
Squish test, 511
Steinmann sign, 612
Sternal compression test, 341
Straight-leg-raising test, 465
Strunsky sign, 655
Thigh circumference test, 614
Thomas test, 561
Turyn sign, 468
Wilson sign, 615

Side-Lying Examination

Femoral nerve traction test, 387
Gaenslen test, 487
Gauvain sign, 546
Iliac compression test, 495
Lewin-Gaenslen test, 500
Matchstick test, 431
Ober test, 556
Sacroiliac resisted-abduction test, 505
Skin pinch test, 459

Prone Examination

Apley compression test, 578
Ely sign, 382
Erichsen sign, 485
Hibbs test, 493
Hoffa test, 644
Hyperextension test, 394
Mannkopf sign, 701
Moses test, 652
Nachlas test, 442
Phelps test, 560
Prone knee-bending test, 448
Sacral apex test, 504
Sponge test, 337
Thompson test, 657
Tinel foot sign, 659
Yeoman test, 514